PHYTOCHEMISTRY

Volume 1

Fundamentals, Modern Techniques, and Applications

PHYTOCHEMISTRY

Volume 1

Fundamentals, Modern Techniques, and Applications

Edited by

Chukwuebuka Egbuna
Jonathan Chinenye Ifemeje, PhD
Stanley Chidi Udedi, PhD
Shashank Kumar, PhD

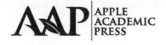

Apple Academic Press Inc.
3333 Mistwell Crescent
Oakville, ON L6L 0A2
Canada

Apple Academic Press Inc.
9 Spinnaker Way
Waretown, NJ 08758
USA

© 2019 by Apple Academic Press, Inc.

First issued in paperback 2021

Exclusive worldwide distribution by CRC Press, a member of Taylor & Francis Group

No claim to original U.S. Government works

Phytochemistry, Volume 1: Fundamentals, Modern Techniques, and Applications
ISBN 13: 978-1-77463-523-0 set
ISBN 13: 978-1-77463-432-5 (pbk)
ISBN 13: 978-1-77188-759-5 (hbk)

Phytochemistry, 3-volume set
ISBN 13: 978-1-77188-762-5 (hbk)

Library and Archives Canada Cataloguing in Publication

Phytochemistry / edited by Chukwuebuka Egbuna, Jonathan Chinenye Ifemeje, PhD, Stanley Chidi Udedi, PhD, Shashank Kumar, PhD.
Includes bibliographical references and index.
Contents: Volume 1. Fundamentals, modern techniques, and applications.
Issued in print and electronic formats.
ISBN 978-1-77188-759-5 (v. 1 : hardcover).--ISBN 978-0-429-42622-3 (v. 1 : PDF)

1. Botanical chemistry. I. Egbuna, Chukwuebuka, editor

QK861.P65 2019	572'.2	C2018-904824-7	C2018-904875-1

....

CIP data on file with US Library of Congress

....

Apple Academic Press also publishes its books in a variety of electronic formats. Some content that appears in print may not be available in electronic format. For information about Apple Academic Press products, visit our website at **www.appleacademicpress.com** and the CRC Press website at **www.crcpress.com**

ABOUT THE EDITORS

Chukwuebuka Egbuna

Chukwuebuka Egbuna is a chartered chemist, a chemical analyst, and an academic researcher. He is a member of the Institute of Chartered Chemists of Nigeria (ICCON), the Nigerian Society of Biochemistry and Molecular Biology (NSBMB), the Royal Society of Chemistry (RSC), United Kingdom, and the Society of Quality Assurance (SQA), USA. He has been engaged in a number of roles at New Divine Favor Pharmaceutical Industry Limited, Akuzor Nkpor, Anambra State, Nigeria, and Chukwuemeka Odumegwu Ojukwu University (COOU), Nigeria. He has attended series of conferences and workshops and has collaboratively worked and published quite a number of research articles in the domain of phytochemistry. He has edited books with top publishers such as Springer Nature and Elsevier. He is a reviewer and an editorial board member for various journals, including serving as a website administrator for the *Tropical Journal of Applied Natural Sciences* (TJANS), a journal of the faculty of Natural Sciences, COOU. His primary research interests are in phytochemistry, food and medicinal chemistry, analytical chemistry, and nutrition and toxicology. He obtained his BSc and MSc degrees in biochemistry at Chukwuemeka Odumegwu Ojukwu University.

Jonathan Chinenye Ifemeje, PhD

Jonathan Chinenye Ifemeje, PhD, is an Associate Professor in the Department of Biochemistry, Faculty of Natural Sciences, Chukwuemeka Odumegwu Ojukwu University, Nigeria. He obtained his PhD in applied biochemistry from Nnamdi Azikiwe University, Awka, Nigeria, and his MSc degree in nutrition and toxicology from the University of Port-Harcourt, Nigeria. He has to his credits over 40 publications in both local and international journals. Dr. Ifemeje is currently the Coordinator, Students Industrial Work Experience Scheme (SIWES), COOU and has served as an external examiner for various institutions. He is the Managing Editor of the Tropical Journal of Applied Natural Sciences and is serving as a reviewer and an editorial board member for various journals. He has worked extensively in the area of phytochemistry, nutrition, and toxicology. He is a member of various institutes, including the Institute of Chartered Chemists of Nigeria (ICCON), the Nigerian Society of Biochemistry and Molecular Biology (NSBMB), and Society of Quality Assurance (SQA).

Stanley Chidi Udedi, PhD

Stanley Udedi Chidi, PhD, is a Full Professor of Biochemistry at the Department of Applied Biochemistry, Nnamdi Azikiwe University, (UNIZIK), Awka, Nigeria. He has taught in various institutions, including Madonna University Okija, Nigeria, and Anambra State University, which is now Chukwuemeka Odumegwu Ojukwu University, Nigeria. He is currently the Dean of Student Affairs at UNIZIK. He has worked extensively in the field of phytochemistry and food and medicinal chemistry and has supervised many MSc and PhD students. He is well published with over 50 publications, which have attracted over 170 citations. He is well traveled and has attended a series of workshops and conferences locally and internationally. He is a member of various professional institutes, which includes the Institute of Chartered Chemists of Nigeria (ICCON), the Nigerian Society of Biochemistry and Molecular Biology (NSBMB), the Nutrition Society of Nigeria, and others. He obtained his PhD and MSc degrees from UNIZIK, Nigeria.

Shashank Kumar, PhD

Shashank Kumar, PhD, is working as Assistant Professor at the Center for Biochemistry and Microbial Sciences, Central University of Punjab, Bathinda, India. He obtained his BSc, MSc, and PhD Biochemistry from the Department of Biochemistry, University of Allahabad, India. He worked as Postdoctoral Fellow at the Department of Biochemistry, King George's Medical University, Lucknow, India. Dr. Kumar has about 60 published scientific papers/reviews/editorial articles/book chapters in various national and international peer-reviewed journals and has been cited more than 1200 times. He has edited several books on topics such as the "concepts in cell signaling," "carbohydrate metabolism: theory and practical approach," and so forth. He has expertise in the areas of free radical biology, cancer biology, characterization of plant natural products, xenobiotic metabolism, and microbiology. He is familiar with many biochemical techniques such as spectrophotometry, enzyme-linked immunosorbent assay, electrophoresis, polymerase chain reaction, real-time polymerase chain reaction, flow cytometry, thin-layer chromatography, high-performance liquid chromatography, liquid chromatography–mass spectrometry, cell culture, and microbiological techniques. He has presented his research findings at more than 25 national/international conferences and attended about 30 workshops at different universities and medical colleges throughout the India. Dr. Kumar is a life time member of Italo-Latin American Society of Ethnomedicine, and the Indian Sciences Congress Association, and member of the Asian Council of Science Editors, Dubai, UAE, and Publication Integrity and Ethics, London. He has been awarded the Junior/Senior and Research Associate Fellowships formulated and funded by various Indian agencies, such as Indian Council of Medical Research, University Grants Commission, Council of Scientific and Industrial Research India. Dr. Kumar laboratory has been funded by the University Grant Commission, India, and the Department of Science and Technology, India, for working on effects of various phytochemicals on cancer cell signaling pathway inhibition.

CONTENTS

Contributors .... *xiii*

Abbreviations .... *xvii*

Foreword .... *xxi*

Preface .... *xxiii*

PART I: Fundamentals of Phytochemistry 1

1. **Introduction to Phytochemistry** 3
   Chukwuebuka Egbuna, Jonathan C. Ifemeje, Toskë L. Kryeziu,
   Minakshi Mukherjee, Hameed Shah, G. M. Narasimha Rao,
   Laurence John Francis J. Gido, and Habibu Tijjani

2. **Biosynthesis of Phytochemicals** 37
   Habibu Tijjani, Chukwuebuka Egbuna, and Luka D. Carrol

3. **Mechanisms of Plant Defense Against Pathogens:**
   Phytoalexins Induction 79
   Hanan M. AL.-Yousef and Musarat Amina

4. **Biological Roles of Phytochemicals** 119
   Peculiar Feenna Onyekere, Chioma Obianuju Peculiar-Onyekere,
   Helen Ogechukwu Udodeme, Daniel Okwudili Nnamani, and
   Christopher Obodike Ezugwu

5. **Phytochemicals as Immunomodulators** 153
   Behnaz Aslanipour

6. **Phytochemicals as Nutraceuticals and Pharmafoods** 179
   Anywar Godwin

7. **Role of Phytochemistry in Plant Classification:**
   Phytochemotaxonomy 197
   Felix Ifeanyi Nwafor and Ifeoma Celestina Orabueze

8. **Plant Metabolomics** 223
   Sagar Satish Datir and Rakesh Mohan Jha

PART II: Methods and Techniques **245**

9. **Phytochemical Extraction, Isolation, and Detection Techniques**............**247**
    Temitope Temitayo Banjo, Paul Akinniyi Akinduti, Temitope Oluwabunmi Banjo,
    and Vinesh Kumar

10. **Techniques in Phytochemotaxonomy**...**261**
    Ifeoma Celestina Orabueze and Felix Ifeanyi Nwafor

11. **Chromatographical Techniques in Phytochemical Research**..................**287**
    Sumera Javad and Shagufta Naz

12. **Ultraviolet/Visible Spectroscopy and HPLC in**
    Phytochemical Analysis: An Introduction **307**
    Ade Kujore

13. **High-Performance Liquid Chromatography and**
    High-Performance Thin-Layer Chromatography as
    Sophisticated Tools in Phytochemical Analysis **343**
    Deepa R. Verma and Rohan V. Gavankar

14. **Analytical Techniques in Elemental Profiling** **367**
    Andrew G. Mtewa and Annu Amanjot

15. **Phytochemical Test Methods: Qualitative, Quantitative**
    and Proximate Analysis **381**
    Chukwuebuka Egbuna, Jonathan C. Ifemeje, Maryann Chinenye Maduako,
    Habibu Tijjani, Stanley Chidi Udedi, Andrew C. Nwaka, and Maryjane Oluoma Ifemeje

16. **Animal Models in Phytopharmacology**.....................................**427**
    Ahmed A. Adedeji, Mulkah O. Ajagun-Ogunleye, and Marta Vicente-Crespo

17. **Toxicological Testing of Plant Products** **463**
    Monica Neagu and Carolina Constantin

18. **Role of Biostatistics in Phytochemical Research:**
    Emphasis on Essential Oil Studies..**481**
    S. Zafar Haider, Gaurav Naik, Hema Lohani, and Nirpendra K. Chauhan

PART III: Computational Phytochemistry....................................... **495**

19. **Computational Phytochemistry in Drug Discovery:**
    Databases and Tools..**497**
    Sugumari Vallinayagam, Karthikeyan Rajendran and Vigneshkumar Sekar

20. **Stemness Modulation by Phytochemicals to**
    Target Cancer Stem Cells...**513**
    Prem Prakash Kushwaha, Pushpendra Singh, and Shashank Kumar

21. **Targeting Cancer Cell Carbohydrate Metabolism
    by Phytochemicals**..**537**

Swastika Dash, Prem Prakash Kushwaha, and Shashank Kumar

22. **Herbal Drug Discovery: The Envision Biotechnology Approach**...........**561**

Aniko Nagy

PART IV: Phytochemical Research **569**

23. **Gas Chromatography–Mass Spectrometry Analysis and
    In Vitro Anticancer Activity of *Tectona grandis*
    Bark Extract Against Human Breast Cancer Cell Line (MCF-7)**..........**571**

Arul Priya R., K. Saravanan, and Umarani B.

24. **Phytochemical Analysis of *Nigella sativa* L. Seeds Aqueous
    Extract by Gas Chromatography–Mass Spectroscopy and
    Fourier-Transform Infrared** **587**

Shaista Jabeen N., Jagapriya L., Senthilkumar Balasubramanian, Devi K., and
Jaison Jeevanandam

25. **Phytochemical Studies on Five Nigerian Indigenous Vegetables**............**605**

Faleyimu, O. I., Solomon T., and Ajiboye John Adebayo

Index *619*

CONTRIBUTORS

Ajiboye John Adebayo
Department of Chemical Sciences, Ondo State University of Science and Technology, Okitipupa, Nigeria

Ahmed A. Adedeji
Department of Pharmacology and Toxicology, Faculty of Medicine and Surgery, University of Gitwe, Rwanda

Mulkah O. Ajagun-Ogunleye
Department of Biochemistry, School of Biomedical Sciences, Kampala International University Western Campus, Uganda

Paul Akinniyi Akinduti
Department of Biological Sciences, Covenant University, Ota, Ogun State, Nigeria

Annu Amanjot
Department of Pharmacology and Therapeutics, Mbarara University of Science and Technology, Mbarara, Uganda

Musarat Amina
Department of Pharmacognosy, College of Pharmacy, King Saud University, Riyadh, Saudi Arabia

Hanan M. AL-Yousef
Department of Pharmacognosy, College of Pharmacy, King Saud University, Riyadh, Saudi Arabia

Behnaz Aslanipour
Department of Bioengineering, Faculty of Engineering, Ege University, Bornova, 35100 İzmir, Turkey

Temitope Oluwabunmi Banjo
Institute for Human Resources Development, University of Agriculture, Abeokuta, Ogun State, Nigeria

Temitope Temitayo Banjo
Department of Biological Sciences, Wellspring University, Irhirhi Road, Benin City, Edo state, Nigeria

Umarani B.
PG and Research Department of Zoology, Nehru Memorial College (Autonomous), Puthanampatti, Tiruchirappalli 621 007, India

Senthilkumar Balasubramanian
Department of Zoology, Thiruvalluvar University, Serkaddu, Vellore, Tamil Nadu, India

Luka D. Carrol
Department of Biochemistry, Faculty of Medical Sciences, University of Jos, Jos, Nigeria

Nirpendra K. Chauhan
Centre for Aromatic Plants (CAP), Industrial Estate Selaqui-248011, Dehradun (Uttarakhand) India

Carolina Constantin
Pathology Department, "Victor Babes" National Institute of Pathology, Colentina University Hospital, Bucharest, Romania

Swastika Dash
Department of Biochemistry and Microbial Sciences, School of Basic and Applied Sciences, Central University of Punjab, Bathinda, Punjab 151001, India

Sagar Satish Datir
Department of Biotechnology, Savitribai Phule Pune University, Pune 411007, Maharashtra, India

Chukwuebuka Egbuna
Department of Biochemistry, Faculty of Natural Sciences, Chukwuemeka Odumegwu Ojukwu University, Anambra State- 431124, Nigeria

Christopher Obodike Ezugwu
Department of Pharmacognosy and Environmental Medicines, University of Nigeria, Nsukka 410001, Enugu State, Nigeria

Rohan V. Gavankar
Department of Biotechnology, VIVA College of Arts, Commerce and Science, Virar, Maharashtra, India

Anywar Godwin
Department of Plant Sciences, Microbiology and Biotechnology, Makerere University, Kampala, Uganda

S. Zafar Haider
Centre for Aromatic Plants (CAP), Industrial Estate Selaqui, Dehradun, Uttarakhand 248011, India

Jonathan C. Ifemeje
Department of Biochemistry, Chukwuemeka Odumegwu Ojukwu University, Anambra State, Nigeria

Maryjane Oluoma Ifemeje
Department of Biochemistry, Chukwuemeka Odumegwu Ojukwu University, Anambra State, Nigeria

Sumera Javad
Department of Botany, Lahore College for Women University, Lahore, Pakistan

Rakesh Mohan Jha
Department of Biotechnology, Savitribai Phule Pune University, Pune, Maharashtra 411007, India

Jaison Jeevanandam
Department of Chemical Engineering, Faculty of Engineering and Science, Curtin University, 98009 Miri, Sarawak, Malaysia

Laurence John Francis J. Gido
Research Center of the College of Medicine, Davao Medical School Foundation, Inc., Davao City, Philippines

Devi K.
Department of Zoology, PG and Research Unit, Dhanabagyam Krishnaswamy Mudaliar College for Women (Autonomous), Sainathapuram, RV Nagar, Vellore, Tamil Nadu 632001, India

Ade Kujore
Cecil Instruments, Milton Technical Centre, Cambridge, UK

Shashank Kumar
School of Basic and Applied Sciences, Department of Biochemistry and Microbial Sciences, Central University of Punjab, Bathinda, Punjab 151001, India

Vinesh Kumar
Department of Sciences, Kids' Science Academy, Roorkee, Uttarakhand, India

Prem Prakash Kushwaha
Department of Biochemistry and Microbial Sciences, School of Basic and Applied Sciences, Central University of Punjab, Bathinda, Punjab 151001, India

Toskë L. Kryeziu
Department of Clinical Pharmacy, University of Pristina, Pristina, Kosovo

Jagapriya L.
Department of Zoology, PG and Research Unit, Dhanabagyam Krishnaswamy Mudaliar College for Women (Autonomous), Sainathapuram, RV Nagar, Vellore, Tamil Nadu 632001, India

Hema Lohani
Centre for Aromatic Plants (CAP), Industrial Estate Selaqui-248011, Dehradun, Uttarakhand India

Maryann Chinenye Maduako
Department of Biochemistry, Chukwuemeka Odumegwu Ojukwu University, Anambra State, Nigeria

Andrew G. Mtewa
Department of Chemistry, Institute of Technology, Malawi University of Science and Technology, Thyolo, Malawi

Minakshi Mukherjee
Department of Biological Sciences, The State University of New York, Buffalo, New York, USA

Aniko Nagy
Envision Biotechnology, Grandville, Michigan, USA

Gaurav Naik
Centre for Aromatic Plants (CAP), Industrial Estate Selaqui, Dehradun, Uttarakhand 248011 India

Shagufta Naz
Department of Biotechnology, Lahore College for Women University, Lahore, Pakistan

Monica Neagu
Pathology Department, "Victor Babes" National Institute of Pathology, Colentina University Hospital, Bucharest, Romania

Shaista Jabeen N.
Department of Zoology, PG and Research Unit, Dhanabagyam Krishnaswamy Mudaliar College for Women (Autonomous), Sainathapuram, RV Nagar, Vellore, Tamil Nadu 632001, India

Daniel Okwudili Nnamani
Department of Pharmacognosy and Environmental Medicines, University of Nigeria, Nsukka 410001, Enugu State, Nigeria

Felix Ifeanyi Nwafor
Department of Pharmacognosy and Environmental Medicines, University of Nigeria, Nsukka, Enugu State, Nigeria

Andrew C. Nwaka
Department of Biochemistry, Chukwuemeka Odumegwu Ojukwu University, Anambra State, Nigeria

Ifeoma Celestina Orabueze
Department of Pharmacognosy, University of Lagos, Lagos State, Nigeria

Peculiar Feenna Onyekere
Department of Pharmacognosy and Environmental Medicines, University of Nigeria, Nsukka 410001, Enugu State, Nigeria

Faleyimu O. I.
Department of Biological Sciences, Ondo State University of Science and Technology, Okitipupa, Nigeria

Chioma Obianuju Peculiar-Onyekere
Department of Microbiology, University of Nigeria, Nsukka 410001, Enugu State, Nigeria

Karthikeyan Rajendran
Mepco Schlenk Engineering College, Sivakasi, Tamil Nadu 626005, India

G. M. Narasimha Rao
Department of Botany, Andhra University, Visakhapatnam, Andhra Pradesh 530 003, India

Arul Priya R.
PG and Research Department of Zoology, Nehru Memorial College (Autonomous), Puthanampatti, Tiruchirappalli 621 007, India

K. Saravanan
PG and Research Department of Zoology, Nehru Memorial College (Autonomous), Puthanampatti, Tiruchirappalli 621 007, India

Vigneshkumar Sekar
Mepco Schlenk Engineering College, Sivakasi, Tamil Nadu 626005, India

Hameed Shah
CAS Key Laboratory for Biomedical effects of Nanomaterials and Nanosafety, National Center for Nanoscience and Technology, University of Chinese Academy of Science, 100049 Beijing, China

Pushpendra Singh
Tumor Biology Laboratory, National Institute of Pathology (ICMR), New Delhi, India

Solomon, T.
Department of Biological Sciences, Ondo State University of Science and Technology, Okitipupa, Nigeria

Habibu Tijjani
Natural Product Research Laboratory, Department of Biochemistry, Bauchi State University, Gadau, Nigeria

Helen Ogechukwu Udodeme
Department of Pharmacognosy and Environmental Medicines, University of Nigeria, Nsukka 410001, Enugu State, Nigeria

Stanley Chidi Udedi
Department of Applied Biochemistry, Nnamdi Azikiwe University, Awka, Nigeria

Deepa R. Verma
Department of Botany, VIVA College of Arts, Commerce and Science, Virar, Maharashtra, India

Sugumari Vallinayagam
Mepco Schlenk Engineering College, Sivakasi, Tamil Nadu 626005, India

Marta Vicente-Crespo
Department of Biochemistry, School of Medicine, St. Augustine International University, Kampala, Uganda DrosAfrica Trust, UK

ABBREVIATIONS

2D	Two-dimensional
3-BP	3-bromopyruvate
3D	Three-dimensional
67LR	67-kDa laminin receptor
AA	Arachidonic acid
AAS	Atomic absorption spectroscopy
AES	Atomic emission spectroscopy
ALA	α-linolenic acid
ANOVA	Analysis of variance
AO/EB	Acridine orange/ethidium bromide
AP-1	Activator protein 1
APE1	Apurinic/apyrimidinic endonuclease-1
ASE	Accelerated solvent extraction
ATM	Ataxia-telangiectasia mutated
ATP	Adenosine triphosphate
BB	Biobreeding
BER	Base excision repair
BSS	Beta-sitosterol
CAGR	Compound annual growth rate
CaOx	Calcium oxalate
CCC	Countercurrent chromatography
CC	Column chromatography
CHI	Chalcone isomerase
CHS	Chalcone synthase
CNS	Central nervous system
CoQ10	Coenzyme Q10
COX-2	Cyclooxygenase-2
CPC	Centrifugal partition chromatography
CPDB	Carcinogenic potency database
CPU	Central processing unit
CSC	Cancer stem cell
DHA	Docosahexaenoic acid
DHTQ	Dihydrothymoquinone
DMAPP	Dimethylallyl diphosphate

DMRT	Duncan's Multiple Range Test
DNA	Deoxyribonucleic acid
DNAPK	DNA-dependent protein kinase
DNP	Dinitrophenylhydrazine
DTH	Delayed-type hypersensitivity
EGCG	Epigallocatechin-3-O-gallate
ent-CDP	Ent-copalyl-diphosphate
EPA	Eicosapentaenoic acid
ER	Estrogen receptor
ERK	Extracellular-signal-regulated kinase
FC	Flash chromatography
FDA	Food and Drug Administration
FTIR	Fourier-transform infrared spectroscopy
GAPDH	Glyceraldehyde 3-phosphate dehydrogenase
GC	Gas chromatography
GC-MS	Gas chromatography–mass spectrometry
GLA	γ-linolenic acid
GLN	Glyceollins
GLUT	Glucose transporter
GPU	Graphics processing unit
GSK-3β	Glycogen synthase kinase-3 β
HIF-1	Hypoxia-inducible factor-1
HIT	Herb ingredients target
HPLC	High-performance liquid chromatography
HR	Homologous recombination
HTS	High-throughput screening
IC$_{50}$	Half maximal inhibitory concentration
ICH	International Conference on Harmonization
ICP-MS	Inductively coupled plasma mass spectroscopy
ICP-OES	Inductively coupled plasma optical emission spectroscopy
IFN	Interferon
IL	Interleukins
IMP	Inosine monophosphate
iNOS	Inducible nitric oxide synthase
IPP	Isopentenyl pyrophosphate
IQ	Installation qualification
IR	Infrared
JA	Jasmonic acid
LC-MS	Liquid-chromatography mass spectrometry
LD50	50% lethal dose

LDH	Lactate dehydrogenase
LDL	Low-density lipoprotein
LGA	Local government area
LOQ	Limit of quantitation
LRP5/6	Lipoprotein receptor-related proteins 5/6
LS	Light scattering
LT	Leukotriene
MAE	Microwave-assisted extraction
MAPK	Mitogen-activated protein kinase
MCT	Monocarboxylate transporter
MD	Molecular dynamics
MEP	Methylerythritol phosphate
MGMT	Mismatch and errors repair
MMR	Mismatch repair
mRNA	Messenger ribonucleic acid
MS	Mass spectrometry
NADH	Nicotinamide adenine dinucleotide
NER	Nucleotide excision repair
NF-κB	Nuclear factor-κB
NHEJ	Non-homologous end joining
NIST	National Institute of Standards and Technology
NK	Natural killer
NMR	Nuclear magnetic resonance
NOD	Nonobese diabetic
NO	Nitric oxide
NP	Nanoparticle
Nrf2	Nuclear factor E2-related factor 2
OECD	Organization for Economic Co-operation and Development
OPLC	Optimum performance laminar chromatography
OQ	Operating qualification
PAL	Phenylalanine ammonia lyase
PA	Pyrrolizidine alkaloid
PCA	Principal components analysis
PDB	Protein Data Bank
PEP	Phosphoenolpyruvate
PFKFB	6-phosphofructo-2-kinase/fructose-2,6-bisphosphatases
PGE2	Prostaglandin E2
PhA	Phytoalexins
PhT	Phytoantipicins
PKA	Protein kinase A

PK	Pyruvate kinase
PM	Plasma membrane
PP	Phenylpropanoid
PQ	Performance qualification
PR	Pathogenesis-related
PRP	Proline-rich protein
PSA	Phytochemical Society of Asia
PSE	Phytochemical Society of Europe
PSNA	Phytochemical Society of North America
PUFA	Polyunsaturated fatty acid
QSAR	Puantitative structure–activity relationship
R_f	Retention factor
RNA	Ribonucleic acid
RNF43	Ring finger 43
ROS	Reactive oxygen species
RP	Reverse phase
SAM	S-adenosyl-L-methionine
SA	Salicylic acid
SD	Standard deviation
SFE	Supercritical fluid extraction
SPE	Solid-phase extraction
SPF	Specific pathogen free
SPSS	Statistical Package for the Social Sciences
SRBC	Anti-sheep red blood cells
STZ	Streptozotocin
syn-CDP	Syn-copalyldiphosphate
TCA	Tricarboxylic acid cycle
TCMID	Traditional Chinese Medicine Integrative Database
TLC	Thin-layer chromatography
TNF	Tumor necrosis factor
UAE	Ultrasound-assisted extraction
UV	Ultraviolet
VDAC	Voltage-dependent anion channel
VEGF	Vascular endothelial growth factor
VLC	Vacuum liquid chromatography
WHO	World Health Organization
XRF	X-ray fluorescence
ZNRF3	Zinc and ring finger 3

FOREWORD

I feel honored for being invited to write the Foreword to the book *Phytochemistry, Volume 1: Fundamentals, Modern Techniques, and Applications*. I am very happy to write this foreword to a book of this kind that has great scope and scholarly contents. A panoramic review of this book indicates that it is well-articulated and written by professionals from diverse academic backgrounds. I congratulate the editors and contributors for their excellent work. The design is exceptional and gives firm background information about modern phytochemistry. The style of grouping the chapters into four parts of fundamentals, methods, computational, and research applications is one that makes it different from other books of phytochemistry. The present book provides a framework starting from the introduction, biosynthesis of phytochemicals to their effects in living systems and to the state-of-the-art modern techniques with insights on the discovery of medicinally active compounds through *in silico* and *in vitro* studies.

As a molecular biologist and a computational chemist with technical and scientific expertise in drug discovery, specialized in network pharmacology, ligand, and structure-based drug design, and with many years of experience in pharmaceutical R&D, biotech, and scientific software development, I will say that the field of phytochemistry is growing at a very astonishing rate because of the renewed interests in the search for safe natural drugs with minor side effects. The plant kingdom, which harbors over 400,000 species of plants, offers the opportunity for the discovery of novel compounds that will be useful for the treatment of diseases. Until today, only about 15% of these plants has been studied closely for their medicinal potentials despite the increasing need for new drugs.

Modern phytochemistry involves the application of high-throughput techniques and modern omics tools. It encompasses the study of plant natural products through metabolic profiling of the various biosynthesis pathways, optimization of the production of plant natural products, and importantly, the utilization of computational docking and simulation tools to identify molecular targets for the discovery of novel therapeutic compounds. Personally, I feel obliged to present this book to the scientific community. I recommend it to teachers, students, researchers, and everyone with interests in phytochemistry. It is with immense pleasure that I sincerely thank the Editor-in-chief, Chukwuebuka Egbuna, for inviting me to write this Foreword.

—Timea Polgar PhD
VP, R&D, Founder
Envision Biotechnology

PREFACE

Phytochemistry is a branch of science that deals with the study of the chemicals produced by plants, particularly the secondary metabolites. It takes into account the synthesis of secondary metabolites, its metabolisms in plants, and their effects in other living organisms. It also encompasses the medicinal, industrial, and commercial applications of plant natural products. Phytochemistry is multifaceted, and this made it complicated and problematic for authors to compose a good book of phytochemistry. Till now, there has been no comprehensive book on phytochemistry other than compendiums of research articles from aftermath of conferences or seminars. They have served a useful purpose, however, and could be excused in times when phytochemistry was without a very clear conceptual framework.

This book *Phytochemistry: Fundamentals, Modern Techniques, and Applications* is a comprehensive book on phytochemistry written by professionals from key institutions around the world. The authors are experts in their academic and research niche. The chapters are drawn carefully and integrated sequentially to aid flow, consistency, and continuity. This book will be very useful to researchers, teachers, students, phytochemists, plant biochemists, food and medicinal chemists, nutritionists and toxicologists, chemical ecologists, taxonomists, analytical chemists, industrialists, and many others.

The chapters are grouped into four parts. Part I covers the fundamentals of phytochemistry. Part II details the state-of-the-art modern methods and techniques in phytochemical research. Part III is an overview of computational phytochemistry and its applications. Part IV presents novel research findings in the discovery of drugs that will be effective in the treatment of diseases. Each chapter has a short abstract that briefly explains the scientific basis of the chapter and what readers should expect. The in-text references ensure that all information is authentic and verifiable.

Chapter 1 by Egbuna et al. is an introductory chapter that discusses the general scope of phytochemistry, its modern history, and the relationship it has with other sciences. It also discusses the prospects for phytochemists and the future projections of phytochemical research. Chapter 2 is a comprehensive description of the biosynthesis of phytochemicals. Tijjani et al. structurally presents the various biosynthetic pathways and the mechanisms involved. Hanan and Musarat present the mechanisms of plants defenses through the induction of phytoalexins (PhA) in Chapter 3. They also discuss the biosynthesis of PhA and its regulation with emphasis on the variations that exist within different plant families. Chapter 4, written by Onyekere et al., is an overview of the biological roles of phytochemicals in animals. Aslanipour presents the immunomodulatory roles of phytochemicals in Chapter 5, while author Anywar discusses phytochemicals as nutraceuticals and pharmafoods in Chapter 6. Nwafor and Orabueze in Chapter 7 details the role of phytochemistry in plant classification. The authors also details the various phytochemical markers of taxonomic importance. Chapter 8 by Datir and Jha is an overview of metabolomics in phytochemistry while highlighting the various high-throughput techniques in modern phytochemistry.

Banjo et al. in Chapter 9 describes the various extraction methods and techniques. Orabueze and Nwafor in Chapter 10 provides an overview of the techniques utilized in phytochemotaxonomy. Chapter 11 by Javad and Naz presents the different chromatographical techniques used for the isolation and characterization of phytochemicals. Kujore of Cecil Instruments in Chapter 12 describes the use of ultraviolet/visible spectroscopy and high-performance liquid chromatography (HPLC) with emphasis on principles, calibrations, and qualifications. Verma and Gavankar in Chapter 13 details the use of HPLC and high-performance thin-layer chromatography as sophisticated tools in phytochemical research. Mtewa and Amanjot discusses the various techniques in the elemental profiling of plant materials in Chapter 14. Egbuna et al. in Chapter 15 presents the various phytochemical tests methods used in the qualitative and quantitative analysis of phytochemicals. The chapter also details reagent preparation and the various calculations commonly encountered in phytochemistry. Adedeji et al. in Chapter 16 details the various animal models in phytopharmacology with emphasis on *Drosophila melanogaster* as a model. Neagu and Constantin in Chapter 17 describes the various protocols involved in the toxicological testing of plant natural products. Chapter 18 by Haider et al. is an overview of the roles of biostatistics in phytochemical research with emphasis on essential oil studies.

Vallinayagam et al. in Chapter 19 presents the various databases and tools utilized in drug discovery under computational phytochemistry. Kushwaha et al. in Chapter 20 presents research findings of the stemness modulation by phytochemicals to target stem cells. In a separate development in chapter 21, Dash et al. presents findings on targeting cancer cell carbohydrate metabolism by phytochemicals through in silico studies. Nagy in Chapter 22 emphasizes herbal discovery through an automated platform capable of establishing a handshake of the ethnobotanical uses of medicinal plants with scientific evidence by the Envision Biotechnology approach.

Priya et al. in Chapter 23 presents cancer research findings on the effects of *Tectona grandis* bark extract on human breast cancer cell line (MCF-7). Authors present a photomicrographs of the anticancer activities of *T. grandis*. Chapter 24 by Shaista et al. is a phytochemical analysis of *Nigella sativa* L. seed aqueous extract by gas chromatography–mass spectrometry and Fourier-transform infrared. Faleyimu et al. in Chapter 25 presents phytochemical studies of five Nigerian indigenous vegetables.

In summary, this book is great in scope and one that is invaluable. The volume took many months to come to completion. I sincerely appreciate the unflinching supports of the chapter contributors, volunteer reviewers, and my co-editors. I also extend my sincere appreciation to my family for their support and patience during the editorial process of this book. My gratitude also goes to Apple Academic Press for their guidance from the onset of this book project and to the management of ResearchGate social platform where the project originated.

I recommend this book to everyone with interests in phytochemistry or related areas. I will welcome reviews, suggestions, and areas that will need improvements with an open heart. Thank you.

—**Chukwuebuka Egbuna**, MNSBMB, MICCON, AMRSC
Department of Biochemistry, Faculty of Natural Sciences
Chukwuemeka Odumegwu Ojukwu University
Anambra State- 431124, Nigeria

PART I
Fundamentals of Phytochemistry

CHAPTER 1

INTRODUCTION TO PHYTOCHEMISTRY

CHUKWUEBUKA EGBUNA[1,*], JONATHAN C. IFEMEJE[1],
TOSKË L. KRYEZIU[2], MINAKSHI MUKHERJEE[3], HAMEED SHAH[4],
G.M. NARASIMHA RAO[5], LAURENCE JOHN FRANCIS J. GIDO[6],
and HABIBU TIJJANI[7]

[1]*Department of Biochemistry, Chukwuemeka Odumegwu Ojukwu
University, Uli, Anambra State, Nigeria, Tel.: +2347039618485*
[2]*Department of Clinical Pharmacy, University of Pristina, Pristina,
Kosovo*
[3]*Department of Biological Sciences, The State University of New York
at Buffalo, Buffalo, New York, USA*
[4]*CAS Key Laboratory for Biomedical Effects of Nanomaterials and
Nanosafety, National Center for Nanoscience and Technology,
University of Chinese Academy of Science, 100049 Beijing, China*
[5]*Department of Botany, Andhra University, Visakhapatnam,
Andhra Pradesh 530003, India*
[6]*Research Center of the College of Medicine, Davao Medical School
Foundation Inc., Davao City, Philippines*
[7]*Natural Product Research Laboratory, Department of Biochemistry,
Bauchi State University, Gadau, Nigeria*
*Corresponding author. E-mail: egbuna.cg@coou.edu.ng;
egbunachukwuebuka@gmail.com; https://egbunac.com
ORCID: https://orcid.org/0000-0001-8382-0693*

ABSTRACT

Phytochemistry is the study of the chemicals produced by plants, particularly
the secondary metabolites, synthesized as a measure for self-defense

against insects, pests, pathogens, herbivores, ultraviolet exposure and environmental hazards. Phytochemistry takes into account the structural compositions of these metabolites, the biosynthetic pathways, functions, mechanisms of actions in the living systems as well as it's medicinal, industrial, and commercial applications. The proper understanding of phytochemical is essential for drug discovery and for the development of novel therapeutic agents against major diseases. This chapter introduces phytochemistry, discusses the history of modern phytochemistry, the relationship of phytochemistry with other sciences and the importance of phytochemistry. It also provides information on the sources and classification of phytochemicals, prospects for phytochemists, the usefulness of computational phytochemistry, biostatistics and the advances in phytochemical research.

1.1 INTRODUCTION

It will be recalled that in the food chain, plants are referred to as the producers because they had the ability to trap energy from sunlight, harness and assemble some basic units which they transform through some chemical process into complex high energy-yielding compounds that are readily available to organisms. Their generosity became overwhelmingly and practically complex to comprehend at a glance. A field has to emerge – "phytochemistry." Phytochemistry is the study of chemicals produced by plants, particularly the secondary metabolites. It takes into account their structural compositions, the biosynthetic pathways, functions, and mechanisms of actions in the living system. The study of phytochemicals has been instrumental in the discovery of new plant natural products which are of commercial values in various industries such as the traditional and complementary medicine systems, pharmaceutical industries, nutraceuticals, and dietary supplement industries. Not left out is the cosmeceuticals industries, clothing and textiles industries, food, wine, and beverage industries, the military among others. Owing to the consistent threat of microorganisms, environmental hazards to public health, the significance of phytochemistry in the medical and pharmaceutical industries for the quest for the discovery of new drugs has overshadowed their essence in other industries.

   Phytochemicals have been in existence since time immemorial and are known to be responsible for the organoleptic properties (color, taste, flavor, aroma, and odor) of plants, such as the smell of garlic, ginger, and the deep purple color of blueberries. The ability of plants to exhibit curative potentials and the characteristic difference that exists within them may also have awakened early interests for the knowledge about their chemical compositions. In the plant kingdom, these variations are quite glaring. One example is the Four O'Clocks plant (*Mirabilis jalapa*), called the marvel-of-Peru, or beauty-of-the-night because of its ability to open in mid-afternoon through the night and closes in the early morning. *Mirabilis*, a Latin word meaning wonder, also radiates some pleasant fragrances and exhibits flowers of different colors such as a white, red, pink, yellow, and some two-toned blooms simultaneously on the same plant. This phenomenal features in their biodiversity can be understood through the study of some chemical networks and interactions within the plants and its external environment. Plants are diverse and widely distributed from lands, rocky hills, mountains to marine environments. There are over 400,000 species of plants in the world (Pitman and Jørgensen, 2002), out of which only a small fraction of about 35,000–70,000 species of plants have been screened for their medicinal use (Veeresham, 2012). The medicinal potentials of phytochemicals are exhibited from the least primitive to higher plants. According to Fabricant and Farnsworth (2001), about 80% of 122 plant-derived drugs are related to their original traditional uses. Reportedly, as at the dawn of 21st century, 11% of the 252 drugs considered as basic and essential by the World Health Organization (WHO) were exclusive of flowering plant origin (Veeresham, 2012).

In the evolutionary study of phytochemicals, it was believed that there was little free oxygen in the atmosphere when plants first evolved. The direct consequence of this is that as plants metabolize, the oxygen concentration in the world increased. This polluted the environment and to deal with it, plants began to synthesize antioxidants molecules to protect it from highly reactive species that are cytotoxic to the plant cells. Moreover, the damaging effects of microbes on the cell structures of plants especially the important biomolecules has left plants with no options than to synthesize more bioactive compounds to protect it (see Chapter 3 for more details). This evolutional theory is supported by recent evidence in the compositional patterns of phytochemicals in plants. For instance, plant parts such as the leaves, flowers, stems, barks, roots, and seeds that are prone to insects, pests, microbial attacks, and the harsh environment have more amounts of phytochemicals than other parts of the plants. Another supportive evidence is the variation that exists in the same species of plants grown in the harsh environment and those in areas with less environmental stress (see Volume 3, Chapter 12 and 13 for more information).

Prior to the in-depth understanding of phytochemicals, the first tool employed by man is the "error and trial tools" which helped man to distinguish between edible and non-edible plants. Many casualties were recorded at that time. Grazing animals are not left out, they graze, identify, and avoid toxic plants through their sense of smell. The study continued and was widely utilized by the oldest medical system, the Chinese and the Indian Ayurvedic medicine, for the treatment of various diseases such as cancer, cardiovascular diseases, and stroke. The knowledge became prominent in the 19th and 20th century due to the extensive research using sophisticated hybrid chromatography and spectroscopy for the extraction, isolation, characterization, and purification of phytochemicals (see Chapter 8–14 for detailed information).

This time around, research is ongoing and individual molecules are constantly been discovered. The search for the discovery of new drugs and repurposing of existing ones have driven the study of phytochemistry to a new era employing in silico study techniques, applying simulation, and molecular docking procedures of bioinformatics and cheminformatics.

1.2 BRIEF HISTORY OF MODERN PHYTOCHEMISTRY

The ethnobotanical studies of medicinal plants for the treatment of diseases have existed since antiquity. For instance, the discovery of quinine marked the first successful use of chemical compounds to treat infectious disease (David and Jacoby, 2005). This was considered as the most important medical discovery of the 17th century (Achan et al., 2011). But in practical terms, the use of the quinine source, that is, the bark of the Cinchona (quinaquina) tree dated back as at the 16th century. However, the beginning of the isolation of plant chemical compounds marked the early stages of modern phytochemistry. One such example is the isolation of alkaloids by the brilliant pharmacist named Friedrich Wilhelm Adam Serturner (1783–1841) in the latter part of 18th century (Krishnamurti and Rao, 2016). This isolation not only led to the synthesis of new drugs but also to the purification of plant extracts used as medicines. It is important to note that apart from being the first to isolate an alkaloid, morphine, Friedrich Wilhelm was the first person to isolate an active ingredient associated with a medicinal plant or herb. Not long enough, his discoveries transformed pharmaceutical chemistry from a state of alchemy to an acknowledged branch of science (Krishnamurti and Rao, 2016).

Under similar circumstance, the scientists Pierre Joseph Pelletier and Joseph Caventou in 1820 isolated quinine from the herb *Cinchona officinalis*, a unique drug with the indication to be used against malaria (Dobson, 2001). Since then (within the last 300 years), many other compounds have been successfully isolated and characterized such as digitalis (1785), picrotoxin (1812–1884), curare (1856–1958), and salicin (1860–1877) (Dikshit, 2017). With the progress in biotechnology during the 1970's, a trend in the synthesis of various derivatives of plant metabolites by mimicking the biosynthetic pathways has led to the production of more stable, consequently, more effective albeit less poisonous compounds which are of commercial value. The in vitro synthesis of phytochemical is detailed in Volume 3 of this book.

Because terpenes represent a diverse nonetheless a problematic class for extraction, the scientists Croteau and Cane in the 1980's became the first to determine terpene-synthesizing enzyme, called terpene synthase which has led to the discovery of alternative pathways for the synthesis of terpenoids, monoterpenes, diterpene, and so forth (Hartmann, 2007). The year 1990 became a significant period for modern phytochemistry because of the development of sophisticated techniques.

1.2.1 STRUCTURE–ACTIVITY RELATIONSHIP

A feature of numerous modern-day drug is that they resemble the natural products from the structural point of view, hence, without the existence of these compounds in nature, scientist would never be able to treat the countless number of diseases. A typical illustration is morphine, a model substance of several anesthetics and salicylic acid, a model for the creation of acetylsalicylic acid (Lydon and Duke, 1989). Another supporting evidence of the stereochemistry of drugs (structural resemblance) which resulted in problems is thalidomide (an analog of glutethimide, a sedative), a sleeping substance administered to pregnant women with little-known aftermath effects. During that period, numerous children born from pregnant mothers who were administered it suffered phocomelia. This led the company to suffer legal issues and has to withdraw the product from the market. In reality, thalidomide contained a racemic mixture of both isomers, ((−) (S) and (+) (R) thalidomide), whereas the isomer (−) (S) thalidomide had teratogenic effects, the other (+) (R) thalidomide doesn't. Eventually, this drug has found usage in cancer therapy (Fabro and Smith, 1967).

1.2.2　TRENDS

During the first decade of the 21st century, there was a decrease in the interest of advancing the knowledge of plant-based chemistry by scientists and pharmaceutical companies for greater interest in synthetic drugs because they were easily mass-produced compared to the natural ones (Schmidt and Ribnicky, 2008). However, due to reported side effects in patients, numerous products were withdrawn from the market. A study has shown that the effect of natural remedies persist higher for patients receiving treatment for their long-lasting diseases. In view of this, there appears to be an increased usage of plant products since 2010, which provides slower effects yet with fewer side effects than synthetic medications. At present, new versions of the pharmacopoeia are also adding recent knowledge about phytochemicals to their volumes as well as gaining extended sophisticated products related to the modification of plant enzymes to easily obtain therapeutic substances. Worthy of note is that some remarkable phytochemicals have been discovered from the marine environment. Marine-derived compounds have recently gained a considerable interest because of the wide variety of pharmacological applications. A detailed overview of marine phytochemistry can be found in Volume 3 of this book.

1.3　RELATIONSHIP WITH OTHER SCIENCES

Phytochemistry is an important part of a number of disciplines. There have been controversies and speculations as to the place of phytochemistry in science. Some scientists consider it as a subfield of botany and chemistry while others believed it should be part of the food and medicinal chemistry because of its wide application in drug discovery. Categorically, phytochemistry is a fulcrum and an aspect of many biosciences and would be difficult to single out as a stand-alone science (Fig. 1.1). For instance, phytochemistry is an important part of Systematic Botany, Taxonomy, Ethnobotany, Conservation biology, Plant Genetic and metabolomics, Evolutionary Sciences and Plant Pathology. The field of Pharmacy and Pharmacognosy, Complementary and Alternative medicine, Ethnomedicine, Biochemistry, Microbiology, Bioinformatics and Computational Chemistry employs the knowledge of phytochemistry in the discovery of bioactive compounds. The field of biotechnology and process engineering, nutrition and food sciences, organic chemistry, employs the knowledge of phytochemistry in the production of natural products with increase phytochemical yields. In the control of environmental pollution, the knowledge of phytochemistry is essential in applying bioremediation techniques such as phytoremediation to mop up harmful substances (detailed in Volume 3).

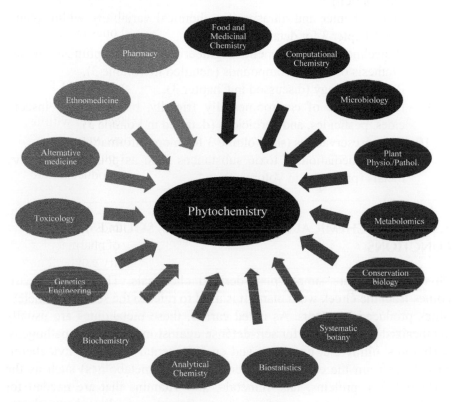

FIGURE 1.1   Some contributing fields to phytochemistry.

1.4   IMPORTANCE OF PHYTOCHEMISTRY

The knowledge of phytochemistry is essential in the:

1. Search for the discovery of new drugs and repurposing of existing ones (see Chapter 20–25 for more information).
2. Characterization and standardization of traditional herbal drugs in the crude form (see Chapter 9–15, 22 for a comprehensive information on the various techniques involved).
3. Assessment of the toxicity levels of plants (see Chapter 16 and 17 for details).

4. Understanding of plant physiology, biosynthetic pathways, and metabolomics (detailed in Chapter 2, 3 and 8).
5. Identification and classification of plants (see Chapter 7 for more information).
6. Study of inter and intraspecific chemical variability within plants (see Chapter 3 for details).
7. Biotechnology and genetic engineering for the optimization and synthesis of classic compounds (detailed in Volume 3).
8. Plant pathology (discussed in Chapter 3).
9. Development of environmentally friendly, biofungicides, insecticides, pesticides, and herbicides (detailed in Volume 3).
10. Food preservations (see Volume 3 for more information).
11. Phytoremediation of toxic substances such as poisons and heavy metals (presented in Volume 3).

1.5 PHYTOCHEMICALS, CLASSIFICATION, SOURCES, AND FUNCTIONS

Phytochemicals are simply plant-derived chemicals. The word "phyto" comes from the Greek word plant. It is used to refer to the secondary metabolites produced by plants. As noted earlier, these metabolites are usually synthesized as a measure for self-defense against insects, pests, pathogens, herbivores, ultraviolet exposure, and environmental hazards. Phytochemicals differ from the essential nutrients (primary metabolites) such as the carbohydrates, proteins, fats, minerals, and vitamins that are needed for the day to day maintenance of the plants. Sometimes, phytochemicals are used to refer to functional foods with antioxidant properties, nutraceuticals, phytonutrients, anti-nutrients, phytotoxins, and so forth.

1.5.1 CLASSIFICATION OF PHYTOCHEMICALS

There are tens of thousands of phytochemicals. So far, there could not have been a consistent classification system because of their numerous number and the pace by which new phytochemicals are discovered. A simple classification system divided phytochemicals into three chemically distinct groups. They are the phenolics, terpenes, N, and S containing compounds (Table 1.1).

TABLE 1.1 Classification of Common Phytochemicals.

Major classes	Subclasses	Representatives
Phenolics	Polyphenols	Flavonoids, isoflavonoids, chalconoids, lignans, stilbenoids (e.g., resveratrol), curcuminoids, tannins (e.g., protocatechuic and chlorogenic acids)
	Aromatic acid	Phenolic acids (e.g., gallic acid, tannic acid, vanillin, ellagic acid), hydroxycinnamic acids (e.g., coumarin)
Terpenes	Monoterpenes (C_{10})	Geraniol, limonene, pyrethroids, myrcene
	Sesquiterpenes (C_{15})	Costunolides
	Diterpenes (C_{20})	Abietic acid, cafestol, gibberellins
	Triterpenes (C_{30})	Azadirachtin, phytoecdysones
	Polyterpenes (C_5)$_n$	Tetraterpenes, for example, carotenoids, rubber
Terpenoids	Carotenoids (tetraterpenoids)	β-carotene, lycopene, phytoene
	Xanthophylls	Lutein, zeaxanthin
	Triterpenoid	Saponins, ursolic acid
	Steroids	Tocopherols (vitamin E), phytosterols (β-sitosterol, campesterol)
N (organonitrides)	Alkaloids	Nicotine, morphine, caffeine, theobromine, theophylline
	Cyanogenic glucosides	
	Nonprotein amino acids	Canavanine, azetidine-2-carboxylic acid
S (organosulfides)	Allicin, alliin, piperine Glutathione, phytoalexins	
Others	Phytic acid, oxalic acid, tartaric acid, malic acid, quinic acid	

1.5.2 SOURCES OF PHYTOCHEMICALS

Phytochemicals are found in fruits, vegetables, whole grains, spices, legumes, herbs, shrubs, and trees (Table 1.2). They get accumulated in plant parts at different concentrations such as in the leaves, fruit, bark, stem, roots, seeds, and flowers. Some phytochemicals are also synthesized by other living organisms such as fungi, although the mechanism by which they synthesize it might differ. However, many foods containing phytochemicals are already part of our daily diet except for some refined foods such as sugar or alcohol. The easiest way to get more phytochemicals is to eat varieties of at least five to nine servings of fruits or vegetable per day representing colors of rainbows. Chapter 6 of this book gave a holistic view of phytochemicals acting as nutraceuticals.

1.5.3   FUNCTIONS OF PHYTOCHEMICALS IN THE LIVING ORGANISMS

Phytochemicals perform quite a number of roles in the living organisms (Table 1.2), and the mechanism by which they accomplish it has not been fully understood. However, phytochemical functions as:

1. Antioxidants by preventing oxidative damage of important biomolecules such as nucleic acids, proteins, and fats (elaborated in Volume 2).
2. Antimicrobial agents: antibacterial, antifungal, antiviral, anti-trypano-cidal agents (discussed in Volume 2).
3. Stimulation of immune system (see Chapter 5 for comprehensive details).
4. Modulation of detoxifying enzymes.
5. Anti-inflammatory functions.
6. Reduction of platelet aggregations.
7. Physiological activities such as interfering with the binding of pathogens to cell receptors.

Others include antimalarial activity, antidiarrheal, antihelminthic, hepatoprotective, anti-atherosclerosis, anti-allergy, antidiabetic, antimuta-genic, wound healing, pain relief, and antihypertension. Phytochemicals are also used in the treatment of a sore throat, cough, toothache, ulcers, menstrual bleeding, improvement of sperm count, dysentery treatment, stomach upset, vertigo, and appetite enhancing. Many other functions of phytochemicals exist depending on the plant. About 80% of the world most useful drugs are from plants. Chapters 4 and 5 of this book gave an overview of the biological functions and immunomodulatory properties of phytochemicals. Volume 2 of this book contains many chapters that discusses the various applications of plant natural products for the treat-ment of diseases.

TABLE 1.2 Types of Phytochemicals, Sources, and its Biological Effects.

Phytochemicals	Sources	Biological effects	References
Carotenes			
α-carotene	Carrots, sweet potatoes and winter squash, pumpkins, maize, tangerine	Antimetastatic agent, provitamin A, immuno-enhancement, cataracts, and macular degeneration	Liu et al. (2015); Rodriguez-Amaya (2015)
β-carotene	Carrots, sweet potatoes and winter squash, dark, leafy greens, red, orange and yellow fruits, and vegetables	Coloring agent and as provitamin A, antimetastatic agent, immuno-enhancement, cataracts, and macular degeneration, anti-autism agent	Avraham et al. (2017); Mehrad et al. (2018); Ravanfar et al. (2018)
Terpenes and Terpenoids			
Triterpenoid	Soybeans, beans, other legumes, maize, alfalfa	Anticancer agents, antidiabetic effect, anti-inflammatory agents, anti-oxidants, and so forth.	Grishko and Galaiko and (2016); Salvador et al. (2017); Xu et al. (2018)
Diterpenes	Mustard, bugleweeds, common skullcap, germanders, and so forth	Antioxidant, antifeedant, antimicrobial, anti-inflammatory	Faiella et al. (2014); Grishko and Galaiko (2016); De Oliveira et al. (2017)
Monoterpenes	Oils of citrus, cherries, spearmint, dill, garlic, celery, maize, rosemary, ginger, basil, citrus oils, caraway, mints	Applications in drugs, flavors, and fragrances, advanced biofuels, enzyme inhibition, effects on bio channels	Zebec et al. (2016); Mewalal et al. (2017); Zhang et al. (2017)
Steroids	Almonds, cashews, peanuts, sesame seeds, sunflower seeds, whole wheat, maize, soybeans, many vegetable oils, avocado, rice bran, wheat germ, corn oils, fennel, peanuts, soybeans, hawthorn, basil, buckwheat	Neuroactive, neuroprotective, and immunomodulatory increase muscle and bone synthesis, regulate many aspects of metabolism and immune function, influence sex differences, and support reproduction	Chrbolka et al. (2017)
Astaxanthin	Salmon, green algae, Krill, arctic shrimp, red snapper	Nutraceuticals, cosmetics, and the food and feed industries, pigmentation, aquaculture, antioxidant, and so forth.	Rodriguez-Amaya (2015)

TABLE 1.2 *(Continued)*

Phytochemicals	Sources	Biological effects	References
β-Cryptoxanthin	Kamut, corn flour, quinoa, noodles, egg	Provitamin A activity, antioxidant, reduces inflammatory disorders, effective against rheumatoid arthritis, antimetastatic potential.	Rodriguez-Amaya (2015)
Lutein	Colorful fruits and vegetables	Reduced risk of age-related macular degeneration and cataracts, found in macular pigment of human retina	Olaf Sommerburg (1998); Rodriguez-Amaya (2015)
Phenolic compounds			
Natural monophenols	Parsley, celery leaf, rosemary, sage, oregano, thyme, pepperwort, wild bergamot	Antimicrobial, antioxidant	Gutiérrez-Larraínzar et al. (2012)
Polyphenols and others			
Flavonoids	Red, blue, purple pigments, tea, strawberries, gooseberries, cranberries, grapefruit, apples, peas, brassicas (broccoli, kale, brussels sprouts, cabbage), chives, spinach, endive, leek, tomatoes	Antioxidant, antimicrobial, enzyme inhibition	Ouédraogo et al. (2018); Xu et al. (2018)
Isoflavonoids	Soy, alfalfa sprouts, red clover, chickpeas, peanuts, kudzu, other legumes	Antimycobacterial agents, estrogenic agents, wound healing agents, antimicrobial potential	Araya-Cloutier et al. (2017); Coronado-Aceves et al. (2017); Ergene Oz et al. (2018);
Aurones	lemons, oranges, and grapefruit	Active against hepatitis C, neuro-generatic agents, antifungal agents, antimicrobial, anticancer, antiviral, antimalarial, antioxidant, anti-inflammatory, anticarcinogenic	Liew et al. (2015); Boucherle et al. (2017); Liew et al. (2017)

TABLE 1.2 *(Continued)*

Phytochemicals	Sources	Biological effects	References
Chalconoids	Licorice root, citrus peel, apple peel	Anticancer, antimalarial, antimicrobial, anti-inflammatory, anti-protozoal, anti-oxidant, antiproliferative agents, enzyme inhibition.	Singh (2014); Mostofi et al. (2015); Mirzaei et al. (2017)
Flavonolignans	Artichokes, milk thistle	Antioxidant agents, antiviral agents, hepato-protective agents, inhibiting blood coagulation	Althagafy et al. (2013); Pyszkova et al. (2016); Bijak et al. (2017);
Lignans	Apricots, strawberries, Broccoli, kale, oats, wheat	Cytotoxic against human tumor cell lines, antioxidant, neuroprotective, cognition enhance-ment, anti-inflammatory, enzyme inhibition	Jiang et al. (2017); Sownd-hararajan et al. (2017); Xu et al. (2017);
Stilbenoids	Grape (skins and seeds, grape wine), nuts, peanuts, Japanese knotweed root	Cytotoxic against human tumor cell lines, antioxidant, phytoalexins activity, anti-inflammatory activity, enzyme inhibition	Basheer et al. (2017); Cao et al. (2016); Hu et al. (2018)
Curcuminoids	Turmeric, mustard.	Anti-turmeric potential, anti-diabetic potential, drug interactive ability, painkiller, anti-microbial agents.	Bahramsoltani et al., (2017); De Meloa et al. (2017); Verma et al. (2017)
Tannins	Tea, berries, horse chestnut (*Aesculus hippocastanum*), cranberry juice, peanut skin	Enzyme inhibition and speed up agents, albumin interactive agents, wound healing promoters, anti-microbial agents,	Adamczyk et al. (2017); Barrett et al. (2018); Sekowski et al. (2018);
Aromatic acid	Peppermint, licorice, peanut, wheat, vanilla beans, cloves, soy	Anti-oxidant agents, anticancerous effect, antibacterial agents	Cvijetic et al. (2018); Zhang et al. (2018)
Glucosinolates	Broccoli, cabbage, kale, cauliflower, turnip, mustard greens	Antioxidant, antitumeric effects, high doses cause toxicity, lower doses stimulate appetite, heart-protective agent	Bieganska-Marecik et al. (2017); Radošević et al. (2017)
Betalains	Beets, chard, Amaranthus tricolor	Antioxidant, anti-tumeric, anti-lipidemic, and antimicrobial activity	Gengatharan et al. (2015); Kumar et al. (2015)

TABLE 1.2 *(Continued)*

Phytochemicals	Sources	Biological effects	References
Chlorophylls	Colorful fruits and vegetables.	Antioxidant, photosensitizers, clastogenic activity, wound healing, anti-inflammatory, photodynamic therapy	Dos Reis et al. (2015); Roca et al. (2016)
Amines	Beetroot	Cytotoxic nature, International Agency for Research on Cancer declared heterocyclic aromatic amines as carcinogenic	Canales et al. (2017); Gu et al. (2018); Papageorgiou et al. (2018)
Carbohydrates	Wheat, barley, rye, oat	Source of energy, maintains cells, tissue, organ structures, some have role in maintaining stomach acidity, additives, role in insulin resistance, brain functions regulator	Arens (2018); Barazzoni et al. (2017); Gerschenson et al. (2017).

1.5.4 ROLE OF PHYTOCHEMICALS IN PLANT DISEASE MANAGEMENT

Plants synthesize a large number of secondary metabolites numbering above 200,000 that do not play a direct role in their growth but help them to survive in the environment especially by providing defense against diseases and pests. The wide variety of secondary compounds is synthesized mainly by the isoprenoid, phenylpropanoid, alkaloid or fatty acid, or polyketide pathways. The biosynthesis of phytochemicals is detailed in the next chapter.

Plant disease management involves the reduction in the economic loss of plants due to diseases caused by pathogens. Plants have evolved several mechanisms which have led to the production of tens of thousands of phytochemicals. Earlier, plant-based chemicals constitute a very small portion which was overlooked. Since the introduction of Food Quality Protection Act of 1996, there has been a vast market opportunity for agro-allied-based chemicals used in plant disease management in the United States and most of North America (Isman, 2000).

A lot of essential oils in plants have shown a high potential for getting rid of insects. A range of essential oils such as cinnamaldehyde, α-pinene, extracts from clove (*Syzygium aromaticum*, major oil being eugenol) and star anise (*Illicium verum*) has been shown to have fumigant and antifeedant effect on red flour beetle (*Tribolium castaneum*), and the maize weevil (*Sitophilus zeamais*) (Ho et al., 1995, 1997; Huang and Ho, 1998; Huang et al., 1998). Eugenol and oils from the holy basil (*Ocimum suave*) have also shown to be effective against *Sitophilus granarius* and *Prostephanus truncatus* (Obeng-Ofori and Reichmuth, 1997). Essential oils of cumin, star anise, oregano, and eucalyptus have been shown to be active against greenhouse pests such as cotton aphid (*Aphis gossypii*) and carmine spider mite (*Tetranychus cinnabarinus*) (Tuni and Sahinkaya, 1998). Volume 3 of this book contains comprehensive chapters on the role of essential oil in pest and disease management.

Plant-derived aldehydes and ketones play key roles against pathogenic fungi. Among aliphatic aldehydes and ketones, cinnamaldehyde has been shown to have the most potent activity against fungi especially two species of *Penicillium* that causes disease in humans (*P. cyclopium* and *P. frequentans*). The effects of perillaldehyde and citral were slightly weaker but potent enough. *Penicillium ulaiense*, an important pathogen causing molds in citrus, and other *Penicillium* spp. causing molds in apple and pear can be targeted using these aliphatic aldehydes that have one or more double bonds conjugated to their carbonyl group. Among aromatic aldehydes, cuminalde-hyde had been shown to have fairly potent antifungal activity (Kurita et al., 1981). The essential oils of *Thymbra spicata* and *Satureja thymbra* plants used as spices in Mediterranean cuisine have been shown to inhibit phyto-pathogenic fungi such as *Fusarium moniliforme*, *Rhizoctonia solani*, and *Phytophthora capsici* at a concentration of 400–800 μg/mL. Thymol and carvacrol have been identified as the major constituents in the essential oils involved in the fungicidal property, followed by monoterpenes γ-terpenin and p-cymene (Muller et al., 1995).

Phenolic compounds play a significant role in plant defense against bacteria and fungi. One important phenolic compound is coumarin. Haloge-nated coumarin, often brominated, chlorinated, or iodinated, is more stable than coumarin. It has been shown to be particularly effective against plant pathogenic fungi such as *Macrophomina phaseolina* (charcoal rot), *Phytoph-thora* spp. (damping off and seedling rot), *Rhizoctonia* spp. (damping off and root rot), and *Pythium* spp. (seedling blight). These four fungi are from different families, showing the broad spectrum activity of halogenated coumarins. In addition, halogenated coumarins have polymer seed coating abilities and less phytotoxicity, making them good candidates for natural pesticide development. In another study, 7-hydroxylated coumarin has been shown to be effective against parasitism of *Orobanche cernua* in sunflower (Serghini et al., 2001).

Tannins are another class of phenolic compounds that provide defensive properties. Though tannins are mostly known to provide defense against herbivores due to their astringent properties, they also play some fungicidal roles. They are active against *Colletotrichum circinans*, a fungus that causes smudge in onions. Tannins are also known to be inhibitory for fungal spore germination. Tannins are also known to be inhibitory for fungal spore germi-nation (Mazid et al., 2011).

Throughout evolution, plants have come up with multiple defense mechanisms against different pathogens and predators. With the develop-ment of high throughput technologies, the understanding of the mechanisms of plant–pathogen interactions has widen. Subsequent chapter address this in details.

1.6 PHYTOCHEMIST, SKILLS, AND FUTURE PROSPECTS

A chemist or chemical scientist is one that is involved in research activi-ties related to chemical analysis, confirmation of elements, elucidation of the structure of chemical compounds for industrial purposes. But a phytochemist is a specialist who is interested in the study of chemical interactions in plants based on the knowledge of chemical science which is employed for a successful isolation of its components and the determination of its molecular structure through the study of its properties. The phytochemists have a good command over medicinal plants through the study of plant physiology, morphology, internal structure elucidation, and metabolic activities. A phytochemist is one who is knowledgeable about the identification, characterization of different natural products by using biochemical analysis to understudy the chemical composition of different plant products. The utilization of plants for medicinal purposes is not a new approach. However, periodically, plants are explored for extraction of chemical compounds which are beneficial to humans in several aspects. Once a plant-derived product is confirmed to exhibit curative potentials, the product will be recommended for drug designing, clinical approach, and finally to pharma industries.

1.6.1   SKILLS AND EXPERTISE REQUIRED OF A PHYTOCHEMIST

A phytochemist is required to be knowledgeable about the basics of plant science, isolation, and identification of molecules from plants. The knowledge and expertise on different analytical techniques for extraction, characterization, and quality assessment is a prerequisite. In addition, a phytochemist should be familiar with natural products induction, metabolomics profiling (nuclear magnetic resonance [NMR], mass spectrometry [MS]), micro-fractionation, natural products database, e-bioprospecting. Expertise in the state-of-art techniques including the various extraction methods, for example, solvent extraction methods, superficial fluid extraction, microwave-assisted extraction, chromatographic fingerprinting, and marker compound analysis is required. Advances in chromatographic techniques (liquid chromatography–MS; liquid chromatography–NMR), gas chromatography–mass spectroscopy, anti-microbial and antioxidant studies will help in a comprehensive analysis of natural product extracts. In the recent years, studies are being conducted in relation to the stress induction of natural products under metabolomics view (plant metabolomics). The use of metabolomics in conjunction with direct NMR profiling approaches is important for the understanding of metabolic reactions in plants. Chapter 8 of this book provides an overview of plant metabolomics and its applications.

1.6.2 FUTURE PROSPECTS FOR PHYTOCHEMISTS

Today, a huge sector of the population is relying on medicinal plants for their preventive and curative properties. WHO stated that those traditional medicine/ethnomedicine are still being used to treat different ailments. Nearly 70% of the populations rely on these medicinal practices. People from remote areas and semi-urban regions of the globe still depend on either crude or purified product from the plant's origin. Standardization and quality control is an important factor in ethnomedicinal formulations. At present, the phytochemists aim to apply modern techniques to preserve and maintain the standard and quality of these plant products. Findings by phytochemists through research investigations are supporting the ethnomedicinal formulations used by the tribal doctors. Several chemical compounds derived from plants are undergoing clinical trials and some of them are in preclinical treatment. Similarly, research is to be focused on the possibility of developing new products in combination with natural compounds from ethnomedicine. They identified the diversity of chemical compounds observed with phytochemicals which have led to the formulations of novel drugs against multidrug-resistant pathogens.

Phytochemists are seriously embarking on research activities involving the extraction of natural compounds present in plants. Some of these phytochemicals have the ability to suppress the activity of cancer cells by encouraging cell cycle inhibition and apoptosis. There is a lot of demand for natural products of plant origin and these by-products are to replace the synthetic products in view of their side effects on human health. Therefore, a lot of attention is needed toward natural products in which a phytochemist plays a key role in this context. Owing to the increasing demand for novel drugs, so many important and vital compounds regularly being manufactured by the industries generate employment opportunities for experts in this field. In addition, the increasing acceptance of the chemical diversity of natural products is well suited to provide the core scaffolds for future drugs. There will be further developments in the use of novel natural products and chemical libraries based on natural products in drug discovery campaigns.

1.7 COMPUTER-AIDED PHYTOCHEMICAL STUDIES

Advances in the knowledge of genome sequencing have led to increase in knowledge of therapeutic targets for pharmaceutics research (de Ruyck et al., 2016). Just as the knowledge of high-throughput crystallography and NMR methods have developed over the time and contributed to the acquisition of atomic structures of proteins and protein–ligand interactions to an increasing level of detail (Gore and Desai, 2014), the knowledge of computational phytochemistry has also grown to give insight into protein interactions with their ligands. Computational phytochemistry method has been utilized by research-based pharmaceutical industries to study structure–activity relationships (Hughes et al., 2011).

This aspect of phytochemistry among other computer-aided drug discovery program have gain extensive use in studies of drug candidates, to increase their efficiency and development pipeline, based on their purpose and required interest (Zhang, 2011). Among such programs are docking techniques. Docking program is a software technique that allows the user to fit a molecule (ligand) into target (protein)-binding sites. It can also be used to predict the structure of the molecular interactions between these pairs (ligand/protein). The ligands are often relatively the smaller molecules which conformations (ligand–receptor complexes), binding energies or affinities, and nature of interactions are assessed in the binding site of their receptors, which are relatively larger macromolecules. The various software, databases, and tools for molecular docking and dynamics simulations are detailed in Chapter 19 of this book. Its applications are discussed further in Volume 2.

Molecular docking studies have diverse applications. It is a powerful and important modeling tool utilized in modern drug discovery. They are cheap, convenient, and not time-consuming, as several samples could be asses in lesser time. Prior to in vivo studies, molecular docking studies are used to access lead compounds for further studies. Its applications to phytochemicals studies are of immense importance, some of which are summarized below;

1. **Identification of natural phytochemical:** Molecular docking tools are used in identifying natural phytochemical as well as in the repurposing of existing commercial drugs that are effective in treating disease. In applying this knowledge to phytochemical studies, the constituents in a particular plant are tested individually for their activities against key enzymes in selected diseases.

2. **Development of phytochemical database:** There exist the importance of means to obtain phytochemicals in the format required for in silico studies. Data-based design for this purpose have been identified (Barlow et al., 2012). The availability of phytochemical dataset with their various two-dimensional/three-dimensional structure, possible target proteins, simplified molecular input line entry

specification, MOL2 files, and chemical class may enable their use in docking studies. This will ease the process of identification of lead compounds from natural products and their development into phytomedicines (Pathania et al., 2015).

3. **Sorting out lead compounds:** Molecular docking studies are applied to a large database, in order to identify hit compounds. The defined program and the various scores obtained from each compound can be compared to identify such hit compounds.

4. **Optimization of lead phytochemicals:** Molecular docking can be used to predict and subsequently develop a more potent, and effective drug candidates from selected phytochemicals. The develop candidate end up with optimized ligand–protein interactions.

5. **Identification of the mechanism of action:** When in search of the mechanism of action of certain active phytochemicals, molecular docking studies may be applied in order to identify the nature of the interaction of the compound with the protein. Their binding affinities and nature of interactions can similarly be analyzed.

1.8   BIOSTATISTICS AS A TOOL FOR PHYTOCHEMISTS

Biostatistics is the application of statistics to topics relating to biology. Biology, is a natural science concerned with life and living organisms, branches out to a handful of other related fields such as ecology, zoology, anatomy, microbiology, biochemistry, and so on. Statistics as the best breed of mathematical analysis provides objective and rational methods that enable research questions to be answered and rational questions to be asked for research after research.

The scope of biostatistics ranges from formulating the research question until the presentation or publication of the results. Biostatisticians and practitioners spend a considerable amount of time in developing research designs, evaluating methodologies, and analyzing statistical results. However, just like how it is used in any other fields, statistics in biology can often be misused. And as the application moves into life applications such as medical and pharmacological studies, statistics must be practiced efficiently and truthfully.

A misconception exists that the role of statistics come into play after data collection – when the analysis is done to determine rationale findings regarding the data. However, statistics should be well accounted all throughout the research process. Good research problems start with simple and measurable objectives. Even for qualitative studies, there must be a clear set of indicators to be used in the research. A sound literature review needs good statistics for the research to gain some traction regarding its significance. Methodologies and data analysis must be systematic and abiding with the fundamentals of the different fields not only biology but most commonly with chemistry and mathematics. Lastly, publication and result dissemination require a grasp of the understanding of how statistics can be used to relay findings in scientific yet technical manner. Essentially, the role of biostatistics is to keep every aspect of a research, from the objectives down to result publication, as efficient and valid as possible.

1.8.1   BIOSTATISTICS IN PHYTOCHEMICAL RESEARCH

Phytochemical research has been able to coexist with biostatistics smoothly. The study of how chemicals from plants may potentially affect humans and other organisms has been objectified and quantified through statistics. Specifically, it is in pharmacology and drug development that biostatistics has been considered not only vital but necessary. The application of biostatistics in pharmacology answers three key notions – validity, significance, and consistency.

The use of biostatistics for validity refers to a sound formulation of objectives, research idea, and importance. One researcher may pick a random plant, derive a concoction, and then test its antimicrobial properties. However, a good phytochemical research involves an assessment of the community needs and formulating measurable objectives. This can only be done by looking into the statistics (statistics in its plural form) related to the plant. This could be about its folkloric use, history, preparation as well as how many studies were done regarding this plant. The validity also comes from the statistics found from these accompanying literature whether future studies can bare fruitful results. Measurable objectives also contribute to validity. Using statistical concepts such as the types of variables and varying levels of the measure will ensure sound objectives and will later on be the basis for statistical analysis.

Testing for significance has been the highlight between the relationship of pharmacology and statistics. To test for significance, treatments (usually in dosages) are compared with a positive treatment (a commercially manufacture drug) and a negative control. This phase of the research is fairly straightforward; nonetheless, the analysis is highly dependent on a sound methodology and appropriate statistical test/analysis. Most often researches do not amount to anything due to bad or mismatched statistical testing. This is where the role of a biostatistician is crucial as they bridge the gap of knowledge between masters of two different fields. A research could only be valid if the statistical methodology on it fits the actual objectives.

With that, consistency allows the public to assess at a glance the research and development that has come through for a specific pharmacological study. For example, ASCOF® Lagundi herbal drug that came from *Vitex negundo* went through almost 42 years of research and development. Summative studies were done to determine the consistency of the findings regarding its anti-inflammatory and anti-histaminic properties before it was commercially made available to the public. Simply, using statistics to evaluate results ensures public safety and protects the best interests of every stakeholder.

1.8.2 ROLE OF A BIOSTATISTICIAN

A lot of statistical tests are utilized for pharma research. A biostatistician must be equipped with three core skills to ensure a productive study. First, he must be equipped with a portfolio of parametric/nonparametric tests and other statistical methods. Sampling or sampling calculations is often an overlooked aspect of pharmacological studies. A practitioner must be able to understand the purpose of the study, the research design, and methodology only then can he start with the sampling technique. A practitioner should at least be equipped with a standard set of parametric and its nonparametric counterpart, with their corresponding post hoc analyses. Classic tests such as analysis of variance, t-tests, and logistic regression analysis have always been effective in pharmacological studies.

Second is that a practitioner must be able, and willing, to understand both sides of the coin – statistics and biology. Compromise has been the key in clinical trials to fit goals with appropriate statistical tests. A practitioner must be able to discuss results on a life science perspective without losing the technicality statistics brings onto the study. Last, practitioners must be able to adapt to technology and developments in the growing field of biostatistics.

1.8.3 TOOLS FOR BIOSTATISTICS

Research and development in biostatistics have always associated with the release of multiple automated software that made the mitigation between biology and statistics easier. Microsoft's Excel spreadsheet has been able to adapt to the increasing demand by publishing downloadable macros that can be used for biostatistics, econometrics, and applied statistics. SPSS and R GUI has been the go-to professional package and academic statistical packages, respectively. SPSS offers user-friendly interface that enables non-practitioners to run data, meanwhile, R GUI has been the most dynamic statistical software tool as it takes advantage of the user's in-depth understanding of statistics to program through codes the different tests. With the increasing demand, specific programs have been made available for commercial usage. OpenEpi and Stata have been widely used in clinical trials. Meanwhile, EpiInfo has been the go-to software for medical professionals, researchers in clinical trials, and even by industrial manufacturers. Chapter 18 of this book detailed the various statistical tools used in phytochemical research with web links to download them while using essential oil studies to make references to the features of few.

1.9 MAJOR PHYTOCHEMICAL SOCIETIES AND FUNDING AGENCIES

There are several phytochemical groups, institutes, research centers all over the world. The activities of Phytochemical Society of North America (PSNA), Phytochemical Society of Europe (PSE), and Phytochemical Society of Asia (PSA) deserves mention.

1.9.1 PHYTOCHEMICAL SOCIETY OF NORTH AMERICA

The PSNA is a nonprofit organization with membership subscription fee. Its membership is open to anyone with an interest in phytochemistry. It aims to promote research on the chemistry and biochemistry of plant constituents, the physiology and pathology effects upon plant and animals, and the industrial applications of phytoconstituents. PSNA transcended from Plant Phenolics Group of North America to this day PSNA with Mabry, T. J. as it is first President as a Society in 1966. PNSA provides professional development opportunities such as research presentations (oral or poster), annual conferences, travel awards, the Frank and Mary Loewus Student Travel Award for undergraduate students, graduate students, and postdoctoral researchers. More information can be accessed from its website: http://www.psna-online.org/index.html.

1.9.2   PHYTOCHEMICAL SOCIETY OF EUROPE

PSE is a membership organization for everyone with the interest in phyto-chemistry. It promotes the advancement of the chemistry and biochemistry of plants constituents and its applications in industry and agriculture. PSE organizes two to three conferences yearly in the United Kingdom and Continental Europe and gives awards to deserving phytochemists. The society metamorphosed from Plant Phenolics Group to Phytochemical Group and to a Society in 1967 and finally adopted its present name in 1977. More information can be accessed from its website: http://phyto-chemicalsociety.org/.

1.9.3   PHYTOCHEMICAL SOCIETY OF ASIA

The PSA was founded in 2007 at Kuala Lumpur, Malaysia with Prof. Yoshinori Asakawa (Japan) elected as the founding President and Prof. Iqbal Choudhary M. (Pakistan) as the Vice President. The aim of the society is to promote collaborative research between scientists and in the growth and advancement of research in the field of natural products from of the region and outside the region. It has different types of membership such as regular membership, student membership, honorary members, life members, insti-tutional membership with different subscription rates. More information can be accessed from its website: http://phytochemsoc-asia.com/.

1.9.4   FUNDING AGENCIES FOR RESEARCHERS IN PHYTOCHEMISTRY

Government funding programs are available in many countries for phytochemical and related investigations. Besides, international organizations such as Intergovernmental Science-Policy Platform on Biodiversity and Ecosystem Services, International Union for Conservation of Nature and WHO are offering funds towards the progress of these investigations.

1.10   ADVANCES IN PHYTOCHEMICAL RESEARCH

So far, a substantial progress has been made for the discovery of new phyto-chemicals which could serve as a lead compounds for the development of new drugs. Drug discovery is capital intensive which usually starts with the screening and identification of active ingredient in traditional plants. According to Business Wire, the global drug discovery informatics market is expected to reach the US \$2.84 Billion in 2022 from the US \$1.67 Billion in 2017 at a CAGR (Compound Annual Growth Rate is the mean annual growth rate of an investment over a specified period of time longer than 1 year) of 11.2%. The discovery of new drugs usually is carried out by pharmaceutical and biotechnology companies with the assistance from the universities. The search for the discovery of new drugs must be continued to stem out the ravaging effects of diseases in plants and animals. Many more phytochemicals abound yet undiscovered in plants because only a small fraction of the plants has been studied. The development of new analytical techniques and validation of the existing ones will greatly help in phytochemical research.

Computer-aided drug discovery is part of the modern drug discovery tool which helps to drive a fast and efficient discovery process through the identification of screen hits by molecular docking, modeling, and dynamics simulations. Target compounds are assessed for their binding affinity to target receptor cells, its selectivity, efficacy or potency, metabolic stability, and oral bioavailability. Once a compound is identified to fulfill the requirements, it will undergo phase I, II, and III clinical trials.

One drawback in the development of new drugs, is that many plant-derived compounds still cannot be synthetized and so are not commercially available. This is why the access to some drugs is quite expensive. More needs to be made in the area of phytochemistry including government and non-governmental agencies for fundings, grants, consultation, and collaboration in research projects and so on. The other way to improve the quality of research output is to establish the field of phytochemistry as a single stand-alone science. Although few institutions have done so there is a need for more tertiary institutions to do so.

Phytochemicals are naturally present in many foods but it is expected that through bioengineering, new plants will be developed, which will contain higher levels. This would make it easier to incorporate enough phytochemicals into the food.

1.10.1 PROGRESS IN PHYTOCHEMICAL RESEARCH

1.10.1.1 AS NANOPARTICLE (NP) SYNTHETIC PRECURSORS

Phytochemicals can act as cheap and raw materials for different classes of nanoparticle (NP) synthesis, which has been discussed in details in Volume 2.

Phytochemicals can be selectively utilized to synthesize the NP of interest, for example, having red emission, having good ability to carry drugs, and so forth.

1.10.1.2 AS A FABRICATING SOURCE OF NPS

Literature goes in favor of the phytochemicals as NPs surface decorating agents for enhancing the phytochemical activity of the related NPs. It is also very interesting that this field of research is nascent, and requires a lot of research which would definitely boost both the areas of phytomedicine and nanotechnology. A lot of reports are available for the applications of phytochemicals as fabricating source (Ahmad et al., 2017).

1.10.1.3 ANTITUMOR EFFECTS

Cancer is a leading cause of deaths worldwide. A lot of research has been done to overcome this notorious disease, while still much is needed to completely haul this disease. Chapters 20, 21, and 23 are research discoveries of potential anticancer drugs. Many chapters in Volume 2 and 3 of this book contain novel research in this direction.

Phytochemicals could contribute to the cancer treatment in the following ways:

a)   Drugs source: certain important chemicals, such as taxol can directly be isolated from plants, and could be potentially used as an anticancer agent (Bo et al., 2016).

b)   Along with a source of drugs isolation, phytochemicals could also be used to obtain NPs having anticancerous effects, as well as NPs using as agents for anticancerous drugs delivery, as well as photoluminescent agents in their treatment (Angelova et al., 2017, Kapinova et al., 2017, Kaur et al., 2017).

1.10.1.4 CUTANEOUS CARCINOMA

The prevention of this heinous disease by phytochemicals is of main concern these days as compared to their chemoprevention. It has been considered that phytochemicals are safely relieving multiple pathological processes, including oxidative damage, epigenetic alteration, chronic inflammation, angiogenesis, and so forth (Wang et al., 2017).

1.10.1.5 OTHER DISEASES

Research outcomes from the study of the pharmacological effects of phytochemicals in the treatment of various diseases are largely being dependent on as interest is growing due to the safety of natural herbal products compared to the synthetic ones with side effects. Many medications for some ravaging diseases remain a mirage despite the enormous work in drug discovery. Diseases such as diabetes, a well-known disease of rich and poor, as well as found in developed and developing nations, have a lot of space to be treated phytochemically. The study of plant-derived chemicals is continuous with many sophisticated techniques being developed to assist in the discovery of compounds which will be of medical significance and to other industries for the betterment of life. An ample discoveries have been made but more is yet to be done.

KEYWORDS

- phytochemistry
- phytochemicals
- terpenes
- flavonoids
- alkaloids

REFERENCES

Achan, J.; Talisuna, A. O.; Erhart, A. et al. Quinine, an Old Anti-Malarial Drug in a Modern World: Role in the Treatment of Malaria. *Malar. J.* **2011,** *10,* 144. DOI: 10.1186/1475-2875-10-144.

Adamczyk, B.; Karonen, M.; Adamczyk, S.; Engström, M. T.; Laakso, T.; Saranpää, P.; Kitunen, V.; Smolander, A. J. Tannins Can Slow-Down but Also Speed-up Soil Enzymatic Activity in Boreal Forest. *Soil. Biol. Biochem.* **2017,** *107,* 60–67.

Ahmad, B.; Hafeez, N.; Bashir, S.; Rauf, A. et al. Phytofabricated Gold Nanoparticles and Their Biomedical Applications. *Biomed. Pharmacother.* **2017,** *89,* 414–425.

Althagafy, H. S.; Graf, T. N.; Sy-Cordero, A. A.; Gufford, B. T.; Paine, M. F.; Wagoner, J.; Polyak, S. J.; Croatt, M. P.; Oberlies, N. H. Semisynthesis, Cytotoxicity, Antiviral Activity, and Drug Interaction Liability of 7-O-Methylated Analogues of Flavonolignans from Milk Thistle. *Bioorg. Med. Chem.* **2013**, *21*(13), 3919–3926.

Angelova, A.; Garamus, V. M.; Angelov, B.; Tian, Z.; Li, Y.; Zou, A. Advances in Structural Design of Lipid-Based Nanoparticle Carriers for Delivery of Macromolecular Drugs, Phytochemicals and Anti-Tumor Agents. *Adv. Colloid Interface Sci.* **2017**, *249*, 331–345.

Araya-Cloutier, C.; Den Besten, H. M.; Aisyah, S.; Gruppen, H.; Vincken, J. P. The Position of Prenylation of Isoflavonoids and Stilbenoids from Legumes (Fabaceae) Modulates the Antimicrobial Activity Against Gram Positive Pathogens. *Food Chem.* **2017**, *226*, 193–201.

Arens, U. Authorised EU Health Claim for Carbohydrates and Maintenance of Normal Brain Function. *Food Nutr. Food Ingredients Authorised EU Health Claims* **2018**, *229*, 236.

Avraham, Y.; Berry, E. M.; Donskoy, M.; Ahmad, W. A.; Vorobiev, L.; Albeck, A.; Mankuta, D. Beta-Carotene as a Novel Therapy for the Treatment of "Autistic Like Behavior" in Animal Models of Autism. *Behav. Brain Res.* **2017**.

Bahramsoltani, R.; Rahimi, R.; Farzaei, M. H. Pharmacokinetic Interactions of Curcuminoids with Conventional Drugs: A Review. *J. Ethnopharmacol.* **2017**, *209*, 1–12.

Barazzoni, R.; Deutz, N. E. P.; Biolo, G.; Bischoff, S.; Boirie, Y.; Cederholm, T.; Cuerda, C.; Delzenne, N.; Leon Sanz, M.; Ljungqvist, O.; Muscaritoli, M.; Pichard, C.; Preiser, J. C.; Sbraccia, P.; Singer, P.; Tappy, L.; Thorens, B.; Van Gossum, A.; Vettor, R.; Calder, P. C. Carbohydrates and Insulin Resistance in Clinical Nutrition: Recommendations from the ESPEN Expert Group. *Clin. Nutr.* **2017**, *36*(2), 355–363.

Barlow, D. J.; Buriani, A.; Ehrman, T.; Bosisio, E.; Eberini, I.; Hylands, P. J. In-Silico Studies in Chinese Herbal Medicines' Research: Evaluation of in-silico Methodologies and Phytochemical Data Sources, and a Review of Research to Date. *J. Ethnopharmacol.* **2012**, *140*, 526–534.

Barrett, A. H.; Farhadi, N. F.; Tracey J. Smith. Slowing Starch Digestion and Inhibiting Digestive Enzyme Activity Using Plant Flavanols/Tannins-A Review of Efficacy and Mechanisms. *LWT Food Sci. Technol.* **2018**, *87*, 394–399.

Basheer, L.; Schultz, K.; Guttman, Y.; Kerem, Z. In Silico and in Vitro Inhibition of Cytochrome P450 3A by Synthetic Stilbenoids. *Food Chem.* **2017**, *237*, 895–903.

Bieganska-Marecik, R.; Radziejewska-Kubzdela, E.; Marecik, R. Characterization of Phenolics, Glucosinolates and Antioxidant Activity of Beverages Based on Apple Juice with Addition of Frozen and Freeze-Dried Curly Kale Leaves (Brassica oleracea L. var. acephala L.). *Food Chem.* **2017**, *230*, 271–280.

Bijak, M.; Szelenberger, R.; Saluk, J.; Nowak, P. Flavonolignans Inhibit ADP Induced Blood Platelets Activation and Aggregation in Whole Blood. *Int. J. Biol. Macromol.* **2017**, *95*, 682–688.

Bo, L.; Cui, H.; Fang, Z.; Qun, T.; Xia, C. Inactivation of Transforming Growth Factor-Beta-Activated Kinase 1 Promotes Taxol Efficacy in Ovarian Cancer Cells. *Biomed. Pharmacother.* **2016**, *84*, 917–924.

Boucherle, B.; Peuchmaur, M.; Boumendjel, A.; Haudecoeur, R. Occurrences, Biosynthesis and Properties of Aurones as High-End Evolutionary Products. *Phytochemistry* **2017**, *142*, 92–111.

Business Wire. $2.84 Billion Drug Discovery Informatics Market 2017 by Function, Solution and End User - Global Forecast to 2022 – Research and Markets. https://www.businesswire.com/news/home/20180108006006/en/2.84-Billion-Drug-Discovery-Informatics-Market-2017. (Accessed Jan 9, 2018).

Canales, R.; Guinez, M.; Bazan, C.; Reta, M.; Cerutti, S. Determining Heterocyclic Aromatic Amines in Aqueous Samples: A Novel Dispersive Liquid-Liquid Micro-Extraction Method Based on Solidification of Floating Organic Drop and Ultrasound Assisted Back Extraction Followed by UPLC-MS/MS. *Talanta* **2017**, *174*, 548–555.

Cao, H.; Jia, X.; Shi, J.; Xiao, J.; Chen, X. Non-Covalent Interaction Between Dietary Stilbenoids and Human Serum Albumin: Structure-Affinity Relationship, and its Influence on the Stability, Free Radical Scavenging Activity and Cell Uptake of Stilbenoids. *Food Chem.* **2016**, *202*, 383–388.

Chrbolka, P.; Paluch, Z.; Hill, M.; Alusik, S. Circulating Steroids Negatively Correlate with Tinnitus. *Steroids* **2017**, *123*, 37–42.

Coronado-Aceves, E. W.; Gigliarelli, G.; Garibay-Escobar, A.; Zepeda, R. E. R.; Curini, M.; Lopez Cervantes, J.; Ines Espitia-Pinzon, C. I.; Superchi, S.; Vergura, S.; Marcotullio, M. C. New Isoflavonoids from the Extract of Rhynchosia Precatoria (Humb. & Bonpl. ex Willd.) DC. and their Antimycobacterial Activity. *J. Ethnopharmacol.* **2017**, *206*, 92–100.

Cvijetic, I. N.; Verbic, T. Z.; Ernesto De Resende, P.; Stapleton, P.; Gibbons, S.; Juranic, I. O.; Drakulic, B. J.; Zloh, M. Design, Synthesis and Biological Evaluation of Novel Aryldiketo Acids with Enhanced Antibacterial Activity Against Multidrug Resistant Bacterial Strains. *Eur. J. Med. Chem.* **2018**, *143*, 1474–1488.

David, B.; Jacoby, R. M. Y. Encyclopedia of Family Health. *Third* **2005**.

De Meloa, I. S. V.; Dos Santosb, A. F.; Buenoc, N. B. Curcumin or Combined Curcuminoids are Effective in Lowering the Fasting Blood Glucose Concentrations of Individuals with Dysglycemia: Systematic Review and Meta-Analysis of Randomized Controlled Trials. *Pharmacol. Res.* **2017**.

De Oliveira, N. A.; Cornclio-Santiago, H. P.; Fukumasu, H.; De Oliveira, A. L. Green Coffee Extracts Rich in Diterpenes–Process Optimization of Pressurized Liquid Extraction Using Ethanol as Solven. *J. Food Eng.* **2017**.

de Ruyck, J.; Brysbaert, G.; Blossey, R.; Lensink, F. M. Molecular Docking as a Popular Tool in Drug Design, an in Silico Travel. *Adv. Appl. Bioinf. Chem.* **2016**, *9*, 1–11.

Dikshit, M. Foreword. In *Herbs for Diabetes and Neurological Disease Management: Research and Advancements*; Kumar, V., Addepalli, V., Eds.; Apple Academic Press: New York, 2017.

Dobson, SMaM. In *Antimalarial Chemotherapy: Mechanisms of Action, Resistance, and New Directions in Drug Discovery*; PJ, R., Ed.; Humana Press: Totowa, New Jersey, The history of antimalarial drugs. **2001**; pp 15–25.

Dos, Reis, L. C. R.; De Oliveira, V. R.; Hagen, M. E. K.; Jablonski, A.; Flôres, S. H.; De Oliveira Rios, A. Carotenoids, Flavonoids, Chlorophylls, Phenolic Compounds and Antioxidant Activity in Fresh and Cooked Broccoli (Brassica Oleracea var. Avenger) and Cauliflower (Brassica Oleracea Var. Alphina F1). *LWT–Food Sci. Technol.* **2015**, *63*(1), 177–183.

Ergene Oz, B.; Saltan Iscan, G.; Kupeli Akkol, E.; Suntar, I.; Bahadir Acikara, O. Isoflavonoids as Wound Healing Agents from Ononidis Radix. *J. Ethnopharmacol.* **2018**, *211*, 384–393.

Fabricant, D. S.; Farnsworth, N. R. The Value of Plants Used in Traditional Medicine for Drug Discovery. *Environ. Health Perspect.* **2001**, *109*, 69–75.

Fabro, S.; Smith, R. L.; Williams, R. T. Toxicity and Teratogenicity of Optical Isomers of Thalidomide. *Nature* **1967**, *215*, 296. https://www.nature.com/articles/215296a0 (accessed Nov 19, 2017).

Faiella, L.; Piaz, F. D.; Bader, A.; Braca, A. Diterpenes and Phenolic Compounds from Sideritis Pullulans. *Phytochemistry* **2014**, *106*, 164–170.

Gengatharan, A.; Dykes, G. A.; Choo, W. S. Betalains: Natural Plant Pigments with Potential Application in Functional Foods. *LWT–Food Sci. Technol.* **2015**, *64*(2), 645–649.

Gerschenson, L. N.; Rojas, A. M.; Fissore, E. N. Carbohydrates. *2017*, 39–101.

Gore, M.; Desai, N. S. Computer-Aided Drug Designing. *Methods Mol. Biol.* **2014**, *1168*, 313–321.

Grishko, V. V.; Galaiko, N. V. Structural Diversity, Natural Sources and Pharmacological Potential of Naturally Occurring A-Seco-Triterpenoids. **2016**, *51*, 51–149.

Gu, J.; Liu, T.; Sadiq, F. A.; Yang, H.; Yuan, L.; Zhang G.; He, G. Biogenic Amines Content and Assessment of Bacterial and Fungal Diversity in Stinky Tofu–A traditional fermented soy curd. *LWT–Food Sci. Technol.* **2018**, *88*, 26–34.

Gutiérrez-Larraínzar, M.; Rúa, J.; Caro, I.; De Castro, C.; De Arriaga, D.; García-Armesto, M.; RosarioDel Valle, P. Evaluation of Antimicrobial and Antioxidant Activities of Natural Phenolic Compounds Against Foodborne Pathogens and Spoilage Bacteria. *Food Control.* **2012**, *26*(2), 555–563.

Hartmann, T. From Waste Products to Ecochemicals: Fifty Years Research of Plant Secondary Metabolism. *Phytochemistry.* **2007**, *68*(22–24), 2831–2846.

Ho, S. H.; Ma, Y.; Goh, P. M.; Sim, K. Y. Star Anise, Illicium Verum Hook F. as a Potential Grain Protectant Against Tribolium Castaneum (Herbst) and Sitophilus Zeamais Motsch. *Postharvest Biol. Technol.* **1995**, *6*, 341–347.

Ho, S. H.; Ma, Y.; Huang, Y. Anethole, a. Potential Insecticide from Illicium Verum Hook F., Against Two Stored Product Insects. *Int. Pest. Control.* **1997**, *39*(2), 50–51.

Hu, H. B.; Liang, H. P.; Li, H. M.; Yuan, R. N.; Sun, J.; Zhang, L. L.; Han, M. H.; Wu, Y. Isolation, Modification and Cytotoxic Evaluation of Stilbenoids from Acanthopanax Leucorrhizus. *Fitoterapia* **2018**, *124*, 167–176.

Huang, Y.; Hee, S. K.; Ho, S. H. Antifeedant and Growth Inhibit- Ory e!ects of -Pinene on the Stored-Product Insects, Tribolium Castaneum (Herbst) and Sitophilus Zeamais Motsch. *Int. Pest Control.* **1998**, *40*(1), 18–20.

Huang, Y.; Ho, S. H. Toxicity and Antifeedant Activities of Cinna- Maldehyde Against the Grain Storage Insects, Tribolium Castaneum (Herbst) and Sitophilus Zeamais Motsch. *J. Stored Prod. Res.* **1998**, *34*, 11–17.

Hughes, J. P.; Rees, S.; Kalindjian, S. B.; Philpott, K. L. Principles of Early Drug Discovery. *Br. J. Pharmacol.* **2011**, *162*, 1239–1249.

Isman, M. B. Plant Essential Oils for Pest and Disease Management. *Crop Prot.* **2000**, *19*, 603–608.

Jiang, Z.; Chai, L.; Liu, Y.; Qiu, H.; Wang, T.; Feng, X.; Wang, Y. et al. Bioactive Lignans from the Stems of Mappianthus Iodoides. Phytochem. Lett. **2017**, *22*, 194–198.

Kapinova, A.; Stefanicka, P.; Kubatka, P.; Zubor, P.; Uramova, S.; Kello, M.; Mojzis, J.; Blahutova, D.; Qaradakhi, T.; Zulli, A.; Caprnda, M.; Danko, J.; Lasabova, Z.; Busselberg, D.; Kruzliak, P. Are Plant-Based Functional Foods Better Choice Against Cancer than Single Phytochemicals? A Critical Review of Current Breast Cancer Research. *Biomed. Pharmacother.* **2017**, *96*, 1465–1477.

Kaur ,V.; Kumar, M.; Kumar, A.; Kaur, K.; Dhillon, V. S.; Kaur, S. Pharmacotherapeutic Potential of Phytochemicals: Implications in Cancer Chemoprevention and Future Perspectives. *Biomed. Pharmacother.* **2017**, *97*, 564–586.

Krishnamurti, C.; Rao, S. C. The Isolation of Morphine by Serturner. *Indian J. Anaesth.* **2016**, *60*(11), 861–862. DOI: 10.4103/0019-5049.193696.

Kumar, S. S.; Manoj, P.; Giridhar, P.; Shrivastava, R.; Bharadwaj, M. Fruit Extracts of Basella Rubra that are Rich in Bioactives and Betalains Exhibit Antioxidant Activity and Cytotoxicity Against Human Cervical Carcinoma Cells. *J. Funct. Foods* **2015**, *15*, 509–515.

Kurita, N.; Miyaji, M.; Kurane, R.; Takahara, Y. Antifungal Activity of Components of Essential Oils. *Agric. Biol. Chem.* **1981**, *45*, 945–952.

Liew, K. F.; Chan, K. L. Lee, C. Y. Blood-Brain Barrier Permeable Anticholinesterase Aurones: Synthesis, Structure-Activity Relationship, and Drug-Like Properties. *Eur. J. Med. Chem.* **2015**, *94*, 195–210.

Liew, K. F.; Hanapi, N. A.; Chan, K. L.; Yusof, S. R.; Lee, C. Y. Assessment of the Blood-Brain Barrier Permeability of Potential Neuroprotective Aurones in Parallel Artificial Membrane Permeability Assay and Porcine Brain Endothelial Cell Models. *J. Pharm. Sci.* **2017**, *106*(2), 502–510.

Liu, Y. Z.; Yang, C. M.; Chen, J. Y.; Liao, J. W.; Hu, M. L. Alpha-Carotene Inhibits Metastasis in Lewis Lung Carcinoma in Vitro, and Suppresses Lung Metastasis and Tumor Growth in Combination with Taxol in Tumor Xenografted C57BL/6 Mice. *J. Nutr. Biochem.* **2015**, *26*(6), 607–615.

Lydon, J.; Duke, S. O. Pesticide Effects on Secondary Metabolism of Higher Plants. *J. Pestic. Sci.* **1989**, *25*(4), 361–373 http://onlinelibrary.wiley.com/woll/doi/10.1002/ps.2780250406/abstract (accessed Nov 17, 2017).

Mazid, M.; Khan, T. A.; Mohammad, F. Role of Secondary Metabolites in Defense Mechanisms of Plants. *Biol. Med.* **2011**, *3*(2), 232–249.

Mehrad, B.; Ravanfar, R.; Licker, J.; Regenstein, J. M.; Abbaspourrad, A. Enhancing the Physicochemical Stability of β-Carotene Solid Lipid Nanoparticle (SLNP) Using Whey Protein Isolate. *Food Res. Int.* **2018**, *105*, 962–969.

Mewalal, R.; Rai, D. K.; Kainer, D.; Chen, F.; Kulheim, C.; Peter, G. F.; Tuskan, G. A. Plant-Derived Terpenes: A Feedstock for Specialty Biofuels. *Trends Biotechnol.* **2017**, *35*(3), 227–240.

Mirzaei, H.; Shokrzadeh, M.; Modanloo, M.; Ziar, A.; Riazi, G. H.; Emami, S. New Indole-Based Chalconoids as Tubulin-Targeting Antiproliferative Agents. *Bioorg. Chem.* **2017**, *75*, 86–98.

Mostofi, M.; Mohammadi Ziarani, G.; Mahdavi, M.; Moradi, A.; Nadri, H.; Emami, S.; Alinezhad, H.; Foroumadi, A.; Shafiee, A. Synthesis and Structure-Activity Relationship Study of Benzofuran-Based Chalconoids Bearing Benzylpyridinium Moiety as Potent Acetylcholinesterase Inhibitors. *Eur. J. Med. Chem.* **2015**, *103*, 361–369.

Muller-Riebau, F.; Berger, B.; Yegen, O. Chemical Composition and Fungitoxic Properties to Phytopathogenic Fungi of Essential Oils of Selected Aromatic Plants Growing Wild in Turkey. *J. Agric. Food Chem.* **1995**, *43*, 2262–2266.

Obeng-Ofori, D.; Reichmuth, Ch. Bioactivity of Eugenol, a Major Component of Essential oil of Ocimum Suave (Wild.) Against four Species of Stored-Product Coleoptera. *Int. J. Pest Manage.* **1997**, *43*, 89–94.

Olaf, S.; Jan, E.; Keunen, E.; Alan, C. B.; Frederik, J G M Van Kuijk. Fruits and Vegetables that are Sources for Lutein and Zeaxanthin: the Macular Pigment in Human Eyes. *Br. J. Ophthalmol.* **1998**, *82*, 907–910.

Ouédraogo, J. C. W.; Dicko, C.; Kini, Félix, B.; Bonzi-Coulibaly, Yvonne L.; Dey, E. S. Enhanced Extraction of Flavonoids from Odontonema Strictum Leaves with Antioxidant Activity Using Supercritical Carbon Dioxide Fluid Combined with Ethanol. *J. Supercrit. Fluids* **2018**, *131*, 66–71.

Papageorgiou, M.; Lambropoulou, D.; Morrison, C.; Kłodzińska, E. Namieśnik, J.; Płotka-Wasylka, J. Literature Update of Analytical Methods for Biogenic Amines Determination in Food and Beverages. *Trends Anal. Chem.* **2018**, *98*, 128–142.

Pathania, S.; Ramakrishnan, S. M.; Bagler, G. Phytochemica: A Platform to Explore Phytochemicals of Medicinal Plants. *Database.* **2015**, 1–8.

Pitman, N. C. A.; Jørgensen, P. M. Estimating the Size of the World's Threatened Flora. *Brevia* **2002**, *298*, 989.

Pyszkova, M.; Biler, M.; Biedermann, D.; Valentova, K.; Kuzma, M.; Vrba, J.; Ulrichova, J.; Sokolova, R.; Mojovic, M.; Popovic-Bijelic, A.; Kubala, M.; Trouillas, P.; Kren, V. V. J. Flavonolignan 2,3-dehydroderivatives: Preparation, Antiradical and Cytoprotective Activity. Free Radic Biol Med **2016**, *90*, 114–125.

Radošević, K.; Srček, V. G.; Bubalo, M. C.; Rimac Brnčić, S.; Takács, K.; Redovniković, I. R. Assessment of Glucosinolates, Antioxidative and Antiproliferative Activity of Broccoli and Collard Extracts. *J. Food Compos. Anal.* **2017**, *61*, 59–66.

Ravanfar, R.; Comunian, T. A.; Dando, R.; Abbaspourrad, A. Optimization of Microcapsules Shell Structure to Preserve Labile Compounds: A Comparison Between Microfluidics and Conventional Homogenization Method. *Food Chem.* **2018**, *241*, 460–467.

Roca, M.; Chen, K.; Pérez-Gálvez, A. Chlorophylls; In *Handbook on Natural Pigments in Food and Beverages*; Woodhead Publishing: Elsevier, **2016**; pp 125–158.

Rodriguez-Amaya, D. B. Carotenes and Xanthophylls as Antioxidants. In *Handbook of Antioxidants for Food Preservatio*; 2015, pp 17–50.

Salvador, J. A. R.; Leal, A. S.; Valdeira, A. S.; Goncalves, B. M. F.; Alho, D. P. S.; Figueiredo, S. A. C.; Silvestre, S. M.; Mendes, V. I. S. Oleanane-, Ursane-, and Quinone Methide Friedelane-Type Triterpenoid Derivatives: Recent Advances in Cancer Treatment. Eur. J. Med. Chem. **2017**, *142*, 95–130.

Schmidt, B.; Ribnicky, D. M.; Poulev, A.; Logendra, S.; Cefalu, W. T.; Raskin, I. A Natural History of Botanical Therapeutics. *Metabolism* **2008**, *57*, S3–S9.

Sekowski, S.; Bitiucki, M.; Ionov, M.; Zdeb, M.; Abdulladjanova, N.; Rakhimov, R.; Mavlyanov, S.; Bryszewska, M.; Zamaraeva, M. Influence of Valoneoyl Groups on the Interactions Between Euphorbia Tannins and Human Serum Albumin. *J. Lumin.* **2018**, *194*, 170–178.

Serghini, K.; de Luque, A. P.; Castejón-Muñoz, M.; García-Torres, L.; Jorrín, J. V. Sunflower (Helianthus annuus L.) Response to Broomrape (Orobanche cernua Loefl.) Parasitism: Induced Synthesis and Excretion of 7-Hydroxylated Simple Coumarins. *J. Exp. Bot.* **2001**, *52*(364), 2227–2234.

Singh, P.; Anand, A.; Kumar, V. Recent Developments in Biological Activities of Chalcones: a Mini Review. *Eur. J. Med. Chem.* **2014**, *85*, 758–777.

Sowndhararajan, K.; Deepa, P.; Kim, M.; Park, S. J.; Kim, S. An Overview of Neuroprotective and Cognitive Enhancement Properties of Lignans from Schisandra Chinensis. *Biomed. Pharmacother.* **2017**, *97*, 958–968.

Tuni, I.; Sahinkaya, S. Sensitivity of Two Greenhouse Pests to Vapours of Essential Oils. *Entomol Exp. Appl.* **1998**, *86*, 183–187.

Veeresham, C. Natural Products Derived from Plants as a Source of Drugs. *J. Adv. Pharm. Technol. Res.* **2012**, *3*(4), 200–201. DOI: 10.4103/2231–4040.104709.

Verma, S.; Mundkinajeddu, D.; Agarwal, A.; Chatterjee, S. S.; Kumar, V. Effects of Turmeric Curcuminoids and Metformin Against Central Sensitivity to Pain in Mice. *J. Tradit. Complementary Med.* **2017**, *7*(2), 145–151.

Wang, S.; Shen, P.; Zhou, J.; Lu, Y. Diet Phytochemicals and Cutaneous Carcinoma Chemoprevention: A Review. *Pharmacol. Res.* **2017**, *119*, 327–346.

Xu, F.; Wang, C.; Wang, H.; Xiong, Q.; Wei, Y.; Shao, X. Antimicrobial Action of Flavonoids from Sedum Aizoon L. Against Lactic Acid Bacteria in Vitro and in Refrigerated fresh Pork Meat. J. *Funct. Foods.* **2018**, *40*, 744–750.

Xu, J.; Cao, J.; Yue, J.; Zhang, X.; Zhao, Y. New Triterpenoids from Acorns of Quercus Liaotungensis and Their Inhibitory Activity Against α -Glucosidase, α -Amylase and Protein-Tyrosine Phosphatase 1B. *J. Funct. Foods.* **2018**, *41*, 232–239.

Xu, Y.; Li, L.; Cong, Q.; Wang, W.; Qi, X. –L..; Peng, Y.; Song, S.-J. Bioactive Lignans and Flavones with in Vitro Antioxidant and Neuroprotective Properties from Rubus Idaeus Rhizome. *J. Funct. Foods.* **2017**, *32*, 160–169.

Zebec, Z.; Wilkes, J.; Jervis, A. J.; Scrutton, N. S.; Takano, E.; Breitling, R. Towards Synthesis of Monoterpenes and Derivatives Using Synthetic Biology. *Curr. Opin. Chem. Biol.* **2016**, *34*, 37–43.

Zhang, L.; Xiao, W. H.; Wang, Y.; Yao, M. D.; Jiang, G. Z.; Zeng, B. X.; Zhang, R. S.; Yuan, Y. J. Chassis and Key Enzymes Engineering for Monoterpenes Production. *Biotechnol. Adv.* **2017**, *35*(8), 1022–1031.

Zhang, S. Computer-Aided Drug Discovery and Development. *Methods Mol. Biol.* **2011**, *716*, 23–38.

Zhang, Y.; Wu, S.; Qin, Y.; Liu, J.; Liu, J.; Wang, Q.; Ren, F.; Zhang, H. Interaction of Phenolic Acids and Their Derivatives with Human Serum Albumin: Structure-Affinity Relationships and Effects on Antioxidant Activity. *Food Chem.* **2018**, *240*, 1072–1080.

Introduction to Phytochemistry

Wang, S.; Alseekh, S.; Fernie, A. R.; Luo, J. The Structure and Function of Major Plant Metabolite Modifications. *Molecular Plant* 2019, *12*, 899–919.

Xu, J.; Wang, C.; Yang, B.; Xiong, C.; Fang, J.; Zhang, S. Antimicrobial Activity of Flavonoids from Plant Sources. *Molecules* 2014, *20*, ...

Xu, Z.; ...

...

CHAPTER 2

BIOSYNTHESIS OF PHYTOCHEMICALS

HABIBU TIJJANI[1], CHUKWUEBUKA EGBUNA[2], and
LUKA D. CARROL[3]

[1]*Natural Product Research Laboratory, Department of Biochemistry, Bauchi State University, Gadau, Nigeria, Tel. +2348037327138*

[2]*Department of Biochemistry, Chukwuemeka Odumegwu Ojukwu University, Anambra State, Nigeria*

[3]*Department of Biochemistry, Faculty of Medical Sciences, University of Jos, Jos, Nigeria*

*Corresponding author. E-mail: tijjanihabibu@basug.edu.ng
ORCID: https://orcid.org/0000-0001-5466-322X.*

ABSTRACT

Phytochemicals are plant secondary metabolites derived from distinct biosynthetic pathways in plants. Their reactions are in some cases complex and require several enzyme catalyses. They are of diverse activities due to their numerous structural biological activities, which are relayed based on their importance in various pharmacological effects. The pentose phosphate, shikimate, malonyl-CoA, nucleotide metabolic, and mevalonate pathways are among the contributing pathways for phytochemical biosynthesis. These biosynthetic pathways, enzymes, and precursors of alkaloids, anthocyanidins, anthraquinones, flavonoids, glycosides, lignans, phenolics, saponins, steroids, and terpenoids are discussed further in this chapter. These pathways have been studied, in some cases to provide alternative means of obtaining phytochemicals in larger quantities with the aim to apply them in bioengineering, pharmaceutics, and nutraceuticals as well as in other fields.

2.1   INTRODUCTION

Phytochemicals are products of plant metabolism devoid of growth and developmental functions in plants. They are required for other functions, which may include their defense and environmental survival. Their roles in photosynthesis, respiration, transport of solute, translocation, nutrient assimilation, and differentiation are not specified (Hartmann, 1998). Thus, they are termed secondary metabolites due to their noninvolvement in major biochemical activities and differentiating them from the primary metabolites, which are necessary for plants growth and survival. Moreover, they are considered nonessential and side products of the primary metabolites (Fig. 2.1). Phytochemicals are of diverse activities due to their numerous structural biological activities (Pandey and Kumar, 2013; Compean and Ynalvez, 2014), making them the important class of compound for drug development. Their biosynthetic pathways are focused on in this chapter, with some pathway discussed in details.

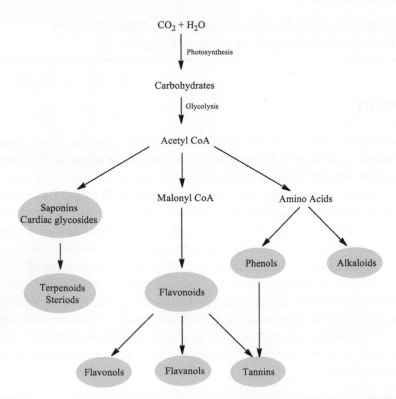

FIGURE 2.1   Interplay between the primary metabolites and the secondary metabolites.

2.1.1 CLASSIFICATION OF PHYTOCHEMICALS

Classifications of phytochemicals are done with no fixed criteria. Several phytochemicals have been identified and classified base on their physical and chemical characteristics (ACS, 2000; Arts and Hollman, 2005; Heneman and Zidenberg-cherr, 2008), while several others are yet to be identified (Zhang et al., 2015). Figure 2.2 attempts the classification of phytochemicals based on their chemical structures. The phenolics, flavonoids, and lignans are the major class from which other phytochemicals are drowned. Flavonoids are further divided into flavonols, flavanols, flavanones, and others as illustrated below. Based on the biosynthetic origins of phytochemicals, they can be classified into three major groups (Mazid et al., 2011): (1) the nitrogen-containing alkaloids or the sulfur-containing compounds such as camalexin; (2) the nonnitrogen-containing saponins, cardiac glycosides, terpenoids, and terpenoid-derived compounds, which include several steroids; and (3) the flavonoids, phenolics, and polyphenolics class of compounds.

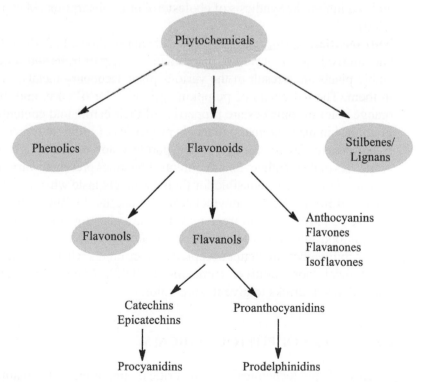

FIGURE 2.2 Simple classification of phytochemicals based on their chemical structures.

2.1.2   IMPORTANCE AND BENEFITS OF PHYTOCHEMICALS

Phytochemicals have diverse importance and relevance in different fields. They are important in pharmaceutical research, providing treatment and management options for different diseases. Phytochemicals are also important in the field of nutraceuticals and the science of food additive (Smetanska, 2008).

1. **Pharmaceutics:** The development of resistance to certain disease has posed many challenges to existing drugs, which have been known for their potent activities. The search for new and potent phytochemicals has provided therapeutic options for several diseases. Several researches on phytochemicals have been done extensively and the outcome is presently used as therapeutic options that are widely accepted and in use (Tijjani et al., 2017). Phytochemicals have beneficial roles in management and treatment of coronary heart disease; they prevent oxidations of low-density lipoprotein (LDL) and can inhibit the synthesis of cholesterol or its absorption (Mathai, 2000).

2. **Nutraceutics:** Phytochemicals have wide applications, both directly and indirectly in nutraceutics. The attractive colors of fruits and some edible plants are a result of the various plant secondary metabolites in them. The red colors of pumpkin, yellow color of corn, and the orange color of tomatoes are properties of their carotenoid contents. Fragrance in many aromatic plants is properties of different terpenes (Laxminarain, 2013). Similarly, the purple color in grapefruits is properties of their anthocyanins contents. Phenolics present in various teas, as tannins are responsible for their astringent taste when taken.

3. **Food additive:** Beside phytochemical benefits in nutraceutics, disease management, and treatment, they are also a good source of several food additives. Their additions improve food palatability and acceptability; they are better accepted by consumers when compared to artificial food additives (Smetanska, 2008). Anthocyanins are applied in soft drinks to give it a red color.

2.2   BIOSYNTHESIS OF PHYTOCHEMICALS

The synthesis of phytochemical is of critical importance to plants. Environmental necessities for survival are believed to trigger this synthesis;

such environmental threats include changes in climate, soil requirements, the presence of herbivores, pollinators, and microorganism (Stepp and Moerman, 2001; Mazid et al., 2011). The various reactions involved in plant biochemical synthesis are said to be generally reversible under the influence of specific enzymatic reactions. In general, plant secondary metabolites are either synthesis in vivo or hydrolyzed.

2.2.1 CONTRIBUTING PATHWAYS FOR THE BIOSYNTHESIS OF PHYTOCHEMICAL

A number of pathways contribute to the biosynthesis of phytochemicals (Fig. 2.3). One or two pathways can also be linked to the synthesis of a particular phytochemical. The contributing pathways include pentose phosphate pathway, a source of various sugar moieties found in the phytochemicals. The shikimic acid pathway generates the amino acids, which are further modified during the biosynthesis of alkaloids, phenolics, flavonoids, and lignins. The malonyl-CoA pathway synthesizes anthraquinone, anthocyanidin, and anthocyanin. Nucleotide metabolic pathway contributes to the synthesis of purine alkaloids, while terpenoids and steroids are biosynthesized majorly through mevalonate and non-mevalonate pathway.

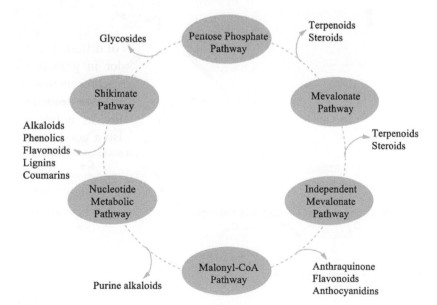

FIGURE 2.3 Contributing pathways to phytochemical biosynthesis.

2.2.1.1 PENTOSE PHOSPHATE PATHWAY

The pentose phosphate pathway provides various sugars, which are conjugated in glycosides. Some of the carbohydrates include arabinose, D-glucose, galactose, glucorhamnose, or L-rhamnose (Pretorius, 2003). The pathway occurs in both plants and animals in two phases (oxidative and nonoxidative) where a hexose phosphate sugar is oxidized to a pentose phosphate sugar with the release of CO_2 (Heldt et al., 2011). The pathway also provides NADPH for biosynthetic reactions. First, the enzyme glucose 6-phosphate dehydrogenase oxidizes glucose 6phosphate to 6-phosphogluconolactone (Fig. 2.4). The reaction is highly exothermic, irreversible, and utilizes $NADP^+$ to generate NADPH. 6-phosphogluconolactone is hydrolyzed by lactonase

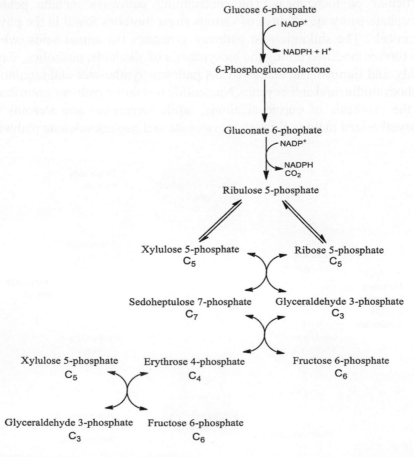

FIGURE 2.4 Pentose phosphate pathway.

to gluconate 6-phosphate (Heldt et al., 2011). Ribulose-5phosphate is formed by the oxidation reaction catalyzed by gluconate 6-phosphate dehydrogenase with the release of NADPH and CO_2. In the oxidative phase, xylulose 5phosphate and ribose 5phosphate are isomerized from ribulose 5phosphate by the enzyme ribulose phosphate epimerase and ribose phosphate isomerase, respectively. While in the nonoxidative phase, xylulose 5phosphate and ribose 5phosphate are converted to sedoheptulose 7phosphate and glyceraldehyde 3-phosphate by a transketolase. The C_{10} compounds, sedoheptulose 7-phosphate, and glyceraldehyde 3-phosphate are converted by a transaldolase to erythrose 4-phosphate and fructose 6-phosphate. Similarly, the C_9 compounds, xylulose 5-phosphate, and erythrose 4-phosphate are converted by a transketolase to glyceraldehyde 3-phosphate and fructose 6-phosphate (Heldt et al., 2011).

2.2.1.2   SHIKIMATE PATHWAY

The shikimic acid pathway located exclusively in plant plastids is for the synthesis of alkaloids, flavonoids, coumarins, lignans, and some cyanogenic glycosides. Others are cinnamates, quinones, and phenolics. The precursors for this pathway are erythrose 4-phosphate and phosphoenolpyruvate, the intermediates from the pentose phosphate pathway and glycolysis, respectively. First, a condensation reaction between erythrose 4-phosphate and phosphoenolpyruvate occurs in two steps catalyzed by dehydroquinate synthase to give rise to a cyclic dehydroquinate compound with the release of two phosphate groups (Fig. 2.5). From the product, a water molecule is removed, which results in the reduction of the carbonyl group to form 3-dehydroshikimate catalyzed by 3-dehydroquinate dehydratase (Heldt et al., 2011). Shikimic acid from which the name of the pathway is derived is then synthesized in the reaction catalyzed by the enzyme shikimate dehydrogenase. The 3' hydroxyl group is then protected by a form of phosphorylation using ATP by shikimate kinase and liberation of ADP to form shikimate 3-phosphate (Heldt et al., 2011). The free hydroxyl group at the 5' carbon reacts with one molecule of phosphoenolpyruvate to form 5'-enolpyruvyl shikimate-3-phosphate. Chorismate is formed thereafter by the hydrolysis of pyrophosphate by chorismate synthase (Heldt et al., 2011).

In another series of enzyme-catalyzed reactions, tryptophan is formed from which alkaloids are synthesized. Also, prephenate and arogenate are formed from which phenylalanine and tyrosine are synthesized. Prephenate is produced by the rearrangement of the side chain from 5' carbon to 1' carbon by chorismate mutase, while arogenate is formed by the transamination of the keto group at the 1' carbon by an amine transferase (Heldt et al., 2011). The removal of water and the decarboxylation of arogenate by prephenate dehydratase give rise to phenylalanine from which phytochemicals such as flavonoids, coumarins, and lignans groups can be synthesized. The oxidation of arogenate by NAD$^+$, followed by its decarboxylation results in the formation of tyrosine from which cyanogenic glycosides and other alkaloids are synthesized.

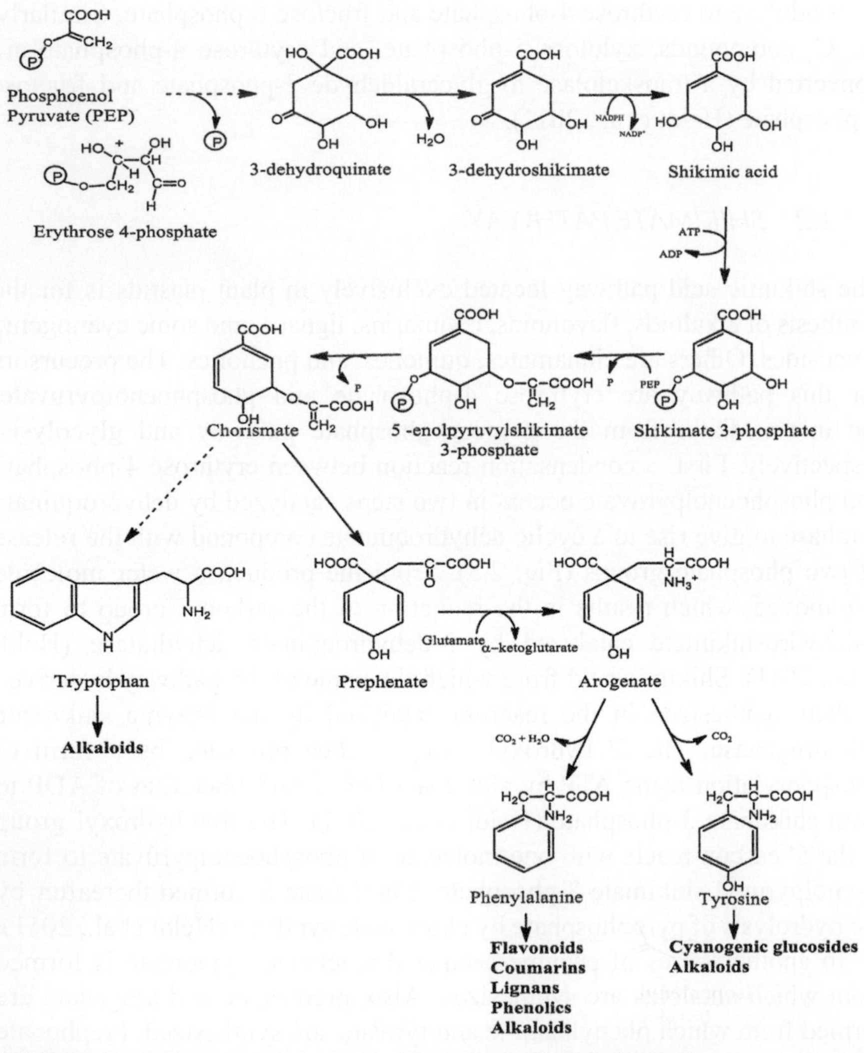

FIGURE 2.5   Shikimate pathway for the biosynthesis of phytochemicals.

2.2.1.3 MALONYL-COA PATHWAY

Malonyl-CoA is synthesized from acetyl-CoA by the action of acetyl-CoA carboxylase which requires biotin as a cofactor (Fig. 2.6). It is an irreversible reaction and the rate-limiting step in fatty acid biosynthesis. Malonyl-CoA is a key metabolite in the synthesis of anthraquinones, anthocyanins, and flavonoids.

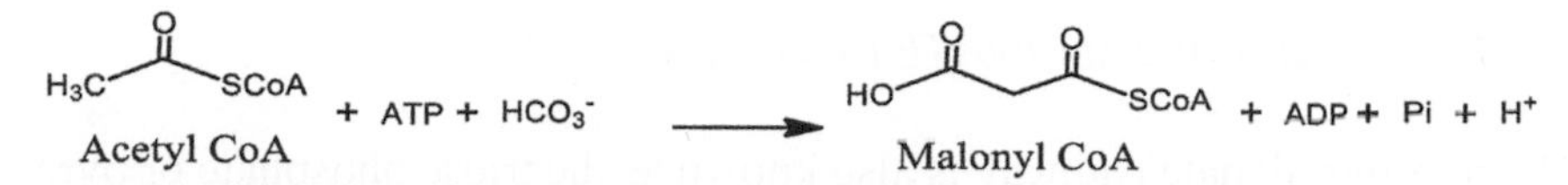

FIGURE 2.6 Malonyl-CoA biosynthesis from acetyl-CoA.

2.2.1.4 MEVALONATE PATHWAY

Mevalonate pathway for the synthesis of terpenes, terpenoids, and steroids is localized in the cytosol. The first reaction in the pathway involves the synthesis of acetoacetyl-CoA catalyzed by the enzyme acetoacetyl-CoA thiolase (Fig. 2.7). HMG-CoA is synthesized from acetoacetyl-CoA catalyzed by the enzyme HMG-CoA synthase. The next reaction is catalyzed by HMG-CoA reductase to produce mevalonic acid and then mevalonic acid phosphate by mevalonate kinase. Mevalonate monophosphate is phosphorylated again by

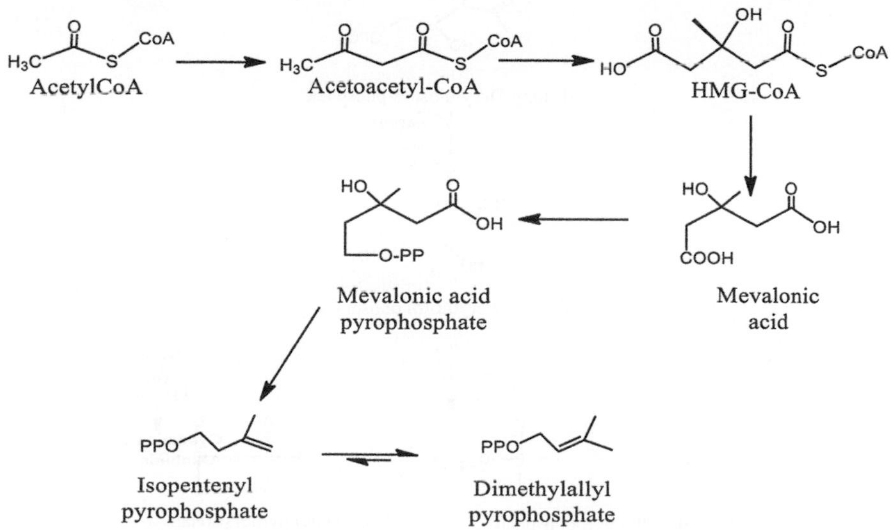

FIGURE 2.7 Mevalonate pathway.

phosphomevalonate kinase where a phosphate group is added. Mevalonate 5-diphosphate decarboxylase catalyzes the formation of isopentenyl pyrophosphate (IPP). A 1,3-allylic rearrangement converts IPP to dimethylallyl diphosphate (DMAPP) in a reaction catalyzed by IPP isomerase. The detailed mechanism of these enzymes has been reported elsewhere by Dewick (Dewick, 2002).

2.2.1.5 NON-MEVALONATE PATHWAY

The non-mevalonate pathway is also known as the triose phosphate or pyruvate pathway. Other names are 1-deoxy-D-xylulose-5-phosphate pathway or the 2C-methyl-D-erythrito-4-phosphate pathway. The pathway has been ascertained in bacteria, algae, and higher plants (Rohmer, 1999). In the reaction steps (Fig. 2.8), glyceraldehyde 3-phosphate condenses with pyruvate to form 1-deoxy-D-xylulose-5-phosphate (Rohmer, 1999; Hunter, 2007). In

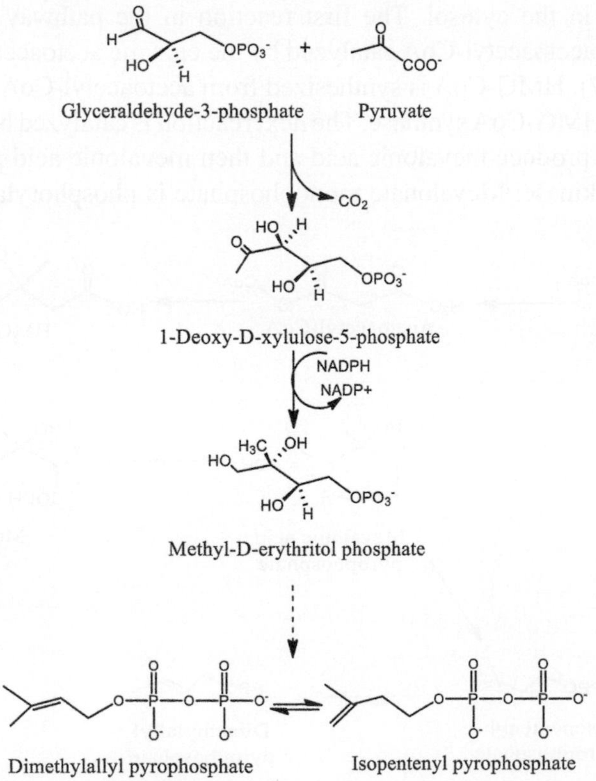

Glyceraldehyde-3-phosphate   Pyruvate

1-Deoxy-D-xylulose-5-phosphate

Methyl-D-erythritol phosphate

Dimethylallyl pyrophosphate   Isopentenyl pyrophosphate

FIGURE 2.8 Non-mevalonate pathway.

the next reaction, which is NADPH dependent, forms the key intermediate 2C-methyl-D-erythritol-4-phosphate, from which IPP and DMAPP are formed (Rohmer, 1999; Hunter, 2007). Enzymes of the non-mevalonate pathway are recently being researched for the development of drugs against infections in pathogenic prokaryotes because the pathway occurs in them rather than in humans (Sassetti et al., 2001; Akerley et al., 2002; Kobayashi et al., 2003). Drugs from such research are targeted at diseases such as malaria and tuberculosis.

2.2.1.6   NUCLEOTIDE METABOLIC PATHWAY

The purine nucleotide metabolic pathway contributes to the biosynthesis of some phytochemicals. These types of phytochemicals, which belong to the alkaloid family, are referred to as the purine alkaloids (Zulak et al., 2006). The reaction pathway has been reviewed extensively by Ashihara et al. (2008). Xanthosine plays a central role and provides the xanthine skeleton frame of caffeine. It is contributed by four different pathways, which include the de novo synthesis of purine metabolism, degradation of adenine nucleotide to form AMP, degradation of guanine nucleotide to form GMP, and the S adenosyl-L-methionine (SAM) cycle of adenosine formation to adenine.

Ribose 5-phosphate through a series of enzyme-catalyzed reactions generates inosine monophosphate (IMP) (Fig. 2.9). IMP dehydrogenase catalyzes the conversion of IMP to xanthosine monophosphate, followed by its conversion to xanthosine. The subsequent steps are reactions leading to the synthesis of caffeine. First, xanthosine is methylated by N-methyltransferase, an SAM depending enzyme to form 7-methylxanthosine catalyzed by 7-methylxanthosine synthase. The product is then hydrolyzed by N-methyl nucleosidase to 7-methylxanthine. Theobromine synthase and caffeine synthase catalyze the last two steps forming theobromine and caffeine, respectively (Ashihara et al., 1996). Several enzymes of this pathway have been isolated from plant sources as well as some of the genes encoding them (Suzuki et al., 1992; Kato et al., 1999; Kato et al., 2000; Mizuno et al., 2003; Uefuji et al., 2003; Ashihara and Suzuki, 2004).

Theobromine (3,7-dimethylxanthine) and caffeine (1,3,7-trimethylxanthine) are examples of purine alkaloid synthesis through this pathway. They are found in tea, coffee, and other nonalcoholic beverages (Ashihara et al., 2008).

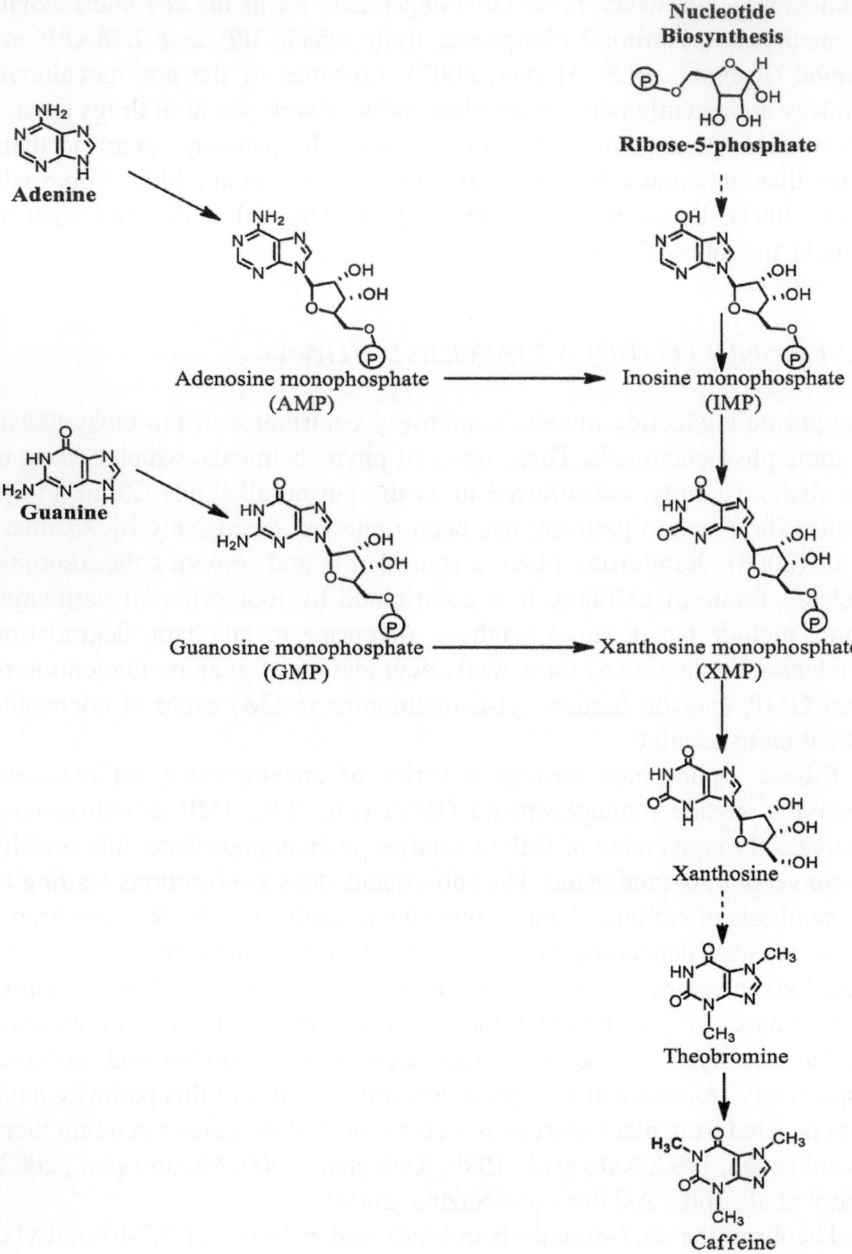

FIGURE 2.9   Nucleotide metabolic pathway for biosynthesis of purine alkaloids.

2.2.2 BIOSYNTHESIS OF FLAVONOIDS

Flavonoids are ubiquitous phytochemicals, existing in a wide range of fruits and plants, including the lower and higher plants (De Groot and Rauen, 1998). They are the most studied plant phenols (Dai and Mumper, 2010). Vegetables, tea, and coffee are other sources rich in flavonoids (Pridham, 1960). Flavonoids are subgrouped into flavonols (kaempferol), flavones (luteolin), flavanone (naringenin), chalcones (butein), and anthocyanidins (pelargonidin) (Harborne et al., 1975).

A common pathway relates biosynthesis of flavonoids. Their precursors are derived from the shikimate and the acetate-malonate pathway (Hahlbrock and Grisebach, 1975; Wong, 1976) with chalcone being the first intermediate from the flavonoid reaction pathway (Fig. 2.10). Several flavonoids are thus generated from reactions involving chalcone (Hahlbrock, 1981). Flavanone, flavone, isoflavone, dihydroflavonol, flavonol, catechin, epicatechin, and anthocyanidin are among the compounds obtained through this pathway.

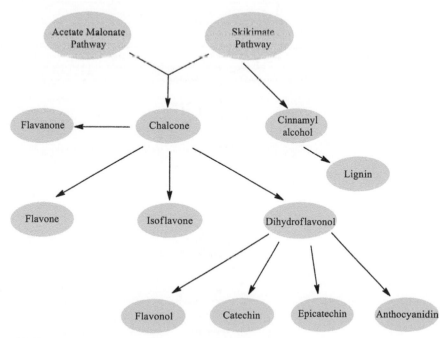

FIGURE 2.10 Biosynthetic pathway of flavonoids.

Flavonoids are a six-member structure linked to a benzene ring to form a pyrone flavone or flavonol. It could also form the dihydro derivatives of pyrone, which are flavanones or flavanols. When the substituted benzene ring is at position 2, a flavanone is formed or when it is at position 3, an isoflavone is formed. Flavonoids may exist in nature as conjugated at position 3 or 7 with several glycosidic linkages. The carbohydrate moieties are derived from the pentose phosphate pathway, and can be L-rhamnose, D-glucose, glucorhamnose, galactose, or arabinose (Pretorius, 2003). Catechin biosynthesis is illustrated in Figure 2.11. The condensation reaction between three molecules of malonyl-CoA and one molecule of cinnamoyl-CoA (Mora-pale et al., 2013) catalyzed by chalcone synthase is the committed step for their biosynthesis. Chalcone formed is then isomerized to a flavanone by chalcone isomerase. The final steps of the reaction is catalyzed by an NADPH-dependent enzyme dihydroflavonol 4-reductase to form leucoanthocyanidins (Martens et al., 2002), which are converted by leucoanthocyanidin reductase to catechin (Tanner et al., 2003).

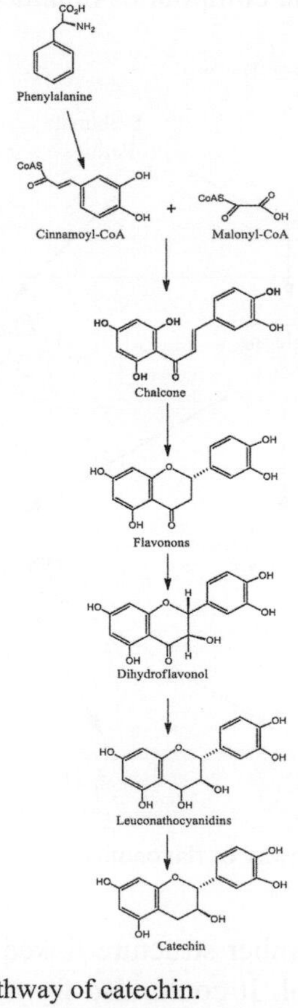

FIGURE 2.11   Biosynthetic pathway of catechin.

2.2.2.1 BIOACTIVITY OF FLAVONOIDS

Biological activities of flavonoids are diverse and well documented. Some of their activities include anti-inflammatory, antimicrobial, anti-allergic, antioxidant, cytotoxic, and antitumor (Tapas et al., 2008). In diabetic treatment, flavonoids have been used to inhibit digestive enzymes with reduced side effects (Bedekar et al., 2010). Specifically, catechin has been reported to trigger the secretion of insulin from pancreatic β-cells (Chemler et al., 2007).

2.2.3 BIOSYNTHESIS OF LIGNAN

Lignans are plant phytochemicals with highly branched polymers. The name (lignan) was first introduced by Haworth (Haworth, 1936), where he describes it as plant compounds with dimeric phenylpropanoids (Fig. 2.12). Dimeric phenylpropanoids are linked through C6–C3 attached by a central carbon at carbon 8 (C8) to form the basic structure of lignans. Another form of linkage that exists through a C5–C5′ is named neolignans (Umezawa, 2003).

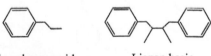

Phenylpropanoid unit   Lignan basic structure

FIGURE 2.12 Basic structure of lignins.

Biosynthesis of lignans is from two aromatic amino acids, phenylalanine or tyrosine by the dimerization of either three of substituted hydroxycinnamoyl alcohols (Fig. 2.13), which are the main precursors of all lignins and lignans. The alcohols are oxidized into free radicals by ubiquitous peroxidase enzymes (Mazid et al., 2011). Through this reaction, the peroxidase induces an electron oxidation of the phenol group, thus causing a delocalization of the unpaired electron through the different resonance forms. Few other steps proceed after the oxidation – formation of a pinoresinol and it is reduced by the enzyme pinoresinol reductase to form lariciresinol. Several lignans are generated from this point onward through this pathway (Fig. 2.14).

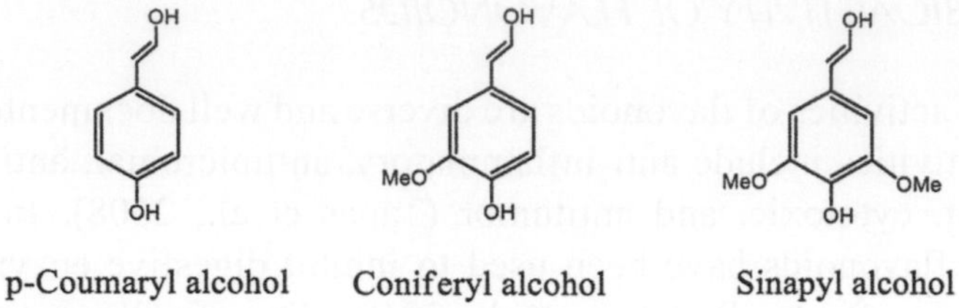
p-Coumaryl alcohol
Coniferyl alcohol
Sinapyl alcohol

FIGURE 2.13 Chemical structures of lignan precursors.

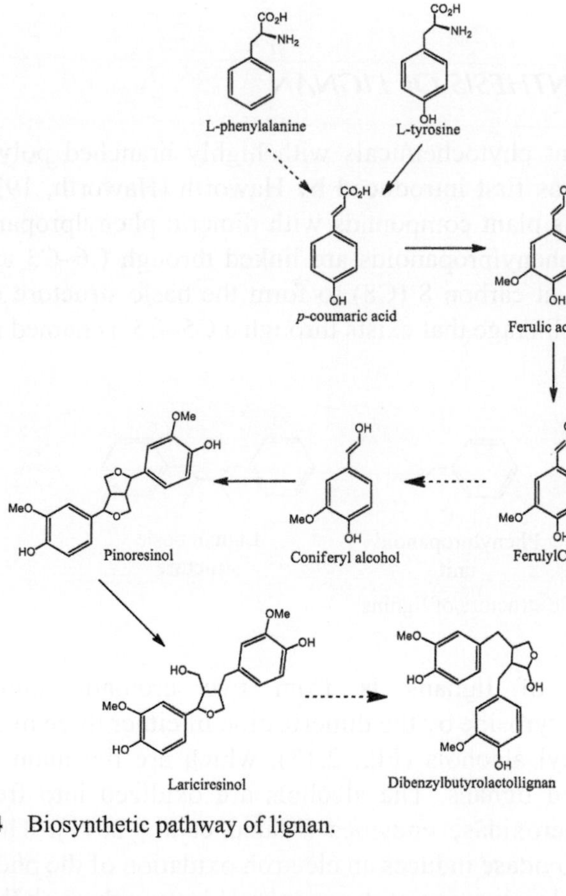
L-phenylalanine
L-tyrosine
p-coumaric acid
Ferulic acid
Pinoresinol
Coniferyl alcohol
FerulylCoA
Lariciresinol
Dibenzylbutyrolactollignan

FIGURE 2.14 Biosynthetic pathway of lignan.

2.2.3.1 BIOACTIVITY OF LIGNANS

Lignans have a wide range of applications. They are applied in cancer therapy for their ability to reduce cell proliferation in colon cancer cells, inhibit metastatic secondary tumors, and decrease the levels of markers in a rat model of colon cancer (Delmas et al., 2006). Lignans are also reported to be anti-inflammatory (Saleem et al., 2005), antimicrobial (Saleem et al., 2005), antioxidant (Fauré et al., 1990; Saleem et al., 2005; Pan et al., 2009), immunosuppressive (Saleem et al., 2005), and hepatoprotective (Negi et al., 2008). Silymarin are flavonolignans formed by the combination of flavonoid and lignan structures by oxidative coupling (Dewick, 2002); they have been used for centuries in the treatment of liver, spleen, and gallbladder disorders (Shaker et al., 2010).

2.2.4 BIOSYNTHESIS OF ANTHOCYANINS

Anthocyanins belong to the water-soluble type of phytochemicals, which provide bright color to many flowers and fruits due to their ability to change color at low pH or pH above neutral scale. Their synthesis is majorly through the phenylpropanoid pathway through the formation of malonyl-CoA, chalcone, and catechin (Fig. 2.15). Finally, following the formation of dihydroflavonols through leucoanthocyanidins, anthocyanidins

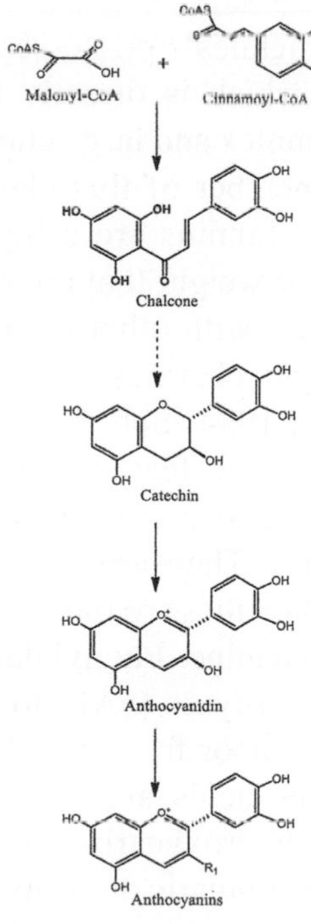

FIGURE 2.15 Biosynthetic pathway of anthocyanins.

are biosynthesized (Mora-pale et al., 2013). Anthocyanin biosynthesis has been recognized as one of the first branches in the general phenylpropanoid pathway, in which their biosynthetic enzymes have been identified (Allen et al., 2008). Enzymes catalyzing the reactions, including chalcone synthase, chalcone isomerase, flavanone 3-hydroxylase, and anthocyanidin synthase (leucoanthocyanidin dioxygenase) have been studied extensively (Shirley et al., 1995; Winkel-Shirley, 2001; Lepiniec et al., 2006).

2.2.4.1   BIOACTIVITY OF ANTHOCYANINS

Anthocyanins are beneficial as antioxidants, anti-inflammatory, anti-carcinogenic, and anti-microbial compounds. They are also reported to be beneficial in preventing cardiovascular and diabetic complications (Ghosh and Konishi, 2007; Toufektsian et al., 2008; Jing et al., 2008; He and Giusti, 2010; Pascual-Teresa et al., 2010).

2.2.5   BIOSYNTHESIS OF PHENOLICS

The phenolic class of phytochemicals possesses a hydroxyl group as part of their chemical structure, which is directly bonded to their aromatic hydrocarbon. They have a complex and large chemical constituent (Walton et al., 2003). The simplest member of this class is the phenol, with the chemical formula (C_6H_5OH). Tannins are a heterogeneous polyphenolic compound with high molecular weight that are capable of forming reversible and irreversible complexes with other compounds such as alkaloids, minerals, nucleic acids, polysaccharides, and proteins (Mueller-Harvey and Mcallan, 1992; Vansoest, 1994; Schofield et al., 2001). Tannins are compounds with the characteristic features similar to tan leather. They are known for their acidic reactions due to the presence of phenolic or carboxylic groups (Kar, 2007). They are categorized as condensed and hydrolyzable tannins. Plant phenolics are biosynthesized from the shikimic acid pathway through phenylalanine. Phenylalanine is deaminated by the enzyme phenylalanine ammonia-lyase (PAL) to cinnamic acid (Fig. 2.16). Cinnamic acid is the first precursor from which several phenolics can be synthesized. Hydroxycinnamic acids are produced from a simple ester formation with a glucose or hydroxycarboxylic acids. Simple phenolics are also synthesized from a ρ-coumaric acid (hydroxycinnamic acid) from the same pathway.

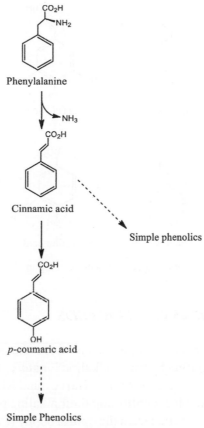

FIGURE 2.16   Biosynthetic pathway of phenolics.

2.2.5.1   BIOACTIVITY OF PHENOLICS

Phenolics are an important class of phytochemicals due to their several beneficial roles in humans. Examples of phenolics with important bioactivities include gallic acid, caffeic acid, cinnamic acid, and vanillic acid (Fig. 2.17). They possess antioxidant defenses against free radical-related diseases. Phenolics reduce toxicity arising from streptozotocin by neutralizing the free radicals generated in the pancreas (Uttara et al., 2009). They are also reported to possess anti-inflammatory, antidepressant, antispasmodic, anti-tumor, antiulcer, and cytotoxic activities (Silva et al., 2007; Ghasemzadeh et al., 2010). The tannins found its usefulness in textile dyes and antioxidants in industries during the production of beer, wine, and fruit juice (Gyamfi and Aniya, 2002).

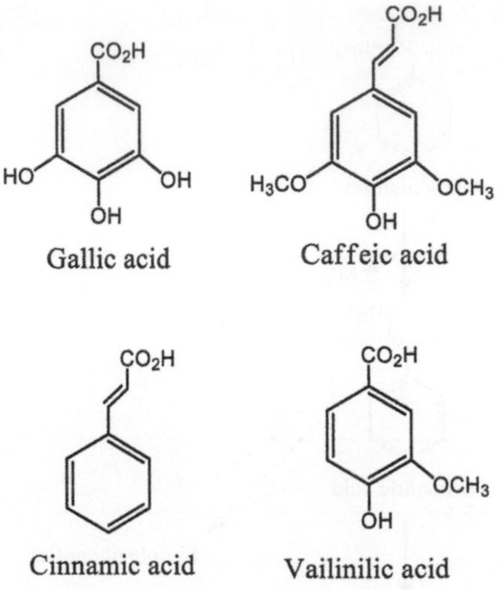

Gallic acid   Caffeic acid

Cinnamic acid   Vailinilic acid

FIGURE 2.17   Structure of some important phenolic compounds.

2.2.6   BIOSYNTHESIS OF ALKALOIDS

Alkaloids derive their name linguistically from the Arabic word *al-qali* (Kutchan, 1995) signifying their "alkaline" nature and describing the presence of a nitrogenous base (Mueller-Harvey and McAllan, 1992). They turn red litmus paper to blue, confirming their alkaline properties. Morphine was the first alkaloid identified from the opium poppy (*Papaver somniferum*) in 1806. More than 10,000 alkaloids have been identified since then with their various structures elucidated (Southon and Buckingham, 1989).

Alkaloids are synthesized from a number of amino acids, which include aspartic acid, lysine, tryptophan, and tyrosine (Pearce et al., 1991). Most of which are aromatic amino acids. Their synthesis was assumed to be from the abnormalities of amino acid synthesis, most likely from a mutation in the control mechanisms, which result to the conversion of excess amino acids to alkaloids as a means of disposal (Waller and Nowacki, 1978).

In the biosynthesis of terpenoid indole alkaloids (Fig. 2.18), tryptophan is first decarboxylated to tryptamine by the enzyme tryptophan decarboxylase (Leete, 1961). Protoalkaloid (tryptamine) serves as the substrate for the first committed step of the reaction catalyzed by strictosidine synthase (Stöckigt and Zenk, 1977). The carbohydrate source, deoxyxylulose is converted to secologanin. Secologanin is then condensed with tryptamine by strictosidine synthase (Stöckigt and Zenk, 1977). Strictosidine synthase is a stereospecific enzyme, which is of biotechnological interest and its product 3α(S)-strictosidine is the first monoterpenoid indole alkaloid in this pathway (O'Connor and Maresh, 2006).

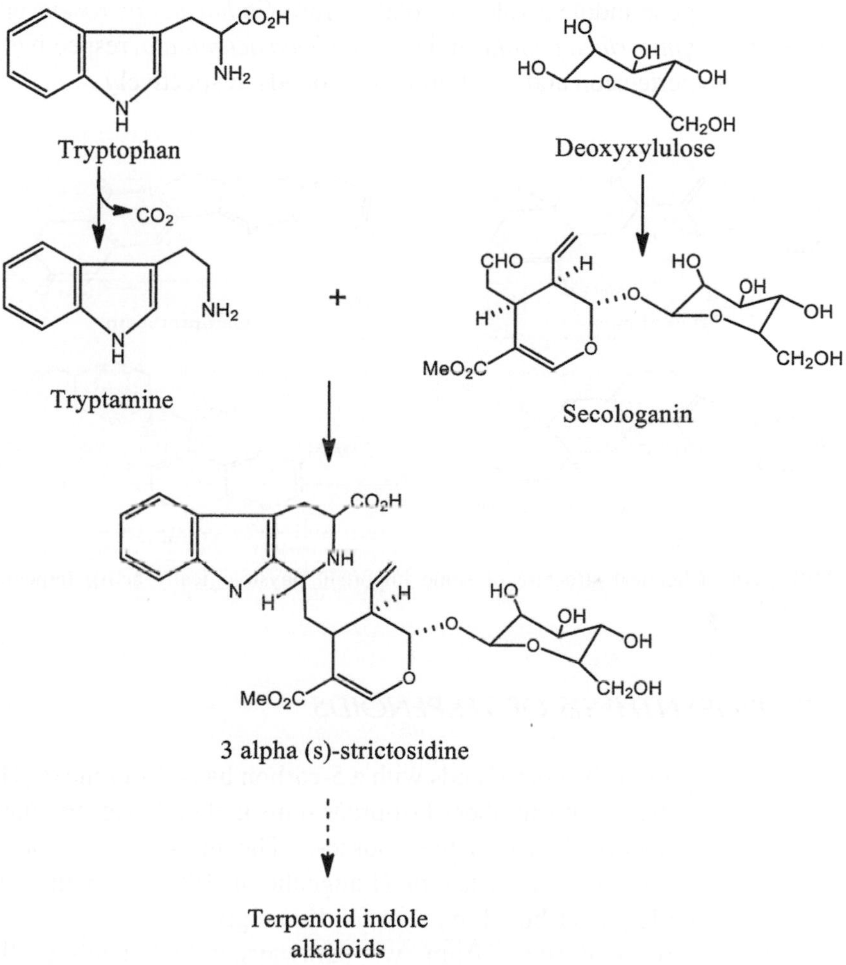

FIGURE 2.18 Biosynthetic pathway of terpenoid indole alkaloids.

2.2.6.1 BIOACTIVITY OF ALKALOIDS

Caffeine, morphine, and nicotine are examples of alkaloids with stimulating properties and are examples of good analgesic (Rao et al., 1978). The alkaloid quinine (Fig. 2.19) is a known antimalarial compound (Rao et al., 1978) obtained from the cinchona plant and it is used in the treatment of symptomatic erythrocyte stages of malaria infection. Yohimbine, an example of terpene indole alkaloids, is an adrenergic receptor blocker, which has been isolated from the plant *Rauvolfia serpentina*. Ajmalicine and camptothecin are other examples of terpene indole alkaloids isolated from *Catharanthus roseus* and *R. serpentina, Ophiorrhiza pumila,* and *Camptotheca acuminata*, respectively. They are antihypertension and anti-tumor compounds, respectively.

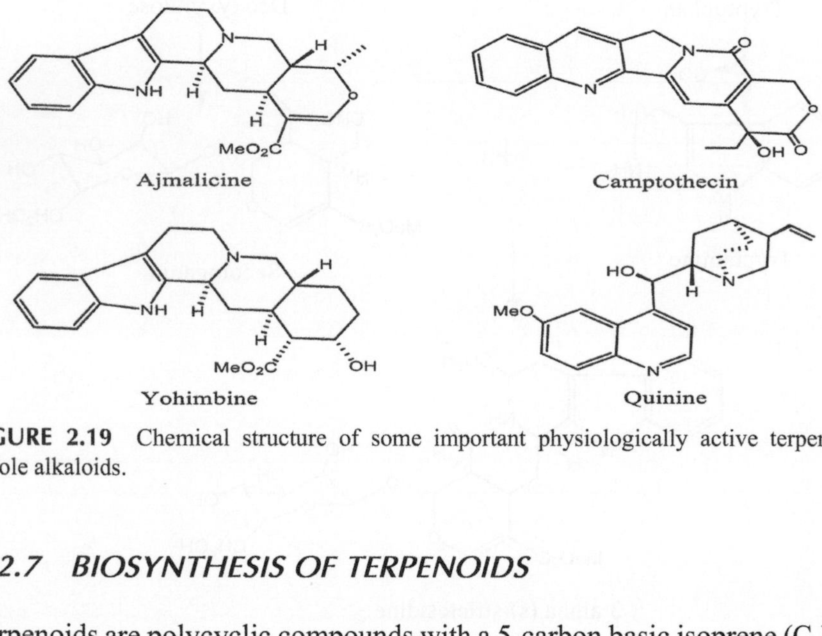

FIGURE 2.19 Chemical structure of some important physiologically active terpenoid indole alkaloids.

2.2.7 BIOSYNTHESIS OF TERPENOIDS

Terpenoids are polycyclic compounds with a 5-carbon basic isoprene (C_5H_8) structure. They differ by the number of isoprene units in their basic structures as well as the functional groups they possess. The number of isoprene units serves as a means of classification (Langenheim, 1994). Terpenes are phytonutrients widely distributed in green foods and grains.

Terpenoids are synthesized from two pathways, which leads to the formation of its two biosynthetic precursors, namely IPP and DMAPP (Chang et al., 2007; Meng et al., 2011). They are the fundamental building blocks in the biosynthesis of biological compounds with isoprenoid units. This includes steroids, carotenoids, saponins, and limonoids. The first pathway for isoprenoid synthesis is through the mevalonic acid pathway (Fig. 2.20). This is specific for some bacteria, plants, and higher eukaryotes (Zurbriggen et al., 2012; Zhou et al., 2012), while the mevalonic independent pathway, also known as the 1-deoxy-d-xylulose-5-phosphate pathway

(Fig. 2.21), is specifically for plants and most bacterial strains (Hoeffler et al., 2002). IPP and DMAPP are restructured by subsequent additions of IPP to form various units of terpenoids. First, hemiterpenes (C_5) and mono-terpenes (C_{10}) are produced and then sesquiterpenes (C_{15}) by the addition of an IPP unit. Triterpenes (C_{30}) are synthesized from two units of triterpenes. Steroids are also generated from triterpene units (Fig. 2.20). Similarly, from the non-mevalonic pathway, terpenoids are synthesized from IPP through geranyl diphosphate and secologanin.

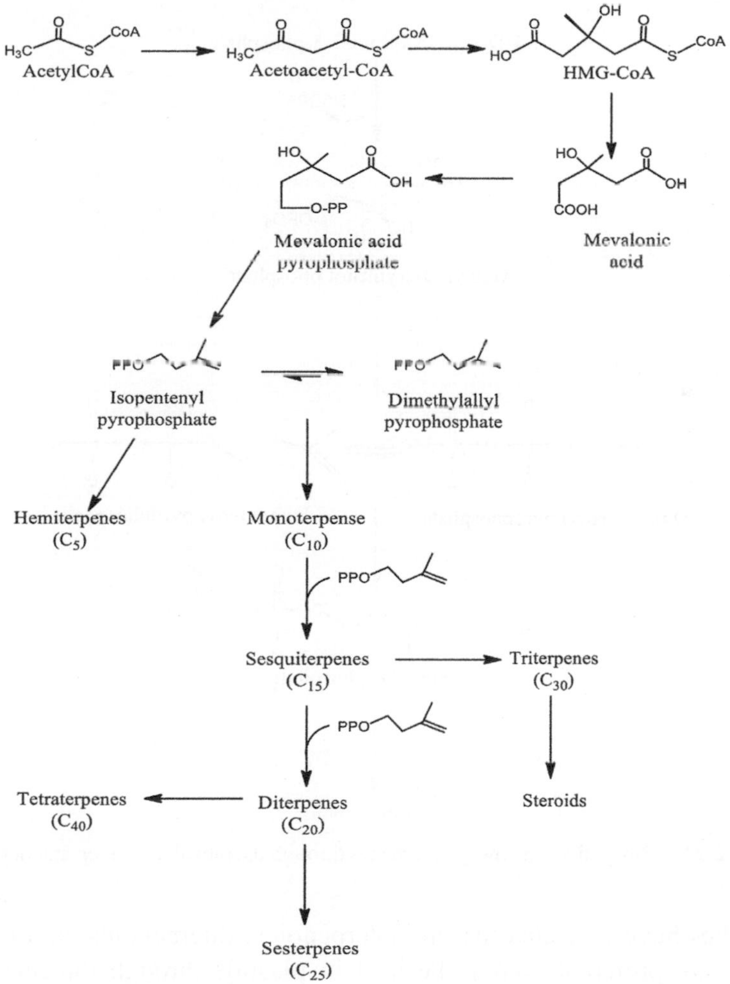

FIGURE 2.20   Biosynthetic pathway of terpenes through the mevalonic pathway.

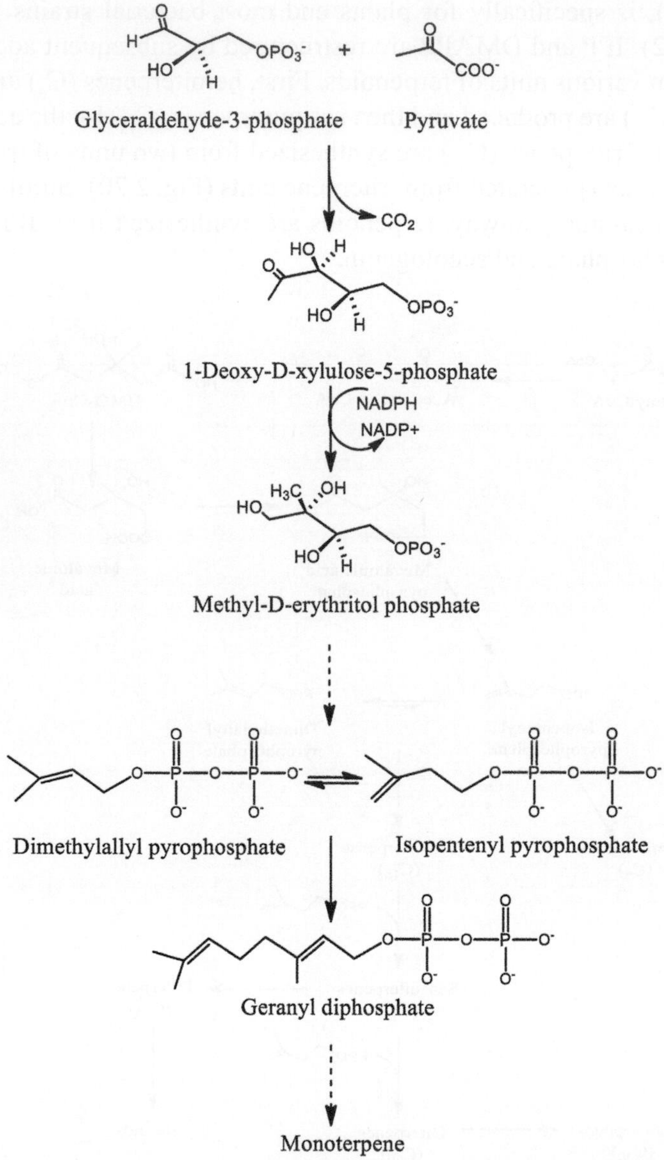

FIGURE 2.21 Biosynthetic pathway of terpenes through the mevalonic independent pathway.

Studies have indicated that monoterpenoids, diterpenoids, and tetraterpenoids are preferably biosynthesized in plastids through the mevalonic independent pathway, while triterpenoids and sesquiterpenes are mostly biosynthesized in the cytosol through mevalonic acid pathway (Sawai and

Saito, 2011). Studies have also indicated that secologanin is derived from the mevalonic independent pathway by feeding ^{13}C-glucose in *C. roseus* cell culture (Contin et al., 1998) and that same mevalonic independent pathway leads to the synthesis of secologanin in *O. pumila* (Yamazaki et al., 2004).

2.2.7.1 BIOACTIVITY OF TERPENOIDS

Terpenoids are of several biological relevances. Their protective role is derived from their bitter taste; hence, they protect some plants from being eaten by animals (Degenhardt et al., 2003). Pyrethroids are a monoterpene ester which exists in the leaves and flowers of the plant *Chrysanthemum*. They are strong insecticidal compound by which *Chrysanthemum* plant protect itself from insects. Lycopene and β-carotene (Fig. 2.22) are two structurally related compounds, transported primarily in LDLs. Their conjugated double bonds enhance their powerful antioxidant nature, thereby protecting LDLs from oxidations during transportation (Goulinet and Chapman, 1997).

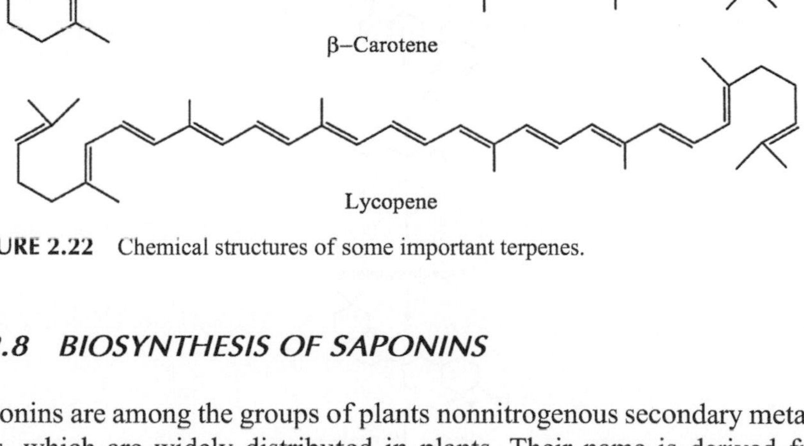

Vitamin A

β–Carotene

Lycopene

FIGURE 2.22 Chemical structures of some important terpenes.

2.2.8 BIOSYNTHESIS OF SAPONINS

Saponins are among the groups of plants nonnitrogenous secondary metabolites, which are widely distributed in plants. Their name is derived from their ability to form stable foam in aqueous solutions when shaken. On hydrolysis, an aglycone moiety called sapogenin is released. Steroidal and triterpenoidal sapogenin are the two known types of sapogenins with a sugar moiety attached to the hydroxyl group on carbon 3. Triterpenoid saponins are examples of saponins synthesized from isoprenoid units (Yendo et al., 2014). Three isopentyl pyrophosphate are combined in an head to tail linkage to form farnesyl pyrophosphate (Fig. 2.23). In the next reaction, catalyzed by squalene synthase, two farnesyl pyrophosphate units are combined with a tail-to-tail manner to form squalene (Vincken et al., 2007). Squalene epoxidase oxidizes the product to 2,3-oxidosqualene. The committed step of the reaction is the cyclization of 2,3-oxidosqualene, a reaction catalyzed by oxidosqualene cyclase followed by oxidation, substitution, and glycosylation to form various triterpenoid saponins.

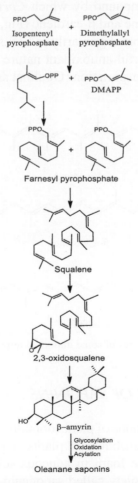

Isopentenyl pyrophosphate + Dimethylallyl pyrophosphate

OPP + DMAPP

Farnesyl pyrophosphate

Squalene

2,3-oxidosqualene

HO β—amyrin

Glycosylation
Oxidation
Acylation

Oleanane saponins

FIGURE 2.23   Biosynthesis of triterpenoid saponins.

2.2.8.1   BIOACTIVITY OF SAPONINS

Saponins have a diverse range of biological activities. Members of this phytochemical group are reported to have anti-inflammatory, antileishmanial, antimutagenic, antiviral, hemolytic, and hepatoprotective properties (Rahimi et al., 2009). Saponins from *Medicago truncatula* (Fig. 2.24) have been studied for their various functions such as antimicrobials, fungicides, insecticides, and other functions (Tava et al., 2011).

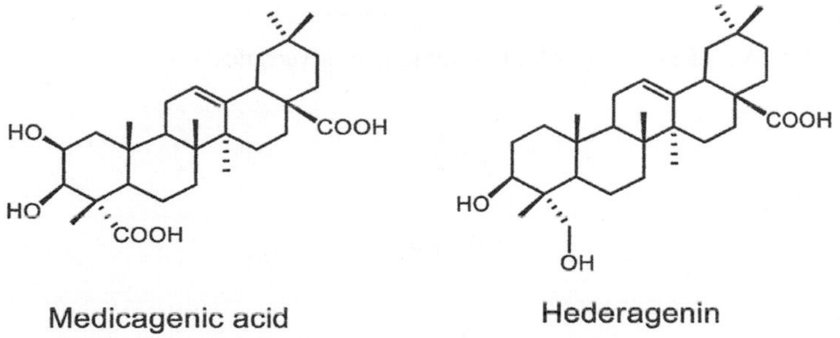

Medicagenic acid   Hederagenin

FIGURE 2.24   Examples of sapogenins from *Medicago truncatula*.

2.2.9   BIOSYNTHESIS OF GLYCOSIDES

Glycosides are products of the condensation of various sugars with different types of organic hydroxyl compounds or few cases in thiol compounds. They are colorless, crystalline carbon, hydrogen or oxygen compounds or nitrogen and sulfur compounds. Due to their nature, glycosides are water soluble. Chemically, they contain a glucose (carbohydrate moiety) and an aglycone (noncarbohydrate moiety) (Kar, 2007; Firn, 2010). The sugar moiety is derived from the pentose phosphate pathway and may be a monosaccharide or disaccharide including either of the following sugars: D glucose, D-xylose, L-rhamnose, L-arabinose, and L-fructose, while the aglycon may be a coumarin, a flavonoid, a lignan, a phenolic, or a terpene compound. Following the various combinations above, aldehyde glycosides, anthraquinone glycosides, cardiac glycosides, cyanogenic glycosides, phenolic glycosides, or saponin glycosides may be formed (Fig. 2.25).

The aglycones are synthesized from the shikimate pathway through phenylalanine or tryptophan. PAL deaminates phenylalanine to cinnamic acid with the release of ammonia from phenylalanine. In the biosynthesis of Arbutin, glucose is conjugate with hydroquinone (Fig. 2.26). Aldoximes

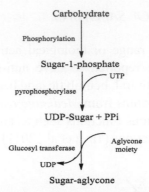

FIGURE 2.25 A typical pathway for biosynthesis of glycosides.

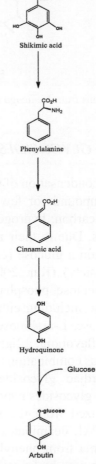

FIGURE 2.26 Biosynthetic pathway of Arbutin.

are important intermediates in the biosynthesis of cyanogenic glycosides (Fig. 2.27) and their reaction is catalyzed by cytochrome-P_{450} enzymes. Cyanogenic glycosides are conjugates of various sugar moieties with an N-protective group from the aldoximes. They release their poisonous compounds like cyanide (HCN) and sulfide (H_2S) when the plant containing them is digested. Therefore, they serve to protect such plants from feeding by insects or animals (Taiz and Zeiger, 1995).

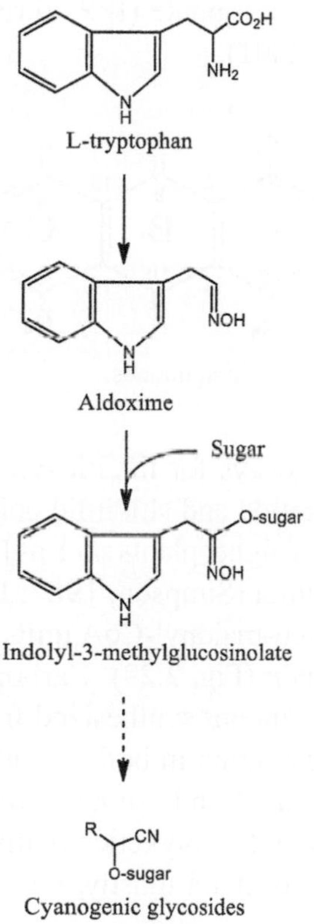

L-tryptophan

Aldoxime

— Sugar

Indolyl-3-methylglucosinolate

Cyanogenic glycosides

FIGURE 2.27 Biosynthesis of the cyanogenic glycoside.

2.2.9.1 BIOACTIVITY OF GLYCOSIDE

Cyanogenic glycosides are themselves not toxic except by the release of their HCN and H_2S contents which are volatile and poisonous. Their primary roles in plants involve the chemical defense and mediating their interactions with insects (Zagrobelny et al., 2004).

2.2.10 BIOSYNTHESIS OF ANTHRAQUINONES

The basic structure of anthraquinones consist of three rings (Fig. 2.28). Ring A is believed to be obtained from the shikimic acid pathway through the synthesis of shikimic acid, chorismic acid, and thiamine diphosphate (Han, et al., 2001). Ring B is derived from tricarboxylic acid pathway through the formation of α-ketoglutarate. The ring closure is achieved by the formation of a succinylbenzoic acid intermediate (Han et al., 2001). The ring C is derived from isopentenyl diphosphate (IPP) through the terpenoid biosynthetic pathway (Han et al., 2001).

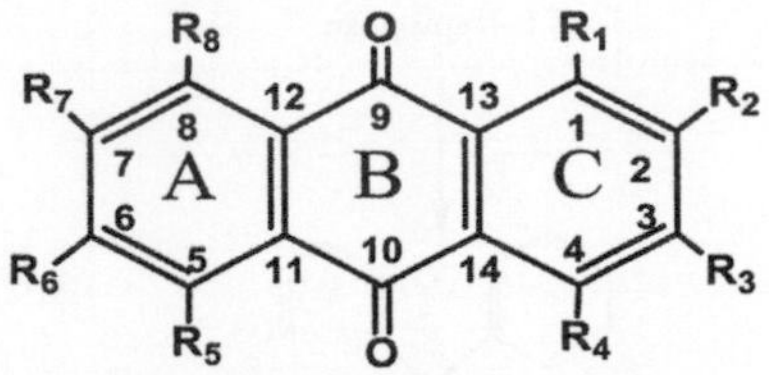

FIGURE 2.28   Basic structure of anthraquinones.

The two distinctive pathways for the biosynthesis of anthraquinones in higher plants are the polyketide and shikimic acid pathway. The polyketide pathway occurs in families of higher plants such as Leguminosae, Rhamnaceae, and Polygonaceae and in fungi (Simpson, 1987; Inouye and Leistner, 1988). The reaction involves a seven-malonyl-CoA units and one acetyl-CoA unit to form an octaketide acyl chain (Fig. 2.29). Carbon dioxide is released in the final reaction step. Anthraquinones synthesized from the polyketide pathway exhibit a characteristic substitution in both A and C rings. For example, the A and C rings in chrysophanol and emodin are typically substituted with hydroxyl groups. Enzymes of the polyketide pathway have been successfully studied and documented in bacteria mostly, with rare occurrences in higher plants (Bernard, 1999).

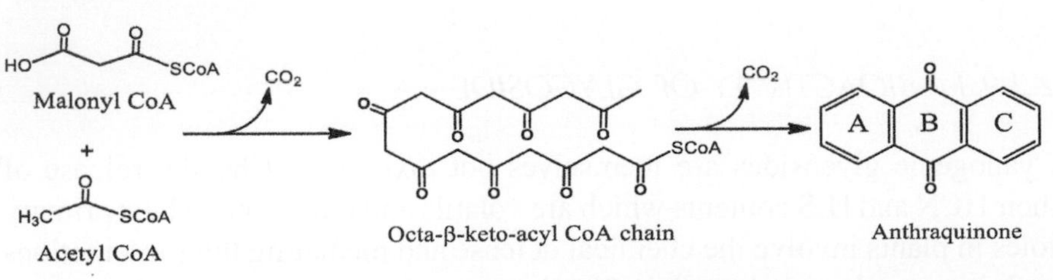

FIGURE 2.29   Polyketide pathway for anthraquinone biosynthesis.

The shikimic acid pathway for the synthesis of anthraquinones also incorporates metabolites from the mevalonic acid pathway (Fig. 2.30). Their A and B rings are derived from chorismic acid and α-ketoglutarate, while the C ring is from IPP (Leistner, 1981; Leistner, 1985) which is a key intermediate in terpenoid biosynthesis. This pathway is used to synthesize anthraquinone with substitutes such as hydroxyl or methyl groups in only one of the rings, while in the polyketide pathway, anthraquinones are synthesized with substitutes in both rings (Han et al., 2001).

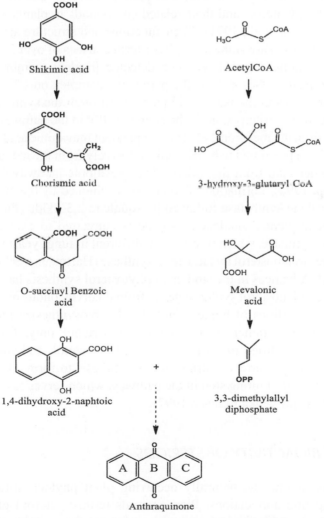

FIGURE 2.30 Shikimic acid pathway for anthraquinone biosynthesis.

2.2.10.1   BIOACTIVITY OF ANTHRAQUINONES

Anthraquinones are of importance to plants. The substituted anthraquinones such as hydroxymethyl anthraquinones protect plants against parasite invasion and protect their seeds from birds (Korulkin and Muzychkina, 2014).

2.2.11   BIOSYNTHESIS OF STEROIDS

Phytosterols are an important aspect of plant physiology and function with over 250 of such sterols and their related compounds in plants and marine materials (Akihisa et al., 1991). Their functions and structure are similar to human cholesterol. Biosynthesis of phytosterol consists of over 30 enzymes-catalyzed reactions, which have been detected in plant membranes (Nes, 1977; Benveniste, 1986) making the pathway a complex one. Their precursors are derived from the isoprenoid pathway through the synthesis of IPP, DMAP, and the C_{30} triterpenoids. The source of IPP in the pathway is argued to be either from the mevalonic acid or independent mevalonic acid pathways. They have been presumed to be derived exclusively from the mevalonic acid pathway rather than from the independent mevalonic pathway (McCaskill and Croteau, 1998). Formation of squalene is achieved by the action of the enzyme squalene synthetase followed by squalene-2,3-oxide (Fig. 2.31). In photosynthetic plants, squalene-2,3-oxide is converted to cycloartenol by cycloartenol synthase, which is, however, different in fungi/yeast where they are converted to lanosterol by lanosterol synthase (Hartmann, 1998; Ohyama et al., 2009). Advances in the studies of phytosterol synthesis have revealed the presence of lanosterol synthase genes from dicotyledonous plant species, indicating the abilities of higher plants to also biosynthesize phytosterols through lanosterol rather than through cycloartenol only. Cycloartenol can be further modified to form campesterol, sitosterol, and stigmasterol. Methylation of cycloartenol during the biosynthesis to form 24-methylene derivative is a rate-limiting step in the pathway, which serves to regulate the pathway (Nes and Venkatramesh, 1997).

2.2.11.1   BIOACTIVITY OF STERIODS

Steriods are among the naturally occurring plant phytoconstituents with great therapeutic applications. Plant steroids termed "steroid glycosides" or "cardiac glycosides" are found to be of great therapeutic applications

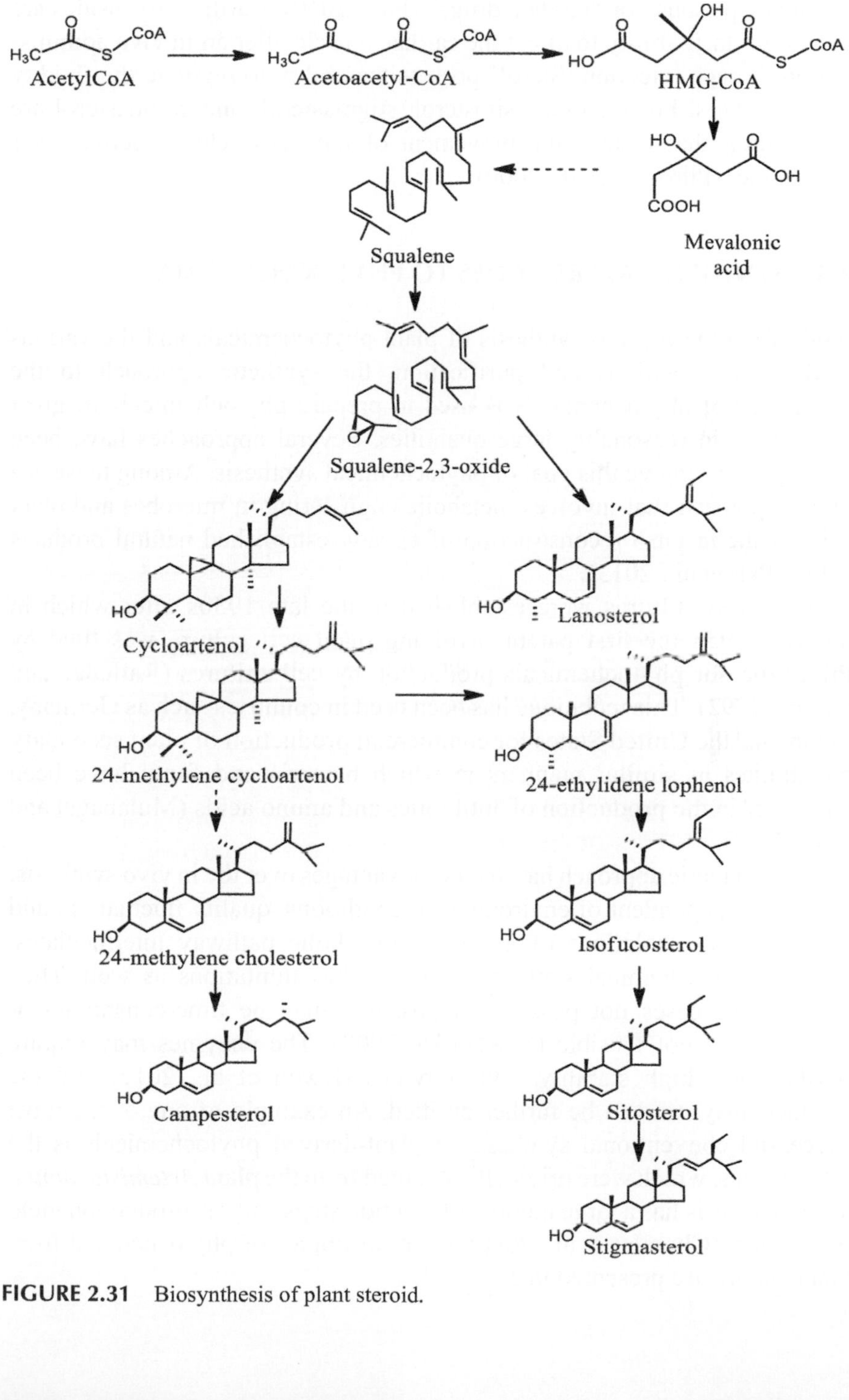

FIGURE 2.31 Biosynthesis of plant steroid.

as "arrow poisons" or "cardiac drugs" (Firn, 2010). Cardiac glycosides are known for their ability to affect the cardiac muscle after an in vivo administration through injection. Sterols possess the ability to regulate the fluidity of membranes. For example, sitosterol, stigmasterol, and campesterol are phytosterols that restrict the movement of fatty acyl chains across their membranes (Piironen et al., 2000).

2.3   SYNTHETIC APPROACHES TO PHYTOCHEMICALS

Aside from the in vivo synthesis of plant phytochemicals and the various methods of isolations and purification, the synthetic approach to the production of phytochemicals is used to prepare phytochemicals of great importance in reasonably large quantities. Several approaches have been employed to achieve this goal of phytochemical synthesis. Among these is a recent approach that involves metabolic engineering in microbes and plant cells or the in vitro reconstruction of already established natural products (Mora-Pale et al., 2013).

Plant cell cultures were established in the late 1930s after which in the year 1956 the first patent involving plant cell culture was filed by Pfizer Inc. for phytochemicals production by cell cultures (Ratledge and Sasson, 1992). This technique has been used in countries such as Germany, Japan, and the United States for commercial production of plant secondary metabolites in similar manners in which bacteria and fungi have been employed in the production of antibiotics and amino acids (Mulabagal and Tsay, 2004).

The synthetic approach has distinct advantages over the in vivo synthesis. They are independent of environmental conditions, quality fluctuation, and allows for the isolations of important metabolic pathway intermediates. However, the chemical synthesis approach has limitations as well. They are in some cases not possible, if possible, may be time-consuming or economically not feasible (Smetanska, 2008). The enzymes may require purifications, high stability, and activities (Kwon et al., 2012) and the products may need to be further purified. An example of one of the most successful conventional synthesis of plant-derived phytochemicals is the artemisinins, which were originally obtained from the plant *Artemisia annua*. Their synthesis has a large number of reaction steps and the production yield is very low (Chemler et al., 2006). Other examples of phytochemical from plant culture are presented in Table 2.1.

TABLE 2.1   Examples of Plant-Culture-Derived Phytochemicals.

Phytochemical	Plant source	References
Shikonin	*Lithospermum erythrorhizon*	Matsubara et al. (1989); Kim and Chang (1990)
Berberine	*Coptis japonica*	Fujita and Tabata (1987), Matsubara et al. (1989)
Sanguinarine	*Papaver somniferum*	Dicosmo and Misawa (1995)
Visnagin	*Chenopodium rubrum*	Berlin et al. (1986)
Diosgenin	*C. rubrum*	Berlin et al. (1986)
Ajmalicine	*Catharanthus roseus*	Lee and Shuler (2000)
Anthraquinones	*Morinda citrifolia*	Zenk (1977)
Caffeic acid	*Vanilla planifolia*	Knorr et al. (1993)
Ginsenoside	*Panax ginseng*	Matsubara et al. (1989)
Nicotine	*Nicotiana tabacum*	Mantell et al. (1983)
Rosmarinic acid	*Coleus blumei*	Petersen and Simmond (2003)
Ubiquinone-10	*N. tabacum*	Fujita and Tabata (1987)

2.4 CONCLUSION

The literature in the present work provides the necessary reaction steps in the biosynthesis of phytochemicals. The various contributing pathways to these syntheses were also reviewed up to the important phytochemicals obtained from each of them. Some biosynthetic pathways are complex and are catalyzed by several enzymes. These pathways were summarized for better presentation and understanding. These pathways have been studied, in some cases, to provide alternative means of obtaining phytochemicals in larger quantities with the aim to apply them in bioengineering, pharmaceutics, and nutraceuticals as well as in other fields.

KEYWORDS

- **phytochemicals**
- **biosynthesis**
- **bioactivities**
- **pathways**
- **enzymes**

REFERENCES

Akerley, B. J.; Rubin, E. J.; Novick, V. L.; Amaya, K.; Judson, N.; Mekalanos, J. J. A Genome-Scale Analysis for Identification of Genes Required for Growth Or Survival of *Haemophilus influenza*. *Proc. Natl. Acad. Sci. USA* **2002**, *99*, 966–971.

Akihisa, T.; Kokke, W.; Tamura, T. Naturally Occurring Sterols and Related Compounds from Plants. In *Physiology and Biochemistry of Sterols;* Patterson, G. W., Nes, W. D. Eds; American Oil Chemists' Society: Champaign, IL, 1991; pp 172–228.

Allen, R. S.; James, M. A. C.; Julie, C. A.; Anthony, F. J. Wayne, G. L.; Philip, L. J. Metabolic Engineering of Morphinan Alkaloids by Overexpression and RNAi Suppression of Salutaridinol 7-Oacetyltransferase in Opium Poppy. *Plant. Biotechnol. J.* **2008**, *6*, 22–30.

American Cancer Society (ACS) Phytochemicals. http://www.cancer.org/eprise/main/docroot/ETO/content/ETO_5_3X_Phytochemicals, 2000 (accessed Oct 13, 2017).

Arts, I. C.; Hollman, P. C. Polyphenols and Disease Risk in Epidemiologic Studies. *Am. J. Clin. Nutr.* **2005**, *81*(1), 317S–325S.

Ashihara, H.; Monteiro, A. M.; Gillies, M. F.; Crozier, A. Biosynthesis of Caffeine in Leaves of Coffee. *Plant Physiol.* **1996**, *111*, 747–753.

Ashihara, H.; Sano H.; Crozier, A. Caffeine and Related Purine Alkaloids: Biosynthesis, Catabolism, Function and Genetic Engineering. *Phytochemistry* **2008**, *69*, 841–856.

Ashihara, H.; Suzuki, T. Distribution and Biosynthesis of Caffeine in Plants. *Front Biosci.* **2004**, *9*, 1864–1876.

Bedekar, A.; Shah, K.; Koffas, M. Natural Products for Type II Diabetes Treatment. *Adv. Appl. Microbiol.* **2010**, *71*, 21–73.

Benveniste, P. Sterol Biosynthesis. *Ann. Rev. Plant Physiol.* **1986**, *37*, 275–308.

Berlin, J.; Sieg, S.; Strack, D.; Bokern, M.; Harns, H. Production of Betalains by Suspension Cultures of *Chenopodium rubrum* L. *Plant Cell, Tissue Organ Cult.* **1986**, *5*, 163–174.

Bernard, J. R. Biosynthesis of Polyketides (Other Than Actinomycete Macrolides). *Nat. Prod. Rep.* **1999**, *16*, 425–484.

Chang, M. C. Y.; Eachus, R. A.; Trieu, W.; Ro, D. K.; Keasling, J. D. Engineering Escherichia Coli for Production of Functionalized Terpenoids Using Plant P450s. *Nat. Chem. Biol.* **2007**, *3*, 274–277.

Chemler, J. A.; Lock, L. T.; Koffas, M. A. G.; Tzanakakis, E. S. Standardized Biosynthesis of flavan-3-Ols with Effects on Pancreatic Beta-Cell Insulin Secretion. *Appl. Microbiol. Biotechnol.* **2007**, *77*, 797–807.

Chemler, J. A.; Yan, Y. J.; Koffas, M. A. G. Biosynthesis of Isoprenoids, Polyunsaturated Fatty Acids and Favonoids in *Saccharomyces cerevisiae*. *Microb. Cell Fact.* **2006**, *5*, 5.

Compean, K. L.; Ynalvez, R. A. Antimicrobial Activity of Plant Secondary Metabolites: a Review. *Res. J. Med. Plants* **2014**, 1–10.

Contin, A.; van der Heijden, R.; Lefeber, A. W. M.; Verpoorte, R. The Iridoid Glucoside Secologanin is Derived from the Novel Triose Phosphate/Pyruvate Pathway in a *Catharanthus roseus* Cell Culture. *FEBS Lett.* **1998**, *434*, 413–416.

Dai, J.; Mumper, R. Plant Phenolics: Extraction, Analysis and Their Antioxidant and Anticancer Properties. *Molecules* **2010**, *15*, 7313–7352.

De Groot, H.; Rauen, U. Tissue Injury by Reactive Oxygen Species and the Protective Effects of Flavonoids. *Fundam. Clin. Pharmacol.* **1998**, *12*, 249–255.

Degenhardt, J.; Gershenzon, J.; Baldwin, I. T.; Kessler, A. Attracting Friends to Feast on Foes: Engineering Terpene Emission to Make Crop Plants More Attractive to Herbivore Enemies. Current Opinion. *Biotechnology* **2003**, *14*, 169–176.

Delmas, D.; Lançon, A.; Colin, D.; Jannin, B.; Latruffe, N. Resveratrol as a Chemopreventive Agent: a Promising Molecule for Fighting Cancer. *Curr. Drug. Targets* **2006**, *7*, 423–442.

Dewick, P. M. *Medicinal Natural Products, A Biosynthetic Approach*. John Wiley and Sons, Ltd: Chichester, UK, 2002.

Dicosmo, F.; Misawa, M. Plant Cell and Tissue Culture: Alternatives for Metabolite Production. *Biotechnol. Adv.* **1995**, *13*, 425–435.

Fauré, M.; Lissi, E.; Torres, R.; Videla, L. A. Antioxidant Activities of Lignans and Flavonoids. *Phytochemistry*. **1990**, *29*(12), 3773–3775.

Firn, R. *Nature's Chemicals*, Oxford University Press: Oxford, 2010; pp 74–75.

Fujita, Y.; Tabata, M. Secondary Metabolites from Plant Cells: Pharmaceutical Applications and Progress in Commercial Production. In *Plant Tissue and Cell Culture;* Green, C. E., Somers, D. A., Hackett, W. P., Biesboer, D. D. Eds.; Alan R. Liss: New York, 1987; pp 169–185.

Ghasemzadeh, A.; Jaafar, H. Z. E.; Rahmat, A. Antioxidant Activities, Total Phenolics and Flavonoids Content in Two Varieties of Malaysia Young Ginger (*Zingiber officinale* Roscoe). *Molecules* **2010**, *15*, 4324–4333.

Ghosh, D.; Konishi, T. Anthocyanins and Anthocyanin-Rich Extracts: Role in Diabetes and Eye Function. *Asia. Pac. J. Clin. Nutr.* **2007**, *16*(2), 200–208.

Goulinet, S.; Chapman, M. J. Plasma LDL and HDL Subspecies are Heterogeneous in Particle Content of Tocopherols and Oxygenated and Hydrocarbon Carotenoids Relevance to Oxidative Resistance and Atherogenesis. *Arterioscler. Thromb. Vasc. Biol.* **1997**, *17*, 786–796.

Gyamfi, M. A.; Aniya, Y. Antioxidant Properties of Thonningianin A, Isolated from the African Medicinal Herb, *Thonningia sanguinea. Biochem. Pharmacol.* **2002**, *63*, 1725–1737.

Hahlbrock, H.; Grisebach, H. Biosynthesis of Flavonoids. In *The Flavonoids*; Harborne, J. B.; Mabry, T. J.; Mabry, H., Eds; Academic Press: San Diego, **1975**; pp 866–915.

Hahlbrock, K. In *The Biochemistry of Plants*, Stumpf, P. K.; Conn, E. E., Eds; Academic Press: NY, 1981; Vol. 7, pp 425–456.

Han, Y. S.; der Heiden, R. V.; Verpoorte, R. Biosynthesis of Anthraquinones in Cell Cultures of the Rubiaceae. *Plant Cell Tissue Organ Cult.* **2001**, *67*, 201–220.

Harborne, J. B.; Mabry, T. J.; Mabry, H. Eds. *The Flavonoids*. Chapman and Hall: London, 1975.

Hartmann, M. A. Plant Sterols and the Membrane Environment. *Plant Cell Tissue Organ Cult.* **1998**, *3*, 170–175.

Haworth, R. D. Natural Resins. *Ann. Rep. Prog. Chem.* **1936**, *33*, 266–279.

He, J.; Giusti, M. M. Anthocyanins: Natural Colorants with Health Promoting Properties. *Annu. Rev. Food Sci. Technol.* **2010**, *1*, 163–187.

Heldt, H.; Piechulla, B.; Heldt, F. Plant Biochemistry, 4th ed.; United Kingdom: London, 2011; pp 172–184.

Heneman, K.; Zidenberg-cherr, S Some Facts about Phytochemicals. UC Cooperative Extension Center for Health and Nutrition Research Nutrition and Health Info Sheet, 2008.

Hoeffler, J. F.; Tritsch, D.; Grosdemange-Billiard, C.; Rohmer, M. Isoprenoid Biosynthesis Via the Methylerythritol Phosphate Pathway. *Eur. J. Biochem.* **2002**, *269*, 4446–4457.

Hunter, W., N. The Non-Mevalonate Pathway of Isoprenoid Precursor Biosynthesis. *J. Biol. Chem.* **2007**, *282*(30), 21573–21577.

Inouye, H.; Leistner, E. Biosynthesis of Quinones. In *The Chemistry of Quinonoid Compounds*; Patai, S., Rappoport, Z., Eds; John Wiley and Sons Ltd.: New York, 1988, Vol. 2, 1293–1349.

Jing, P.; Bomser, J. A.; Schwartz, S. J.; He, J.; Magnuson, B. A.; Giusti, M. M. Structure-Function Relationships of Anthocyanins from Various Anthocyanin-Rich Extracts on the Inhibition of Colon Cancer Cell Growth. *J. Agric. Food Chem.* **2008**, *56*(20), 9391–9398.

Kar, A. Pharmacognosy and Pharmacobiotechnology (Revised-Expanded Second Edition). New Age International Limited Publishers: New Delhi; **2007**, pp 332–600.

Kato, M.; Mizuno, K.; Crozier, A.; Fujimura, T.; Ashihara, H Caffeine Synthase Gene from Tea Leaves. *Nature* **2000**, *406*, 956–957.

Kato, M.; Mizuno, K.; Fujimura, T.; Iwama, M.; Irie, M.; Crozier, A.; Ashihara, H Purification and Characterization of Caffeine Synthase from Tea Leaves. *Plant Physiol.* **1999**, *120*, 579–586.

Kim, D. J.; Chang, H. N. Enhanced Shikonin Production from *Lithospermum erythrorhizon* by in Situ Extraction and Calcium Alginate Immobilization. *Biotechnol. Bioeng.* **1990**, *36*(5), 460–466.

Knorr, D.; Caster, C.; Dörnenburg, H.; Dorn, R.; Gräf, S.; Havkin-Frenkel, D.; Podstolski, A.; Werrmann, U. Biosynthesis and Yield Improvement of Food Ingredients from Plant Cell and Tissue Culture. *Food Technol.* **1993**, *47*(12), 57–63.

Kobayashi, K.; Ehrlich, S. D.; Albertini, A.; Amati, G.; Andersen, K. K.; Arnaud, M.; Asai, K. et al. Essential *Bacillus subtilis* Genes. *Proc. Natl. Acad. U S A.* **2003**, *100*(8), 4678–4683.

Korulkin, Y. D.; Muzychkina, A. R. Biosynthesis and Metabolism of Anthraquinone Derivatives. *Int. Scholarly Sci. Res. Innovation* **2014**, *8*(7), 454–457.

Kutchan, T. M. Alkaloid Biosynthesis: The Basis for Metabolic Engineering of Medicinal Plants. *Plant Cell* **1995**, *7*, 1059–1070.

Kwon, S. J.; Mora-Pale, M.; Lee, M. Y.; Dordick, J. S. Expanding Nature's Small Molecule Diversity Via in Vitro Biosynthetic Pathway Engineering. *Curr. Opin. Chem. Biol.* **2012**, *16*, 186–195.

Langenheim, J. H. Higher Plant Terpenoids: a Phytocentric Overview of Their Ecological Roles. *J. Chem. Ecol.* **1994**, *20*, 1223–1280.

Laxminarain, M. Traditional Phytomedicinal Systems, Scientific Validations and Current Popularity as Nutraceuticals. *Int. J. Tradit. Nat. Med.* **2013**, *2*(1), 27–75.

Lee, C. W. T.; Shuler, M. L. The Effect of Inoculum Density and Conditioned Medium on the Production of Ajmalcine and Catharanthine from Immobilized *Catharanthus roseus* Cells. *Biotechnol. Bioeng.* **2000**, *67*, 61–71.

Leete, E. Biogenesis of the Rauwolfia Alkaloids Alkaloids—II : the Incorporation of Tryptophan Into Serpentine and Reserpine. *Tetrahedron* **1961**, *14*, 35–41.

Leistner, E. Biosynthesis of Chorismate-Derived Quinones in Plant Cell Cultures. In *Primary and Secondary Metabolism of Plant Cell Cultures*; Neumann, K. H., Barz, W., Reinhard, E., Eds.; Springer-Verlag: Berlin, New York, **1985**; pp 215–224.

Leistner, E. Biosynthesis of Plant Quinones. In *The Biochemistry of Plants*; Conn, E. E, Ed.; Academic Press: London, 1981; Vol. 7, pp 403–423.

Lepiniec, L.; Debeaujon, I.; Routaboul, J. M.; Baudry, A.; Pourcel, L.; Nesi, N.; Caboche, M. Genetics and Biochemistry of Seed Flavonoids. *Annu. Rev. Plant Biol.* **2006**, *57*, 405–430.

Mantell, S. H.; Pearson, D. W.; Hazell, L. P.; Smith, H. The Effect of Initial Phosphate and Sucrose Levels on Nicotine Accumulation in Batch Suspension Cultures of *Nicotiana tabacum* L. *Plant Cell Rep.* **1983**, *2*, 73–83.

Martens, S.; Teeri, T.; Forkmann, G. Heterologous Expression of Dihydroflavonol 4-Reductases from Various Plants. *FEBS Lett.* **2002**, *531*, 453–458.

Mathai, K. Nutrition in the Adult Years. In *Krause's Food, Nutrition, and Diet Therapy*; Mahan, L. K., Escott-Stump, S. Eds., 10th Edn.; 2000; pp, 274–275.

Matsubara, K.; Shigekazu, K.; Yoshioka, T.; Fujita, Y.; Yamada, Y. High Density Culture of Coptis Japonica Cells Increases Berberine Production. *J. Chem. Technol. Biotechnol.* **1989**, *46*, 61–69.

Mazid, M.; Khan, T. A.; Mohammad, F. Role of Secondary Metabolites in Defense Mechanisms of Plants. *Biol. Med.* **2011**, *3*(2), 232–249.

McCaskill, D.; Croteau, R. Some Caveats for Bioengineering Terpenoid Metabolism in Plants. *Trends Biotechnol.* **1998**, *16*, 349–355.

Meng, H.; Wang, Y.; Hua, Q.; Zhang, S.; Wang, X. In Silico Analysis and Experimental Improvement of Taxadiene Heterologous Biosynthesis in Escherichia Coli. *Biotechnol. Bioprocess Eng.* **2011**, *16*, 205–215.

Mizuno, K.; Kato, M.; Irino, F.; Yoneyama, N.; Fujimura, T.; Ashihara, H. The First Committed Step Reaction of Caffeine Biosynthesis: 7-Methylxanthosine Synthase is Closely Homologous to Caffeine Synthases in Coffee (*Coffea arabica* L.). *FEBS Lett.* **2003**, *547*, 56–60.

Mora-Pale, M.; Sanchez-Rodriguez, S. P.; Linhardt, R. J.; Dordick, J. S.; Koffas, M. A. G. Metabolic Engineering and in Vitro Biosynthesis of Phytochemicals and Non-Natural Analogues. *Plant Sci.* **2013**, *210*, 10–24.

Mueller-Harvey, I.; McAllan, A. B. T. Their Biochemistry and Nutritional Properties. In *Advances in Plant Cell Biochemistry and Biotechnology*; Morrison, I. M. Ed.; JAI Press Ltd.: London, UK, 1992, Vol. 1, pp 151–217.

Mulabagal, V.; Tsay, H. Plant Cell Cultures as a Source for the Production of Biologically Important Secondary Metabolites. *Int. J. Appl. Sci. Eng.* **2004**, *2*, 29–48.

Negi, A. S.; Kumar, J. K.; Luqman, S.; Shanker, K.; Gupta, M. M.; Khanuja, S. P. Recent Advances in Plant Hepatoprotectives: a Chemical and Biological Profile of Some Important Leads. *Med. Res. Rev.* **2008**, *28*(5), 746–772.

Nes, W. D. The Biochemistry of Plant Sterols. *Adv. Lipid Res.* **1977**, *15*, 233–324.

Nes, W. D.; Venkatramesh, M. Enzymology of Phytosterol Transformations, in Biochemistry and Function of Sterols; Parish, E. J., Nes, W. D., Eds.; CRC Press: Boca Raton, FL, **1997**; pp 111–122.

O'Connor, E. S.; Maresh, J. J. Chemistry and Biology of Monoterpene Indole Alkaloid Biosynthesis. *Nat. Prod. Rep.* **2006**, *23*, 532–547.

Ohyama, K.; Suzuki, M.; Kikuchi, J.; Saito, K.; Muranaka, T. Dual Biosynthetic Pathways to Phytosterol Via Cycloartenol and Lanosterol in Arabidopsis. *PNAS.* **2009**, *106*(3), 725–730.

Pan, J. Y.; Chen, S. L.; Yang, M. H.; Wu, J.; Sinkkonen, J.; Zou, K. An Update on Lignans: Natural Products and Synthesis. *Nat. Prod. Rep.* **2009**, *26*(10), 1460–4752.

Pandey, A. K.; Kumar, S. Perspective on Plant Products as Antimicrobials Agents: a Review. *Pharmacologia.* **2013**, *4*(7), 469–480.

Pascual-Teresa, D. S.; Moreno, D. A.; Garcia-Viguera, C. Flavanols and Anthocyanins in Cardiovascular Health: a Review of Current Evidence. *Int. J. Mol. Sci.* **2010**, *11*(4), 1679–1703.

Pearce, G.; Strydom, D.; Johnson, S.; Ryan, C. A. A Polypeptide from Tomato Leaves Induces Wound Inducible Proteinase Inhibitor Proteins. *Science* **1991**, *253*, 895–898.

Petersen, M.; Simmonds, M. S. Rosmarinic Acid. *Phytochemistry* **2003**, *62*(2), 121–125.

Piironen, V.; Lindsay, G. D.; Miettinen, A. T.; Toivo, J.; Lampi, A. Plant Sterols: Biosynthesis, Biological Function and Their Importance to Human Nutrition. *J. Sci. Food Agric.* **2000**, *80*, 939–966.

Pretorius, J. C. Flavonoids: a Review of Its Commercial Application Potential as Anti-Infective Agents. *Curr. Med. Chem. Anti-Infective Agents* **2003**, *2*, 335–353.

Pridham, J. B. In *Phenolics in Plants in Health and Disease*; Pergamon Press: New York, **1960**; pp 34–35.

Rahimi, R.; Ghiasi, S.; Azimi, H.; Fakhari, S.; Abdollahi, M. A Review of the Herbal Phosphodiesterase Inhibitors. Future Perspective of New Drugs. Cytokine. **2009**, *49*(2), 123–129.

Rao, R. V. K.; Ali, N.; Reddy, M. N. Occurrence of Both Sapogenins and Alkaloid Lycorine in *Curculigo orchioides*. *Indian J. Pharma. Sci.* **1978**, *40*, 104–105.

Ratledge, C.; Sasson, A. *Production of Useful Biochemical by Higher-Plant Cell Cultures: Biotechnological and Economic Aspects*; Cambridge University Press: Cambridge, **1992**, p 402.

Rohmer, M. The Discovery of a MevalonateIndependent Pathway for Isoprenoid Biosynthesis in Bacteria, Algae and Higher Plants. *Nat. Prod. Rep.* **1999**, *16*(5), 565–574.

Saleem, M.; Kim, H. J.; Ali, M. S.; Lee, Y. S. An Update on Bioactive Plant Lignans. *Nat. Prod. Rep.* **2005**, *22*(6), 696–716.

Sassetti, C. M.; Boyd, D. H.; Rubin, E. J. Comprehensive Identification of Conditionally Essential Genes in Mycobacteria. *Proc. Natl. Acad. Sci. U S A* **2001**, *98*, 12712–12717.

Sawai, S.; Saito, K. Triterpenoid Biosynthesis and Engineering in Plants. *Front. Plant Sci.* **2011**, *2*, 25.

Schofield, P.; Mbugua, D. M.; Pell, A. N. Analysis of Condensed Tannins: a Review. *Anim. Feed Sci. Technol.* **2001**, *91*, 21–40.

Shaker, E.; Mahmoud, H.; Mnaa, S Silymarin, the Antioxidant Component and *Silybum marianum* Extracts Prevents Liver Damage. *Food Chem. Toxicol.* **2010**, *48*, 803–806.

Shirley, B. W.; Kubasek, W. L.; Storz, G.; Bruggemann, E.; Koornneef, M.; Ausubel, F. M.; Goodman, H. M. Analysis of Arabidopsis Mutants Deficient in Flavonoid Biosynthesis. *Plant J.* **1995**, *8*(5), 659–671.

Silva, E. M.; Souza, J. N. S.; Rogez, H.; Rees, J. F.; Larondelle, Y. Antioxidant Activities and Polyphenolic Contents of Fifteen Selected Plant Species from the Amazonian Region. *Food Chem.* **2007**, *101*, 1012–1018.

Simpson, T. J. The Biosynthesis of Polyketides. *Nat. Prod. Rep.* **1987**, *4*, 339–376.

Smetanska, I. Production of Secondary Metabolites Using Plant Cell Cultures. *Adv. Biochem. Engin/Biotechnol.* **2008**, *111*, 187–228.

Southon, I. W., Buckingham, J., Eds. *Dictionary of Alkaloids*. Chapman and Hall Ltd.: London, 1989.

Stepp, J. R.; Moerman, D. E. The Importance of Weeds in Ethnopharmacology. *J. Ethnopharmacol.* **2001**, *75*, 19–23.

Stöckigt, J.; Zenk, Y. H. Strictosidine (Isovincoside): the Key Intermediate in the Biosynthesis of Monoterpenoid Indole Alkaloids. *J. Chem. SOC Chem. Commun.* **1977**, 912–914.

Suzuki, T.; Ashihara, H.; Waller, G. R. Purine and Purine Alkaloid Metabolism in Camellia and Coffea Plants. *Phytochemistry* **1992**, *31*, 2575–2584.

Taiz, L.; Zeiger, E. *Plant Physiology Edition*; Panima Publishing Corporation: New Delhi, Bangalore, 1995.

Tanner, G. J.; Francki, K. T.; Abrahams, S.; Watson, J. M.; Larkin, P. J.; Ashton, A. R. Proanthocyanidin Biosynthesis in Plants Purification of Legume Leucoanthocyanidin Reductase and Molecular Cloning of Its cDNA. *J. Biol. Chem.* **2003**, *278*, 31647–31656.

Tapas, A. R.; Sakarkar, D. M.; Kakde, R. B. Flavonoids as Nutraceuticals: a Review. *Trop. J. Pharm. Res.* **2008**, *7*, 1089–1099.

Tava, A.; Scotti, C.; Avato, P. Biosynthesis of Saponins in the Genus *Medicago. Phytochem. Rev.* **2011**, *10*(4), 459–469.

Tijjani, H.; Mohammed, A.; Idris, Z. L.; Adegunloye, P. A.; Luka, C. D.; Alhassan, A. J. Current Status of Antidiabetic Plants in the Lamiaceae Family; Omniscriptum GmbH and Co. KG: Germany, 2017.

Toufektsian, M. C.; De Lorgeril, M.; Nagy, N.; Salen, P.; Donati, M. B.; Giordano, L.; Mock, H. P.; Peterek, S.; Matros, A.; Petroni, K.; Pilu, R.; Rotilio, D.; Tonelli, C.; de Leiris, J.; Boucher, F.; Martin, C Chronic Dietary Intake of Plant-Derived Anthocyanins Protects the Rat Heart Against Ischemia-Reperfusion Injury. *J. Nutr.* **2008**, *138*(4), 747–752.

Uefuji, H.; Ogita, S.; Yamaguchi, Y.; Koizumi, N.; Sano, H. Molecular Cloning and Functional Characterization of Three Distinct N-Methyltransferases Involved in the Caffeine Biosynthetic Pathway in Coffee Plants. *Plant Physiol.* **2003**, *132*, 372–380.

Umezawa, T. Diversity in Lignan Biosynthesis. *Phytochem. Rev.* **2003**, *2*(3), 371–390.

Uttara, B.; Singh, A. V.; Zamboni, P.; Mahajan, R. T. Oxidative Stress and Neurodegenerative Diseases: a Review of Upstream and Downstream Antioxidant Therapeutic Options. *Curr. Neuropharmacol.* **2009**, *7*, 65.

Vansoest, P. J. *Nutritional Ecology of the Ruminant*, 2nd ed.; Cornell University Press: Ithaca, NY, 1994, p 476.

Vincken, J. P.; Heng, L.; de Groot, A.; Gruppen, H. Saponins, Classification and Occurrence in the Plant Kingdom. *Phytochemistry* **2007**, *68*(3), 275–297.

Waller, R. G.; Nowacki, K. E. *Alkaloid Biology and Metabolism in Plants: Alkaloids in Chemotaxonomic Relationships*; Plenum Press. New York and London, 1978, p 294.

Walton, N. J.; Mayer, M. J.; Narbad, A. Molecules of Interest: Vanillin. *Phytochemistry* **2003**, *63*, 505–515.

Winkel-Shirley, B. Flavonoid Biosynthesis. a Colorful Model for Genetics, Biochemistry, Cell Biology and Biotechnology. *Plant Physiol.* **2001**, *126*, 485–493.

Wong, E. Biosynthesis of Flavonoids. In *Chemistry and biochemistry of plant pigments*; Goodwin, T. W. Ed.; Academic Press: NY, London, 1976; Vol. 1, pp 464–526.

Yamazaki, Y.; Kitajima, M.; Arita, M.; Takayama, H.; Sudo, H.; Yamazaki, M.; Aimi, N.; Saito, K. Biosynthesis of Camptothecin. in Silico and in Vivo Tracer Study from [1–13C] Glucose. *Plant Physiol.* **2004**, *134*, 161–170.

Yendo, C. A. A.; de Costa, F.; Da Costa, T. C.; Colling, C. L.; Gosmann, G.; Fett-Neto, G. A. Biosynthesis of Plant Triterpenoid Saponins: Genes, Enzymes and Their Regulation. *Mini-Rev. Org. Chem.* **2014**, *11*, 292–306.

Zagrobelny, M.; Bak, S.; Rasmussen, A. V.; Jorgensen, B.; Naumann, C. M.; Lindberg Moller, B. L. Cyanogenic Glucosides and Plant-Insect Interactions. *Phytochemistry* **2004**, *65*, 293–306.

Zenk, M. H. Plant Tissue Culture and its Biotechnological Application. Springer: Berlin, Heidelberg, 1977, p 27.

Zhang, Y. J.; Gan, R. Y.; Li, S.; Zhou, Y.; Li, A. N.; Xu, D. P.; Li, H. B. Antioxidant Phytochemicals for the Prevention and Treatment of Chronic Diseases. *Molecules* **2015**, 27–20(12), 21138–21156.

Zhou, Y. J.; Gao, W.; Rong, Q.; Jin, G.; Chu, H.; Liu, W.; Yang, W.; Zhu, Z.; Li, G.; Zhu, G.; Huang, L.; Zhao, Z. K. Modular Pathway Engineering of Diterpenoid Synthases and the Mevalonic Acid Pathway for Miltiradiene Production. *J. Am. Chem. Soc.* **2012**, *134*, 3234–3241.

Zulak, K. G.; Liscome, D. K.; Ashihara, H.; Facchini, P. J. Alkaloids. In *Plant Secondary Metabolites: Occurrence Structure and Role in the Human Diet*; Crozier, A., Clifford, M. N., Ashihara, H. Eds.; Blackwell: Oxford, 2006, pp 102–136.

Zurbriggen, A.; Kirst, H.; Melis, A Isoprene Production Via the Mevalonic Acid Pathway in *Escherichia coli* (Bacteria). *Bioenergy Res.* **2012**, *5*, 814–828.

CHAPTER 3

MECHANISMS OF PLANT DEFENSE AGAINST PATHOGENS: PHYTOALEXINS INDUCTION

HANAN M. AL-YOUSEF[1,*] and MUSARAT AMINA[1]

[1]Department of Pharmacognosy, College of Pharmacy, King Saud University, Riyadh, Saudi Arabia, Tel.: 966555287629

*Corresponding author. E-mail: halyousef@ksu.edu.sa
ORCID: https://orcid.org/0000-0002-2607-0918

ABSTRACT

Crops are usually attacked by many pathogens and they respond by the activation and production of defense genes, the formation of ROS, the synthesis of pathogenesis-related proteins, localized cell wall enforcement and the induction of antimicrobial compounds. Plants use innate defense mechanisms toward pathogens, including the induction of substances that have antimicrobial activity which are known as phytoalexins (PhA). PhA production is now considered as an important defense mechanism toward microbial infection through a broad spectrum of various secondary metabolites induced. Molecular approaches are helping to resolve some mechanisms and the complexity of these bioactive PhA compounds. This chapter focuses on the biosynthesis and regulation of various PhA compounds and its role in plant defense. Moreover, this chapter also discusses some of the PhA induced by plants from different families. This includes the very recently identified kauralexins and zealexins induced by maize, and the biosynthesis and regulation of PhA induced by rice.

3.1   INTRODUCTION

Terrestrial plants produce antimicrobial compounds which are called phyto-alexins (PhA) following invasion by different microbial infections. They possess an inhibitory activity against bacteria, fungi, nematodes, insects and can be toxic to the animals and to the plant itself (Braga, 1991). PhA described as "stress compounds" are stimulated by different kind of factors capable of causing damage or poison to plant tissues, such as ultraviolet (UV) light (Bridge et al., 1973), exposure to heat or cold (Rahe et al., 1975), heavy metals (Rathmell et al., 1971), fungicides (Oku et al., 1973), and antibiotics (Cruickshank et al., 1974). The synthesis of PhA in response to pathogen invasion could be influenced by so many factors such as temperature, humidity, and water availability. Several parts of the plant could produce PhA such as leaves, flowers, stems, seeds, and root tubers (Mikkelsen et al., 2003). The majority of PhA are lipophilic constituents that have an ability to pass through plasma membrane (PM) and enter the cell. Smith (1996) has reported that PhA toxicity occurs in the plant as a function of their acidic character due to the presence of hydroxyl group. The pivotal role of PhA in plant disease resistance has been described earlier (Hans and Jurgen, 1978; Hain et al., 1992).

3.2   PHYTOALEXIN (PhA) CONCEPT

The PhA concept started from ancient years from the findings that *Solanum tuberosum* (a tuber tissue of potato) had previously been infected with an incompatible race of *Phytophthora infestans* which promoted resistance to a compatible race of *P. infestans* (Muller and Borger, 1940). It was presumed that the tuber tissue of potato in response to the incompatible interaction-induced compounds that prevented the pathogen and protected the tissue against infectious attack by other compatible races of the pathogen (Muller and Borger, 1940; Coleman et al., 2011; Pedras et al., 2011). Later studies have evolved not only to investigate the roles of PhA in defense against pathogens, but also to their health improving effects (Boue et al., 2009; Holland and O'keefe, 2010; Ng et al., 2011; Smoliga et al., 2011; Jahangir et al., 2009; Yang et al., 2009). For example, indole PhA from *Brassica* vegetables possesses an antioxidant, anticarcinogenic, and cardiovascular protective activities (Jahangir et al., 2009; Pedras et al., 2011). A peanut *Arachis hypogaea* PhA have antidiabetic, anticancer, and vasodilator effects (Holland and O'keefe, 2010). The glyceollin PhA from soybean (*Glycine max*) has many biological activities such as antiproliferative and antitumor actions (Ng et al., 2011). The sorghum PhA, (*Sorghum bicolor*), 3-deoxy-anthocyanins, may have a potential effect against gastrointestinal cancer (Yang et al., 2009). Resveratrol PhA from the grapevine, *Vitis vinifera*, has anti-aging, anticancer, anti-inflammatory, and antioxidant properties that may promote the longevity of life (Smoliga et al., 2011).

Plant pathogens have evolved various strategies for getting nutritious materials from plants and then preformed chemical and physical barriers such as the immune system to fight the pathogen invasion. Antimicrobial substances from plants are classified into two broad categories: phytoantipicins (PhT) and PhA (Mansfield, 1999). PhT is defined as "low molecular weight, antimicrobial substances that are found in plants before microorganisms invasion, or are induced after infection only, from prerequisite precursors" (which are constitutive in plants). On the other hand, PhA are described as "low molecular weight, anti-microbial substances that are both synthesized and accumulated in plants after exposure to biotic or abiotic agents" (increased markedly in response to infection attack) (Paxton, 1980; Braga and Dietrich, 1987; Van Etten et al., 1994; Grayer and Kokubun, 2001; Zhang et al., 2013). Plants usually produce more than 100,000 compounds of low molecular weight – the secondary metabolites, which differ from the primary metabolites because they are not essential to plant life (Domingo and López-Brea, 2003). Some metabolites act as antimicrobials, working in defense against plant pathogens. Although fungi are the most commonly used in the study of induction of PhA, bacteria, viruses, nematodes, and stimuli from abiotic origin might also induce the accumulation of these defense compounds in plants. PhA represents one of the potential component-induced defense mechanisms used by lytic enzymes in plants as chitinases and glucanases, oxidizing agents, cell wall lignification and numbers of pathogenesis-related (PR) proteins, and transcripts of unknown functions (Lamb et al., 1989; Dixon and Lamb, 1990).

Genetic changes in plants might enhance PhA production and thus increase its resistance to stress or diseases. These genes degradation might be exploited for transforming microbial pathogens to plants (Turgeon and Yoder 1985; Van Etten et al., 1989). However, PhA degradative enzyme inhibitors (PhA synergists) may be used to control plant diseases (Van Etten et al., 1989). It has been stated that the mechanisms of PhA on fungi may include fracture of the PM, cytoplasmic granulation, cellular contents disorganization, and fungal enzymes suppression, which leads to seed germination inhibition and germ tube elongation, and mycelial growth inhibition (Cavalcanti et al., 2005).

Numerous reports have revealed a significant role of PhA in the resistance of plants against stress/diseases. Several PhA compounds with similar structure were not produced only as a response to infection but also, on exposure to any of stress mechanisms; they are not specific toxins. Specificity is depended on the way in which the plants react (resistance or susceptibility) in certain host–parasite combinations (Hans and Jurgen, 1978).

Sometimes, the pathogenic fungi are insensitive to the PhA of their hosts, whereas nonpathogenic fungi are sensitive to the same PhA. The in vitro tolerance of fungi toward PhA might be related to the ability of the fungi to convert the PhA into nontoxic compounds. The host–parasite system is affected by many factors in vivo. This system consisting of several cultivars (varieties) of the host plant and numerous pathogenic races of microbes, therefore, some varieties of host plant are susceptible for and some are resistance to (varietal specific resistance). On the other hand, the resistance reaction in such system is usually accompanied by the hypersensitivity reaction in which many cells at the site of infected plant tissue rapidly die, necrosis cells are formed and PhA accumulates (Hans and Jurgen, 1978). The system of host–parasite combinations consisted of many species of fungus, for example, *Colletotrichum lindemuthianum* and many varieties of bean (*Phaseolus vulgaris*), fungus *Phytophthora megasperma* var *sojae* and soybean (*Glycine max*), also of the fungus *P. infestans* and potato (*S. tuberosum*) (Bailey and Deverail, 1971; Keen, 1971; Keen et al., 1971; Bailey, 1974; Cramer et al., 1985; Kessmann et al., 1990). In spite of many species of the pathogenic agents, they are almost evenly sensitive to the PhA of their host (Keen et al., 1971; Bailey, and Deverail, 1971; Bailey, 1974) and the host cultivars produced the same PhA (Keen, 1971), some cultivars of the host plant are susceptible for and others are resistance. This dissimilar behavior might be owing to the PhA synthesis commenced after varying lag periods, a conduct at different rates and which lead to different concentrations. These have shown that higher concentrations of PhA were more rapidly accumulated in incompatible combinations of host cultivars and parasite species (i.e., with resistance) than in compatible combinations (i.e., susceptible). Thereby in incompatible interactions, PhA accumulation inhibit or kill pathogen growth, thereby allowing resistance to the plant. In compatible interactions, the pathogen might either tolerate the accumulated PhA, detoxifies them, decreases PhA accumulation, or avoids eliciting PhA production (Mansfield, 1982).

Furthermore, many compounds may act as PhA in a plant organ and be substantial in another part of the same plant, for example, momilactone A, which is substantially present in rice husks, and rice stems (Lee et al., 1999), but is a PhA in rice leaves (Cartwright et al., 1981). Moreover, it has been reported that momilactone A is substantially produced and exuded from the root. Therefore, PhA are identified as dynamics of their function and biosynthesis, not by the class of chemical structure to which they belong, or biosynthetic pathway through which they were formed (Toyomasu et al., 2008). Nevertheless, the biosynthesis of the most PhA and the regulatory networks, as well as the molecular mechanisms beyond their cytotoxicity, are largely unknown.

3.3 ELICITORS OF PhA

Enhancement of PhA level in a plant (biotic or abiotic elicitors) is utilized which always activate mRNA transcripts and enzymes translation needed in PhA biosynthesis. Moreover, genes encoding elicitor-releasing proteins such as β-1,3-endoglucanase of one plant may be transferred to another for more potent resistant. Transgenic plant shows higher β-1,3-glucanase activity than an untransformed plant. PhA biosynthetic genes might also be converted to the desired plant which will impact resistance. Besides, biosynthetic pathways of PhA can be successfully changed by recombinant deoxyribonucleic acid (DNA) technology for enhancing PhA accumulation (Purkayastha, 1995). Many studies on PhA biosynthetic genes will actively contribute to our knowledge of the molecular biology of the host cells. The techniques of plant molecular biology have been applied successfully to establishing the role of PhA in plant resistance. However, the elicitation of the marked concentration of PhA by genetic manipulation is not always useful but may be more harmful to the host plant. Therefore, the understanding of PhA inhibitor/suppressor or degradation/detoxification mechanisms will be an aid in the regulation of excess PhA accumulation in plants and to comprehend the molecular basis of pathogenicity. PhA degradation by a pathogen metabolite makes the plant more vulnerable to invasion. Therefore, PhA inhibitors detoxifying enzymes should be exploited for enzymes inactivation and for keeping PhA level at the site of infection. Genes encoding PhA detoxifying enzymes and PhA suppressors has been determined in many virulent fungal pathogens. Although, extensive work has been done on PhA during the last century (Purkayastha, 1995), but some fundamental issues has remained yet to be elucidated.

Tissues from whole parts of terrestrial plants might produce PhA in response to infection by pathogenic and nonpathogenic fungus (Keen and Harsch, 1972), bacteria (Stholasuta et al., 1971, Keen and Kennedy, 1974), viruses (Bailey et al., 1975; 1976), and nematodes (Abawi et al., 1971; Rich et al., 1977). The production of PhA is induced "elicited" not only by living microbes but also by different extracts (Varns et al., 1971). Compounds released from microbes which stimulate the induction of PhA synthesis in plants has been claimed as elicitors (Keen et al., 1972). However, the PhA might remain ineffective if the pathogenic agent does not get in contact with them during its development in the plant. Biotic elicitors might contribute to the interaction between plants and pathogens, whilst abiotic elicitors may not contribute to these interactions. Exogenous biotic elicitors might be in the attack of the organism, whilst endogenous elicitors are of plant origin and they are induced by the interaction of both microorganism and plant (Darvill and Albersheim, 1984).

Substances with elicitor activity have been detected along with a wide range of chemical structural types including polysaccharides, glycoproteins, lipids, lipopolysaccharides, oligosaccharides, and even enzymes, though their activity can be contributed to their effect in producing elicitor-active substances from the cell walls of the host or pathogen (Anderson, 1989; Blein et al., 1991; Hahn et al., 1992; Alghisi and Favaron, 1995). Abiotic elicitors form a numerous collection of substances that are not derived from natural sources, such as the tissues of the host or pathogen. Under normal conditions, they would not be produced by the plant, this includes substances such as fungicides, heavy metals (Cu^{2+} and Hg^{2+}), detergents, polylysine, histone, and reagents that intercalate a DNA (Dixon et al., 1983; Darvill and Albersheim, 1984). The exposure the plant tissues with factors that cause stress such as freezing, wounding, or exposure to UV light can also induce PhA synthesis (Kodama et al., 1988; Kodama et al., 1992a,b,c; Mert-Türk et al., 1998).

PhA consists of various groups of natural products. The only compounds considered were those which satisfied the standard of PhA concept (compounds which only detect in high amounts after infection and which prohibit the growth of microbes). There is a relationship between the chemical nature of the PhA and plant families, such as Legumes, Solanaceae, Fabaceae, and Orchidaceae produces isoflavonoids, diterpenes, polyacetylenes, and dihydrophenanthrenes, respectively (Ingham and Harborne, 1976; Harborne, 1999; Cavalcanti, 2005; Ahuja et al., 2012; Ejike et al., 2013). Table 3.1 is a list of the major PhA of various plant families. PhA include isoflavonoids, sesquiterpenes, furanoterpenoids, polyacetylenes, dihydrophenanthrenes, and so forth. Pisatin was the first natural product PhA characterized from pea plants. After this, other PhA were isolated from various crops such as beans, rice, barley, banana (Braga, 1991), and more than 300 types of PhA have been identified. *Poaceae* plants have also been studied for the induction of

TABLE 3.1 Phytoalexin from Different Plant Families.

Plant families	Types of phytoalexins (PhA)/examples	References
Amaryllidaceae	Flavans	Coxon et al. (1980)
Brassicaceae (Cruciferae)	Camalexin sulfur-containing/indole PhA/ brassinin	Browne et al. (1991)
Compositae	Safynol/polyacetylenes	Geigert et al. (1973)
Chenopodiaceae	Flavanones/betagarin Isoflavones/betavulgarin	Pedras et al. (2000)
Convolvulaceae	Ipomeamarone/Furano sesquiterpenes	Allen et al. (1971)
Euphorbiaceae	Diterpenes/casbene	Uritani et al. (1960); Sitton et al. (1975)
Linaceae	Coniferyl alcohol/phenylpropanoids (PP)	Keen et al. (1975)
Leguminosae	Isoflavans, isoflavones, isoflavanones, coumestans, pterocarpans/pisatin, glyceollin, phaseolin, maiackiain, wyerone/furano acetylenes, stilbenes/resveratrol pterocarpens	Jeandet et al. (2013)
Moraceae	Furano pterocarpans/moracins A-H	Takasugi et al. (1979)
Malvaceae	Gossypol/terpenoids naphtaldehydes	Kumar et al. (2006)
Orchidaceae	Loroglossol/dihydrophenanthrenes	Ward et al. (1975)
Poaceae	Diterpenoids: oryzalexins; momilactones; phytocassanes; zealexins; kauralexins; apigeninidin flavanones/sakuranetin phenylamides and deoxyanthocyanidins/ luteolinidin	Poloni et al. (2014); Park et al. (2013); Jeandet et al. (2013)
Rutaceae	Xanthoxylin/methylated phenolic compounds	Hartmann et al. (1974); Harding et al. (1981)
Rosaceae	Cotonefurans/biphenyls/auarperin dibenzofurans	Kokubun et al. (1995)
Solanaceae	PP-related compounds; steroid glycoalkaloids; norsequi and sesquiterpenoids coumarins; polyacetylenic derivatives	Jeandet et al. (2013)
Umbelliferae	Falcarinol phenolics: xanthotoxin 6-methoxymellein/polyacetylenes	Johnson et al. (1973); Condon et al. (1963)
Vitaceae	Stilbenes/resveratrol	Langcake et al. (1979)

Source: Reprinted from Arruda et al., 2016. With permission via the Creative Commons Attribution License, https://creativecommons.org/licenses/by/4.0/

a variety of PhA (Ahuja et al., 2012). They have a great diversity of classes of chemical compounds, members of family Poaceae produces mainly diterpenoid PhA. Corn produces kauralexins diterpenoids and zealexins acid sesquiterpenoids C and D PhA. The elicitors of PhA in corn include pathogens such as *Aspergillus flavus, Aspergillus sojae, Cochliobolus heter-ostrophus, Colletotrichum sublineolum, Fusarium graminearum, Ostrinia nubilalis, Rhizopus microspores*, and *Ustilago maydis* (Huffaker et al., 2011, Rejanne et al., 2016). The rate of PhA production is considered a key factor for the establishment of the pathogen infection. Therefore, in some cases, PhA could be used as taxonomic markers.

3.4 PhA IN DISEASE RESISTANCE

The regulation and mechanisms of PhA in plants defense response are important in the resistance to infection in plants. Many work has been carriedout with the aim of exploring the PhA induced in different parts of plants families in the defense against pathogenic invasion and to detect the use of substances isolated from these plants to enhance the synthesis of PhA (Ejike et al., 2013). It follows that PhA induction or accumulation in a host plant might be regulated in many ways owing to promote its resistance to diseases. The biotic elicitors, which are characterized by viable or inactivated microbes, plant extracts have been used to enhance the induction of resistance, once these compounds have the advantages of not being phytotoxic and are readily biodegradable (Devaiah, 2009). Otherwise, when they are not pathogenic organisms, their mechanism of action is enhanced systemic resistance, which not causing symptoms as necrosis and might activate the defense response of plants by induction of PhA.

The suppressor sometimes acts as both suppressor of PhA biosynthesis and a determinant of pathogenicity by suppressing other defense reaction (Oku and Shiraishi, 1995). Resistance or susceptibility of plants growing under physiological stress conditions depends on several factors and not on PhA alone. There is evidence that sometimes plants under physiological stress are unable to produce an adequate amount of PhA and become more susceptible to disease.

Moreover, the pathogenic organisms might prevent the plant from synthesizing PhA. It has been established whether the PhA produced by pathogenic microbes (Strobel, 1977) may be termed as effectors for such mechanism. Another mechanism could be by the inhibition of elicitor action by competitive factors (Ayers et al., 1976) or inactivation of the elicitors before they reach their site of action in the plant cells.

The original response of plant defense is activated through two mechanisms, which are triggered immunity (PTI) known as nonhost defense and effector-triggered immunity known as host-specific resistance. The PTI defense mechanism occurs when in contact with the pathogen, and is determined as the first line of innate immunity in plants (Zhang and Zhou, 2010). Scientific evidence that PhA are effective in providing plants with disease resistance has been confirmed by transferring foreign PhA expression from one plant to another. Stilbene PhA, which include resveratrol (1) (Fig. 3.1) need only stilbene synthase, to link the two present precursors, malonyl-CoA and p-coumaryl-CoA, for their synthesis. Pathogen resistance has thus been engineered into tobacco plants by the transfer of stilbene synthase genes from grapevine, *V. vinifera*, a resveratrol inducer. The regenerated tobacco plant proved to have improved pathogenic resistance to *Botrytis cinerea*. It not only accumulates its usual sesquiterpenoid PhA on inoculation but also rapidly synthesizes up to 40 μg resveratrol/g fresh weight (Hain et al., 1993). According to the gene for gene theory, it depends on the highly specific interaction between the pathogen and R gene products (Boller and Felix, 2009). Based on the signaling pathway, which might lead to the expression of defenses, enhancement of resistance can be divided into induced (ISR), that is activated by nonpathogenic microbes and mediated by jasmonate and ethylene, and that acquired (SAR), which is activated by pathogenic microbes, and is a salicylate-dependent induction (Pieterse et al., 2001; Zhang et al., 2015). The understanding of these pathways is important for selecting the most suitable elicitor agent which cause the desired defense system and thus obtain the highest expression of these antimicrobial substances.

Camalexin (3-thiazol-2'-yl-indole) and rapalexin A are a major PhA in *Arabidopsis* (Browne et al., 1991; Pedras and Adio, 2008), which has also been detected in *Arabidopsis* and *Brassicaceae* species (Bednarek et al., 2011). Many studies on the major pathways controlling the production of camalexin in Arabidopsis indicated that their participation may depend on the pathogenic attack. Other studies searching for the response of *Arabidopsis* jasmonic acid (JA) signaling mutants to *Alternaria brassicicola* infection led to the summary that camalexin synthesis is under the control of a JA-independent pathway (Van Wees et al., 2003; Thomma et al., 1999). Innovative studies with *B. cinerea* have concluded that JA signaling controls camalexin synthesis to a substantial extent (Thomma et al., 1999). Other studies have suggested that camalexin induction is controlled by salicylic acid (SA)-independent (Nawrath and Metraux, 1999; Roetschi et al., 2001) and SA-dependent (Denby et al., 2005) signaling pathways. Reactive oxygen species are also combined with camalexin induction, as shown by oxidative stress-inducing chemicals such as paraquat and acifluorfen (Zhao et al., 1998; Tierens et al., 2002). Nevertheless, it has been suggested that both hydrogen peroxide and SA are required for the production of camalexin (Chaouch et al., 2010).

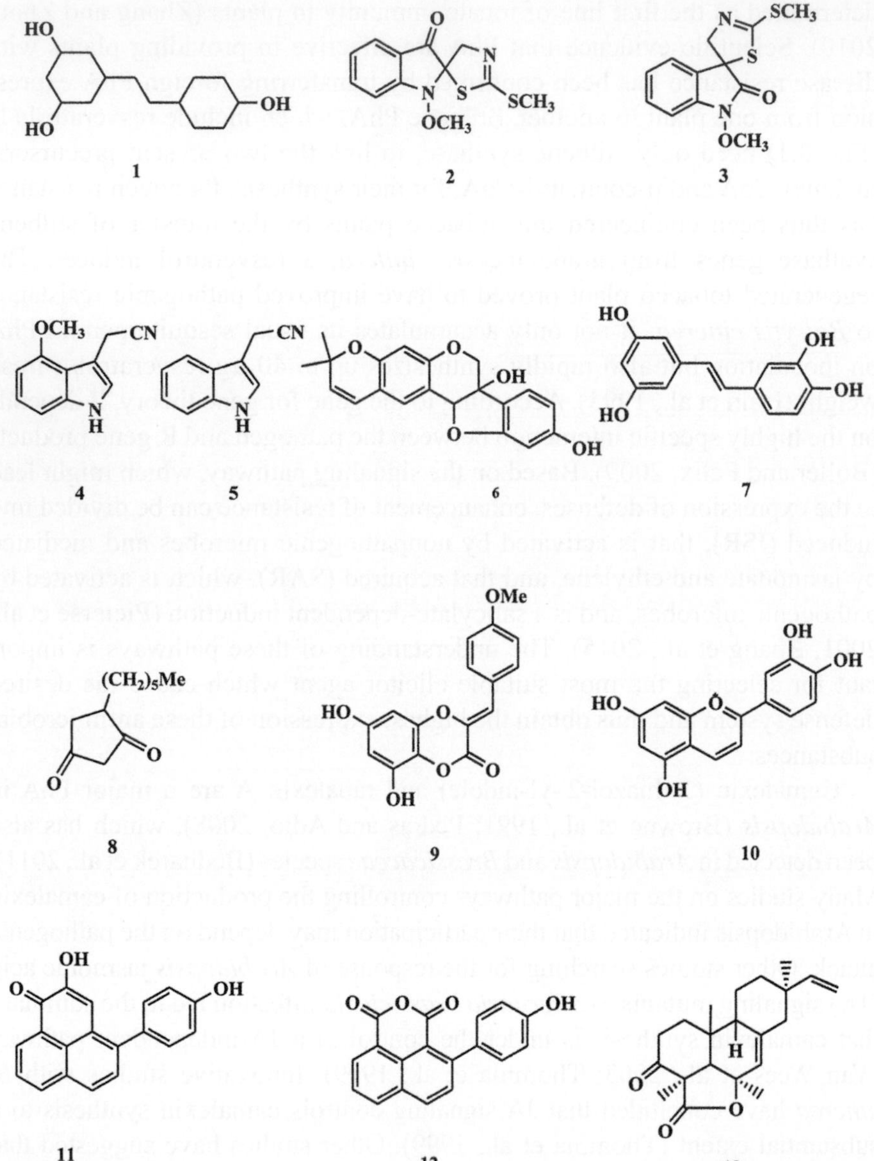

FIGURE 3.1 Chemical structures of isolated phytoalexin (PhA).

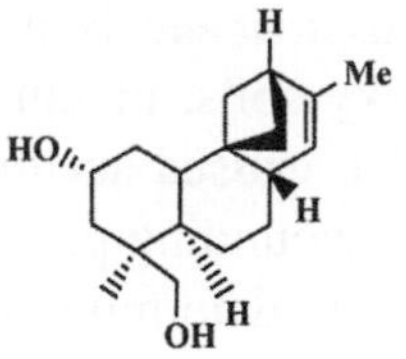

14 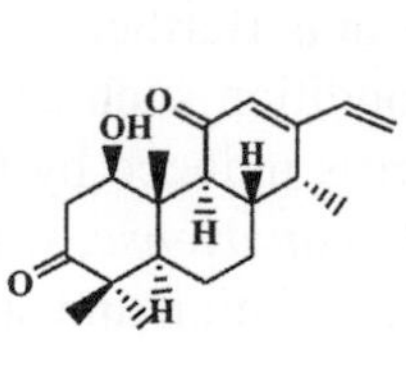   15 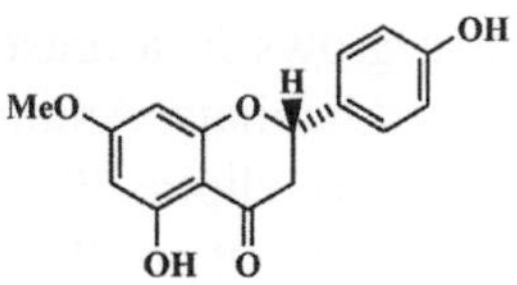   16

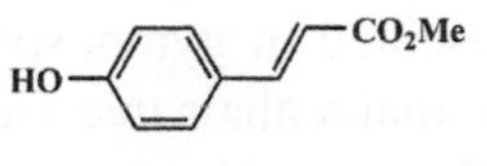

17 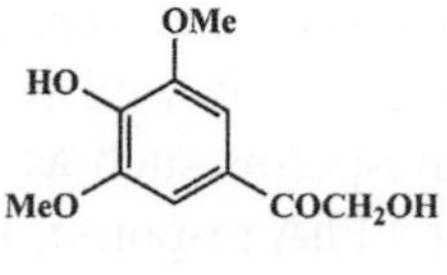   18 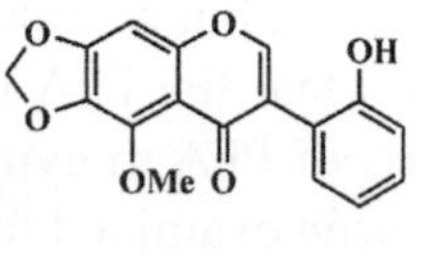   19

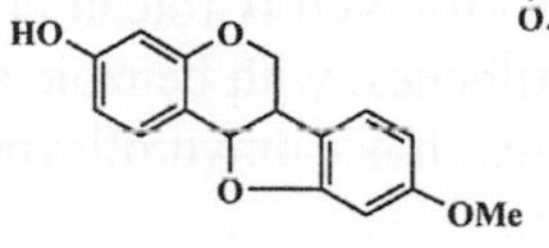

20 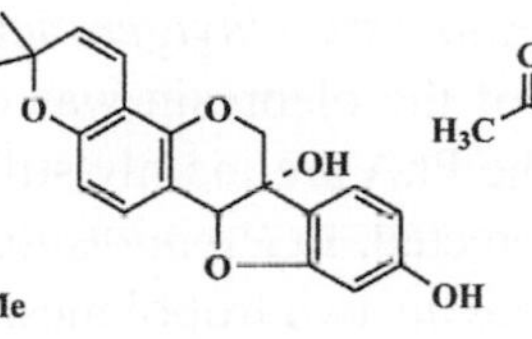   21 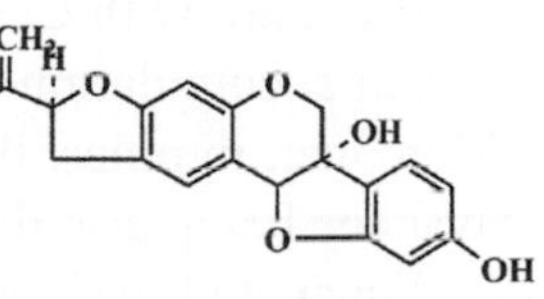   22

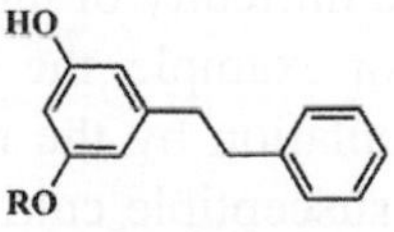

23 R = H
24 R = Me   25

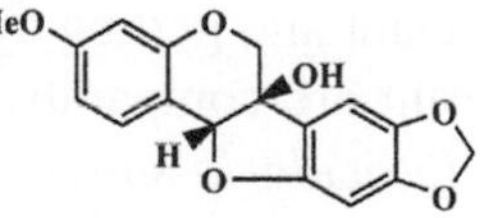

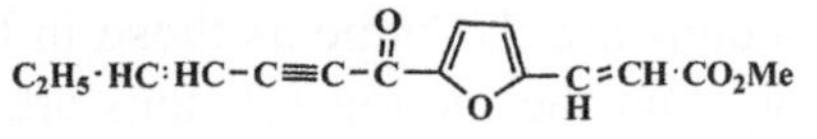

26

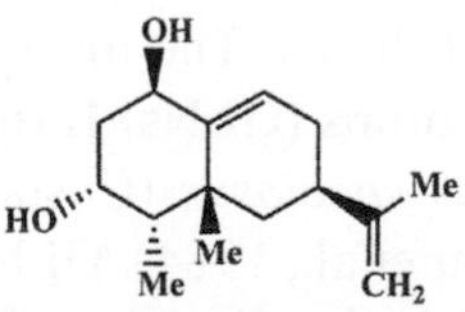

27 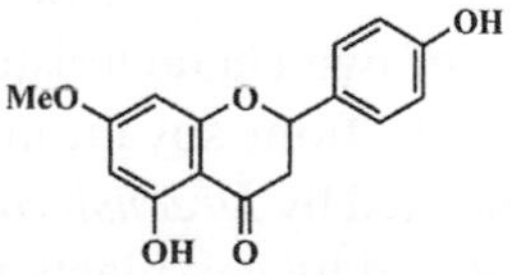   28

FIGURE 3.1   *(Continued)*

Erucastrum canariense Webb and Berthel F. *Brassicaceae* is a wild crucifer that grows in a drastic condition such as rocky soils, in salt, and water-stressed habitats. Abiotic stress induced by $CuCl_2$ caused accumulation of galacto-oxylipins PhA in *E. canariense*, whilst wounding produced galacto-oxylipins but not PhA. The isolation and structure determination of compounds isolated from the leaves of *E. canariense* revealed the presence of erucalexin (2), 1-methoxyspirobrassinin (3), arvelexin (4) and indolyl-3-acetonitrile (5), but no galactooxylipins were detected (Fig. 3.1).

It appears that the PhA response is well represented in gymnosperms. Many reports of PhA in gymnosperms such as the maidenhair tree *Ginkgo biloba*, has been examined for a PhA response. In fact, infection by *Botrytis allii* successfully produced substances, which inhibited fungal penetration into the leaf (Christensen, 1972). Other report about the treatment of *Pinus contorta* bark with *Ceratocystis clavigera* lead to enhanced terpenoid synthesis and accumulation of the oleoresin was observed (Croteau et al., 1987). Moreover, in pines, the PhA are mainly stilbenes, with benzoic acid and a flavanone being also detected. In *Pseudotsuga*, it is a dihydroflavonol, in *Picea* a lignan and in *Cupressus* two tropolones.

There are about 46 PhA that have been identified in 17 monocot species. Some are listed in Table 3.2. One of the major obstacles in progressing PhA research in monocotyledonous families is the difficulty of inoculating tissues of plant and getting a necrotic reaction. For example, the leaves of the rice plant are comparatively resistant to inoculation by the rice blast organism *Pyricularia sativa*, even when using a susceptible cultivar. This can be overcome by employing UV irradiation or by using punch inoculation to mimic pathogen attack (Dillon et al., 1997). Many PhA types that are present in the monocotyledons are the same as those in the dicotyledons, and this support the theory that the monocotyledons are thought to have evolved from within the dicotyledons. However, there are some astonishing equivalent in PhA production between mono- and dicots. The most noteworthy is of two characteristic legume PhA, glyceollins (GLNs) II (6) and III (Fig. 3.1) from soyabean *Glycine max*, *Costus speciosus* (Costaceae) leaves infected by *Drechslera longirostrata* (Kumar et al., 1984). GLNs are PhA produced by soy plants in response to stressful stimuli such as fungal infections, UV exposure, or changes in temperature. GLNs have demonstrated antiestrogenic activity both in in vitro and in vivo, suppressing estrogen-responsive tumors through action at estrogen receptors (ERs). Recent evidence suggests that GLNs might also possess estrogenic properties or might have exhibited their effects through non-ER-mediated mechanisms. In addition to antitumor effects, GLNs possess antimicrobial and antioxidant activity, along with effects on glucose and lipid metabolism (Bamji, 2017).

TABLE 3.2 Phytoalexin Compounds Isolated from Monocotyledons Plant Families.

Plant families	Chemical classes	Compounds isolated	References
Alliaceae	Cyclic dione*	5-Hexylcyclopenta-1,3-dione	Tverskoy et al. (1991)
Amaryllidaceae	Flavan	7,4'-Dihydroxyflavan	Coxon et al. (1980)
Costaceae	Isoflavonoid	Glyceollin II	Harborne (1999)
Dioscoreaceae	Bibenzyl	Batatasin IV	Hashimoto et al. (1972)
Gramineae	Flavanone	Sakuranetin	Ogawa et al. (2017);
	Stilbene	Resveratrol	Shrikanta et al. (2015);
	Deoxyanthocyanidin	Luteolinidin	Viswanathan et al. (1996)
	Diterpene*	Momilactone A	
	Anthranilic acid	HDIBOA glucoside	
Liliaceae	Stilbene	Resveratrol	Shrikanta et al. (2015)
Musaceae	Phenalenone*	Musanolone C	Holscher et al. (2014)

*Chemical classes from monocotyledons plant families.

Other parallel findings are of the stilbene resveratrol (1) in *Festuca versuta* leaf (Powell et al., 1994) and of the related piceatannol (7) (Fig. 3.1) in the leaf of sugarcane, *Saccharum officinarum* (Brinker and Seigler, 1991). Resveratrol is a PhA found in the dicots of both the peanut *Arachis hypogaea* (Leguminosae) and the vine, *V. vinifera* (Vitaceae), and in the gymnosperms of *Pinus* sapwoods.

However, in many cases, PhA produced is entirely distinctive of a particular monocot genus, Table 3.2. Such as infected bulbs of the onion *Allium cepa* induce two aliphatic diones, 5-hexylcyclopenta-1,3-dione (8) (Fig. 3.1) and the 5-octyl analogue (Tverskoy et al., 1991). In spite of onion and other *Alliums* species that are rich in sulfur compounds, some of which are antimicrobial, it is remarkable that the PhA of onion is not only sulfur. It has an individual structure PhA which is yurinelide (9) (Fig. 3.1) and a benzodioxin-2-one synthesized by *Lilium maximowiczii* in the bulb (Monde et al., 1992). Moreover, monocots have the ability to synthesize PhA pigments such as red 3-desoxyanthocyanidin. Apigeninidin and luteolinidin (10) (Fig. 3.1) pigments were identified in sorghum tissues after response to infection by a fungus (Nicholson et al., 1987). Apigeninidin 5-caffeoyl-glucoside and luteolinidin 5-methyl ether have also been identified in inoculated sorghum tissue (Lo et al., 1996). Sugarcane (*Saccharum offi-cinarum*) also accumulates luteolinidin and piceatannol (7) in response to fungal infection (Brinker and Seigler, 1991). In the the banana plant, *Musa acuminata* (Musaceae), phenalenone-type structures are accumulated after fungal infection *Colletotrichum musae* such as irenolone (11) and naphthalic anhydride (12) (Fig. 3.1) from leaves and fruit peels (Hirai et al., 1994; Luis et al., 1993).

Sixteen (16) PhA have been reported in rice, *Oryza sativa* (Gramineae), 14 are diterpenoids, ranging from momilactones A (13) and B (Cartwright et al., 1981) and oryzalexin S (14) to phytocassanes (15) (Koga et al., 1997). Two flavanones reported are naringenin and its 7-methyl ether sakuranetin (16) (Fig. 3.1) (Kodama et al., 1992a,b,c). Experiments with susceptible and resistant rice cultivars suggest that sakuranetin, momilactone A, and oryzalexin S are produced in suitable amounts to support such resistance (Dillon et al., 1997).

Maize (*Zea mays*) is Poaceae crop plant. The PhA which accumulate in the plant in response to pathogen attack are kauralexins and zealexin (Fig. 3.2). It has recently been disclosed that maize stem invaded by fungi *Rhizopus microsporus* and *Colletotrichum graminicola* stimulates the accumulation of six ent-kaurane-related diterpenoids, termed kauralexins (Huffaker et al., 2011). A physiologically relevant amount of kauralexins inhibited the growth of these pathogens. Accumulation of the fungal-induced kaurene synthase 2 (An2) transcripts preceded highly localized kauralexin induction, and a combination of JA and ethylene application detected their synergistic role in kauralexin regulation. Other maize PhA, termed zealexins, have also been recently discovered following an attack by *F. graminearum* (Schmelz et al., 2011). The characterization of these recently discovered kauralexins and zealexins should be required in the identification of the roles of nonvolatile terpenoid PhA in maize disease resistance (Huffaker et al., 2011; Schmelz et al., 2011).

About 24 families of the dicotyledons are listed in Table 3.3. PhA production may yield one or more of the same structural class, while other species can give rise to multiple unrelated structures. PhA in the dicotyle-dons are classified into four main chemical classes as phenolics, acetylenics, terpenoids, and nitrogen-containing compounds. In phenolics, they have free hydroxyl groups masked by o-methylation and this might enhance their lipophilicity. Phenylpropanoids (PPs) have been reported in the Linaceae and Scrophulariaceae, Table 3.3. Moreover, p-coumaric acid methyl ester (17) (Fig. 3.1) has been isolated from cucumber leaves, *Cucumis sativus* infected by powdery mildew (Daayf et al., 1997).

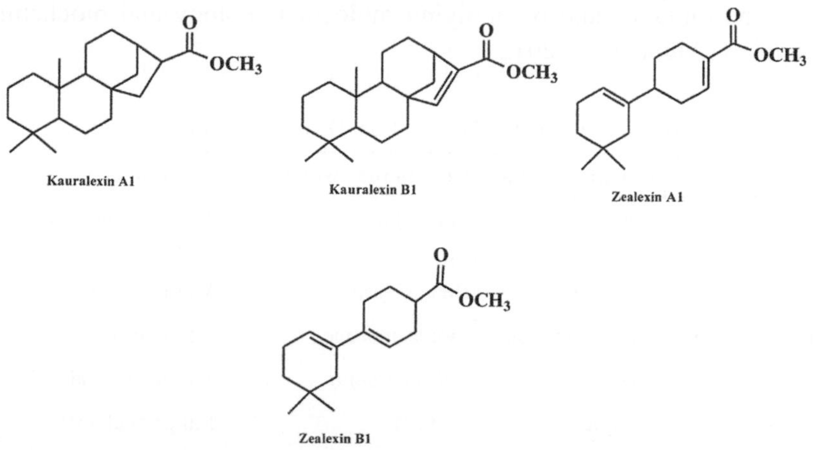

Kauralexin A1

Kauralexin B1

Zealexin A1

Zealexin B1

FIGURE 3.2 Structure of PhA in maize plants.

Xanthoxylin (phloracetophenone 4,6-dimethyl ether) is PhA from *Citrus limon* (Afek and Sztejmberg, 1988), while danielone (18) (Fig. 3.1) is a PhA from papaya fruit, *Carica papaya* (Caricaceae) (Echeverri et al., 1997), whereas 4-hydroxy- and 3,4-dihydroxyacetophenone, are PhA in cocoa *Theobroma cacao* (Sterculiaceae) (Resende et al., 1996). In the cocoa plant, they also accumulate arjunolic acid triterpene. Moreover, many reports of coumarin PhA such as aesculetin 6,7-dimethyl ether are found in *C. limon* (Rutaceae) (Afek and Sztejnberg, 1988) and furanocoumarin, xanthyletin from the same plant (Khan et al., 1985). Furthermore, coumarin scopoletin PhA is reportedly found in the rubber tree *Hevea brasiliensis* (Euphorbiaceae) leaves (Giesemann et al., 1986) and from a plant tree, *Platanus acerifolia* (Platanaceae) leaves (El Modafar et al., 1993). Isoflavones PhA are accumulated in legume leaves and are formed in the unrelated *Beta vulgaris* of the Chenopodiaceae, Table 3.3. Betavulgarin (19) (Fig. 3.1) a major isoflavone of *B. vulgaris*, also occurs as the 2'-xyloside and as the 2'-glucoside. It has been suggested that these glycosides have a role in promoting resistance (Elliger and Halloin, 1994). Acetylenics are presented in Umbelliferae and Compositae families. They have also been determined in the Solanaceae, a family where sesquiterpenoids are the main PhA. Occasionally, various terpenoid have been reported also from Convolvulaceae, Euphorbiaceae, Malvaceae, Phytolaccaceae, Tiliaceae, and Ulmaceae (Table 3.3). Finally, to develop disease protection strategies, plant pathogen research in the field of PhA has concentrated on interpreting their biosynthesis pathways and regulation in different crop plants by using different cultivars, transgenic plants, and mutants, and by applying molecular biology and biochemical approaches (Ahuja et al., 2012).

TABLE 3.3   Phytoalexin Compounds Isolated from Dicotyledons Plant Families.

Plant families	Chemical classes	Compounds isolated	References
Cercidiphyllaceae	Biphenyl	Magnolol	Takasugi and Katui (1986)
Chenopodiaceae	Isoflavone	Betavulgarin	Marti (1977)
Convolvulaceae	Furanoterpenoid	Ipomeamorone	Coxon et al. (1975)
Cruciferae	Indole*	Spirobrassinin	Mezencev et al. (2009)
Compositae	Acetylenic*	Safynol	Ranga et al. (1977)
Cactaceae	Aurone	4,5-methylenedioxy-6-hydroxyaurone	Paul et al. (1991)
Euphorbiaceae	Diterpene	Casbene	Sitton and West (1975)
Linaceae	PP	Coniferyl alcohol	Hano et al. (2006)
Leguminosae	Isoflavonoid*	Pisatin	Perrin and Bottomley (1962)
Moraceae	Stilbene	Oxyresveratrol	Chung et al. (2003)
Malvaceae	Sesquiterpene	Gossypol	Stipanovic et al. (2005)
Phytolaccaceae	Saponin	Phytolaccoside	Kanzaki et al. (1999)
Papaveraceae	Alkaloid	Sanguinarine	Cline et al. (1988)
Rubiaceae	Anthraquinone	Purpurin 1-methyl ether	Wijnsma et al. (1984)
Rutaceae	Acetophenone	Xanthoxylin	Hartmann et al. (1974)
Rosaceae	Biphenyl*	Aucuparin	Widyastutfi et al. (1992).
Solanaceae	Sesquiterpene*	Rishitin	Komaraiah et al. (2003)
Scrophulariaceae	PP	Acteoside	Chun et al. (2002)
Tiliaceae	Sesquiterpene	7-Hydroxycalamenene	Burden and Kemp (1983)
Umbelliferae	Furanocoumarin*	Xanthotoxin	Al-Barwani et al. (2004)
Ulmaceae	Diterpene	Mansonone A	Meier et al. (1997)
Vitaceae	Stilbene	Pterostilbene	Langcake et al. (1979)
Verbenaceae	Naphthofuranone	Naphtho [1,2-b] furan-4,5-dione	Tsai et al. (2014)

*Chemical classes from dicotyledons plant families.

3.5 ELICITATION OF PhA BY INDUCING/STIMULATION mRNA TRANSCRIPTION AND ENZYMES TRANSLATION SOUGHT IN PhA BIOSYNTHESIS

It has been known that both biotic and abiotic elicitors give similar PhA accumulation. Addition of fungal elicitors (e.g., elicitor, heat released from cell walls of the pathogenic fungus, *C. lindemuthianum*, was added to a final concentration of 60 µg of glucose equivalent/ml) to bean cell suspension cultures results in inducing PhA synthesis (Cramer et al., 1985). The elicitors stimulate the formation of messenger ribonucleic acids (mRNAs) encoding the enzymes of PP metabolism. These enzymes are synthesized prior to PhA synthesis and might be noticed within 20 min after elicitor was added and reaches its maximum level within 3–4 h. Most of the PhA are derived from the PP biosynthetic pathways. The PPs are involved in many functions and play a pivotal role in the interaction between the plant and its surrounding. Various secondary metabolites contribute in the plant diseases resistance and enzymes that catalyze the biosynthesis of PhA are phenylalanine ammonia lyase (PAL), cinnamate-4-hydrolase, and coenzyme 4-cumarascligase (Mateos and Leal, 2013). The understanding of the PhA biosynthetic pathways and the required enzymes has lead to the knowledge of the expression of plant response to pathogens infection.

Terpenoid PhA exists in a variety of species such as tobacco (*Nicotiana tabacum*), cotton (*Gossypium hirsutum*), sweet potato (*Ipomoea batatas*), and elm (*Ulmus americana*) (Harborne, 1999). In plants, the isopentenyl diphosphate and dimethylallyl pyrophosphate isoprenoid precursors can be derived from the mevalonate or metileritritol phosphate. The methylerythritol phosphate (MEP) pathway leads to the biosynthesis of geranylgeranyl diphosphate and the diterpenoid biosynthesis pathway (Okada, 2007). The diterpene cyclases catalyzes the conversion of ent-copalyl-diphosphate (ent-CDP) or syn-copalyldiphosphate (syn-CDP) in four key hydrocarbons in the PhA biosynthesis in rice, which are entcassa-12,15-diene; ent-sandaracopimara-8,15diene; 9β-pimara-7,15-diene; and stemar-13-ene. The geranylgeranyl diphosphate production in rice probably occurs in the plastids by MEP pathway, whereas sesquiterpenes and triterpenes are usually synthesized in the cytoplasm through the mevalonate pathway (Toyomasu 2008 , Vranova et al., 2013). Diterpenoid PhA are expected to be formed through the diphosphate geranylgeranyl methylerythritol.

In the biosynthesis of isoflavanoid PhA, medicarpin (20) (Fig. 3.1) several reactions are involved. Activation of enzymes by elicitors to enhance PhA production. Soybean plants synthesize and accumulate isoflavonoid derived

PhA, GLNs in the plant's tissues after exposure to pathogens (Bailey et al., 1975). Synthesis of GLNs can be produced in soy plants after exposure to fungal strains such as *A. sojae* (Boué et al., 2000), which elicits induction of a trace to moderate amounts of GLNs mixture, I (21), II (6) and III (22) (Fig. 3.1) in response to the pathogenic attack (Eromosele et al., 2013; Isaac et al., 2017). Many studies have been established that GLNs have antibacterial, antioxidant, antifungal, anti-inflammatory, antitumor, and insulinotropic actions both in vitro and in vivo (Salvo et al., 2006; Kim et al., 2010a,b; Park et al., 2010; Kim et al., 2011; Ng et al., 2011).

GLNs biosynthesis (Fig. 3.3) includes enzymes that are used in the synthesis of isoflavonoids and PhA (Ebel, 1986). Phenylalanine is first converted to trans-cinnamic acid by the action of enzyme PAL, followed by a hydroxylation reaction catalyzed by cinnamate 4-hydroxylase (C4H) that converts the trans-cinnamic acid to *p*-coumaric acid (Dixon and Paiva, 1995). A series of subsequent reactions involving enzymes 4CL, chalcone synthase (CHS), CHR, chalcone isomerase (CHI), and IFS, leads to the formation of 2,7,40-trihydroxyisoflavone, which then leads to the production of the isoflavonoid daidzein (Dixon and Paiva, 1995; Yoneyama et al., 2016). Daidzein undergoes cyclization and hydroxylation reactions to glycinol, (non-prenylated precursor for GLNs) (Dixon and Paiva, 1995). Two separate prenylated transferases, G4-DT and G2-DT, then prenylated glycinol to GLNs I and II, respectively (Akashi et al., 2009). The final steps of GLNs biosynthesis are the cyclization of glyceollidins by GS to convert glyceollidin I to glyceollin I, and glyceollidin II to GLNs II and III (Welle and Grisebach, 1988).

Moreover, CHS is the key enzyme of the flavonoid/isoflavonoid biosynthetic pathway. The amount of CHS mRNA increased significantly in soybean leaves when inoculated with an avirulent race of *Pseudomonas syringae* pv. *glycinea* (*Psg*) but not with a virulent race. In contrary, the increase in CHS mRNA was similar in roots inoculated with zoospores from an avirulent or a virulent race of *P. megasperma* f. sp. *glycinea* (*Pmg*) (Dhawale et al., 1989). The major elicitor releasing an enzyme in soybean is β-1,3-endoglucanase. This enzyme could release PhA elicitors from *Pmg* cell walls. Antiserum raised against the purified enzyme was detected to be specific for soybean releasing enzyme. The antiserum inhibited β-1,3-glucanase, the elicitor-releasing activity of the purified enzymes and soybean crude extracts (Takeuchi et al., 1990, Yoshioka et al., 1993). This observation indicated that host enzymes play a pivotal role in the production of PhA by releasing PhA-elicitors from fungal cell walls. It disclosed that β-1,3-endoglucanase was a key enzyme involved in elicitor signal induction. It was found that transgenic tobacco plants, expressing the soybean glucanase gene were resistant to fungal diseases. These results interpreted that disease-resistant transgenic tobacco plants might be developed which would promote the release of active elicitor molecules from fungal cell walls (Yoshioka et al., 1993).

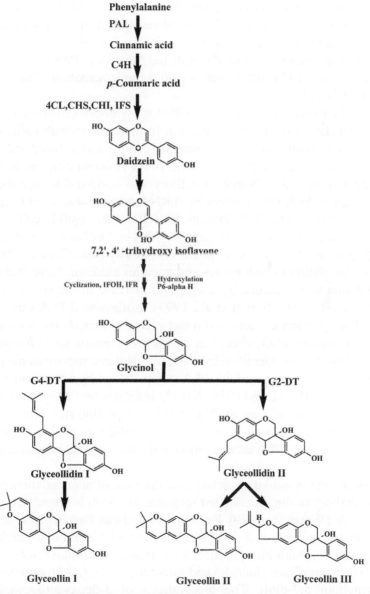

FIGURE 3.3   Biosynthetic pathway of glyceollins in soybeans.

Elicitor enhances metabolic changes in cell cultures of both resistant and susceptible chick pea (*Cicer arietinum* L.cvs) were established by Daniel et al. (1990). Cell suspension cultures of resistant (cv. ILC 3279) and susceptible (cv. ILC 1929) cultivars were compared to their elicitor enhance accumulation of pterocarpan PhA and activities of enzymes. The treatment of cell cultures with a polysaccharide elicitor from *Ascochyta rabiei* afforded 5-fold higher concentrations of PhA medicarpin and maackiain in the cells of the resistant than in the susceptible cultivar. Daniel and Barz noticed a differential accumulation of Medicarpin and Maackiain PhA in *C. arietinum* cvs. and enhance CHS-mRNA activity after implementation of an *A. rabiei* derived elicitor (1990).

The CHS involved in the first step of PhA biosynthesis showed a maximum activity between 8–12 h after elicitation in the cells of both cultivars. An approximately 5-fold higher concentration of PhA and a 2-fold increase in CHS activity was determined in the cells of the resistant cvs. The highest of the elicitor produced CHS-mRNA activity was noticed 4 h after the onset of induction in both the cultivars by mRNA activity was 2-fold higher in resistant cultivar (ILC 3279) than in the cells of susceptible cultivar (ILC 1929). Elicitation mechanism of isoflavan PhA in *Agrobacterium rhizogenes* transformed root of *Lotus corniculatus* cultures by glutathione (GSH) leads to the accumulation in both tissues and in callus medium. Nevertheless, the accumulation was preceded by a temporal increase in the activity of PAL (Robbins et al., 1991, Seifert et al., 1993). Isoflavonoid PhA was isolated from cell suspension cultures and intact plants of *Ornithopus sativus* after using of yeast or $CuSO_4$ elicitor or a spore suspension of *Colletotrichum trifolii*. Glabridin was identified by using physical and spectroscopic properties, the transient increase of this PhA was preceded by a transient increase in the activities of PAL and CHS. A study indicates that exogenous JA also enhances the accumulation of PAL, CHS and proline-rich protein (PRP) transcripts in soybean cells (Gundlach et al., 1992), as well as, it might be enhanced to activate PhA accumulation and other defense responses (Dixon et al., 1994).

CHS change in activity is relative to the time of accumulation of PhA, 3-deoxyanthocyanidin, in etiolated sorghum mesocotyls inoculated with *C. graminicola* (Wei et al., 1989). Results revealed that PhA began to accumulate in the tissue between 3 and 6 h. after the initial increase in the level of the enzyme. Sorghum PhA produces known as apigeninidin (2-(4-hydroxyphenyl) benzopyrilium chloride) and luteolinidin (2-(3,4-dihydroxyphenyl) chromenylium 5,7-diol). The biosynthesis of 3-deoxyanthocyanidin is independent of light, it happens in the dark (Wharton and Nicholson, 2000).

Huang and Backhouse (2004), have reported that the production of 3-deoxy-anthocyanidin is not the first line of defense by sorghum against pathogens. They noticed that sorghum inoculated with *Fusarium proliferatum,* and *Fusarium thapsinum*, enhanced the levels of apigeninidin and luteolinidin, also the amounts of the resistance-related proteins peroxidases, β-1,3 gluca-nases and chitinases.

Stress responses in alfalfa (*Medicago sativa* L.) has been conducted. It was noticed that cell suspension cultures accumulated high amount of the pterocarpan PhA medicarpin after treatment with an elicitor prepared from cell walls of *C. lindemuthianum*. A maximum accumulation was detected within 24 h after treatment. This was preceded by an increase in the extract-able biosynthetic enzymes of isoflavonoid for example L- PAL, Cinnamic acid 4-hydroxylase (CA4H), 4-coumarate COA ligase (4CL), CHS, CHI and Isoflavone O-methyl transferase, Isoflavone hydroxylase, Isoflavone reduc-tase, and pterocarpan synthase. Pectic polysaccharides are weak elicitors of PAL, therefore could enhance medicarpin concentration (Dalkin et al., 1990).

Some serious diseases on rice (*Oryza sativa*) as blast, which is caused by the fungus *Pyricularia oryzae*, lead to losses in productivity (Grayer and Kokubun, 2001). In fact, studies have been done to improve more resistant cultivars. The manipulation of defense mechanisms is one of the potential strategies to impart resistance in rice plants, which can be induced by a variety of biotic and abiotic factors (Li et al., 2014). Several diterpenoids, Momilactone A and B and Oryzalexins A–D (Fig. 3.4) were detected in rice tissue infected by *Pyricularia oryzae* and casbene was extracted from *Rhizopus stolonifera*, infected castor bean seedlings. Seven enzymes were found to be involved in casbene (from mevalonate to casbene) biosynthetic pathway, enhanced activities of casbene synthetase and farnesyl transferase were noticed in cell free extracts of castor bean seedlings after infection with *R. stolonifera* (Charles et al., 1990). The changes in enzymes activities after fungus exposure indicate that the elicitors released by the fungus are recognized by the host cells to trigger the defense response of the host.

Ajuha *et al*, have been also indicated that many diterpenoids such as momilactone A, B, and phytocassane A-E as well as flavonoids such as sakuranetin (5,4'-dihydroxy-7-methoxyflavanone) were isolated from infected rice (2012). The sakuranetin is an antifungal agent present in the rice leaves. it is produced at the moment of the pathogen invasion (Kodama et al., 1992a,b,c). Okada (2007) has been reported that the diterpenoid PhA are classified into four distinct types of polycyclic diterpenes based on the structure of their hydrocarbon diterpene precursors: phytocassanes A-E, A-F oryzalexins, momilactones A and B and oryzalexin S (Fig. 3.4). Two diterpenoids PhA has been reported; phytocassane F and ent-10-oxode-pressin (Inoue, 2013; Horie, 2015). The Momilactones A and B are potent antifungal agents against *Magnaporthe oryzae, Botrytis cinerae, Fusarium solani, Fusarium oxysporum, Colletrotichum gloesporides*. These PhA have potential antibacterial activity against *Escherichia coli, Pseudomonas ovalis, Bacillus pumilus* and *Bacillus cereus* (Fukuta et al., 2007).

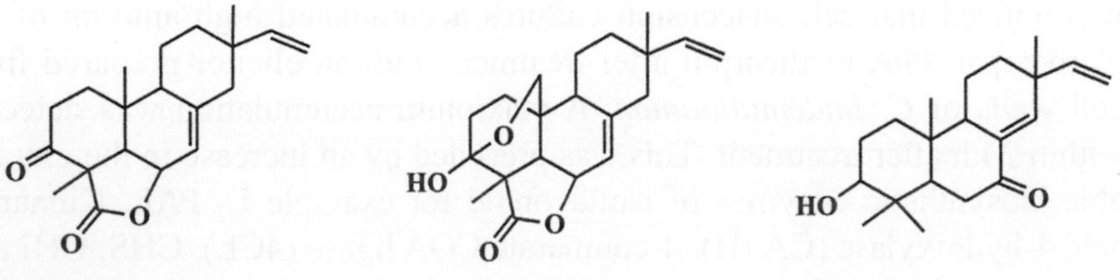

Mamlactone A	Mamlactone B	Oryzalexin A
Oryzalexin B	Oryzalexin C	Oryzalexin C
Oryzalexin D	Oryzalexin E	Oryzalexin S

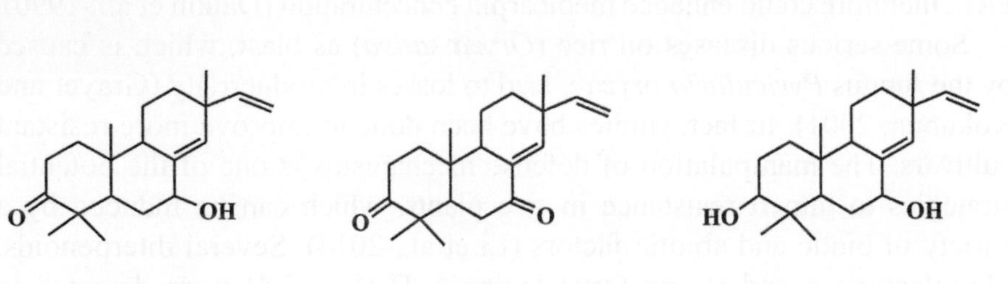

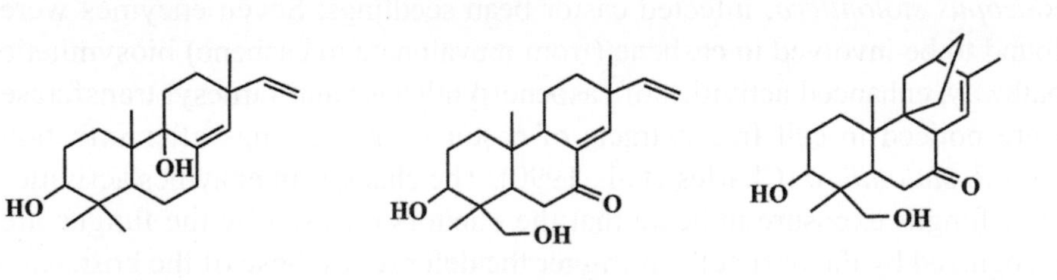

FIGURE 3.4 Chemical structure of PhA isolated from rice plants.

Diterpene PhA biosynthesis pathway of Momilactone and Oryzalexins in rice was postulated by Charles et al. (1990). Many authors suggested that geranylgeranyl-PP is considered to be an acyclic precursor of all cyclic diter-penes. Two modes of cyclization of geranylgeranyl-PP have been operated to afford bicyclic pyrophosphorylated intermediates 9βH-labdadienyI-PP and copalyl-PP as precursors of the Momilactone and Oryzalexin respectively. The cyclization activity was enhanced greatly by UV-irradiation (an abiotic PhA elicitor) of rice leaves. Diterpene products are accumulated in UV-irradiated rice leaf extract from geranylgeranyl-PP and copalyl-PP as substrates (Charles et al., 1990).

The production of stilbene PhA in various plants has also been reported. The heartwood of pine tree contains large amounts of stilbene, pinosylvin (23) and pinosylvin monomethyl ether (24) (Fig. 3.1). In young plants of *Pinus sylvestris*, the concentrations of these stilbenes were difficult to detect. However, at stress conditions, stilbene content is dramatically increased. Pinosylvin was considered to be the predominant PhA formed by pines and may be responsible for resistance. Only synthase acting upon cinnamoyl-CoA was the key enzyme for the formation of stilbenes. Pinosylvin was formed by Stilbene synthase which was isolated from UV light-treated 4 weeks of the old plants, purified and identified by Gehlert et al. (1990). The inoculation of pine seedlings with *B. cinerea* owing to a 38-fold high in stilbene synthase activity within a day. The rapid response might be measured prior to any detectable lesion, sclerotia or blight. Melchior and Kindl have also studied the mechanisms controlling the production of stilbene synthase and PAL "key regulatory enzymes of the biosynthetic pathway of stilbene PhA." The enzymes were induced in cell suspension cultures of grape (*Vitis cv* optima) by fungal (*Phytophthora cambivora*) cell wall. Both PAL and stilbene synthase mRNA were produced within 1 h by adding fungal cell wall preparations to the cell cultures. The majority of activity was reached within a maximum of 6 h and then declined (1991).

Similarly, the addition of *Phytophthora* sp. cell wall fragments or *Trichoderma viride* cellulase to tobacco cv. KY 14 cell suspension cultures enhanced the accumulation of the extracellular sesquiterpenoid PhA "capsidiol" and also enhance activities of both 3-hydroxy-3-methyl glutaryl coenzyme A reductase and sesquiterpene cyclase. These enzymes were involved in sesquiterpene biosynthetic pathway (Chappell et al., 1991). It appears from the above information that many key enzymes of PhA biosynthetic pathways played a pivotal role in PhA-regulation mechanisms.

3.6 INHIBITION/SUPPRESSION OF PhA PRODUCTION BY DIFFERENT MICROBIAL METABOLITES

It has been reported that infection of two carnation varieties, highly and moderately resistant to *Fusarium wilt* (caused by *F. oxysporum* f. sp. *dianthi*) stimulate the accumulation of PhA and aromatic acids. Pretreatment of plants with phenyl serine or SA diminished the PhA production and their resistance to infection (Niemann and Baayen, 1989). Etiolated hypocotyls of a resistant soybean cv. Harosoy 63 were susceptible to *P. megasperma* sp. *glycinea* race I after treated with abscisic acid. The susceptibility was manifested by increments in lesion size and a dramatic decrement in the accumulation of isoflavonoid PhA glyceollin. Nevertheless, PAL activity and accumulation of mRNA of this enzyme rapidly increased after infection in untreated hypocotyls. These increases were suppressed after treating the hypocotyls with abscisic acid. It has been suggested that the possibility of glyceollin biosynthesis in the resistance response of soybean may be controlled at the transcriptional level by changes in abscisic acid amount (Ward et al., 1989). Johal and Rahe noticed that *P. vulgaris* (bean plants) treated with glyphosate (2.5 µg), decreased the accumulation of PhA. The spreading lesions caused by *C. lindemuthianum* coalesced and rolled the entire hypocotyl. In contrast, the normal levels of PhA have been detected at infection sites in bean plants pretreated with a PAL. In addition to, lesions didn't spread. These results support the interpretation of the ability of glyphosate to decrease the accumulation of PhA that depends on the availability and demand for precursors such as PAL (1990).

Yoshioka et al., have been studied the effects of elicitor and suppressor of pisatin (25) (Fig. 3.1) released by *Mycosphaerella pinodes* (pea pathogen) on ATPase activity in the PM of etiolated pea epicotyls. They noticed that pisatin concentration induced by the elicitor was delayed for 3–6 h in the presence of orthovanadate or verapamil (100 PM). It was unaffected by the elicitor but was dramatically inhibited by suppressor from *M. pinodes* or verapamil. This result suggests that the ATPase played a pivotal role in pisatin accumulation (1990).

Yoshioka and Sugimoto (1993) demonstrated that soybean pathogen might induce an intracellular, branched β-1,3-glucan with suppressor activity with the cell wall-associated elicitors. This is a unique interaction at the site of receptor binding. The intracellular branched β-1,3- glucan claimed "mycolaminaran" was isolated and purified from the cytosol of *P. mega sperma* f. sp. *glycinea* which acted as a suppressor of glyceollin production in soybean cotyledons. The assumed mechanism of suppression of the PhA accumulation by mycolaminaran was suggested that the possibility to compete for the elicitor binding to the putative receptor in soybean membranes. Pisatin biosynthesis was also determined in pycnospore germination fluid of *M. pinodes*. The elicitor was detected as a polysaccharide and two suppressors were found to be glycopeptides. Eight species of pea (non-pathogens) established infection on pea leaves in presence of suppressor (Oku and Shiraishi, 1995).

A model system has been established to detect suppression of defense responses in bean by the compatible bacterium *P. syringae* pv. *phaseolicola*. Bean plants infiltrated with *P.s. phaseolicola* failed to induce transcript for a PAL. CS or CHI up to 120 h after infiltration and CHT (chitinase transcript) concentration was also significantly delayed when compared to the incompatible *P. syringae* strains. Bean plants infiltration with 10^8 cells/ml of *P.s. phaseolicola* NPS 3121, 8 h precede to infiltration with an equal amount of incompatible *P.s. pv. taba* Pt 11,528 significantly decreased the typical profile of defense transcript accumulation when compared to plants infiltrated with Pt 11,528 alone. Suppression of PhA concentration was also noticed. NPS 3121 suppressed PAL, CS, CHI, and CHT transcript concentrations and PhA accumulation induced by *Escherichia coli* or by the elicitor GSH. Heat-killed cells of both cells treated with protein synthesis inhibitors or NPS 3121, lost the suppressor activity. These findings suggested that NPS 3121 had an active mechanism to suppress the production of defense transcripts and PhA biosynthesis in bean (Jakobek et al., 1993).

Specific biosynthesis suppression of PhA (shikimate pathway in *Cassia obtusifolia*) by a sublethal dose (50 mM) of glyphosate has been shown to increase the susceptibility to the *Alternaria cassia* (mycoherbicide). Glyphosate utilized the conidia suppressed PhA synthesis at 12 h. Five times less inoculum was needed for the induction of disease symptoms after used with glyphosate. The PhA synthesis elicited by fungal inoculation was suppressed also by darkness (Sharon et al., 1992.

3.7   DEGRADATION OF PhA BY MICROBIAL ENZYMES

Virulence of organisms may depend upon its ability to degrade PhA (Desjardins et al., 1989; Miao and Van Etten, 1992). It is obvious that the control of degradation by using PhA-detoxifying enzymes inhibitors could promote plant disease resistance. Wyerone (26) (Fig. 3.1), is the predominant PhA induced by *Vicia faba*. Wyerone degradation by *Rhizobium leguminosarum* has been reported by George and Werner (1991). HPLC analysis of the medium during bacterial growth obviously indicated that *R. leguminosarum* was able to metabolize Wyerone, identified as hydroxyester wyerol.

N. haematococca on pea, virulence of *Gibberella pulicaris* on potato tubers and its association with a gene for rishitin metabolism were studied by Desjardins and Gardner (1991). The ability of field strains of *G. pulicaris* to trigger dry rot of potato tubers is relevant to their ability to metabolize rishitin (potato PhA). Genetic analysis of one potato pathogenic field strain R-6380 postulated that multiple loci may counter rishitin metabolism. More studies has disclosed that rishitin metabolism in str. R-6380 is controlled by genes at two or more loci but high virulence of *G. pulicaris* on a potato is related to only one of these loci, as Rim I (Desjardins and Gardner 1991). The ability of *B. cinerea* to degrade stilbenes produced by grapes has also been discussed in detail by Pezet et al. (1992).

3.8 PhA DETECTION METHODS

Shimizu et al., have been explored a protocol for precise quantification of phytocassanes and momilactones PhA compounds in rice, using HPLC and mass spectrometry (MS) with electrospray ionization as an analytical method. These PhA are commonly analyzed by using gas chromatography (GC). The authors confirm that use of HPLC method is more benefit than GC especially when HPLC coupled with MS in tandem which does not require sophisticated methods for purification and also no required high temperatures (2008).

Nugroho et al. (2002) have been investigating the accumulation of PhA produced in tobacco plants and they have shown that an efficient analytical method in the determination of sesquiterpene PhA, Capsidiol (27) (Fig. 3.1) is the use of a GC equipped with an autosampler and flame ionization detector. The detection of these PhA was done after the extraction process using ethanol, MeOH and chloroform and liquid nitrogen for plant maceration. Sakuranetin compound (28) (Fig. 3.1) was analyzed by injecting the leaf extract of rice using HPLC (RP-18 column) eluted with benzene-ethyl acetate-formic acid (10:1:1). The sakuranetin was detected by UV at λ 285 nm (Kodama et al., 1992a,b,c). Pedras et al. (2008) reported the identification of 23 cruciferous PhA by HPLC and MS using diode array detection.

Detection of PhA in a specific plant species supports the prospective findings of elicitors of active substances in plant defense against biotic stresses. The search for potential molecules might be extracted in large scale and be used to enhance other plants producing these substances, which is an effective mechanism that can give high protection to these plants. Plant extracts contain a diversity of secondary metabolites, which act synergistically to protect the plant against pathogens and can be used as a matrix for the isolation and synthesis of selective potent molecules, facilitating enormous amounts used. The synthesis of PhA mechanism has not been established yet and therefore the means of obtaining this is restricted to the process of isolation and determination, which requires a time, effort and lower yield, due to the lack of specific standards for such determination. The research also need to find the best elicitors for each species studied.

3.9 CONCLUSION AND SUMMARY

PhA are considered important for plant resistance toward pathogens, although the PhA of most plants are yet to be characterized. Recent studies on the PhA of some crop plants from different families have created information on basic parts of plant defenses, including how to improve control of the diseases. More importantly, efforts put in studying the regulation of PhA compound biosynthesis which led to the new description of possible signaling pathways. Nevertheless, the roles of each of these pathways under specific inducing conditions, as well as their interactions, needs to be well understood and one which requires more investigation. Moreover, the ways in which compounds act upon pathogens and the different mechanisms that some pathogens have developed to detoxify other compounds are also still poorly understood. PhA study has focused on both dicot species (e.g. Arabidopsis, peanut, and grapevine) and monocots (e.g. rice, maize, and sorghum), which has promoted our understanding of plant resistance mechanisms.

Moreover, PhA are components of the multiple mechanisms for disease resistance in plants. Studies on PhA have contributed to molecular biology and plant biochemistry. The study on the PhA should be integrated with genetical analyses in which the biochemical and physiological evidence are a key role for PhA in resistance. The study of molecular biology is a strategy that has been strongly analyzed due to the understanding of expressed genes which facilitates the elucidation of species with similar defense response characteristics that allows the extraction and elucidation of these PhA through a bank of genomic information. The use of more advanced techniques such as metabolomics and proteomics which are intended to qualify and quantify the set of metabolites induced by plant, are tools available that might be relevant to a complete process of the analysis of PhA. Research to detect the different mechanisms regulating PhA in various crop plants should have high potential in developing strategies to enhance and manipulate disease resistance in these plants. Novel approaches, such as genome-wide analyses, should start for studies of the regulatory networks controlling the metabolism of PhA and support for a better knowledge of the role of PhA in defense toward pathogens.

Prospects for further studies to evaluate the discovery of novel PhA identification mechanisms, and research that prove their activities and the application process for this mechanism to reduce production losses of important crops for human consumption. Obviously, future studies on these compounds will permit the researcher to investigate and evaluate plant-pathogen interactions and provide new techniques to control the diseases. All efforts in molecular biology and biotechnology should be geared toward the introduction of novel approaches to disease control that are environmentally friendly.

KEYWORDS

- phytoalexins
- plant defense
- pathogens
- antimicrobials
- disease resistance

REFERENCES

Abawi, G. S; VanEtten, H. D; Mai, W. F; J. Phaseollin Production Induced by Pratylenchus Pene- Trans in Phaseolusv Ulgaris. *J. Nematol.* **1971,** *3,* 301.

Afek, U; Sztejnberg, A. Scoparone, a phytoalexin Associated with Resistance of Citrus to *Phytophthora Citrophora. Phytopathology.* **1988,** *78,* 1678–1682.

Ahuja, I. et al., Phytoalexins in Defense Against Pathogens. *Trends Plant Sci.* **2012,** *17*(2), 73–90.

Akashi, T; Sasaki, K; Aoki, T; Ayabe, S; Yazaki, K. Molecular Cloning and Characterization of a cDNA for Pterocarpan 4-dimethylallyltransferase Catalyzing the Key Prenylation Step in the Biosynthesis of Glyceollin, a Soybean Phytoalexin. *Plant Physiol.* **2009,** *149*(2), 683–693. http://dx.doi.org/10.1104/pp.108.123679.

Al-Barwani, F. M.; Elated, E. A. Xanthotoxin and Other Furanocoumarins as Phytoalexins in Pastinaca sativa L. Roots. *SAQ J. Sci.* **2004,** *9,* 7–17.

Alghisi, P.; Favaron, F. Pectin-degrading Enzymes and Plant Parasite Interactions. *Euro. J. Plant Pathol.* **1995,** *101,* 365–375.

Allen, E. H.; Thomas, C. A. Trans-trans-3,11-tridecadiene-5,7,9-triyne-1,2-diol, an Antifungal Polyacetylene from Diseased Safflower (*Carthamus tinctorius*). *Phytochem.* **1971,** *10,* 1579–1582.

Anderson, A. J. The Biology of Glycoproteins as Elicitors. In *Plant Microbe Interactions*; Kosege, T., Nester, E. W., Ed.; McGraw-Hill: New York, 1989; Vol. 3.

Arruda, R. L.; Paz, A. T. S.; Bara, M. T. F.; Côrtes, M. V. C. B.; Filippi, M. C. C.; Conceição, E. C. An Approach on Phytoalexins: Function, Characterization and Biosynthesis in Plants of the Family Poaceae. *Ciência Rural.* **2016,** *46*(7), 1206–1216. https://dx.doi.org/10.1590/0103-8478cr20151164.

Ayers, A. R.; Valent B.; Ebel, J.; Albersheim P. Host-pathogen Interactions. XI. Composition and Structure of Wall-Released Elicitor Fractions. Plant Physiol. 1976, 57, 766.

Bailey, J. A.; Deverail B. J. Formation and Activity of Phaseollin in the Interaction between Bean Hypocotyls (*Phaseolus vulgaris*) and Physiological Races of *Colletotrichum Lindemuthianum* Physiol. *Plant. Pathol.* **1971,** *1,* 435–449.

Bailey, J. A. The Relationship between Symptom Expression and Phytoalexin Concentration in Hypocotyls of Phaseolu s Vulgaris Infected with Colletotrichum Lindemuthianum. Physiol. Plant Pathol. **1974,** 4, 477–488.

Bailey, J. A.; Burden, R. S.; Vincent, G. G. The Antifungal Activity of Glutinosone and Capsidiol and Their Accumulation in Virus-Infected Tobacco Species. *Physiol. Plant. Pathol.* **1976,** *8*(1), 35–41.

Bailey, J. A; Burden, R. S.; Vincent, G. G. Capsidiol: An Antifungal Compound Produced in Nicotiana Tabacum and N. Clevelandii Following Infection with Tobacco Necrosis Virus. *Phytochemistry.* **1975,** *14,* 597.

Bamji, S. F; Cynthia, C. Glyceollins: Soybean Phytoalexins that Exhibit a Wide Range of Health-Promoting Effects. *J. Funct. Foods.* **2017,** *34,* 98–110.

Bednarck, P. et al., Conservation and Clade-Specific Diversification of Pathogen-Inducible Tryptophan and Indole Glucosinolate Metabolism in Arabidopsis Thaliana Relatives. *New Phytol.* **2011,** *192,* 713–726.

Blein, J. P.; Mitat, M. L.; Ricci, P. Responses of Cultured Tobacco Cells to Cryptogein, a Proteinaceaus Elicitor from Phytophthora Cryptogea. *Plant Physiol.* **1991,** *95,* 486–491.

Boller, T.; Felix, G. A. Renaissance of Elicitors: Perception of Microbe-Associated Molecular Patterns and Danger Signals by Pattern-Recognition Receptors. *Annu. Rev. Plant Biol.* **2009,** *60,* 379–406.

Boue, S. M. et al., Phytoalexin-Enriched Functional Foods. *J. Agric. Food Chem.* **2009,** *57,* 2614–2622.

Boué, S. M.; Carter, C. H.; Ehrlich, K. C.; Cleveland, T. E. Induction of the Soybean Phytoalexins Coumestrol and Glyceollin by Aspergillus. *J. Agric. Food Chem.* **2000,** *48*(6), 2167–2172. http://dx.doi.org/10.1021/ jf9912809.

Braga, M. R. et al., Phytoalexins Induction in Rubiacea. *J. Chem. Ecol.* **1991,** *17,* 1079–1090.

Braga, M. R.; Dietrich, S. M. C. Defesas Químicas de Plantas: Fitoalexinas. *Acta Bot. Bras.* **1987,** *1*(1), 3–16.

Bridge, M. A; Klarmam, W. L. Soybean Phytoalexin, Hydroxyphaseollin, Induced by UV-Irradiation. *Phytopathology* **1973,** *63,* 606.

Brinker, A. M.; Seigler, D. S. Identification of Piceatannol as a Phytoalexin from Sugar Cane. *Phytochemistry* **1991,** *30,* 3229–3232.

Browne, L. M. et al., The Camalexins: New Phytoalexins Produced in the Leaves of Camelina Sativa (Cruciferae). *Tetrahedron* **1991,** *47,* 3909–3914.

Burden, R. S.; Bailey, J. A. Structure of the Phytoalexin from Soybean. Phytochemistry **1975,** *14*(5), 1389–1390. http://dx.doi.org/10.1016/S0031-9422(00) 98633-3.

Burden, R. S.; Kemp, M. S. (−)-7-hydroxycalamenene, a Phytoalexin from Tilia Europea. *Phytochem* **1983,** *22,* 1039–1040.

Cartwright, P. Isolation and Characterization of Two Phytoalexins from Rice as Momilactones A and B. Phytochemistry **1981,** *20,* 535–537.

Cavalcanti, L. S. et al., Aspectos Bioquímicos e Moleculares da Resistência Induzida. In *Indução de resistência em plantas a patógenos e insetos;* Cavalcanti, L. S. et al., Eds.; FEALQ: Piracicaba, 2005; pp 81–124.

Chaouch, S. et al., Peroxisomal Hydrogen Peroxide is Coupled to Biotic Defense Responses by Isochorismate Synthase1 in a Daylength-Related Manner. *Plant Physiol.* **2010**, *153,* 1692–1705.

Chappell, J.; Von Lanken, C.; Vogeli, U. Elicitorinducible 3-hydroxy-3-methylglutaryl Coenzyme A Reductase Activity is Required for Sesquiterpene Accumulation in Tobacco Cell Suspension Cultures. *Plant Physiol.* **1991,** *97,* 693–698.

Charles, A. W.; Augusto, F. L.; Karen, A. W.; Yue-Ying, R. Diterpenoid Phytoalexins: Biosynthesis and Regulation. In *Biochemistry of Mevalonic Acid Pathway to Terpenoids*; Neil Tower, G. H., Stafford, H. A., Eds.; Plenum: New York, 1990; pp 219–248.

Christensen, T. G. The Resistance of *Ginkgo biloba* to Fungi: Phytoalexin Production Induced by *Botrytis allii*. *Diss. Abstr. Int. B.* **1972**, *32,* 4340.

Chun, J. C.; Kim, J. K.; Hwang, I. T.; Kim, S. E. Acteoside from Rehmannia Glutinosa Nullifies Paraquat Activity in Cucumissativu. *Pestic. Biochem. Phys.* **2002**, *72,* 153–159.

Chung, K.-O.; Kim, B.-Y.; Lee, M.-H. et al. In-vitro and in-vivo anti-inflammatory effect of oxyresveratrol from Morus alba L. *J. Pharm. Pharmaco.* **2003**, *55,* 1695–1700.

Cline, S. D.; Coscia, C. J. Stimulation of Sanguinarine Production by Combined Fungal Elicitation and Hormonal Deprivation in Cell Suspension Cultures of Papaver Bracteatum. *Plant Physiol.* **1988**, *86,* 161–165.

Coleman, J. J. et al., An ABC Transporter and a Cytochrome P450 of Nectria Haematococca MPVI are Virulence Factors on Pea and are the Major Tolerance Mechanisms to the Phytoalexin Pisatin. *Mol. Plant Microbe Interact.* **2011**, *24,* 368–376.

Condon, P. et al., Production of 3-methyl-6-methoxy-8-hydroxy-3, 4-dihydroisocoumarin by Carrot Root Tissue. *Phytopathology.* **1963**, *53,* 1244–1250.

Coxon, D. T., et al. Identification of Three Hydroxyflavan Phytoalexins from Daffodil Bulbs. *Phytochem* **1980**, *19,* 889–891.

Coxon, D. T.; Curtis, R. F.; Howard, B. Ipomeamorone, a Toxic Furanoterpenoid in Sweet Potatoes (Ipomoea batatus) in the United Kingdom. *Food Cosmet. Technol.* **1975**, *13,* 87–90.

Cramer, C. L.; Ryder, T. B.; Bell, J. N.; Lamb, C. J. Rapid Switching of Plant Gene Expression Induced by Fungal Elicitor. *Science.* **1985**, *277,* 1240–1242.

Croteau, R.; Gurkewitz, S.; Johnson, M. A.; Fisk, H. J. Monoterpene and Diterpene Biosynthesis in Lodgepole Pine Saplings Infected with *Ceratocystis clavigera*. *Plant Physiol.* **1987**, *85,* 1123–1128.

Cruickshank, I. A. M.; Biggs, D. R.; Perrin, D. R.; Whittle, C. P. Phaseollin and phaseollidin relationships in infection-droplets on endocarp of *Phaseolus vulgaris*. *Physiol. Plant. Pathol.* **1974**, *4,* 261–276.

Daayf, F.; Schmidt, A.; Belanger, R. R. Phytoalexins in Cucumber Leaves Infected with Powdery Mildew. *Plant Physiol.* **1997**, *113,* 719–727.

Dalkin, K.; Edwards, R.; Edington, B.; Dixon, R. A. Stress Responses in Alfalfa (Medicago sativa L.). I. Induction of Phenyl Propanoid Biosynthesis and Hydrolytic Enzymes in Elicitor-Treated Cell Suspension Cultures. *Plant Physiol.* **1990**, *92,* 440–446.

Daniel, S.; Barz, W. Elicitor-induced Metabolic Changes in Cell Cultures of Chick Pea (Cicer Arietinum Cultivars Resistant and Susceptible to Ascochyta Rabiei. Il. Differential Induction of Chalconesynthase–mRNA Activity and Analysis of in Vitro Translated Protein Patterns. *Planta* **1990**, *82,* 279–286.

Daniel, S.; Tiemann, K.; Wittkampf, U.; Bless, W.; Hinderer, W.; Barz, W. Elicitor-induced Metabolic Changes in Cell Cultures of Chick Pea (Cicer Arietinum L) Cultivars Resistant and Susceptible to Ascochyta Rabiei. I. Investigations of Enzyme Activities Involved in Isoflavone and Pterocarpan Phytoalexin Biosynthesis. *Planta.* **1990**, *82,* 270–278.

Darvill, A. G.; Albersheim, P. Phytoalexins and their Elicitors-A Defense Against Microbial Infection in Plant. *Annu. Rev. Plant Physiol.* **1984**, *35,* 243–275.

Denby, K. J. et al., Ups1, an Arabidopsis thaliana Camalexin Accumulation Mutant Defective in Multiple Defence Signalling Pathways. *Plant J.* **2005**, *41,* 673–684.

Desjardins, A. E.; Gardner, H. W.; Plattner, R. D. Virulence of Gibberella Pulicaris on Potato Tubers and its Relationship to the Gene for Rishitin Metabolism. *Phytopathology* **1991**, *81,* 429–435.

Desjardins, A. E.; Gardner, H. W.; Plattner, R. D. Detoxification of the Potato Phytoalexin Lubimin by Gibberella Pulicaris. *Phytochemistry* **1989**, *28,* 431–437.

Devaiah, S. P. et al., Induction of Systemic Resistance in Pearl Millet (*Pennisetum glaucum*) Against Downy Mildew (*Sclerospora graminicola*) by *Datura metel* Extract. *Crop. Protection.* **2009**, *28*(9), 783–791. DOI: 10.1016/j.cropro.2009.04.009. http://www.sciencedirect.com/science/article/pii/S0261219409000982. (accessed: Out. 01, 2015).

Dhawale, S.; Sonciet, G.; Kuhn, D. N. Increase of Chalcone Synthase mRNA in Pathogen Inoculated Soybeans with Race-Specific Resistance is Different in Leaves and Roots. *Plant Physiol.* **1989**, *91,* 911–916.

Dillon, V. M; Overton, J; Grayer, R. J; Harborne, J. B. Differences in Phytoalexin Response Among Rice Cultivars of Different Resistance to Blast. *Phytochemistry* **1997**, *44,* 599–603.

Dixon, R. A.; Harrison, M. J.; Lamb, C. J. Early Events in the Activation of Plant Defense Responses. *Annu. Rev. Phytopathol.* **1994**, *32,* 479–501.

Dixon, R. A; Paiva, N. L. Stress-induced Phenylpropanoid Metabolism. *Plant Cell.* **1995**, *7*(7), 1085–1097.

Dixon, R. A.; Dey, P. M.; Lamb, C. J. Phytoalexins: Enzymology and Molecular Biology. *Adv. Enzymol. Relat. Areas Mol. Biol.* **1983**, *53,* 1–36.

Dixon, R. A.; Lamb, C. J. Molecular Communication in Interaction between Plants and Microbial Pathogens. *Annu. Rev. Plant Physiol Plant Mol. Biol.* **1990**, *41,* 339–367.

Domingo, D.; Lopez-Brea, M. Plantas Com Acción Antimicrobiana. *Revista Española de Quimioterapia* **2003**, *16*(4), 385–393.

Ebel, J. Phytoalexin Synthesis: The Biochemical Analysis of the Induction Process. *Annu. Rev. Phytopathol.* **1986**, *24*(1), 235–264. http://dx.doi.org/ 10.1146/annurev.py.24.090186.001315.

Echeverri, F.; Torres, F.; Cardana, W. Q. G; Archbold, R.; Roldan, J.; Brita, I.; Luis, J. G.; Lahlen. Danielone, a Phytoalexin from Papaya Fruit, *Carica papaya. Phytochemistry* **1997**, *44,* 255–256.

Ejike, C. E. C. C. et al., Phytoalexins from the Poaceae: Biosyntesis, Function and Prospects in Food Preservation. *Food Rev. Int.* **2013**, *52*(1), 167–177.

El Modafar, C.; Clerivet, A.; Fleuriet, A.; Macheix, J. J. Inoculation of *Platanus acerifolia* with *Ceratocystis fimbriata. Phytochemistry* **1993**, *34,* 1271–1276.

Elliger, C. A.; Halloin, J. M. Phenolics Induced in *Beta vulgaris* by *Rhizoctonia solani* Infection. *Phytochemistry* **1994**, *37,* 691–693.

Eromosele, O.; Bo, S.; Ping, L. Induction of Phytochemical Glyceollins Accumulation in Soybean Following Treatment with Biotic Elicitor (Aspergillus oryzae). *J. Funct. Foods.* **2013**, *5*(3), 1039–1048. http://dx.doi.org/10.1016/ j.jff.2013.02.010.

Fukuta, M. et al., Comparative Efficacies in Vitro of Antibacterial, Fungicidal, Antioxidant, and Herbicidal Activities of Momilactones A and B. *J. Plant Interact.* **2007**, *2,* 245–251.

Gehlert, R.; Schoppner, A.; Kindl, H. Stilbene Synthase from Seedlings of Pinus Sylvestirs: Purification and Induction in Response to Fungal Infection. *Mol. Plant Microbe Interact.* **1990,** *3,* 444–449.

Geigert, J. et al. Two Phytoalexins from Sugarbeet (Beta vulgaris) Leaves. *Tetrahedron 1973,* *29,* 2703–2706.

George, E.; Werner, D. Degradation of Wyerone, the Pnytoalexin of Faba Bean Rhizobium Leguminosarum. *Curr. Microbiol.* **1991,** *23,* 153–157.

Giesemann, A.; Biehl, B.; Lieberii, R. Identification of Scopoletin as a Phytoalexin of the Rubber Tree *Hevea brasiliensis. J. Phytopathol.* **1986,** *117,* 373.

Grayer R. J.; Kokubun, T. Plant-fungal Interactions: the Search for Phytoalexins and Other Antifungal Compounds from Higher Plants. *Phytochemistry 2001,* *56,* 253–263.

Gundlach, H.; Muller, M. J.; Kutchan, T. N.; Zenk, M. H. Jasmonic Acid is a Signal Transducer in Elicitor-induced Plant Cell Cultures. *Proc. Natl. Acad. Sci. U. S. A.* **1992,** *89,* 2389–2393.

Hahn, M. G.; Darvill, A.; Albersheim, P.; Bergmann, C.; Cheong, J. J.; Koller, A.; Lo, V. M. Preparation and Characterization of Oligosaccharide Elicitors of Phytoalexin Accumulation. In *Molecular Plan Pathology: A Practhical Approach*; Gurr, S. J.; McPherson, M. J.; Bowles, D. J. Eds.; IRL Press: Oxford, New York, Tokyo, 1992, Vol. 2.

Hain, M. G.; Darvill A.; Albersheim, P.; Bergamann, C.; Cheong, J.-J.; Koller, A.; Lo V.-M. Preparation and Characterization of Oligosaccharide Elicitors of Phytoalexin Accumulation. In *Molecular Plant Pathology: A Practical Approach*; Gurr, S. J.; Mcpherson, M. J.; Bowles, D. J. Eds.; OIRL Press: Oxford, 1992; Vol. 11, pp 103–147, 304.

Hain, R.; Reif, H. J.; Krause, E.; Langebartels, R.; Kindl, H.; Vernau, B.; Weise, W.; Schmatzer, E.; Schreier, P. H. Disease Resistance Results from Foreign Phytoalexin Expression in a Novel Plant. *Nature* **1993,** *361,* 153–156.

Hano, C.; Addi, M.; Bensaddek, L.; Crônier, D. et al., Differential Accumulation of Monolignol-Derived Compounds in Elicited Flax (Linumusitatissimum) Cell Suspension Cultures. *Planta: An Integr. J. Plant Biol.* **2006,** *223,* 975–989.

Hans, G.; Jurgen, E. Phytoalexins, Chemical Defense Substances of Higher Plants? *Angew. Chem. Int. Ed. Engl.* **1978,** *17,* 635–647.

Harborne, J. B. The Comparative Biochemistry of Phytoalexins Induction in Plants. *Biochem. Syst. Ecol.* **1999,** *27,* 335–367. DOI: 10.1016/S0305-1978(98)00095-7.

Harding, V. K.; Heale, J. B. The Accumulation of Inhibitory Compounds in the Induced Resistance Response of Carrot Root Slices to Botrytis Cinerea. *Physiol. Plant Pathol.* **1981,** *18,* 7–15.

Hartmann, G., Nienhaus, F. The Isolation of Xanthoxylin from the Bark of Pbytophthora- and Hendersonula-infected Citrus limon and its Fungitoxic Effect. *J. Phytopathol.* **1974,** *81,* 97–113.

Hashimoto, T., Hasegawa, K., Kawarada, A. Batatasins: New Dormancy-inducing Substances of Yam Bulbils. *Planta (Berl.)* **1972,** *108,* 369–374.

Hirai, N.; Ishida, H.; Kashimizu, K. A Phenalenone-type Phytoalexin from *Musa Accuminata. Phytochemistry* **1994,** *37,* 383–385.

Holland, K. W.; O'Keefe, S. F. Recent Applications of Peanut Phytoalexins. *Recent Pat. Food Nutr. Agric.* **2010,** *2,* 221–232.

Holscher, D.; Dhakshinamoorthy, S.; Rony, L. S. Phenalenone-type Phytoalexins Mediate Resistance of Banana Plants (Musa spp.) to the burrowing nematode Radopholussimilis. *Proc. Natl. Acd. Sci.* **2014,** *111,* 105–110.

Horie, K. et al., Identification of UV-induced Diterpenes Including a New Diterpene Phytoalexin, Phytocassane F, from Rice Leaves by Complementary GC/MS and LC/ MS Approaches. *J. Agric. Food Chem.* **2015,** *63*(16), 4050–4059. DOI: 10.1021/acs. jafc.5b00785.

Huang, L. D; Backhouse, D. Effects of *Fusarium* Species on Defence Mechanisms in Sorghum Seedlings. *N. Z. Plant Prot.* **2004,** *57,* 121–124. DOI: 10.1111/j.1439-0434.2005.01013.x.

Huffaker, A. et al., Novel Acidic Sesquiterpenoids Constitute a Dominant Class of Pathogen-induced Phytoalexins in Maize. *Plant physiol.* **2011,** *156,* 2082–2097. DOI: 10.1104/ pp.111.179457.

Ingham, J. L.; Harborne, J. B. Phytoalexin Induction as a New Dynamic Approach to the Study of Systematic Relationships Among Higher Plants. *Nature* **1976,** *260,* 241–243.

Inoue, Y. et al., Identification of a Novel Casbane-Type Diterpene Phytoalexin, ent-10-Oxodepressin, from Rice Leaves. *Biosci. Biotechnol. Biochem.* **2013,** *77*(4), 760–765. DOI: 10.1271/bbb.120891.

Isaac, I. C.; Johnson, T. J.; Berhow, M.; Baldwin, E. L.; Karki, B.; Woyengo, T.; Gibbons, W. R. Evaluating the Efficacy of Fungal Strains to Stimulate Glyceollin Production in Soybeans. *Mycol. Prog.* **2017,** *16*(3), 223–230. http://dx.doi.org/10.1007/s11557-017-1269-1.

Jahangir, M. et al., Health-affecting Compounds in Brassicaceae. *Compr. Rev. Food. Sci. Food Saf.* **2009,** *8,* 31–43.

Jakobek, J. L.; Smith, J. A.; Lindgren, P. B. Sup- pression of Bean Defense Responses by Pseudomonas Syringae. *Plant Cell.* **1993,** *5,* 57–63.

Jeandet, P. et al., Modulation of Phytoalexin Biosynthesis in Engineered Plants for Disease Resistance. *Int. J. Mol. Sci.* **2013,** *14,* 14136–14170. DOI: 10.3390/ijms140714136.

Johal, G. S.; Rahe, J. E. Role of Phytoalexins in the Suppression of Resistance of Phaseolus Vulgaris to Colletotrichum Lindemuthianum by Glyphosate. *Can. J. Pl. Pathol.* **1990,** *12,* 225–235.

Johnson, N. C. et al. Xanthotoxin: A phytoalexin of Pastinaca sativa root. *Phytochem.* **1973,** *12,* 2961–2962.

Kanzaki, H.; Kagemori, T.; Yamachika, Y.; Nitoda, T.; Kawazu, K. Inhibition of Plant Transformation by Phytolaccoside B from Phytolaccaamericana Callus. *Biosci. Biotechnol. Biochem.* **1999,** *63,* 1657–1659.

Keen, N. T. Hydroxyphaseollin Production by Soybeans Resistant and Susceptible to Phytophthora Megasperma var. sojae. *Physiol. Plant. Pathol.* **1971,** *1,* 265–275.

Keen, N. T.; Littlefield, L. J. The Possible Association of Phytoalexins with Resistant Gene Expression in Flax to Melamspora Lini. *Physiol. Plant Pathol.* **1975,** *14,* 275–280.

Keen, N. T; Horsch, R. Hydroxy-phaseollin Production by Various Soybean Tissues: a Warning Against the Use of "unnatural" Hostparasite Systems. *Phytopathology* **1972,** *62,* 439–442.

Keen, N. T; Kennedy, B. W. Surface Glycoproteins: Evidence that they May Function as the Race Specific 'phytoalexin. *Physiol. Plant. Pathol.* **1974,** *4,* 173–185.

Keen, N. T.; Partridge, J. E.; Zaki, A. I. Pathogen-produced Elicitor of a Chemical Defense Mechanism in Soybean Mono-genically Resistant to Phytophthora Megasperma var. sojae. *Phytopathology* **1972,** *62,* 768.

Keen, N. T.; Sims, J. J.; Erwin, D. C.; Rice, E.; Partridge, J. E. 6-a-Hydroxyphaseollin, an Antifungal Chemical Induced in Soybean Hypocotyls by Phytophthora Megasperma Var. sojae. *Phytopathology* **1971,** *61,* 1084–1089.

Kessmann, H.; Choudhury, A. D.; Dixon, R. A. Stress Responses in Alfalfa (Medicago sativa L.). Ill. Induction of Medicarp in and Cytochrome P450 Enzyme Activities in Elicitor Treated Cell Suspension Cultures and Protoplasts. *Plant Cell Rep.* **1990,** *9,* 38–41.

Khan, A. J.; Kunesch, G.; Chuilan, S.; Revise, A. Xanthyletin, a New Phytoalexin of Citrus. *Fruits (Paris)* **1985**, *40,* 807–811.

Kim, H. J.; Suh, H. J.; Kim, J. H.; Park, S.; Joo, Y. C.; Kim, J. S. Antioxidant Activity of Glyceollins Derived from Soybean Elicited with Aspergillus Sojae. *J. Agric. Food Chem.* **2010a,** *58*(22), 11633–11638. http://dx.doi.org/10.1021/jf102829z.

Kim, H. J.; Suh, H. J.; Lee, C. H.; Kim, J. H.; Kang, S. C.; Park, S.; Kim, J. S. Antifungal Activity of Glyceollins Isolated from Soybean Elicited with Aspergillus Sojae. *J. Agric. Food Chem.* **2010b,** *58*(17), 9483–9487. http://dx. doi.org/10.1021/jf101694t.

Kim, H. J.; Sung, M. K.; Kim, J. S. Anti-inflammatory Effects of Glyceollins Derived from Soybean by Elicitation with Aspergillus Sojae. *Inflammation Res.* **2011,** *60*(10), 909–917. http://dx.doi.org/10.1007/s00011-011-0351-4.

Kodama, O. et al., Sakuretin, a Flavanone Phytoalexin from Ultraviolet–Irradiated Rice Leaves. Phytochemistry **1992c,** *31*(11), 3807–3809. DOI: 10.1016/S0031-9422(00)97532-0.

Kodama, O.; Li, W. X.; Tamogami, S.; Akatsuka, T. Oryzalexin S, a Novel Stemarane-type Diterpene Rice Phytoalexin. *Biosci. Biotech. Biochem.* **1992b,** *56,* 1002–1003.

Kodama, O.; Miyakawa, J.; Akatsuka, T.; Kiyosawa, S. Sakuranetin, a New Flavonoid-Type Rice Phytoalexin from Ultraviolet-irradiated Rice Leaves. *Phytochemistry* **1992a,** *31,* 3807–3813.

Kodama, O.; Suzuki, T.; Miyokawa, J.; Akatsuka, T. Ultraviolet Induced Accumulation of Phytoalexines in Rice Leaves. *Agr. Biol. Chem.* **1988,** *52,* 2469–2473.

Koga, J.; Ogawa, N.; Yamauchi, T.; Kikuchi, M.; Ogasawara, N.; Shimura, M. Functional Moiety for the Antifungal Activity of Phytocassene, a Diterpene Phytoalexin from Rice. *Phytochemistry* **1997,** *44,* 249–254.

Kokubun, T.; Harbrone, J. B. Phytoalexin Induction in the Sapwood of Plants of the Maloideae (Rosaceae): Biphenyls or Dibenzofurans. *Phytochemistry* **1995,** *40,* 1649–1654.

Komaraiah, P.; Reddy, G. V.; Reddy, P. S.; Raghavendra, A. S.; Ramakrishna, S. V.; Reddanna, P. Enhanced Production of Antimicrobial Sesquiterpenes and Lipoxygenase Metabolites in Elicitor-treated Hairy Root Cultures of Solanum Tuberosum. *Biotech. Lett.* **2003,** *25,* 593–597.

Kumar, S. G. Engineering Cottonseed for use in Human Nutrition by Tissue-specific Reduction of Toxic Gossypol. *Proc. Nat. Acad Sci.* **2006,** *103,* 18054–18059.

Kumar, S; Shukla, R. S; Singh, K. P; Paxton, J. D; Husain, A. Glyceollin: a Phytoalexin in Leaf Blight of *Costus speciosus*. *Phytopathology* **1984,** *74,* 1349–1352.

Lamb, C. J.; Lawton, M. A.; Dron, M.; Dixon, R. A. Signals and Transduction Mechanisms for Activation of Plant Defenses Against Microbial Attack. *Cell.* **1989,** *56,* 215–224.

Langcake, P.; Cornford, C. A.; Pryce, R. J. Identification of Pterostilbene as a Phytoalexin from Vitis vinifera Leaves. *Phytochem* **1979,** *18,* 1025–1027.

Lee, C. W. et al., Momilactones A and B in Rice Straw Harvested at Different Growth Stages. Bioscience Biotechnology and Biochemisty. **1999,** *63,* 1318–1320, DOI: 10.1271/ bbb.63.1318, http://www.tandfonline.com/doi/abs/10.1271/bbb.63.1318. (accessed: Ago. 23, 2015).

Li, Y. et al., Comparative Proteomic Analysis of Methyl Jasmonate Induced Defense Responses in Different Rice Cultivars. *J. Proteomics* **2014,** *14*(9), 1088–10101. DOI: 10.1002/pmic.201300104.

Lo, S. C; Weiergong, I; Bonham, R; Hipskind, J; Wood, K; Nicholson, R. L. Phytoalexin Accumulation in Sorghum, Identification of a Methyl Ether of Luteolinidin. *Physiol. Mol. Plant Pathol.* **1996,** *44,* 21–31.

Luis, J. G; Echeverri, F; Quinones, W; Brito, I; Lopez, M; Torres, F. Irenolane and Emenolone: Two New Types of Phytoalexin from *Musa paradisiaca*. *J. Org. Chem.* **1993**, *58*, 4306–4308.

Mansfield, J. W. Antimicrobial Compounds and Resistance: the Role of Phytoalexins and Antianticipins. In *Mechanisms of Resistance to Plant Diseases;* Slusarenko, A. J., Fraser, R. S. S, Van Loon, L. C., Ed.; Kluwer: Amsterdam, 1999.

Mansfield, J. W. Role of Phytoalexins in Disease Resistance. In *Phytoalexins*; Mansfield, J. W., Bailey, J., Ed.; Blackie: Glasgow, 1982.

Marti, S. S. Accumulation of the Flavonoids Betagarin and Betavulgarin in Beta Vulgaris Infected by the Cercosporabeticola. *Physiol. Plant Pathol.* **1977**, *11*, 297–303.

Mateos, R. G; Leal, R. P. Fitoalexinas: Mecanismo de Defense de Las Plantas. *Rev. Chapingo Ser. Cie.* **2003**, *9*(1), 5–10.

Meier, F. G.; Remphrey, W. R. Accumulation of Mansonones in Callus Cultures of Ulmusamericana L. in the Absence of a Fungal-derived Elicitor. *Canad J. Bot.* **1997**, *75*, 513–517.

Mert-Türk, F.; Bennett, M. H.; Glazebrook, J.; Mansfield, J.; Holub, E. Biotic and Abiotic Elicitation of Camalexin in Arabido Psisthaliana. *7th International Congress of Plant Pathology.* Edinburgh, Scotland, UK, 1998.

Mezencev, R.; Gailzzi, M.; Kutschy, P.; Docampo, R. Trypanosoma Cruzi: Antiproliferative Effect of Indole Phytoalexins on Intracellular Amastigotes in Vitro. *Exp. Parasitol.* **2009**, *122*, 66–69.

Miao, V. P. W.; Van Etten, H. D. Three Genes for Metabolism of the Phytoalexin Maackiain in the Plant Pathogen Nectria Haematococca: Meiotic Instability and Relationship to a New Gene for Pisatin Demethylase, *Appl. Environ. Microbiol.* **1992**, *58*, 801–808.

Mikkelsen, M. D. et al., Modulation oh CYP79 Genes and Glucosilate Profiles in Arabidopsis by Defense Pathways. *Plant physiol.* **2003**, *131*, 298–308. DOI: 10.1104/pp.011015.

Monde, K.; Kishimoto, M.; Takasugi, M. Yurinelide, a Novel 3-benzylidene-1,4-Benzodioxin-2(3H) One Phytoalexin from *ilium maximowiezii*. *Tetrahedron Lett.* **1992**, *33*, 5395–5398.

Muller, K. O.; Börger, H. Experimentelle Untersuchungen über die Phythophthora-Resistenz der Kartoffel. Zugleich ein Beitrag zum Problem der 'erworbenen Resistenz' im Pflanzenreich. Arbeiten der Biologischen Reichsanstalt für Land- und Forstwirtschaft. **1940**, *23*, 189–231.

Nawrath, C.; Métraux, J. P. Salicylic Acid Inductiondeficient Mutants of Arabidopsis Express PR-2 and PR-5 and Accumulate High Levels of Camalexin After Pathogen Inoculation. *Plant Cell.* **1999**, *11*, 1393–1404.

Ng, T. B; Ye, X. J; Wong, J. H; Fang, E. F; Chan, Y. S; Pan, W.; Wang, H. X. Glyceollin, a Soybean Phytoalexin with Medicinal Properties. *Appl. Microbiol. Biotechnol.* **2011**, *90*(1), 59–68. http://dx.doi.org/10.1007/ s00253-011-3169-7.

Nicholson, R. L; Kollipara, S. S; Vincent, J. A; Lyons, P. C; Gomez, G. C. Phytoalexin Synthesis by the Sorghum Mesocotyl in Response to Infection by Pathogenic and Non-Pathogenic Fungi. *Proc. Nat. Acad. Sci.* **1987**, *84*, 5520–5524.

Niemann, G. J.; Baayen, R. P. Inhibitory Effects of Phenylserine and Salicylic Acid on Phytoalexin Accumulation in Carnations Infected by Fusarium Oxysporum f. sp. Dianthi. *Mededelingen Van de Faculteit Land bouwwetens chappen Rijksuni; Versiteit Gent.* **1989**, *54*, 435–438.

Nugroho, L. H. et al., It is the Accumulation of Sesquiterpenephytoalexins Induced in Plants Tobacco Constitutively Producing Salicylic Acid? *Plant Sci.* **2002**, *162*(6), 989–993. DOI: 10.1016/S0168-9452(02)00049-3.

Ogawa, S.; Miyamoto, K.; Nemoto, K.; Sawasaki, T.; Yamane, H.; Nojiri, H.; Okada, K. OsMYC2, an Essential Factor for JA-inductive Sakuranetin Production in Rice, Ineracts with MYC2-like Proteins that Enhance its Tranactivation Ability. *Sci. Rep.* **2017,** *7,* 40175.

Okada, A. et al., Elicitor Induced Activation of the Methylerythritol Phosphate Pathway Toward Phytoalexins Biosynthesis in Rice. *Plant Mol. Biol.* **2007,** *65,* 177–187. DOI: 10.1007/s11103-007-9207-2.

Oku, H.; and Shiraishi, T. Phytoalexins and Host Specificity. In *Handbook of Phytoalexin Metabolism and Action*; Daniel, M., Purkayastha, R. P. Eds.; Marcel Dekker, Inc.: New York, 1995; pp 41–60.

Oku, H; Nahanishi, T; Shiraishi, T; Ouchi, S. Phytoalexin Induction by Some Agricultural Fungicides and Phytotoxic Metabolites of Pathogenic Fungi. *Sci. Rep. Fac. Agric. Okayama Univ.* **1973,** *42,* 17.

Park, S.; Ahn, I. S.; Kim, J. H.; Lee, M. R.; Kim, J. S.; and Kim, H. J. Glyceollins, One of the Phytoalexins Derived from Soybeans Under Fungal Stress, Enhance Insulin Sensitivity and Exert Insulinotropic Actions. *J. Agric. Food Chem.* **2010,** *58*(3), 1551–1557. http://dx.doi.org/10.1021/jf903432b.

Park, H. L. et al., Transcriptomic Analysis of UV-treated Rice Leaves Reveals UV-induced Phytoalexin Biosynthetic Pathways and their Regulatory Networks in Rice. *Phytochem* **2013,** *96,* 57–71.

Paul, W. P.; Dmitrieva, N.; Tom, J. M. Phytoalexinaurone Induced in Cephalocereussenilis Liquid Suspension Culture. *Phytochem* **1991,** *30,* 1133–1135.

Paxton, J. D. Phytoalexins a Working Redefinition. *Phytopathol* **1980,** *132,* 1–45.

Pedras, M. S. C. et al., Phytoalexins from Crucifers: Synthesis, Biosynthesis and Biotransformation. *Phytochem* **2000,** *53,* 161–176.

Pedras, M. S. C. et al., The Phytoalexins from Cultivated and Wild Crucifers: Chemistry and Biology. *Nat. Prod. Rep.* **2011,** *28,* 1381–1405.

Pedras, M. S. C.; Adio, A. M. Phytoalexins and Phytoanticipins from the Wild Crucifers Thellungiella Halophila and Arabidopsis Thaliana: Rapalexin A, Wasalexins and Camalexin. *Phytochemistry* **2008,** *69,* 889–893.

Perrin, D. R. P.; Bottomley, W. Studies on Phytoalexins. V. The Structure of Pisatin from Pisumsativum L. *J Am. Chem. Soc.* **1962,** *84,* 1919–1922.

Pezet, R.; Pont, V.; Hoang-Van, K. Enzymatic Detoxification of Stilbenes by Botrytis Cinerea and Inhibition by Grape Berries Proanthocyanidins; in Recent Advances in Botrytis Research; *Proc. 10th Int. Botrytis symp*; Verhoeff, K.; Malathrakis, N. E.; Williamson, B. Eds.; Pudoc Sc. Publishers: Netherlands, 1992; pp 87–92.

Pieterse, C. M. J. et al., Rhizobacteria-mediated Induce Systemic Resistance: Triggering, Signaling, and Expression. *Eur. J. Plant Pathol.* **2001,** *107,* 51–61. DOI: 10.1023/A:1008747926678.

Poloni, A., Schirawski, J. Red card for pathogens: Phytoalexins in sorghum and maize. *Molecules.* **2014,** *19,* 9114–9133.

Powell, R. G; Tepaske, M. R; Plattner, R. D; White, J. F; Clement, S. L. Isolation of resveratrol from *Festuca versuta* and evidence for its widespread occurrence in the Poaceae. *Phytochemistry.* **1994,** 35, 335.

Purkayastha, R. P. Progress in Phytoalexin Research During the Past 50 Years. In *Handbook of Phytoalexin Metabolism and Action*; Daniel, M., Purkayastha, R. P., Eds.; Marcel Dekker, Inc.: New York, 1995; pp 1–39.

Rahe, J. E; Arnold, R. M. *Phytopathology.* **1975,** 53, 921.

Ranga, R. V.; Ramachanddram, M., Arunachalam, V. An Analysis of Association of Components of Yields and Oil in Safflower (Carthamustinctorius). *Theor. Appl. Genet.* **1977**, *50*, 185–91.

Rathmell, W. G.; Bendall, D. S; *Physiol. Plant, Patholo.* **1971**, 1, 351.

Rejanne, L. A; Andressa, T. S. P; Maria, T. F. B.; Márcio, V. C. B. C.; Marta, C. C. F.; Edemilson, C. C. An Approach on Phytoalexins: Function, Characterization and Biosynthesis in Plants of the Family Poaceae. *Ciência Rural, Santa Maria.* **2016**, *46*(7), 1206–1216.

Resende, M. L. V.; Flood, J.; Ramsden, J. D.; Rowan, M. G.; Beal, M. H.; Cooper, R. M. Novel Phytoalexins Including Elemental Sulphur in Resistance of Cocoa (*Theotroma cacao.*) to *Verticillium* wilt (*Verticillium dahliae* Kleb.). *Physiol. Mol. Plant Pathol.* **1996**, *48*, 347–355.

Rich, J. R; Keen, N. T; Thomason, I. J; *Physiol. Plant. Pathol.* **1977**, *10*, 105.

Robbins, M. P.; Hartnoll, J.; Morris, P. Phenyl Propanoid Defense Responses in Transgenic Lotus Corniculatus. 1. Glutathione Elicitation of Isoflavan Phytoalexins in Transformed Root Cultures. *Plant Cell. Rep.* **1991**, *10*, 59–62.

Roetschi, A. et al., Characterization of an Arabidopsis–Phytophthora Pathosystem: Resistance Requires a Functional PAD2 Gene and is Independent of Salicylic Acid, Ethylene and Jasmonic Acid Signalling. *Plant J.* **2001**, *28*, 293–305.

Salvo, V. A; Boue, S. M.; Fonseca, J. P.; Elliott, S.; Corbitt, C.; Collins-Burow, B. M.; Burow, M. E. Antiestrogenic Glyceollins Suppress Human Breast and Ovarian Carcinoma Tumorigenesis. *Clin. Cancer Res.* **2006**, *12*(23), 7159–7164. http://dx.doi.org/10.1158/1078-0432.CCR-06-1426.

Schmelz, E. A. et al., Identity, Regulation, and Activity of Inducible Diterpenoid Phytoalexins in Maize. *Proc. Natl. Acad. Sci. U. S. A.* **2011**, *108*, 5455–5460.

Seifert, K.; Hartling, S.; Porzel, A.; Johne, S.; Krauss, G. Phytoalexin Accumulation in Ornithopus Sativus as a Response to Elicitor Treatment. *Z. Naturforsch. Sect. C. Biosci.* **1993**, *48*, 550–558.

Sharon, A.; Amsellen, Z.; Gressel, J. Glyphosate Suppression of an Elicited Defense Response Increased Susceptibility of Cassia Obtusifolia to a Mycoherbicide. *Plant Physiol.* **1992**, 98, 654–689.

Shimizu, T. et al., Effects of a Bile Acid Elicitor, Acid Cholic, on the Biosynthesis of Diterpenoid Phytoa Lexin in Suspension Cultured Rice Cells. *Phytochemistry.* **2008**, *69*(4), 973–981.

Shrikanta, A.; Kumar, A.; Govindaswamy, V. Resveratrol Content and Antioxidant Properties of Underutilized Fruits. *J. Food Sci. Tech.* **2015**, *52*, 383–390.

Sitton, D., West, C. A. CASBENE: an antifungal diterpene produced in cell-free extracts of Ricinus communis seedlings. *Phytochem.* **1975**, *14*, 1921–1925.

Smith, C. J. Accumulation of Phytoalexins: Defense Mechanism and Stimulus Response System. *New Phytol.* **1996**, *132*(1), 1–45.

Smoliga, J. M. et al., Resveratrol and Health – a Comprehensive Review of Human Clinical Trials. *Mol. Nutr. Food Res.* **2011**, *55*, 1129–1141.

Stholasuta, S.; Bailey, J. A.; Severin, V.; Deverall, B. J. Effect of Bacterial Inoculation of Bean and Pea Leaves on the Accumulation of Phaseollin and Pisatin. *Physiol. Plant. Pathol.* **1971**, *1*, 177–183.

Stipanovic, R. D.; Puckhaber, L. S.; Bell, A. A.; Percival, A. E.; Jacobs, J. Occurrence of (+)- and (−)-Gossypol in Wild Species of Cotton and in Gossypiumhirsutum Var. Marie-Galante (Watt) Hutchinson. *J. Agric. Food Chem.* **2005**, *53*, 6266–6271.

Strobel G. A. Bacterial Phytotoxins. *Annu. Rev. Microbiol.* **1977,** *31,* 205–224.

Takasugi, M. et al., Structures of Moracins E, F, G and H, New Phytoalexins from Diseased Mulberry. *Tetrahedron Lett.* **1979,** *28,* 4675–4678.

Takasugi, M.; Katui, N. A Biphenyl Phytoalexin from Cercidiphyllum Japonicum. *Phytochem.* **1986,** *25,* 2751–2752.

Takeuchi, Y.; Yoshikawa, M.; Horino, O. Immunological Evidence that B-l,3-Endoglucanase is the Major Elicitor-Releasing Factor in Soybean. *Am. Phytopathol. Soc. Jen.* **1990,** *56,* 523–531.

Thomma, B. P. H. J. et al., Deficiency in Phytoalexin Production Causes Enhanced Susceptibility of Arabidopsis Thaliana to the Fungus Alternaria Brassicicola. *Plant J.* **1999,** 19, 163–171.

Tierens, K. F. M. J. et al., Esa1, an Arabidopsis Mutant with Enhanced Susceptibility to a Range of Necrotrophic Fungal Pathogens, Shows a Distorted Induction of Defense Responses by Reactive Oxygen Generating Compounds. *Plant J.* **2002,** *29,* 131–140.

Toyomasu, T. et al., Diterpene Phytoalexins are Biosynthesized in and Exuded from the Roots of Rice Seedlings. *Biosci. Biotechnol. Biochem.* **2008,** *72*(2), 562–567.

Tsai, P. C.; Chu, C. L.; Fu, Y. S.; Tseng, C. H.; Chen, Y. L.; Chang, L. S.; Lin, S. R. Naphtho[1,2-b]furan-4,5-dione Inhibits MDA-MB-231 Cell Migration and Invasion by Suppressing Src-Mediated Signaling Pathways. *Mol. Cell Biochem.* **2014,** *387,* 101–111.

Turgeon, G.; Yoder, O. Genetically Engineered Fun S for Weed Control. In *Biotechnology Applications and Research*; Cheremisinoff, P. N., Quellette, R. P., Eds.; Technomic Publ.: Lancaster, 1985; pp 221–230.

Tverskoy, L.; Dmitriev, A.; Kozlovsky, A.; Grodzinsky, J. Two Phytoalexins from *Allium cepa* Bulbs. *Phytochemistry* **1991,** *30,* 799–800.

Uritani, I. et al., Similar Metabolic Alterations Induced in Sweetpotato by Poisonous Chemicals and by Ceratostomella Fimbriata. *Phytopathology* **1960,** *50,* 30–34.

Van Etten, H. D.; Matthews, D. E.; Matthews, P. S. Phytoalexin Detoxification; Importance for Pathogenicity and Practical Implications. *Annu. Rev. Phytopath.* **1989,** *27,* 143–164.

Van Etten, H. D.; Mansfield, J. W.; Bailey, J.; Farmer, E. E. Letter to the Editor: two Classes of Plant Antibiotics: Phytoalexins Versus Phytoanticipins. *Plant Cell.* **1994,** 1191–1192.

Van Wees, S. C. et al., Characterization of the Early Response of Arabidopsis to Alternaria Brassicicola Infection Using Expression Profiling. *Plant Physiol.* **2003,** *132,* 606–617.

Varns, J. L.; Currier, W. W.; Kuc, J. Specificity of Rishitin and Phytuberin Accumulation by Potato. J. *Phytopathol.* **1971,** *71,* 968–971.

Viswanathan, R.; Mohanraj, D.; Padmanaban, P.; Alexander, K. C. Accumulation of 3-Deoxyanthocyanidin Phytoalexins Luteolindin and Apigeninidin in Sugarcane in Relation to Red Rot Disease. *Indian Phytopathol.* **1996,** *49,* 174–175.

Vranova, E. C. D.; Gruissem, W. Network Analysis of the MVA and MEP Pathways for Isoprenoid Synthesis. *Rev. Plant Biol.* **2013,** *64,* 665–700.

Ward, E. W. B. et al., Loroglossol: an Orchid Phytoalexin. *Phytopathology.* **1975,** *65,* 632–633.

Ward, E. W. B.; Cahill, D. M.; Bhattacharyya, M. K. Abscisic Acid Suppression of Phenylalanine Ammonia Lyase Activity and mRNA and Resistance of Soybeans to Phytophthora Megasperma f. sp. Glycinea. *Plant Physiol.* **1989,** *91,* 23–27.

Wei, L. L.; Kuhn, D.; Nicholson, R. L. Chalcone Synthase Activity in Sorghum Mesocotyls Inoculated with Colletotriclnon Graminicola. *Physiol. Mol. Pl. Pathol.* **1989,** *35,* 413–422.

Welle, R.; Grisebach, H. Induction of Phytoalexin Synthesis in Soybean: Enzymatic Cyclization of Prenylated Pterocarpans to Glyceollin Isomers. *Arch. Biochem. Biophys.* **1988,** *263*(1), 191–198. http://dx.doi.org/10.1016/ 0003-9861(88)90627-3.

Wharton, P.; Nicholson, R. Temporal Synthesis and Radio Labelling of the Sorghum 3-Deoxyanthocyanidin Phytoalexins and the Anthocyanin, Cyanidin 3-dimalonyl Glucoside. *New Phytopatol.* **2000,** 145, 457–469.

Widyastutfi, S. M.; Nonaka, F.; Watanabe, K.; Sako, N.; Tanaka, K. Isolation and Characterization of Two Aucuparin-Related Phytoalexins from Photiniaglabra Maxim. *Ann. Phytopathol. Soc. Japan.* **1992,** 58, 228–233.

Wijnsma, R.; Verpoorte, R.; Mulder-Krieger, T.; Svendsen, A. B. Anthraquinones in Callus Cultures of Cinchona Ledgeriana. *Phytochem* **1984,** 23, 2307-2311.

Yang, L. et al., Sorghum 3-deoxyanthocyanins Possess Strong Phase II Enzyme Inducer Activity and Cancer Cell Growth Inhibition Properties. *J. Agric. Food Chem.* **2009,** 57, 1797–1804.

Yoneyama, K.; Akashi, T.; Aoki, T. Molecular Characterization of Soybean Pterocarpan 2-dimethylallyltransferase in Glyceollin Biosynthesis: Local Gene and Whole-Genome Duplications of Prenyltransferase Genes Led to the Structural Diversity of Soybean Prenylated Isoflavonoids. *Plant Cell Physiol.* **2016,** 57(12), 2497–2509. http://dx.doi. org/10.1093/pcp/pcw178.

Yoshioka, M.; Sugimoto, K. A Fungal Suppressor of Phytoalexin Production Competes for the Elicitorreceptor Binding. *Naturwissenschaften* **1993,** 80, 374–376.

Yoshioka, H.; Shirarishi, T.; Yamada, T.; Ichinose, Y.; Oku, H. Suppression of Pisatin Production and ATPase Activity in Pea Plasma Membranes by Orthovanadate, Verapamil and Supiressor from *Mycosphaerella Pinodes. Plant Cell Physiol.* **1990,** 31, 1139.

Zhang, H. et al., *Arabidopsis* At ERF15 Positively Regulates Immunity Against *Pseudomonas syringae* pv. tomato DC3000 and *Botrytis Cinerea. Front. Plant Sci.* **2015,** 6, 686–699.

Zhang, J.; Zhou, J. M. Plant Immunity Triggered by Microbial Molecular Signatures. *Mol. Plants* **2010,** 3(5), 783–793.

Zhang, Y. et al., The Genetic and Molecular Basis of Plant Resistance to Pathogens. *J. Genet. Genomics* **2013,** 40(1), 23–35.

Zhao, J. M. et al., Induction of Arabidopsis Tryptophan Pathway Enzymes and Camalexin by Amino Acid Starvation, Oxidative Stress, and an Abiotic Elicitor. *Plant Cell.* **1998,** 10, 359–370.

CHAPTER 4

BIOLOGICAL ROLES OF PHYTOCHEMICALS

PECULIAR FEENNA ONYEKERE[*,1],
CHIOMA OBIANUJU PECULIAR-ONYEKERE[2],
HELEN OGECHUKWU UDODEME[1],
DANIEL OKWUDILI NNAMANI[1], and
CHRISTOPHER OBODIKE EZUGWU[1]

[1]Department of Pharmacognosy and Environmental Medicines, University of Nigeria, Nsukka, 410001, Enugu State, Nigeria

[2]Department of Microbiology, University of Nigeria, Nsukka, 410001, Enugu State, Nigeria

*Corresponding author. E-mail: peculiar.onyekere@unn.edu.ng
ORCID: https://orcid.org/0000-0001-8063-1301

ABSTRACT

Globally, there is a growing need for the search of chemical compounds from natural sources for the treatment of human chronic diseases such as diabetes, microbial infections, cancer, and so forth. Over the years plants have become a major source of such chemical compounds known as phytochemicals with different medicinal and biological activities. The aim of this topical study is to provide a succinct knowledge on the biological roles of phytochemicals. This would serve as a veritable resource in the area of phytochemistry. There are many phytochemicals that can be found in plants. This chapter focuses on eight major phytochemicals found in most plants; tannins, saponins, alkaloids, flavonoids, glycosides, oxalates, protease inhibitors, and amylase inhibitors. Most phytochemicals are obtained from the seeds, fruits, bark, and leaves of different medicinal plants or legumes. Their different biological roles such as antioxidant, antibacterial, antitumor, antidiabetic, antiviral activities, and so forth, have been discussed.

4.1   INTRODUCTION

Generally, phytochemicals are plant-derived chemical compounds that thrive or thwart predators, competitors, or pathogens (Kaufman et al., 2000). They are broadly categorized into primary and secondary metabolites. The secondary metabolites function in a defensory capacity against herbivores, insects, pathogens, or adverse growing conditions. They are present naturally in plants and are necessary for its conventional cellular and physiological functions (Horvath, 1981), hence they must be supplied from the diet (Ashutosh, 2008; Evans, 2009).

These phytochemicals can be obtained from different sources of plants and plant parts such as bark, leaves, fruits, seeds, and so forth. They are known to have various biological roles in man and animals. This ranges from antibacterial, antioxidant, anticancer effects, and so forth (Ashutosh, 2008).

Due to the diverse chemical properties of individual compounds, the biological effects of the various phytochemicals differ remarkably (Kaufman et al., 2000). The diverse structures and properties and their essential biological roles are discussed in this chapter.

4.2   MAJOR PHYTOCHEMICALS OF PLANT ORIGIN

The major phytochemicals mostly found in plant sources are listed below: tannins, saponins, alkaloids, glycosides, oxalates, protease inhibitors, and amylase inhibitors.

4.2.1   TANNINS

Tannins (Fig. 4.1) are complex substances that are ubiquitously distributed among plants and localized in the leaves, fruits, barks, or stems of plants. They combine with protein and precipitate them out of solution which is their main characteristic property. They are also complex with organic compounds such as amino acids, alkaloids, and some essential metals like iron and calcium to form insoluble tannates which are extremely valuable in the antidotal treatment of alkaloid, iron, and calcium poisoning. Tannins have a bitter taste which helps prevent damage to plants by insects and fungi (Ashutosh, 2008).

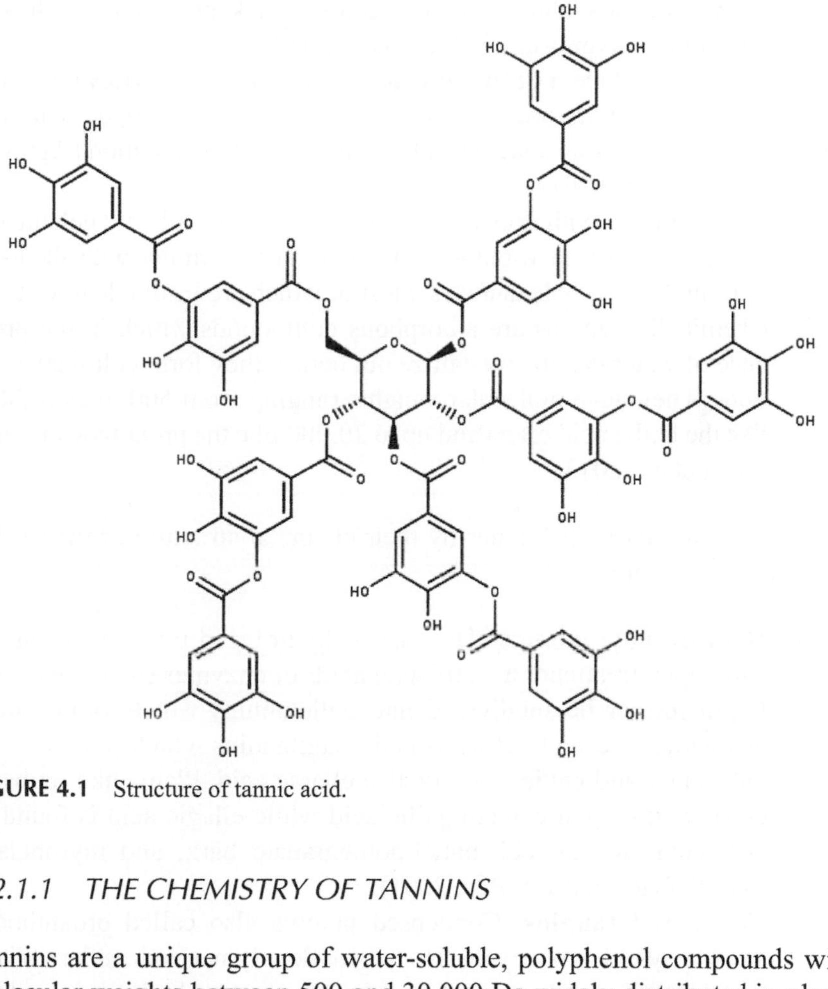

FIGURE 4.1 Structure of tannic acid.

4.2.1.1 THE CHEMISTRY OF TANNINS

Tannins are a unique group of water-soluble, polyphenol compounds with molecular weights between 500 and 30,000 Da widely distributed in plants as defined by Bate-Smith and Swain (1962). They can complex strongly with carbohydrates, proteins, and alkaloids. Some of its physical and chemical properties are:

1. Tannins appear as light yellow or white amorphous powders or shiny, nearly colorless masses.
2. Tannins are known to have characteristic bitter (astringent) taste and strange smell.
3. Tannins are freely soluble in water, glycerol, alcohol, acetone, and dilute alkalis. They are sparingly soluble in chloroform, ethyl acetate, and other organic solvents.

4. They give dark-blue color or greenish-black precipitate with iron compounds (Agrawal and Paridhavi, 2012).
5. Tannins produce a deep red color with potassium ferricyanide and ammonia and are precipitated by metallic salts of copper, lead, tin, and also by strong aqueous potassium dichromate solution (Agrawal and Paridhavi, 2012).
6. They combine with skin and hide to form leather and with gelatin and isinglass to form an insoluble compound. They combine with alkaloids to form the insoluble tannates, most of which are insoluble in water.
7. Chemically, tannins are amorphous compounds which in the presence of water cannot crystallize out hence, they form colloidal solutions. They have molecular weights ranging from 500 to over 3000 like the gallic acid esters and up to 20,000 like the proanthocyanidins (Teng et al., 2013).

Tannins can be divided either by their chemical structure or their solubility and extractability.

a) **Hydrolyzable tannins:** This can be hydrolyzed into simpler molecules upon treatment with mineral acids or enzymes such as tannase. It can further be subdivided into gallotannins which yields sugar and gallic acid on hydrolysis and ellagitannins which produces not only sugar and gallic acid but also ellagic acid. Plants like rhubarb, clove, and nutgall contain gallic acid while ellagic acid is found in eucalyptus leaves, oak bark, pomegranate bark, and myrobalans (Khanbabaee and van Ree, 2001).

b) **Condensed tannins**: Condensed tannins also called proanthocyanidins, yield anthocyanidins when depolymerized under oxidative conditions. They are, however, resistant to hydrolysis and do not contain sugar moiety (Khanbabaee and van Ree, 2001). Their building blocks include catechins and flavonoids which are esterified with gallic acid. This class of tannins differs from the hydrolyzable tannins in that on treatment of acids or enzymes, they are converted to red complex insoluble compounds called phlobaphenes, which give a characteristic red color to many drugs such as red cinchona bark that contains phlobatannins and their composition products. They are also sometimes called catechol tannins because on dry distillation, they yield catechol as the end product. Examples of plants containing condensed tannins are: cinchona bark, male fern, tea leaves, wild cherry bark, and cinnamon bark.

c) **Complex tannins:** This is a combination of either gallotannin or ellagitannin unit from the hydrolyzable tannins and the catechin unit of condensed tannins. The monomers of this class have been isolated in some plant families like Combretaceae, Fagaceae (e.g., *Quercus robur, Castanea sativa*) Mytarceae, Polygonaceae, and Theaceae (Ashutosh, 2008).

d) **Pseudotannins**: These are phenolic compounds of lower molecular weight than the true tannins. They differ from the hydrolyzable and condensed tannins since they do not change color during the Gold-beater's skin test and so cannot be used as tanning compounds. Some examples of pseudotannins and their sources are gallic acid found in rhubarb crystallizable catechins found in catechu, cutch; chlorogenic acid found in cocoa, coffee, nux vomica, and ipecacuanha tannins found in ipecacuanha root (Ashutosh, 2008).

4.2.1.2   SOURCES OF TANNINS

Food rich in tannins include:

1. Beverages such as red wine, tea, apple juice, beer, and so forth.
2. Chocolates and coffee powder which have the high-tannin content unlike milk and white chocolate that have less.
3. Legumes such as chickpeas, beans, black-eyed peas, and lentils that have high protein and low-fat content also contain high levels of tannins. Those with darker colors such as red or black beans are known to contain more tannin as compared with light-colored legumes like white beans (Horvath, 1981).
4. Fruits such as apples, grapes, pomegranates, and berries (blueberries, blackberries, cherries, and cranberries) have tannins concentrated in their peels.
5. Vegetables like squash, rhubarb, and herbs and spices such as cinnamon, thyme, cumin, tarragon, cloves, and vanilla (Ashutosh, 2008).

4.2.1.3   BIOLOGICAL ROLES OF TANNINS

A number of observable biological actions and pharmacological activities have been attributed to tannin-containing food and plant extract due to their astringent, hemostatic, and antiseptic properties (Ashutosh, 2008):

1. **Antimicrobial activity:** Tannins are capable of disrupting the extracellular microbial enzymes, thereby depriving the microbes the necessary substrates required for microbial growth. Tannins also act directly on the microbial metabolism through inhibition of oxidative phosphorylation (Akiyama, 2001; Scalbert, 1991).

2. **Anti-inflammatory activity:** Tannins are useful remedies for toothache, pain, and inflammation. Food rich in tannins has been helpful in controlling all indications of gastritis, esophagitis, enteritis, and irritating bowel disorders (Chamakuri, 2015).

3. **Antioxidant activity:** Both hydrolyzable and condensed tannins are potentially very important biological antioxidants as they scavenge free radicals in the body. The polyphenolic nature of tannic acid, its relatively hydrophobic "core" and hydrophilic "shell," as well as the tannin-protein complexes formed, are the features responsible for its antioxidant action (Gunnars and Lars, 2009; Parmar, 2015).

4. **Anticancer activity:** The ability of tannins to inhibit active oxygen, scavenge free radicals, and inhibit the growth of tumors has made it a useful compound in cancer therapy (Ashutosh, 2008; Parmar, 2015; Yamada, 2012).

5. **Anti-allergic activity:** Studies have shown that tannins are capable of inhibiting allergic reactions and may be useful for the treatment or prevention of allergic diseases (Gunnar and Lars, 2009; Kojima, 2000).

4.2.2 SAPONINS

Saponins are structurally complex glycosidic compounds with diverse physical, chemical, and biological functions. They are amorphous in nature with high-molecular weight and are widely recognized for their soapy lather when agitated in water, hence, the name "saponins." This ability to froth is a distinguishing feature for their identification in plant species. They have other properties that are peculiar to particular types of saponins such as their hemolytic activity, bitterness, and cholesterol-binding properties.

The hydrolysis of saponin yields an aglycone (sapogenin) and aglycone (sugar). Saponins are classified based on the nature of their aglycone, which includes those bearing a steroidal aglycone and those bearing a triterpenoid aglycone. Steroidal saponins are present in vast amounts in nature especially among plants such as tomato, yam, pepper, oat, allium, and so forth (Oakenfull, 1981). Triterpenoid saponins are present in *Solanum* spp., potato, peppers, and tomatoes and have been reported to have toxic effects. The structural and unique diversity of saponins is reflected in their diverse biological and physicochemical properties which have been harnessed for a number of traditional applications such as the production of soaps, molluscicides, and fish poison. There had been limited application of saponins in food due to its bitter taste which erroneously leads to its removal by early researchers in a bid to facilitate human consumption. However, recent research highlighted the increasing health benefits of saponins in lowering cholesterol as well as its anticancer properties. Also, the health benefits of foods such as soybeans and garlic have been attributed to their saponin content (Guclu-Ustundag and Mazza, 2007).

4.2.2.1   CHEMISTRY OF SAPONINS

Saponins (Figs 4.2 and 4.3) are glycosidic compounds that contain one or more sugar chains (pentoses, hexoses, or uronic acid) on either a triterpenoid or a steroidal aglycone backbone (He et al., 2010). The aglycone nature, the functional group on its backbone, and the number and nature of its sugar varies greatly; hence, it is widely diverse (Guclu-Ustundag and Mazza, 2007).

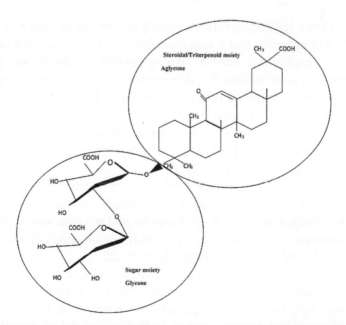

FIGURE 4.2   General structure of saponins showing its steroidal and sugar moieties.

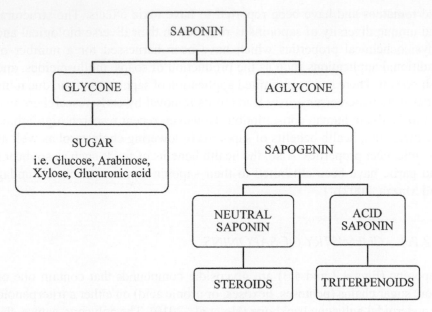

FIGURE 4.3   Diagrammatic representation of saponins.

The physical and chemical properties of saponins are as follows:

1. Saponins are amphiphilic in nature due to the presence of a lipid-soluble aglycone and a water-soluble sugar chain in their structure. Their amphiphilic attribute is responsible for its diverse physical properties such as its ability to act as surface active agents/surfactants, emulsifying agents, and form stable foams (He et al., 2010).

2. They also have a strong hemolytic activity and can form micelles just like detergents. This diversity of physical properties has been exploited technologically in the manufacturing of carbonated drinks and shampoo (Negi et al., 2013).

3. The physicochemical and biological properties of saponins are modified by their interaction with sterols, proteins, and minerals. The interaction of sterols (cholesterol and phytosterols) with steroid (saponins, alfalfa saponins and triterpenoid saponins) form water-insoluble additional products (He et al., 2010).

4. Saponins undergo chemical transformations during storage and processing, which has a significant effect on their pharmacological properties. Heating in the presence of water, acids/alkali, enzymes, and microbial activity causes hydrolysis of the glycosidic (bond

between the sugar chain and aglycone) and interglycosidic bonds (bond between the sugar residues) leading to the formation of aglycones, sugar residues, monosaccharides, and prosapogenins (Negi et al., 2013). Acid hydrolysis yields aglycone and monosaccharides while alkaline hydrolysis yields prosapogenins (Guclu-Ustundag and Mazza, 2007).

4.2.2.2   SOURCES OF SAPONINS

Foods rich in saponins include the following (Oakenfull, 1981):

- Legumes and beans such as kidney beans, chickpeas, soybeans, navy beans, and so forth, are very rich in saponins. Soybeans are actually one of the major sources of dietary saponins and can be prepared in various ways. Another notable source of dietary saponins is chickpeas.
- The rhizome and root of liquorice (*Glycyrrhiza glabra*) are important sources of saponin and thus used as a condiment/flavoring agent in cooking. They are also used in the tobacco industry.
- Oats, quinoa, and amaranth are rich sources of saponins.
- Garlic and vegetables such as alfalfa sprouts, peas, yucca, and asparagus are rich sources of saponin.
- Red wine is also a rich source of saponin, although the type of wine determines the quantitative content of the saponin. The saponin content of wine is derived from the coating on the skin of the grapes that are used in wine production.
- The bark of *Quillaja saponaria* (soap tree) are rich sources of saponin (about 10%) and are used as a medium for extracting saponin for commercial purposes. The saponin from *Quillaja* is used as foaming agent in the food industry.
- Animals like sea cucumber (marine invertebrate) also contain saponins; however, the amount of saponin depends on the type of the animal. These animals can be either be eaten raw, for example, sushi or cooked in different ways (Sparg et al., 2004).

4.2.2.3   BIOLOGICAL ROLES OF SAPONINS

Saponins possess an extremely diverse range of biological activities ranging from its role as an adjuvant, anti-inflammatory agent, antioxidant, antiparasitic, antispasmodic, antiphlogistic, antipsoriatic, antiprotozoal, antipyretic, antimutagenic, anti-allergic, anti-edematous to its effect on absorption of minerals and vitamins, cognitive behavior, animal growth, and reproduction (Das et al., 2012; Egbuna and Ifemeje, 2015)

a) **Hemolytic activity:** Saponins are capable of lysing erythrocytes. They do this by forming pores on the cell membrane thereby increasing its permeability and subsequent bursting. This has been attributed to the affinity between the aglycone moiety (in the saponin) and the phospholipids on the cell membrane which leads to the formation of insoluble complexes. The deleterious effect of saponin on the lipid bilayers is irreversible as saponin-lysed erythrocytes are incapable of resealing. Escin saponins present in *Aesculus hippocastanum* L. (Hippocastanaceae) and jujuboside saponins from *Zizyphus jujuba* Mill. (Rhamnaceae) have strong hemolytic activity.

b) **Immunological adjuvant:** Saponins improve the effectiveness of vaccines administered orally by enhancing the immune response to antigens. They also enhance assimilation of large molecules and have immunostimulatory effects. *Q. saponaria* is mainly used for the industrial production of saponin adjuvants (Das et al., 2012).

c) **Cholesterol-lowering effect:** The cholesterol-lowering effect of saponin has been observed in human and animal studies. Animals fed with saponin-rich diets (soybean, chickpea, alfalfa, etc.) had lower plasma and liver cholesterol levels. This attribute is based on the ability of saponin to inhibit the absorption of cholesterol from the small intestine and the reabsorption of bile acids (Guclu-Ustundag and Mazza, 2007).

d) **Anticancer effect:** Triterpene and steroidal saponins have been reported to have anticancer activities. The National Cancer Institute has identified protoneodioscin, protodioscin (furastanol saponins isolated from the rhizomes *of Dioscorea collettii*) methyl proto-neogracillin, and methyl protogracillin (steroidal saponins extracted from the rhizomes of *D. collettii*), as potential anticancer agents (Thakur et al., 2011).

e) **Antimicrobial effects:** Oleanolic acid (the most common triterpene saponin aglycone) has been reported to possess antiviral and anti-bacterial activities. When surgical site infections were stimulated in a wound model using BALB/c mice, Diosgenyl 2-amino-2-deoxy-β-D-glucopyranoside was reported to be effective against

Enterococcus faecalis and *Staphylococcus aureus.* Saponins from *Q. saponaria* have been reported to have antiviral activity against the rhesus rotavirus in BALB/c mice. CAY-1 (a steroidal saponin) extracted from the fruit of *Capsicum frutescens* L. (Solanaceae) was observed to be a potent antifungal agent as well as having anti-yeast properties (Das et al., 2012).

f) **Tumor-suppressive effects:** Saponin has been observed to have anti-tumor suppressive effects. They are capable of enhancing the specificity of target cells such as the reported observation in increasing the toxicity and synergism of specific ribosome-inactivating proteins at sub-micellar levels (Das et al., 2012).

4.2.3 ALKALOIDS

Alkaloids are an enormously large and diverse family of naturally occurring nitrogen-containing compounds. They are secondary metabolites produced by a wide variety of plants (i.e., potato, tomato, etc.), animals (i.e., shellfish), and even microorganisms such as mushroom and bacteria. They have diverse pharmacological applications and can be used as recreational drugs, medications (i.e., quinine, the antimalarial drug), as well as an analgesic. Some alkaloids are bitter, that is, caffeine and can be purified from crude extracts by simple acid–base extractions (Edeoga and Eriata, 2001; Babbar, 2015).

Alkaloids can be broadly classified according to four different schemes namely:

1. **Taxonomy:** Alkaloids are classified exclusively based on taxa such as family, genus, specie, subspecie. Examples of plant families (i.e., natural order) and their associated species are:

   • Solanaceous alkaloids, for example, *Atropa belladonna, Mandragora officinarum, Capsicum annuum* L., *Solanum dulcamara,* and so forth.
   • Cannabinaceous alkaloids, for example, *Cannabis sativa.*
   • Rubiaceous alkaloids, for example, *Mitragyna speciosa, Cinchona* sp.
   • Based on genus, we have *Ephedra, Cinchona,* coca, and so forth.

2. **Pharmacology**: Alkaloids are classified based on their pharmacological activity as they exhibit a wide range of pharmacological

characteristics such as analgesics (morphine), antimalarial (quinine), oxytocic (ergonovine), neuaralgia (aconitine), choleretics, and laxatives (boldine), reflex excitability (lobeline), antiglaucoma agent (pilocarpine), bronchodilator (ephedrine), and so forth (Babbar, 2015). The alkaloids in this group do not have any chemical or structural similarity.

3. **Biosynthesis:** Here, alkaloids are classified based on the precursors utilized by plants to synthesize the compound regardless of their pharmacological characteristics and taxonomic distribution. Examples include:

   • Indole alkaloids from tryptophan.
   • Imidazole alkaloids from histidine.
   • Piperidine alkaloids from lysine.
   • Phenylethylamine alkaloids from tyrosine.
   • Pyrrolidine alkaloids from ornithine.

4. **Chemical classification:** Alkaloids are classified into two major categories based on their basic ring structure, that is, the presence or absence of a heterocyclic nucleus.

4.2.3.1   NON-HETEROCYCLIC ALKALOIDS

As the name implies, they lack a heterocyclic ring in their nucleus. It includes:

   • Phenylethylamine: The alkaloids contain phenylethlamine as their basic ring structure (Fig. 4.4). Examples are narceine (*Papaver somniferum*), ephedrine (*Ephedra vulgaris*), mescaline (*Laphophora williamsii*), hordenine (*Hordeum vulgare*), capsaicin (*Capsicum annunum*), and so forth.

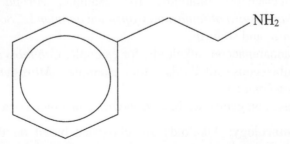

FIGURE 4.4   Phenylethylamine.

4.2.3.2 HETEROCYCLIC ALKALOIDS

Heterocyclic alkaloids (Fig. 4.5) contain a heterocyclic ring in their nucleus (Babbar, 2015). They include:

- Pyrrolidine: They contain pyrrolidine as their basic ring structure. Examples are hygrine (*Erythroxylon coca*), stachydrine (*Stachys tuberifera*).
- Pyridine: They contain pyridine as their basic ring structure. Examples are arecoline (*Areca catechu*), ricinine (*Ricinus communis*).
- Piperidine: They contain piperidine as their basic ring structure. Examples are coniine (*Conium maculatum*), lobeline (*Lobelia inflata*).
- Tropane (piperidine–pyrrolidine): Tropane is their basic ring structure. Examples are atropine (*Atropa belladonna*), cocaine (*E. coca*) (Griffin and Lin, 2000).
- Quinoline: Here, quinoline is the basic ring structure. Examples are quinine and quinidine (*Cinchona officinalis*), cuspareine (*Cusparia trifoliata*).
- Isoquinoline: The basic ring structure is isoquinoline. Examples are berberine (*Hydrastis canadensis*), Papaverine (*P. somniferum*).
- Aporphine (reduced isoquinoline): Here, the alkaloids contain a reduced isoquinoline ring in their nucleus. Example is boldine (*Peumus boldus*).
- Norlupinane: They contain norlupinane as their basic ring structure. They are present in leguminosae plants. Examples are sparteine (*Lupinus luteus*), Lupinine (*Anabasis aphylla*).
- Indole (benzopyrrole): They contain an indole ring in their nucleus. Examples are ergotamine (*Claviceps purpurea*), reserpine (*Rauvolfia serpentina*).
- Imidazole: They contain an imidazole basic ring structure. Examples are pilocarpine (*Pilocarpus jaborandi*).
- Purine: These contain a purine ring in their nucleus. Examples are caffeine (*Thea sinensis, Coffea arabica, Theobroma cacao*) (Zrenner et al., 2006).
- Tropolone: They contain a tropolone ring as their basic structure. Examples are colchicine (*Colchicum autumnale*).
- Steroid: They contain a steroidal ring in their nucleus. Examples are funtumine (*Funtumia latifolia*), solanidine (*Solanum sp.*).
- Pyrrolizidine: Alkaloids in this group contain a pyrrolizidine ring as their basic structure. Examples are Senecionine (*Senecio vulgaris*) (Mattock, 1986).

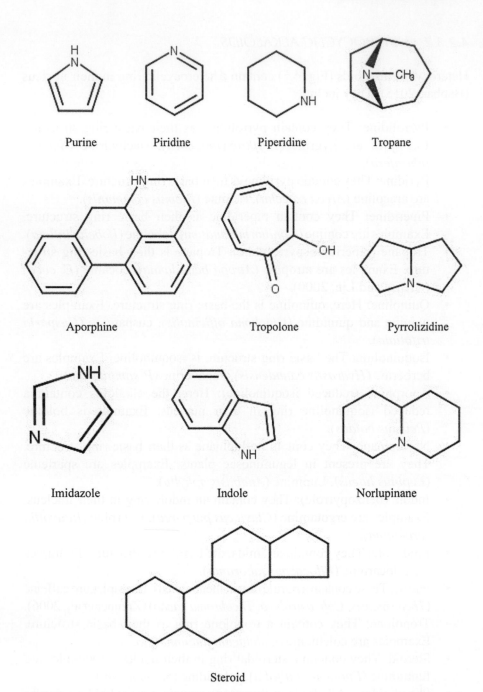

FIGURE 4.5   Basic structures of some alkaloids.

4.2.3.3   CHEMISTRY OF ALKALOIDS

The physical and chemical properties of phytochemicals are as follows:

Physical properties

- Alkaloids are solid crystalline compounds except for coniine and nicotine which are liquid. Emetine is amorphous.
- They are colorless with the exception of berberine and betaine, which are yellow and red, respectively.
- The presence of a nitrogen atom makes them basic which depends on the availability of free electrons, as well as the type of hybridization and aromaticity.
- They are insoluble in water except for liquid alkaloids like nicotine that are soluble in water.

Chemical properties

- They are present in plants in diverse forms such as esters, quaternary compounds, salts, N-oxide, and so forth.
- They are unstable when exposed to heat or light.
- They have a characteristic bitter taste.
- They are soluble in an aqueous solution of sodium carbonate or ammonia on treatment with alcohol, thus forming an ester.

4.2.3.4   SOURCES OF ALKALOIDS

Alkaloids are found in the tissues (i.e., stems, leaves, roots, seeds, and barks) of a vast variety of higher plants such as Apocynaceae (the richest source by a large margin), Papaveraceae (a particularly rich source though less than the Apocynaceae), Rubiaceae, Asteraceae, Rutaceae, Boraginaceae, Berberidaceae, Ranunculaceae, Fabaceae, Rutaceae, and Solanaceae. Foods such as tea, coffee, cocoa, honey, as well as nightshade fruits like potatoes, eggplant, honey, hot peppers are sources of alkaloids (Ranjitha and Sudha, 2015).

4.2.3.5   BIOLOGICAL ROLES OF SOME SELECTED ALKALOIDS

Alkaloids have diverse pharmacological and biochemical properties. For instance; ajmaline is reported to be antiarrhythmic. Codeine is used as cough medicine and an analgesic. Colchicine is used as a remedy for gout, ergot alkaloids serve as vasodilator and antihypertensive drugs. Quinidine is antiarrhythmic, quinine antipyretics is useful as an antimalarial agent. Reserpine is also antihypertensive. Tubocurarine serves as a muscle relaxant. Vinblastine and vincristine are antitumor agents. Yohimbine is a stimulant and an aphrodisiac (Hesse, 2000; Babbar, 2015).

Atropine

Biological function
- Ophthalmic functions: The application of atropine topically aids in dilating the pupils by temporarily paralyzing the accommodation reflex. Hence, it serves as a therapeutic mydriatic.
- Resuscitation: Atropine injections are useful in treating extremely low heart rate conditions as well as pulse-less electrical activity in patient under cardiac arrest.
- Secretions and bronchoconstriction: The action of atropine on the parasympathetic nervous system prevents the formation of secretions such as saliva, sweat, mucus, and so forth. This is particularly useful in treating hyperhidrosis.
- Treatment of chemical poisoning: Due to its ability to block acetylcholine receptors, atropine is given as a prophylactic for the salivation, lacrimation, urination, diaphoresis, gastrointestinal motility, emesis symptoms that occur as a result of poisoning by organophosphate-containing insecticide.

Cocaine

Biological functions
- It is a potent central nervous system stimulant and an appetite suppressant.
- It is applied topically as anesthetic in ophthalmology as it is quickly absorbed from the mucous membrane.

Purine

Biological functions

- Paraxanthine, a caffeine metabolite helps in elevation of plasma levels of glycerol and free-fatty acids.
- Theophylline, another metabolite of caffeine is used to treat asthmatic patients as it relaxes the smooth muscles of the bronchi.
- Caffeine consumption increases vigor and mental alertness while reducing the sensation of tiredness.
- Theobromine, a caffeine metabolite facilitates dilation of the blood vessels.
- Caffeine has been shown to increase one's capacity for mental and physical labor.
- Caffeine citrate is reported to be invaluable in treating breathing disorders and bronchopulmonary dysplasia in premature babies (Zrenner et al., 2006)

Pyrrolizidine

Biological functions

- They are used as a cough suppressant.
- They can be used in treating obstructive lung diseases such as asthma, bronchitis, and emphysema.
- Pyrrolizine alkaloids have been observed to have a significant antimicrobial activity such as its capacity to inhibit the growth of *Escherichia coli, S. aureus, Bacillus subtilis, Bacillus anthracis*.
- Saturated pyrrolizidine alkaloid (PA) has spasmolytic, antihistaminic, anti-HIV, antiviral activities, as well as acting as an inhibitor of glucosidase (Mattocks, 1986).

4.2.4 GLYCOSIDES

Glycosides are chemical organic compounds that on hydrolysis by mineral acids or enzymes yield sugars. They are usually of plant origin and composed of sugar portion linked to a non-sugar portion via a glycosidic bond. The sugar portion is known as the glycone while the non-sugar moiety is referred to as the aglycone or genin of the glycoside. The aglycone portion may either be a flavonoid, saponin, terpene, coumarin, or any other natural product.

Glycosides are stored in the vacuole, protected from hydrolytic enzymes of the cytoplasm. They exist as solid bitter compounds and belong to different secondary metabolites.

4.2.4.1   CHEMISTRY OF GLYCOSIDES AND SOURCES

The general chemical properties of glycosides are:

- Glycosides are colorless, crystalline amorphous, nonvolatile chemical compounds (except flavonoid which gives yellow color and anthraquinone with red color)
- Except for populin, glycyrrhizin, and stevioside, others exist as bitter compounds.
- They are insoluble in organic solvents but soluble in water.
- They can easily be hydrolyzed by mineral acids, water, or enzymes except for C-glycosides that require ferric chloride for hydrolysis.
- On hydrolysis, glycosides give positive test to Molisch's test and Fehling's solution.
- In their pure state, they are optically active (levorotatory) in nature.
- The aglycone portion is responsible for the biological or pharmacological activity of the glycosides.

Glycosides are classified on the basis of the type of aglycone linked to them and the type of glycosidic bond involved in the bond formation.

Table 4.1 shows classification of glycosides on the basis of the chemical structure of the aglycone or pharmacological activity and their sources:

TABLE 4.1   Classification of Glycosides and Various Sources.

Aglycone portion	Sources
Anthraquinone glycosides	Aloe, buckthorn, senna, rhubarb
Anthocyanosides	Blueberry, currant
Cardiac glycosides	Digitalis, strophanthus, lily of the valley, squill
Coumarin glycosides	Bergamot, sweet woodruff
Cyanogenic glycosides	Almond, cherry, apricot
Flavonoid glycosides	Hyssop, liquorice
Hydroquinone glycosides	Arbutus
Saponin glycosides or saponosides	Liquorice, horse chestnut
Iridoid glycosides	Plantain, devil's claw
Salicylic glycosides	White willow, poplar

Based on the nature of the glycone; if it is a glucose, then the molecule is a glucoside; if it is fructose, then the molecule is a fructoside. Hence, the terminal -e- of the name of the corresponding cyclic form of the monosaccharide is replaced by -ide-. Also, if it is glucuronic acid, then the molecule is a glucuronide.

Chemically, the sugar moiety of a glycoside can be joined to the aglycone via a nucleophilic atom such as (Fig. 4.6):

- Oxygen atom (O-glycosides)
- Carbon atom (C-glycosides)
- Nitrogen atom (N-glycosides)
- Sulfur atom (S-glycosides)

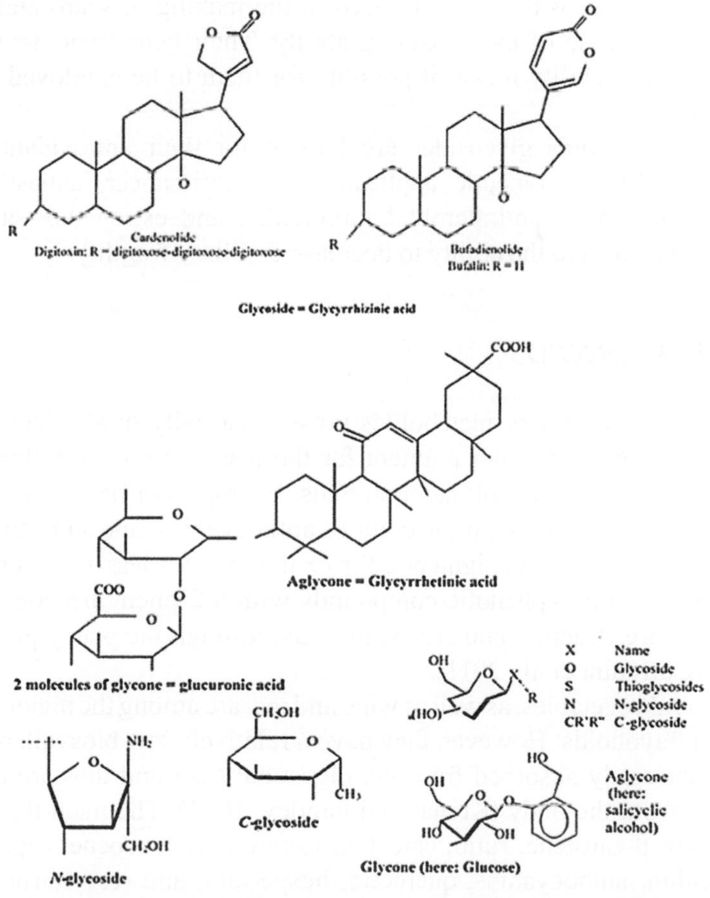

FIGURE 4.6 Chemical nature of glycosides.

4.2.4.2   BIOLOGICAL ROLES OF GLYCOSIDES

- Glycosides-containing plants defend themselves against herbivores becoming less attractive or palatable.
- Anthracene glycosides are used as cathartics and exert their action by increasing the tone of the smooth muscle in the wall of the colon and stimulate the gastric secretion of water and electrolytes into the large intestine.
- Cardiac glycosides, for example, digitoxin from *Digitalis purpurea* are known to exert powerful effect on the heart muscle and heart rhythm leading to myocardial contraction.
- Many glycosides are extremely active compounds but toxic at the same time (e.g., digitoxin)
- Saponin glycosides are employed in the making of soaps and detergents because of their foaming ability. Their hemotoxic nature and hemolytic ability makes it possible for them to be employed as fish poisons.
- The flavonoids glycosides are known for their antioxidant effect hence find therapeutic applications as anti-cancer, antiasthmatic, antispasmodic, antimicrobial, fungicidal, and estrogenic activities. They also have the ability to decrease capillary fragility.

4.2.5   FLAVONOIDS

Flavonoids are secondary metabolites present virtually in all plants. They are the most important color pigment for the leaves, fruits, and flowers of plants designed to attract pollinator animals. Examples of flavonoids are the yellow color of chalcones, purple color of anthocyanins, and so forth. When not visible, they act as copigments, for example, colorless flavones. They are hydroxylated polyphenolic compounds with a 2-phenylbenzopyranone ring as the core structure and are synthesized through the phenylpropanoid pathway (Corradini et al., 2011).

Foods and vegetables, as well as wine and tea, are among the major dietary sources of flavonoids. However, they have a relatively low bioavailability as they are not easily absorbed from the digestinal tract and thus are quickly eliminated from the body (Kumar and Pandey, 2013). The main flavonoids in plants are β-carotene, rutin, catechin, α-carotene, lycopene, capsanthin, cryptoxanthin, anthocyanins, quercetin, hesperidin, and resveratrol (Tapas et al., 2008).

Flavonoids have versatile physiological and biochemical functions in all forms of life. In higher plants, they serve as combatants of oxidative stress, growth regulators, and inhibitors of the cell cycle as well as chemical messengers amongst others. In humans, they can scavenge free radicals and chelate metal ions due to the presence of functional OH groups (i.e., anti-oxidation activities). They play roles in protecting the body against cardio-vascular diseases, cancer, as well as other age-related diseases. They are anti-inflammatory, hepatoprotective, and have antiviral attributes (Ghasemzadeh and Ghasemzadeh, 2011, Øyvind and Markham, 2006; Ververidis et al., 2007).

4.2.5.1   CHEMISTRY OF FLAVONOIDS

The general structure of flavonoids is based on a 15-carbon skeleton made up of two benzene rings connected by a heterocyclic pyrane ring (Fig. 4.7). Flavonoids can exist both as glycosidic conjugates and free aglycones (the basic structure). The former increases polarity of the flavonoid as well as decreasing its reactivity, which is vital for preventing cellular cytoplasmic damage (Kumar and Pandey, 2013). C-linkage bond between aglycone and sugar is quite strong; therefore, a mixture of concentrated HCl and acetic acid (Killian's agent) is used to carry out the hydrolysis of C-glycosides (Corradini et al., 2011).

There are eight major classes of flavonoids based on the degree of unsaturation and oxidation of the three-carbon segment (Kumar and Pandey, 2013). They are:

- Flavones, for example, luteolin, apigenin, tangeritin, and so forth.
- Isoflavones, for example, genistein, daidzein, glycitein.
- Anthocyanidins, for example, cyanidin, delphinidin, malvidin, pelargonidin, peonidin, petunidin.
- Flavanones, for example, hesteretin, naringenin, eriodictyol.
- Flavanols, for example, catechins and epicatechins.
- Flavonols, for example, quercetin, kaempferol, myricetin, isorhamnetin, pachypodol.
- Chalcones, for example, butein.
- Aurones, for example, isoliquiritigenin and hispidol.

Flavonoids are crystalline in nature. Flavones, chalcones, aurones are bright yellow while catechins, flavanones form colorless crystals. Generally,

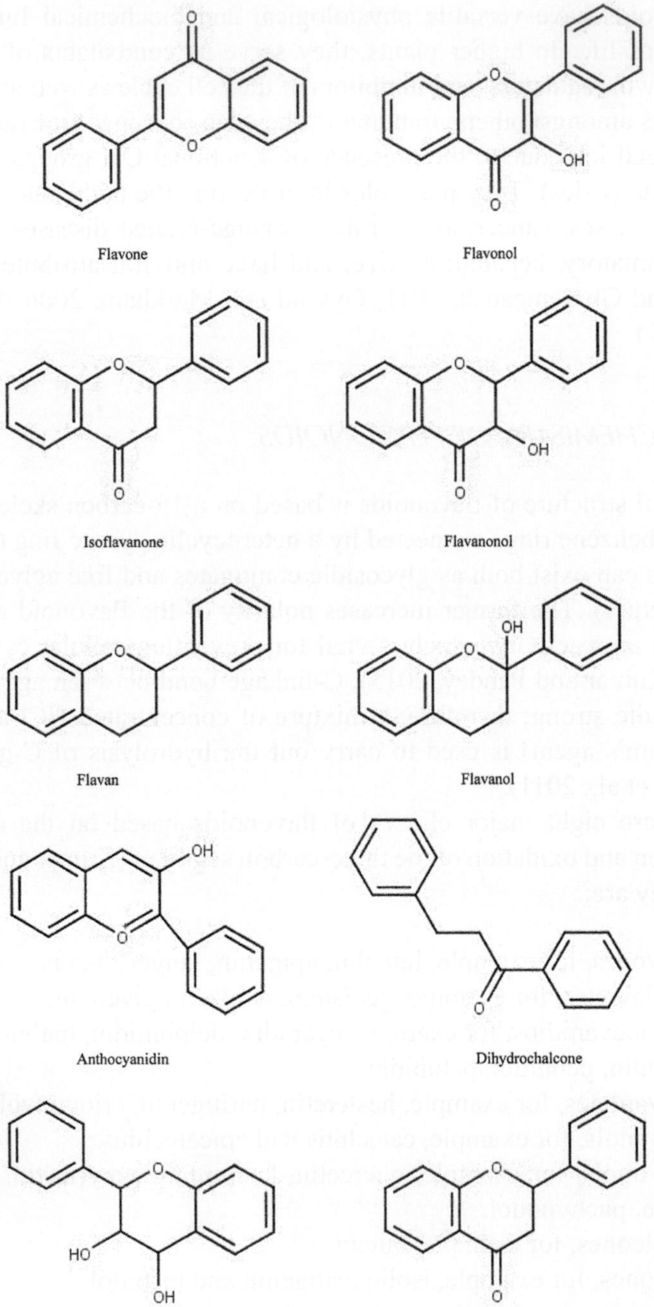
O
O
Flavone
O
OH
O
Flavonol
O
O
Isoflavanone
O
OH
O
Flavanonol
O
Flavan
OH
O
Flavanol
OH
O+
Anthocyanidin
O
Dihydrochalcone
O
HO
OH
Flavan-3,4-diol
O
O
Flavanone

FIGURE 4.7 Flavonoid subgroups

glycosides are soluble in water and alcohol; however, flavonoid glycosides are soluble in hot water and diluted alcohols. Aglycones are soluble in alkaline hydroxide solutions and apolar organic solvent due to the presence of a free phenolic group; however, flavonoid aglycones are soluble in diethyl ether, alcohols, acetone, but practically insoluble in water (Kumar and Pandey, 2013).

The color of sap pigments (which are anthocyanins) is determined by the pH of the sap, that is, in acid medium, they turn red while in alkaline medium, they turn blue. Also the red color of roses and blue color of cornflower is as a result of the presence of the same glycosides (Corradini et al., 2011).

Catechins are optically active. When flavononones and flavanones are treated with oxidants, they yield leucocyanidins and chalcones, respectively. Hence, they are very unstable compounds.

4.2.5.2 SOURCES OF FLAVONOIDS

All fruits and vegetables contain one or more flavonoids. Common food sources for anthocyanidins are red, blue, and purple berries and grapes as well as red wine; for flavanols, teas, chocolate, grapes, berries, apples, red grapes, red wine, and so forth are the major dietary sources. Citrus fruits (oranges, grapefruits, lemons) are the major sources of flavanones. Onions, scallions, broccoli, teas, apples, berries, and kales are the major food sources. For flavones, parsley, thyme, hot peppers, and celery are the sources while soybeans, legumes, and soy foods are the major sources (Tapas et al., 2008; Kumar and Pandey, 2013).

4.2.5.3 BIOLOGICAL ROLES OF FLAVONOIDS

Flavonoids are known for their prominent antioxidant functions as they help in preventing coronary heart diseases as well as cancer. They also have antimicrobial, antidiabetic, antihistamine, mood boosting, as well as memory-enhancing properties (Agrawal, 2011; Friedman, 2007; Tapas et al., 2008). Some specific biological roles of flavonoids are highlighted below:

- **Effect on cholesterol:** Flavonoid-containing chocolate/cocoa helps in reducing blood pressure. They also have significant positive effects on low-density lipoprotein and high-density lipoprotein cholesterol levels in the body (Ghasemzadeh and Ghasemzadeh, 2011; van Dam et al., 2013).

- **Anticancer agents:** Flavonoid-containing celery, artichokes have cytotoxic effects on cancer cells. However, they should not be administered with the chemotherapeutic drug as it may be counterproductive but instead should be given as pretreatment.
- **Effect on menopause**: Isoflavones in soybean reduces the sensation of hot flash that is so common among perimenopausal and postmenopausal women. It also helps in increasing the bone mineral density thereby reducing the risk of bone fracture as well as postmenopausal osteoporosis.
- **Therapeutic effect on rheumatoid arthritis**: The antioxidation activity of grape seed proanthocyanidin extract scavenges the hydrogen peroxide product of oxidative stress thereby reducing the destruction of collagens by the hydrogen peroxide. This aids in the treatment of collagen-induced rheumatoid arthritis.
- **Prevention of gum disease:** Proanthocyanidins in cranberry has anti-inflammatory activity thereby preventing the development of gum disease. It can also be used to cure the disease.
- **Improved cognitive functions**: Anthocyanidins in blueberries and strawberries improves cognitive functions of elderly people as it effectively slows down the rate of cognitive decline. It also improves body movements and slows down irritability, fatigue, and depression (Spencer, 2008).

4.2.6 OXALATES

Oxalates (ethanedioate) is a dianion salt with a molecular formula $C_2O_4^{2-}$ (Fig. 4.8). It is a salt of oxalic acid a strong dicarboxylic acid found in many plants; oxalate is produced in the body by metabolism of glyoxylic acid (from glycine) or ascorbic acid; it is not metabolized but excreted in the urine.

Oxalate is a bidentate ligand (having two teeth) and can form complexes with metal ions and some nutrients. A high intake of oxalate can sometimes cause a deficiency, since calcium oxalate is insoluble. Some disease states are associated with oxalate metabolism, for example, urolithiasis, nephrolithiasis; hyperoxaluria is a primary risk factor of urolithiasis because virtually all oxalate consumed is excreted via urine.

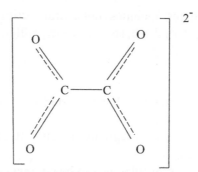

FIGURE 4.8   Structure of the oxalate anion.

4.2.6.1   CHEMISTRY OF OXALATES

Physical properties:

- Oxalate is an odorless white solid with a sour taste and a density of 1.9 g/cm³.
- Oxalate has a melting point temperature of 189.5°C.
- Oxalate is soluble in ethanol but slightly soluble in ether and insoluble in benzene, chloroform, and petroleum ether.

Chemical properties:

- Oxalate is a strong reducing agent.
- Oxalic acid can bind with minerals as iron and calcium to form iron oxalate and calcium oxalate, respectively.
- Oxalate forms acid chloride (oxalyl chloride).
- Oxalate is a conjugate base of oxalic acid and a ligand (bidentate) for metal ions.
- Oxalate undergoes autocatalytic reaction in which it is oxidized by permanganate.

4.2.6.2   SOURCES OF OXALATES

Oxalate is found in many food substances; oxalate is also present in the body as metabolites of glycine and ascorbic acid metabolism.

Foods rich in oxalates includes nuts, cranberries, coffee, chocolate, spinach, berries, oranges, rhubarb, sesame seeds, millet, soybeans, black tea, wheat bran, and beans.

4.2.6.3   BIOLOGICAL ROLES OF OXALATES

- Oxalate (calcium oxalate) regulates calcium (Ca) and aids protection against herbivores.
- Oxalates help to confer tolerance to heavy metals on plants.
- Oxalate (oxalic acid) is required in the formation of orotic acid and uracil: a component of ribonucleic acid.
- Oxalate helps decrease the risk of cancer: oxalate is a competitive inhibitor of lactate dehydrogenase (an enzyme that catalyzes the conversion of pyruvate to lactic acid). Cancer cells use anaerobic metabolism hence, inhibition of lactate dehydrogenase leads to the inhibition of tumor formation and growth.

4.2.7   PROTEASE INHIBITORS

Proteases are important enzymes that aid the regulation of cellular processes, they are ubiquitous and present in all cells and tissues. Upon lysing of the cell, cell proteases are released into the lysate. Proteases catalyze the hydrolysis of peptide bonds. Release of these enzymes in large quantities may impede biochemical analysis and may be potentially destructive to cells and tissues, hence the need for its regulation by the body. Protease inhibitors are a group of low-molecular-weight protein present in cells and tissues that regulate the effects of proteases; these enzymes may act endogenously or exogenously as defense mechanisms against proteolytic degradation and regulation of many biological processes (Vijaya and Gandreddi, 2014). They do this by forming inactive complexes or complexes with lesser activity when they bind to cognate enzymes; the mode of this inhibition may be direct blockage of the active site, indirect blockage of the active site, adjacent or exosite binding, and allosteric inhibition (Huma and Khalid, 2007). Protease inhibitors occur widely in nature and are found in plants, animals, and microbes where they regulate biological processes; some other functions other than regulation of proteases have been observed for protease inhibitors, functions as regulation of growth activities, receptor clearance signaling, regulate inflammation, extracellular matrix synthesis, and tissue repair (Huma and Khalid, 2007).

4.2.7.1 CHEMISTRY OF PROTEASE INHIBITORS

There has been an initial classification of protease inhibitors and this classification was based on the protease inhibited but more recently classification is based on the similarities of primary amino acid sequence and based on the nature of binding of the inhibitor to its enzyme. The classification given below is based on primary amino acid sequence (Aberoumand, 2012; Meenu and Murugan, 2016; Vijaya and Gandreddi, 2014).

1. Serine protease inhibitors (Serfins) pathogenesis-related proteins
    - Bowman–Birk (trypsin/chymotrypsin)
    - Kunitz (trypsin; others)
    - Potato I (trypsin; chymotrypsin)
    - Potato II (chymotrypsin; trypsin)
    - Curcubit (trypsin)
    - Cereal superfamily (amylase, trypsin)
    - Ragi I-2 family (amylase, protease)
    - Maize 22 kDa/thaumatin/Pathogenesis related proteins (amylase, trypsin)

2. Cysteine protease inhibitor (cystatins and stefin)
    - Cystatin superfamily
    - Cystatin family
    - Stefin family
    - Fitocystatin family

3. Metalloprotease inhibitor
    - Carboxypeptidase

4.2.7.2 SOURCES OF PROTEASE INHIBITORS

Protease inhibitors are found occurring naturally in fungi, bacteria, viruses, Kingdom Animalia and Kingdom Plantae. It is found in a wide variety of edible plant (Vijaya and Gandreddi, 2014).

Soybeans and other legumes: These are abundant source of protease inhibitors and this is reported to be the reason for its anticancer activity. Two types of protease inhibitors found in soy are Kunitz trypsin inhibitor which is present in large concentration and Bowman–Birk inhibitor.

Potatoes: Protease inhibitors are present as small proteins in the tubers and stem of potato where they are induced in response to attack or injury caused by pathogenic microorganisms or insects. Protease inhibitors suppress tumor growth in clinical setting.

Green tea: This contains epigallocatechin gallate a catechin that possesses antioxidant properties and inhibits proteases. It also contains vitamins, minerals, theanine, and saponins.

Blue-green algae: The blue-green algae are rich in nutrients and supplements. It is also a rich source of protease inhibitors.

4.2.7.3   BIOLOGICAL ROLES OF PROTEASE INHIBITORS

Protease inhibitors have been shown to elicit antimicrobial, antiviral, antineoplastic, insecticidal, and defense mechanism and anti-inflammatory properties (Hiestra, 2002; Whitaker, 1997).

a) **Antiviral property:** Viruses replicate by proteolytic cleavage of protein precursors essential for the production of viral particles; protease inhibitors bind to viral proteases thereby preventing the proteolytic cleavage of protein precursors necessary for the production of infectious viral particles.

b) **Antimicrobial property:** Certain phytopathogenic fungi are known to produce proteases extracellularly; these proteases play an important role in the pathogenesis of diseases. Plant protease inhibitors suppress these enzymatic activities in response to attack by proteases produced by the fungi.

c) **Insecticidal property and defense mechanism:** It has been observed that protease inhibitors are capable of inhibiting the growth of insect larvae; wounded plants produce protease inhibitors; hence, the presence of these enzymes prevents absorption of proteins and disrupts the activities of some essential proteases in the insect thus discouraging the insect from consuming them.

d) **Antineoplastic agent:** Protease inhibitors affect the expression of certain oncogenes, hence suppression of carcinogenesis.

c) **Anti-inflammatory property:** Protease inhibitors regulate the proteolytic activity of proteases implicated in inflammation and it also modulates signal transduction, cytokine expression, and tissue remodeling thus preventing inflammation (Hiestra, 2002).

4.2.8 AMYLASE INHIBITORS

Amylase (α-1,4-glucan-4-glucanohydrolase, EC 3.2.1.1) catalyze the hydrolysis of the α-1,4 glycosidic linkages in oligosaccharides, that is, starch. Amylase inhibitors are proteinaceous molecules that delay the breakdown of these oligosaccharides. They are often referred to as "starch blockers." The necessity of delaying the breakdown is to allow for a consistent level of glucose in the blood. This controlled kinetics in the breakdown and absorption of carbohydrate is invaluable in controlling disorders associated with carbohydrate uptake such as obesity, periodontal diseases, diabetes, as well as hyperlipidemia and hyperproteinemia (Alagesan et al., 2012).

The smaller the molecular weight of the amylase inhibitors, the more effective the compound as they can be easily absorbed into the bloodstream from the gut. They are generally heat labile and are active over a pH range of 4.5–9.5.

4.2.8.1 SOURCES OF AMYLASE INHIBITORS

Amylase inhibitors are found in over 800 genera of plants, all of which are relevant in treating type II diabetes. Amylase inhibitors are either of plant (legumes and cereals) or microbial origin (*Streptomyces* spp.). Plant sources are widely considered to be safer and more effective compared to microbial sources. Also, spices such as chili, garlic, rosemary, clove, sage, basil, parsley, and onion have significant amylase inhibition activities. Pigeon pea also contains amylase inhibitors. Catechins from black teas have also been implicated in the inhibition of salivary amylases (Sales et al., 2012).

4.2.8.2 BIOLOGICAL ROLES OF AMYLASE INHIBITORS

The aqueous extracts of *Syzygium cumini* seeds and *Psidium guajava* leaves are reported to show a dose-dependent inhibitory effect on the activity of amylase. *S. cumini* extract was notably reported to have significantly reduced the blood glucose levels in diabetic rats. Also, the hexane, methanol, and ethyl acetate extracts of the seeds of *Amaranthus caudatus* were reported to have significant amylase inhibition activity (>80% inhibition rate at dose concentrations of 0.25–1 mg/mL) (Archana and Jeyamanikandan, 2015).

In a cohort study with healthy and type II diabetic subjects, it was observed that natural amylase inhibitors of plant origin (wheat and white bean) markedly reduced the peak of postprandial glucose (Alagesan et al., 2012).

Quite a number of natural compounds also have excellent amylase inhibitor activities such as flavonols, flavanone, proanthocyanidin, tannins, cinnamic acid derivatives (chlorogenic acids, rosmarinic acids, isochlorogenic acids), and terpenes. Tannins carry out their inhibitory effect due to their ability to bind strongly to carbohydrates and proteins as well as its free OH groups that facilitate hydrogen bonding.

Acarbose is a product of the microbial fermentation of *Actinoplanes* spp. It is an oligosaccharide inhibitor and is commonly used for treating type II diabetes (diabetes mellitus) (Khacheba et al., 2014). It competitively inhibits amylase due to its unsaturated cyclohexene ring as well as its glycosidic nitrogen linkages that mimics the transition state for the enzymatic cleavage of the glycosidic linkages. Acarbose is hence metabolized by the intestinal carbohydrases to yield acarviosine glucose and glucose (Elya et al., 2015; Prabhakar et al., 2013).

4.3   CONCLUSION

Phytochemicals found in plants and other food sources contain essential substances that exert various biological functions in the human body. Alkaloids, saponins, tannins, and flavonoids are among the major sources of essential phytochemicals. The tannins and flavonoids due to their polyphenolic nature serve as antioxidants, antimutagenic, and anticholesterol activities. It is important to know that the biological roles of the different phytochemicals are linked to their plant sources, structural properties, as well as the severity of the diseased state, the age of the patient, and the quantity taken of the phytochemical.

KEYWORDS

- **phytochemicals**
- **flavonoids**
- **alkaloids**
- **saponins**
- **tannins**

REFERENCES

Agrawal, A. Pharmacological Activities of Flavonoids: A Review. *Int. J. Pharm. Sci. Nanotechnol.* **2011,** *4*(2), 1394–1398.

Agrawal, S. S.; Paridhavi, M. Ed.; *Herbal Drug Technology: Tests for Tannins;* 2nd ed.; University Press Private Limited: India, 2012.

Akiyama, H. Antibacterial Action of Several Tannins against *Staphylococcus aureus. J. Antimicrob. Chemother.* **2001,** *48*(4), 487–491.

Alagesan, K.; Raghupathi, P.; Sankarnarayanan, S. Amylase Inhibitors: Potential Source of Anti-Diabetic Drug Discovery from Medicinal Plants. *Int. J. Pharm. Life Sci.* **2012,** *3*(2), 1407–1412.

Archana, K.; Jeyamanikandan, V. *In Vitro* Antibacterial, Antioxidant and α-Amylase Inhibition Activity of Medicinal Plants. *J. Chem. Pharm. Res.* **2015,** *7*(4), 1634–1639.

Ashutosh, K. *Pharmacognosy and Pharmacobiotechnology; Cyanogenic glycosides*; New Age International (P) Ltd. and Anshan Ltd.: UK, 2008.

Babbar, N. An Introduction to Alkaloids and their Applications in Pharmaceutical Chemistry. *Pharma Innov. J.* **2015,** *4*(10), 74–75.

Bate-Smith, E. C.; Swain, T. Flavonoid Compounds. In *Comparative Biochemistry*; Mason, H. S., Florkin, A. M. Eds.; Academic Press: New York. 1962; pp 755–809.

Chamakuri, S. R. Pharmacological Anti-inflammatory Activity of *Psidium guajava* Linn. Leaves and Bark by Tannin Fractions. *J. Pharmcogn. Phytochem.* **2015,** e-ISSN: 2321–6182 p-ISSN: 2347–2332.

Corradini, E.; Foglia, P.; Giansanti, P.; Gubbiotti, R.;Samperi, R.;Laganà, A. Flavonoids: Chemical Properties and Analytical Methodologies of Identification and Quantitation in Foods and Plants. *Nat. Prod. Res.* **2011,** *25*(5), 469–495.

Das, T.; Banerjee, D.; Chakraborty, D.; Pakhira, M.; Shrivastava, B.; Kuhad, R. Saponin: Role in Animal system. *Vet.World.* **2012,** *5*(4), 248–254.

Edeoga, H.; Eriata, D. Alkaloid, Tannin and Saponin Contents of Some Nigeria Medicinal Plants. *J. Med. Aromat. Plant Sci.* **2001,** *23,* 344–349.

Egbuna, C.; Ifemeje, J. Biological Functions and Anti-nutritional Effects of Phytochemicals in Living System. *IOSR J. Pharm. Biol. Sci.* **2015,** *10*(2), 10–19.

Elya, B.; Handayani, R.; Sauriasarim, R. Antidiabetic Activity and Phytochemical Screening of Extracts from Indonesian Plants by Inhibition of Alpha Amylase, Alpha Glucosidase and Dipeptidyl Peptidase IV. *Pak. J. Biol. Sci.* **2015,** *18*(6), 279–284.

Evans, W. C., Ed. *Trease and Evans Pharmacognosy*; 16th Ed.; St Louis Syndey Toronto, Saunders Elsevier: Edinburgh London New York Philadelphia, 2009.

Friedman, M. Overview of Antibacterial, Antitoxin, Antiviral, and Antifungal Activities of Tea Flavonoids and Teas. *Mol. Nutr. Food Res.* **2007,** *51*(1), 116–134.

Ghasemzadeh, A.; Ghasemzadeh, N. Flavonoids and Phenolic Acids: Role and Biochemical Activity in Plants and Human. *J. Med. Plant Res.* **2011,** *5*(31), 6697–6703.

Griffin, W.; Lin, G. Chemotaxonomic and Geographical Relationship of Tropane Alkaloid Producing Plants. *Phytochemistry* **2000,** *53,* 623–637.

Guclu-Ustundag, O.; Mazza, G. Saponins: Properties, Applications and Processing. *Crit. Rev. Food Sci. Nutr.* **2007,** *47,* 231–258.

Gunnar, S.; Lars, B., Eds. *Drugs of Natural Origin: Gallic acid and Tannins;* 6th Ed.; Swedish Pharmaceutical Press: Stockholm Sweden, 2009.

He, L.; Guoying, Z.; Huaiyun, Z.; Yuanhao, H. Chemical Constituents and Biological Activities of Saponin from the Seed of Camellia Oleifera. *Sci. Res. Essays* **2010,** *5*(25), 4088–4092.

Hesse, M. Alkaloids: Nature's Curse or Blessing? Wiley-VCH: Zurich, Switzerland, 2002.

Hiestra, P. S. Novel Roles of Protease Inhibitors in Infection and Inflammation. *Biochem. Soc. Trans.* **2002,** *2*(30), 116–118.

Horvath, P. J. The Nutritional and Ecological Significance of Acer-tannins and Related Polyphenols. Cornell University: Ithaca, NY, USA, 1981.

Huma, H.; Khalid, M. F. Plant Protease Inhibitors: A Defense Strategy in Plants. *Biotech. Mol. Biol. Rev.* **2007,** *2*(3), 68–70.

Kaufman, P. B.; Cseke, L. J.; Warber, S.; Duke, J. A.; Brielmann, H. L. Natural Products from Plants: Chemical Defence Strategies. CRC Press LLC: USA, 2000.

Khacheba, I.; Djeridane, A.; Yousfi, M. Twenty Traditional Algerian Plants used in Diabetes Therapy as Strong Inhibitors of α-Amylase Activity. *Int. J. Carbohydr. Chem.* **2014,** Article ID 287281.

Khanbabaee, K.; van Ree, T. Tannins: Classification and Definition. Nat. Prod. Rep. **2001,** *18,* 641–649.

Kojima, T. Anti-allergic Effect of Apple Polyphenol on Patients with Atopic Dermatitis: A Pilot Study. *Allerg. Int.* **2000,** *49*, 69–73.

Kumar, S.; Pandey, A. Chemistry and Biological Activities of Flavonoids: An Overview. *Sci. World J.* **2013,** Article ID 162750.

Mattocks, A. *Chemistry and Toxicology of Pyrrolizidine Alkaloids*; Academic Press: London, New York, 1986.

Meenu, K. V.; Murugan, K. Solanum Protease Inhibitors and their Therapeutic Potentialities: A Review. *Int. J. Pharm. Pharm. Sci.* **2016,** *8*(12), 14–18.

Negi, J.; Negi, P.; Pant, G.; Rawat, M.; Negi, S. Naturally Occurring Saponins: Chemistry Biology. *J. Poison Med. Plant Res.* **2013,** *1*(1), 001–006.

Oakenfull, D. Saponins in Food–A Review. *Food Chem.* **1981,** *6,* 19–40.

Øyvind, A.; Markham, K. *Flavonoids: Chemistry, Biochemistry and Applications*, 1st Ed.; CRC Press: New York, 2006.

Parmar, F. *In vitro* Antioxidant and Anticancer Activity of *Mimosa pudica*linn Extract and l-mimosine on Lymphoma Daudi Cells. *Int. J. Pharm. Pharm. Sci.* **2015,** *7*(12), 100–104.

Prabhakar, V.; Jaidka, A.; Singh, R. *In Vitro* Study on α-Amylase Inhibitory Activity and Phytochemical Screening of Few Indian Medicinal Plant Having Anti-Diabetic Properties. *Int. J. Sci. Res. Pub.* **2013,** 3(8)

Ranjitha, D.; Sudha, K. Alkaloids in Food. *Int. J. Pharm. Chem. Biol. Sci.* **2015,** *5*(4), 896–906.

Sales, P.; Souza, P.; Simeoni, L.; Dâmaris, S. α-Amylase Inhibitors: A Review of Raw Material and Isolated Compounds from Plant Source. *J. Pharm. Pharm. Sci.* **2012,** *15*(1), 141–183.

Scalbert, A. Antimicrobial Properties of Tannins. *Phytochemistry* **1991,** *30* (12), 3875–3883.

Sparg, S.; Light, M.; van Staden, J. Biological Activities and Distribution of Plant Saponins. J. Ethnopharmacol. **2004,** *94,* 219–243.

Spencer, J. Flavonoids: Modulators of Brain Function? *Br. J. Nutr.* **2008,** *99,* ES60–E77.

Tapas, A.; Sakarkar, D.; Kakde, B. Flavonoids as Nutraceuticals: A Review. *Trop. J. Pharm. Res.* **2008,** *7*(3), 1089–1099.

Teng, B.; Zhang, T.; Gong, Y.; Chen, W. Molecular Weights and Tanning Properties of Tannin Fractions from the Acacia Mangium Bark. *Afr. J. Agric. Res.* **2013,** *8*(47), 5996–6001.

Thakur, M.; Melzig, M.; Fuchs, H.; Weng, A. Chemistry and Pharmacology of Saponins: Special Focus on Cytotoxic Properties. *Bot.: TargetsTher.***2011,***1,*9–29.

vanDam, R.; Naidoo, N.; Landberg, R. Dietary Flavonoids and the Development of Type 2 Diabetes and Cardiovascular Diseases. *Curr. Opin. Lipidol.* **2013,** *24*(1), 25–33.

Ververidis, F.; Trantas, E.; Douglas, C.; Vollmer, G.; Kretzschmar, G.; Panopoulos, N. Biotechnology of Flavonoids and other Phenylpropanoid-Derived Natural Products. Part I: Chemical diversity impacts on plant biology and human health. *Biotechnol. J.* **2007,** *2*(10), 1214–1234.

Vijaya, R.; Gandreddi, S. A. Review of Protease Inhibitors from Different Sources. *Int. J. Appl. Phys. Bio-Chem. Res.* **2014,** *4*(2), 1–9.

Whitaker, J. R. Protease and α-Amylase Inhibitors of Higher Plants. Antinutrients and Phytochemicals in Food ACS Symposium Series; Amer. Chem. Soc: Washington, DC, **1997,** 10–15.

Yamada, P. Inhibitory Effect of Tannins from Galls of *Carpinus tschonoskii* on the Degranulation of RBL-2H3 Cells. *Cytotechnology* **2012,** *63*(3), 349–356.

Zrenner, R.; Stitt, M.; Sonnewald, U.; Boldt, R. Pyrimidine and Purine Biosynthesis and Degradation in Plants. *Annu. Rev. Plant Biol.* **2006,** *57,* 805–836.

CHAPTER 5

PHYTOCHEMICALS AS IMMUNOMODULATORS

BEHNAZ ASLANIPOUR

Department of Bioengineering, Faculty of Engineering, Ege University, 35100 Bornova, Izmir, Turkey, Mob: +905466848406

Corresponding author. E-mail: Behnaz_Aslanipour@yahoo.com
ORCID: https://orcid.org/0000-0002-6183-9745

ABSTRACT

Immunomodulators are substances capable of weakening or suppressing the immune system. They are considered to have fewer side effects than existing drugs, including less potential for creating resistance when treating microbial infections. Immunomodulators could be classified as either immunostimulants, immunoadjuvants, or immunosuppressants. Some plant-derived chemicals such as those from alkaloids, phenolics, flavonoids, anthocyanins, terpenoids, saponins, sterols, polysaccharides, and lectins have been established as having an immunomodulating property. Phytochemicals are good immunomodulatory candidates as they are considered to be safer than synthetic drugs. This chapter details the immunomodulating functions of plant-derived chemicals with supporting evidence. Background information was laid on the phytochemicals discussed and plant families and extracts confirmed to have immunomodulating properties were presented in tables.

5.1 INTRODUCTION

Homeostasis is a well-organized feature of a healthy living organism in which the immune system maintains a stable internal environment. Numerous endogenous and exogenous factors affect the immune system's function, which by some mechanism results in either immunostimulation or immunosuppression. Medically, immunomodulators are classified as either immunostimulants, immunoadjuvants or immunosuppressants. The efficacy of a vaccine can be enhanced by immunoadjuvants that are known as specific immune stimulators. Immunostimulants are agents that have the capacity to activate or induce the mediators or components of an immune system, while immunosuppressants are a class of drugs that suppress, or reduce the strength of the body's immune system. However, these agents can be useful for treating hypersensitivity reactions, infection-associated immunopathology, and autoimmune diseases. Some plant-derived chemicals such as those from alkaloids, phenolics, flavonoids, anthocyanins, terpenoids, saponins, sterols, polysaccharides, and lectins have been established as having an immunomodulating property. In this regards, research is constantly ongoing and some extracts of plants origin have been reported to possess some immunomodulatory activity (Table 5.1). The process of discovering a single chemical metabolite with the requisite affinity, selectivity, and low toxicity is quite challenging. However, the designing and development of plant-derived drugs have been a major focus for many years. In this chapter, the effect of some naturally synthetized phytochemicals in preventing and treating some diseases, indirectly through immunomodulatory effects, will be discussed.

5.2 ALKALOIDS

Alkaloids, an assemblage of naturally occurring chemical composites mostly contain basic nitrogen atoms, encompass the biggest class of secondary plant materials. They are all synthesized from amino acids and have low molecular weight (Harborne, 1991). Alkaloids originated from either botanical or fungal sources, and are present in many beverages, foods, and supplements. They are also present in fungi, bacteria, and animals (Cushnie et al., 2014). Although some animal-based molecules such as adrenaline (epinephrine) and 5-hydroxytryptamine (serotonin) structurally fit alkaloids, they are not considered as alkaloids due to being obtained only from animals (Senchina et al., 2012). Alkaloids are a rich source for performance enhancement and improving immune function (Table 5.2). A diverse class of biological properties such as anticholinergic, antitumor, diuretic, antiviral, antihypertensive, antiulcer, analgesic, and anti-inflammatory properties of alkaloids have been stated so far. Alkaloids are arranged in three different classes as true alkaloids, protoalkaloids, and pseudoalkaloids. A heterocyclic ring with nitrogen forms the main structure of true alkaloids while the N atom derived from

TABLE 5.1 Some Plant Extracts with Immunomodulatory Effects.

Plant's name	Family	Part	Extract type	Immunomodulatory activity	References
Picrorhiza kurrooa	Plantaginaceae	Root and rhizome	Iridoid glycoside fraction	Enhancement of antibody and delayed-type hypersensitivity (DTH) response	Puri et al. (1992)
Nyctanthes arbor-tristis	Oleaceae	Seeds	Ethanolic	Antigen-specific and nonspecific immunity stimulator, macrophage migration activator	Puri et al. (1994)
Platycodon grandiflorus	Campanulaceae	Roots	Aqueous	Immunostimulatory	Choi et al. (2001)
Saussurea lappa	Compositae	Roots	Aqueous	Immunostimulant	Kulkarni and Desai (2001)
Trigonella foenum graecum	Leguminosae	Whole plant	Aqueous	Immunostimulant	Bin-Hafeez et al. (2003)
Uncaria tomentosa	Rubiaceae	Bark	Aqueous	Anti-inflammatory	Aguilar et al. (2002)
Echinacea angustifolia	Asteraceae	Flowers	Aqueous/Ethanolic	Immunomodulator	Senchina et al. (2005)
Salicornia herbacea	Chenopodiaceae	Herb	Methanolic	Immunomodulator	Im et al. (2006)
Oreochromis mossambicus	Cichlidae	Leaf	Aqueous extract	enhancing the nonspecific immune responses	Christybapita et al. (2007)
Haussknechtia elymatica	Apioideae	Herb	Methanolic	Immunomodulator	Amirghofran et al. (2007)
Rhodiola imbricata Gray	Crassulaceae	Rhizomes,	Aqueous extract	Immunostimulating	Mishra et al. (2008)
Byrsonima crassa Nied	Malpighiaceae	Leaves	Chloroform/methanolic	Antimicrobial, antioxidant activities	Bonacorsi et al. (2009)
Hibiscus rosa sinensis	Malvaceae	Flowers	Hydro-alcoholic Extract	Inhibiting the proinflammatory mediator such as Nitric oxide (NO) and Tumor necrosis factor (TNF)-α	Kandhare et al. (2012)
Nigella sativa	Ranunculaceae	Seeds	Ethanolic	Immunomodulator	Al-Sa'aidi et al. (2012)
Asparagus racemosus	Liliaceae	Leaves, seeds	Aqueous extract	immunomodulatory potential	Veena et al. (2014)

TABLE 5.2 In vitro and in vivo Immunomodulatory Effects of Some Alkaloids.

Source	Isolated part	Phytochemical	Dose/day	Treatment case	Mechanism of action	References
Berberis Vulgaris	Root	Alkaloids (pure berberine)	2 mg/kg	anti-sheep red blood cells (SRBC)	Effecting anti-SRBC antibody	Ivanovska and Philipov, (1996)
Han-Fang Chi	Herb	Alkaloid (Tet)	10 μM	Human peripheral blood T cell	Having antirheumatic activity through downregulating IκBα kinases–IκBα Nuclear factor (NF-κB) signaling pathway	Ho et al. (2004)
Berberis Vulgaris	Root	Alkaloids (pure berberine)	28 mg/kg	Endotoxemic mice	Modulating cytokine secretion, inhibiting of pro-inflammatory mediator production and upregulating of interleukin (IL)-10 release	Li et al. (2006)
Chelidonium majus	Whole plant	Alkaloids (methyl 20-(7,8-dihydrosanguinarine-8-yl) acetate, stylopine, protopine, norchelidonine, chelidonine, berberine	50 μM	RAW264.7 cells	Inhibition of LPS-induced NO production	Park et al. (2011)
Stephania tetrandra Moore	Whole plant	Bisbenzylisoquinoline alkaloid (Tet)	Optimal doses of 0.1 μM, 0.5 μM or 1 μM	BV2 Cells	Inhibiting NF-kB and extracellular-signal-regulated kinase (ERK) signaling pathways	Dang et al. (2014)
Chelidonium majus	Root	Alkaloid (Chelidonine)	50 mg/mL	Asthmatic mice	Improving allergic asthma and weakens eosinophilic airway inflammation in mice through suppressing IL-4, eotaxin-2	Kim et al. (2015)

TABLE 5.2 *(Continued)*

Source	Isolated part	Phytochemical	Dose/day	Treatment case	Mechanism of action	References
Chelidonium majus L.	Whole plant	Alkaloid (Chelerythrine)	1 mg/kg	Treatment against endotoxic shock in mice	Anti-inflammatory activity through the synthesis of MCP-1, IL-6, TNF-α, prostaglandin E2 (PGE2) and NO	Li et al. (2012)
Chelidonium majus L.	Whole plant	Alkaloid (Sanguinarine)	10 mg/kg	Treatment against acetic acid-induced ulcerative colitis in mice	Anti-inflammatory activity decreased the expression of MCP-1, IL-6, TNF-α, and NF-κB genes	Niu et al. (2013)
Chelidonium majus L.	Whole plant	Alkaloid (Sanguinarine)	6.21 μM	Treatment in human peripheral blood nectrophil	Immunomodulatory effect through inhibition of degranulation and phagocytosis of polymorphonuclear leukocytes	Agarwal et al. (1991)

amino acids does not exist in the heterocyclic ring of protoalkaloids. While, some alkaloids-like, terpene-like, purine-like, and steroid-like alkaloids that do not originate from amino acids are known as pseudoalkaloids (Aniszewski, 2007). Up till now, more than 20,000 alkaloids have been identified and many of them have shown significant role in clinical practice (Staniek et al., 2013). More than a few studies have represented the anti-inflammatory property of alkaloids comprising regulation or inhibition of essential mediators of inflammation such as nuclear factor-κB (NF-κB), cyclooxygenase-2 (COX-2), and inducible nitric oxide synthase (iNOS) (Yang et al., 2006; Matheus et al., 2007; Zhao et al., 2015). Souto et al. (2011) reported in a published review that 40 alkaloids have been confirmed to possesans anti-inflammatory activities.

5.3   PHENOLIC COMPOUNDS

Secondary metabolism of plants derives a heterogenic group of compounds namely phenolic compounds with at least one aromatic ring on which there can be one or maybe more hydroxyl groups attached to aromatic or aliphatic structures. Flavonoids and non-flavonoids are two major groups of phenolic compounds from which flavonoids, subcategorized as flavones, isoflavones, anthocyanins, flavonols, flavanols, flavanones, and so forth consists of two aromatic rings attached to an oxygen heterocycle, whereas non-flavonoids are generally identified as phenolic acids with two demonstrative subunits called benzoic and cinnamic acid (Bravo, 1998). There has been a huge interest in the investigation of phenolic compounds because of their importance in the food industry and health care. Phenolic compounds have shown many effects upon some diseases such as cardiovascular diseases, Alzheimer, diabetes, Parkinson, and inflammation (Bravo, 1998; Mohamed, 2014). Anti-inflammatory properties of phenolic compounds are exceedingly deliberated. Apart from the dearth of information regarding the mechanisms of anti-inflammatory activities of phenolic compounds, there is a relationship between the amount of food intake rich in phenolic compounds and inflammatory response's downregulation in a positive way (Alarcón de la Lastra and Villegas, 2005). In both inflammatory and antioxidant pathways, phenolic compounds can cause an up/downregulation in transcriptional factors such as NF-κβ or Nrf-2 (Sergent et al., 2010). There are some theories regarding the anti-inflammatory activities of phenolic compounds from which pro-inflammatory mediator's synthesis inhibition, alteration of eicosanoid synthesis, activated immune cells inhibition, or nitric oxide synthase and COX-2 inhibition through its inhibitory properties upon nuclear factor NF-κβ are determined thus far. A diversity of inhibitory activities of pro-inflammatory mediators and/or gene expression are two main mechanisms of actions for phenolic compounds (Alarcón de la Lastra and Villegas, 2005; Chuang and McIntosh, 2011). Therefore, it is obvious that phenolic compounds are widespread and diverse group possessing an extraordinary anti-inflammatory potential regarding their manifold inhibitory properties of pro-inflammatory mediators. The immune modulatory effects of some phenolic compounds were presented in Table 5.3.

5.4 FLAVONOIDS

Flavonoids are known as natural materials being present in both vegetables and fruits. So far, almost 4000 various flavonoids have been recognized and they take part in our regular diet. Flavonoids are known as one of the most broadly dispersed natural products found in plants existing as both glycosides and free-state. These compounds are chiefly water-soluble and their chemical structure is composed of the C6 C3 C6 skeleton of carbon. Flavonoids have potential in the prevention of oxidative cell damage as well as anti-cancer activity and protection upon carcinogens; besides, they are able to prohibit all processes of initiation, promotion, and tumor progression (Okwu, 2004). Regarding the structure baseline, flavonoids are well-ordered into diverse categories such as flavanones, flavones, isoflavone, flavanols, catechin, chalcones, and anthocyanin. Many enzyme system activities' enhancement is one of the most beneficial actions of flavonoids on cells of human body. Flavonoids are considered because of possessing anti-oxidant activities as well as having immunomodulatory mechanisms (Erlund, 2004; Table 5.4). They cause a decrease in activity of inflammatory cells by modulation of secretory mechanisms and results in the immunomodulation of inflammatory cells, which is a regular occurrence in body cells (Middleton and Kandaswami, 1992). Immunomodulation of pro-inflammatory enzymes can also occur by both the inhibition of nitric oxide (NO) synthase activity and arachidonic acid pathways, which causes a reduction in the assembly of inflammatory mediators, NO, prostaglandins, and leukotrienes (LTs) (Bindoli et al., 1977). Reduction in inflammatory cytokine production, TNF-α and interleukins (ILs) through flavonoids immunomodulation of pro-inflammatory mediators. Flavonoids are also responsible for lessening pro-inflammatory gene transcription by which immunomodulation of

TABLE 5.3 In vitro and in vivo Immunomodulatory Effects of Some Phenolic Compounds.

Source	Isolated part	Phytochemical	Dose/day	Treatment case	Mechanism of action	References
Green tea	Leaves	Phenolic compound (Gallic acid)	–	SRBC	Proliferation of B-cell and inhibition of mast cell degranulation	Hu et al. (1992)
Punica granatum	Fruit	Phenolic compound (ellagic acid)	100 μg/mL	Colon cell lines including HT-29 and HCT116	Both antiproliferative and apoptotic activities	Seeram et al. (2005)
Plantago major	Leaves	Phenolic compound (chlorogenic acid)	100 μL/well	PBMC	Enhancing lymphocyte proliferation and interferon (IFN) secretion	Chiang et al. (2003)
Plantago major	Leaves	Phenolic compound (ferulic acid)	100 μL/well	PBMC	Enhancing lymphocyte proliferation and IFN secretion	Chiang et al. (2003)
Plantago major	Leaves	Phenolic compound (p-Coumaric acid)	100 μL/well	PBMC	Enhancing lymphocyte proliferation and IFN secretion	Chiang et al. (2003)
Plantago major	Leaves	Phenolic compound (vanillic acid)	100μL/well	PBMC	Enhancing lymphocyte proliferation and IFN secretion	Chiang et al. (2003)
Curcuma longa	Rhizome	Phenolic compound (curcumin)	Dose-independent	Mouse macrophage cells, RAW-264.7	Bone marrow cellularity enhancement, activating α esterase positive cells and phagocytic and finally Inhibiting both IL-2 expression and NF-κB	Yadav et al. (2005)

TABLE 5.4 In vitro and in vivo Immunomodulatory Effects of Some Flavonoids.

Source	Isolated part	Phytochemical/ molecule name	Dose/day	Treatment case	Mechanism of action	References
Ziziphus lotus	Root bark	Flavonoid (flavonoid fraction)	200 mg/kg	Carrageenan-induced rat paw edema and the algesia induced in mice	Inhibiting the DTH induced by oxazolone	Borgi et al. (2008)
Bidens pilosa	Whole plant	Flavonoid (centaurein)	75 µg/ml	Jurkat cells	Aiming the induction of nuclear factor of activated T-cells activity and NF-κB enhancers	Chang et al. (2007)
Jatropha curcas	Leaves	Flavonoid (Apigenin 7-o-β-D-Neohesperidoside)	0.5, and 1 mg/kg BW	One-day-old specific pathogen free (SPF) chicks	Stimulating humoral and cell-mediated immune response	Abd-Alla et al. (2009)
Jatropha curcas	Leaves	Flavonoid (Apigenin 7-O-β-D-Galactoside)	0.25 mg/kg BW	One-day-old SPF chicks	Stimulating humoral and cell-mediated immune response	Abd-Alla et al. (2009)
Jatropha curcas	Leaves	Flavonoid (Orientin)	0.25 mg/kg BW	One-day-old SPF chicks	Stimulating humoral and cell-mediated immune response	Abd-Alla et al. (2009)
Jatropha curcas	Leaves	Flavonoid (Vitexin)	0.5, and 1 mg/kg BW	One-day-old SPF chicks	Stimulating humoral and cell-mediated immune response	Abd-Alla et al. (2009)
Cedrus deodara	The aerial parts	Flavonoid (Dihydroquercetin)	Increasing doses of 0.1, 0.5 and 1% of dihydroquercetin	Dietary application of immune status of gilthead seabream	Increasing the immune status of gilthead seabream in lower concentration	Awad et al. (2015)

pro-inflammatory gene expression is initiated. Furthermore, reactive oxygen species (ROS) formation inhibition by flavonoids in prooxidant enzymes radical scavenging mechanism is a remarkable antioxidant activity of flavonoids (Torel et al., 1986; Clemetson, 1989; Yilma et al., 2012).

5.5   ANTHOCYANINS

Anthocyanins, the water-soluble pigments, are subunits of polyphenol class that can have color alteration from red to blue seen in numerous fruits and vegetables. There have been many reports regarding the activities of anthocyanins in in vitro and in vivo investigations (Bagchi et al., 2004; Table 5.5). The pigments of anthocyanins are anthocyanidin glycosides. Their aglycone structure contains a central skeleton of 2-phenylbenzopyrylium known as flavylium cation (Kong et al., 2003; da Silva et al., 2014).

The percentage of anthocyanins in foods are estimated by the following percentages; cyaniding with 50% availability as the highest amount of anthocyanin in comparison to pelargonidin (12%), delphinidin and peonidin (both 12% of each), petunidin and malvidin (7% of each) (Kong et al., 2003). Studies have shown that anthocyanins have a notable role in modulating inflammation (Table 5.5), and oxidative stress as well as reducing the peril of developing chronic diseases. Furthermore, regarding the phenolic structure of anthocyanins, they can reduce the number of ROS by giving or removing electrons from hydrogen atoms. The anti-inflammatory, antiestrogenic, and cell proliferation inhibitory effects of anthocyanins make them very interesting areas for further studies. They also have a high anti-inflammatory potential to inhibit the initiation of the signaling pathway mediated by NF-κB. Despite showing a regular anti-inflammatory effect in the in vitro and in vivo, the mechanisms of action of anthocyanins are currently being clarified (Neyrinck et al., 2013; Esposito et al., 2014).

Anthocyanins have also been considered to hinder the expression and activity of iNOS in some *in vitro* studies. There have been many *in vivo* studies referring to evaluation on anthocyanin's bioactivity including the ability of lowering inflammatory cytokine concentrations, expression of several tissues, expression and activity of stress-induced iNOS and COX-2 as well as affecting both NF-κB and mitogen-activated protein kinase pathways (Mauray et al., 2010). Anthocyanins do not only lessen the pro-inflammatory mediators' expression but also increase the concentration of anti-inflammatory molecules.

TABLE 5.5 In vitro and in vivo Immunomodulatory Effects of Some Anthocyanin Compounds.

Source	Isolated part	Phytochemical/molecule name	Dose/day	Treatment case	Mechanism of action	References
Blackberry	Fruit	Anthocyanin (cyanidin-3-glycoside)	0.1 μM	Platelets (P-selectin expression) ex vivo studies in humans	Mechanism of anti-inflammatory	Rechner and Kroner (2005)
Blackberry	Fruit	Anthocyanin (peonidin)	0.1 μM	Platelets (P-selectin expression) ex vivo studies in humans	Mechanism of anti-inflammatory	Rechner and Kroner (2005)
Blueberry	Fruit	Anthocyanins (cyanidins, peonidins, malvidins, and delphinidins)	1.29 mg/g b	Mice (C57BL/6)	Inflammatory response via reducing high fat-diet and glucose	DeFuria et al. (2009)
Jaboticaba peel	Peel	Anthocyanins (delphinidin and cyaniding)	0.6598 mg/g b	Swiss inbred mice	Reduction of TNF-α and IL-6	Dragano et al. (2013)

5.6 TERPENOIDS

Terpenes, secondary metabolites, categorized into hemi, mono, sesqui, di, sester, or tri-based depends on the number of isoprene units they contain. Terpenoids, the biggest group of phytochemicals, are usually found in higher plants. They are recently being investigated as anticancer activators in clinical trials (Singh and Sharma, 2015). Terpenoids occur in most of the organisms, especially plants. A huge number of terpenoids numbering more than 40,000 of which are known in nature; and the number of them increases every year. More than a few terpenoids have cytotoxic activity against several tumors and cancer cells along with anticancer effects in preclinical animal models (Sacchettini and Poulter, 1997). Although most of the terpenoids known are those of plant origin, there are some other organisms such as bacteria and yeast, which are rich sources for terpenoids. Their carbon skeleton is structured into six isoprene units which result from the cyclic C_{30} hydrocarbon, squalene. Isoprenoid, the building blocks of terpenoids are a basic form to classify terpenoids as the number of building blocks structures differ. Some examples of terpenoids are monoterpenes (e.g., carvone, perillyl alcohol), diterpenes (e.g., retinol and trans-retinoic acid), triterpenes (e.g., betulinic acid, lupeol), and tetraterpenes (e.g., α-carotene, β-carotene). It is clear that terpenoids possess anti-inflammatory, immunomodulatory, antiviral, anti-allergenic, antispasmodic, and anti-hyperglycemic properties (Rabi and Bishayee, 2009). Triterpenoids, saponins, steroids, and cardiac glycosides, are well-known compounds with highly active effects and are present in leaves or fruit's waxy part (for instance apple and pear). Triterpenoids are responsible for defensive function in repelling insects and microbial attack (Harborne, 1973). Some immunomodulatory effects of specific terpenoids are presented in Table 5.6. The effects of these compounds over immune system can be occurred through either antibody production enhancing or T-cell response suppression (Venkatalakshmi et al., 2016).

5.7 SAPONINS

Saponins, steroid, or triterpenoid glycosides, are commonly found in a huge quantity of plants and plant products. Although triterpenoid saponins are originated in cultivated crops, steroid saponins are usual in plants, which are used as herbs. They are considered as significant compounds in human and animal diets. It is obvious that saponins obtained from plants

TABLE 5.6 In vitro and in vivo Immunomodulatory Effects of Some Terpenoids.

Source	Isolated part	Phytochemical/ molecule name	Dose/day	Treatment case	Mechanism of action	References
Andrographis paniculata	Leaves	Terpenoid (andrographolide)	100 µM	RAW 264.7 cells	Immunostimulatory and anti-inflammatory effects through Inhibiting inducible NO synthase (iNOS) protein expression and NO production	Chiou et al. (2000)
Boswellia serrata	Gum resin	Terpenoid (boswellic acid)	0.25 mg/paw	Rat paw edema modeling	Having anti-arthritic potential and inhibiting pro-inflammatory mediators	Singh et al. (2008)
Mycobacterium tuberculosis	Leaves	Terpenoid (ursolic acid)	10 g/ml	Alveolar epithelial A549 cells	Reducing the cytotoxic role of NO	Podder et al. (2015)

retain a potential utility as immunoadjuvant and they have the ability to induce the immunogenicity of numerous vaccines. Saponins are potent compounds capable of inducing the production of cytokines including ILs and interferons (IFN) that may interpose their immunostimulant efficacies. Probably, the induction of these responses happens through their interaction with antigen-presenting cells (Jie et al., 1984, Kensil, 1996; Aslanipour et al., 2017a,b). Structurally, saponins comprise a steroidal or triterpenoid aglycone to which one or maybe more sugar residues are adjoined (Oda et al., 2003). The utilization of saponins as adjuvants, a pharmacological or immunological agent, for modulating the cell-mediated immune system and enhancing antibody production is considered as one of the most outstanding activities of saponins (Table 5.7). The advantageous approach for saponins used as adjuvants is the low dose usage (Oda et al., 2000). Saponins have a strong adjuvant effect on both T-dependent and T-independent antigens; besides, two other responses of saponins referring to cytotoxic $CD8^+$ lymphocyte and mucosal antigens are subject of recent research. Although saponins have been studied in causing hemolysis of red blood cells in vitro through their surface-active mechanism, hemolysis does not emerge to be in relationship with adjuvant activity. Several saponins can affect tumor cell growth inhibition through apoptosis and cell cycle arrest with IC_{50} standards up to 0.2 mM. (Kensil, 1996; Oda et al., 2000).

5.8   STEROLS AND STEROLINS

The main phytosterol in advanced plants known as beta-sitosterol (BSS) is found in healthy individual's serum and tissues almost 800–1000 times less than that of endogenous cholesterol. BSSG, glycoside form of BSS, can similarly be found in serum even with lower concentrations. They are both synthesized in plants but not animals; therefore, animals gain them through diet (Pegel, 1997). There have been some in vitro and ex vivo studies reported regarding the immunomodulatory effects of BSS:BSSG in various ratios such as affecting cellular proliferation of T-lymphocytes and enhancing response to mitogens as well as increasing lytic ability of the natural killer (NK) cells to a cancer cell line. Besides, BSS:BSSG mixture could enhance IL-2 and IFN-γ secretion and inhibit the secretion of IL-4. The above-mentioned mixture could have anti-inflammatory activities through inhibition of IL-6 and TNF-α in a dose-dependent manner (Myers and Bouic, 1998). Sterols with specific ratio may possibly

TABLE 5.7 In vitro and in vivo Immunomodulatory Effects of Some Saponins.

Source	Isolated part	Phytochemical/molecule name	Dose/day	Treatment case	Mechanism of action	References
Asiaticoside *Centella asiatica*	Root	Saponin	100 mg/kg bw	PBMCs	Enhancement of phagocytic index and total WBC number	Punturee et al. (2005)
Glycyrrhizin *Glycyrrhiza glabra*	Root	Saponin (water-soluble constituent glycyrrhizin)	1.0 mg/ml	Rat liver microsomes	Classical complement pathway Inhibition	Ablise et al. (2004)
Astragalus trojanus (for Ast VII) *Astragalus oleifolius* (for Mac B)	Root	Saponin (Ast VII and Mac B)	156 µg/ml.	6–8 week old male Swiss albino mice	Having immunoregulatory effects without inflammatory cytokine stimulation	Nalbantsoy et al. (2012)
Calendula officinalis	Whole plant	Saponin (*C. officinalis*) Saponins L3 (GlcUAOA)	100 µg×mL⁻¹	BALB/c mice	cytokine production induction in mice	Doligalska et al. (2013)
Albizia julibrissin	Stem bark	Saponin (AJS₇₅)	2.53 µg/ml	0.5% rabbit red blood cell suspensions	Improving antigen cellular and humoral immune responses, inducing cytokine release and eliciting a Th1/Th2 response	Sun et al. (2014)
Chinese ginseng	Herb	Saponin (PDS-C)	1400 mg/kg	The BALB/c mouse model with ITP	Proliferation and differentiation of megakaryocytes, modulating immune function	Lin et al. (2015)
Ginseng	Stem–leaf	Saponin (GSLS)	100 mg/kg BW	Chickens vaccinated with live infectious bursal disease	Improving vaccination in immunosuppressed chickens.	Yu et al. (2015)
Quillaja brasiliensis	Leaves	Saponin (purified saponin fraction) (QB-80, QB-90)	(50 µg or 100 µg)	Female Swiss mice	Having immunological adjuvants in vaccines against a lethal through Challenging a chief live-stock pathogen	Yendo et al. (2016)

TABLE 5.7 (Continued)

Source	Isolated part	Phytochemical/molecule name	Dose/day	Treatment case	Mechanism of action	References
Smilax davidiana	Rhizomes	Saponin (Davidianoside F)	In both concentration of 10.2 and 4.3 µM	Human tumor cell lines (MCF-7 and HELA cell lines)	Evaluating anti-inflammatory and cytotoxic activities in vitro, anti-inflammatory effects to IL-1β suppression	Zhou et al. (2017)
Ilex pubescens	Roots	Saponin (Ilexsaponin I and b-D-glucopyranosyl 3-b-[b-Dxylopyranosyl-(1/2)-b-D-glucopyranosyloxy]-olea-12-en-28-oate)	30 or 10 mM	LPS-stimulated RAW 264.7 cells	Having potent anti-inflammatory properties through inhibiting LPS-induced NO and PGE2 production through suppressing the expression of iNOS and cyclooxygenase-2	Wu et al. (2017)
Astragalus karjaginii BORISS and *Astragalus brachycalyx* FISCHER	Roots	Saponins	3 and 6 µg	Human whole blood	Inductions of cytokine release	Aslani-pour et al. (2017a,b)

stabilize equilibrium between the Th1–Th2 cells, which is a very important achievement for the final result of the immune response. Even in very low concentrations, the phytosterols, β-sitosterol, and its glycoside could enhance the proliferative in vitro response to T-cells stimulation (Bouic, 2001). Murine macrophages activation, lysosomal, and phagocytosis enzymes activity induction was reported by Ghosal et al. (1989) when 100–400 µg/mouse leaves extract of *Withania somnifera* which contains withanolide, a sterol.

5.9 POLYSACCHARIDES

Polysaccharides are bioactive macromolecule substances that consist of several monosaccharides, 10 or more, which are attached to glycoside bonds (Kui et al., 2010). There are three main sources of polysaccharides which include the animals, plants, and fungus. The plant-derived polysaccharides display many valuable therapeutic properties by mechanisms of taken part in the innate immunity modulation, more precisely the function of macrophage. Some specific polysaccharides are supposed to have a notable immunomodulatory effect as well (Anderson et al., 1994). Various facts suggest that saccharide is an informational molecule in organism participating in physiological reactions and pathological procedures including immune regulations, intercellular material transport, and intercellular recognitions. They have been considered to support standard bowel function and blood glucose and lipid levels for many years. Plant polysaccharides have inclusive bioactivities containing antitumor, anticancer, and so on, especially in enhancing immunity of organisms from which their effect upon immunity has been focused on activation and stimulation of macrophage proliferation as well as reduction of some cytokines such as IL-6 and TNF-α serum levels and induction of some other cytokines including IL-2, IL-4, and IL-10 serum levels (Kui et al., 2010). Consequently, the methodical estimation of the above-mentioned polysaccharides is a rare chance for the detection of original therapeutic agents and adjuvants containing advantageous immunomodulatory agent (Schepetkin and Quinn, 2006). Many studies suggest a link of polysaccharides on immune system function from which the capability of oral polysaccharides in immune system stimulation is highly considered. Besides, the abilities of some polysaccharides on inflammation and cancer metabolism have been of interests to scientist still present (Chan et al., 2009).

5.10 LECTINS

Lectins and C-type lectins, known as a heterogeneous non-enzymatic group of proteins are present in almost all of the organisms from viruses, bacteria, and yeast to plants and animals (Gupta et al., 2012). They are also well-known as a class of proteins with various functions and possess a distinctive structural motif.

Carbohydrate recognition domain, the singular structural signature of lectins, provides a binding capability of attaching specific carbohydrates to lectins. Lectins, the nonimmune origin of carbohydrate-binding proteins, are involved in various biological processes such as cell–cell recognition, cell proliferation, and migration as well as extracellular matrix adhesion (Van Damme et al., 1998). C-type lectins, known as calcium-dependent lectins, are found to have an essential role in immunological fields of natural killer gene complex, LLT1, and CD161 (Zelensky et al., 2005). Glycan's moieties existed on the external part of immune cells and are responsible for immunomodulatory activities of plant-derived lectins through an interaction resulting in the production of specific cytokines and induction of effective immune responses counter to microbial infections or tumors.

Lectins with immunomodulatory effects (Table 5.8) partake in pharmaceutical applications or can support the detection of sugar targets for novel therapeutic approaches. A number of 15 distinct structural families have been listed in animal lectins category from which group five has been highlighted for its immunological prominence and it includes a variety of NK cell receptors. Although the effect of lectin family members is chiefly related to the compilation of NK cell activity, the exact role of some subunits of the family leftovers remains unidentified (Zelensky et al., 2005).

KEYWORDS

- **immune system**
- **phytochemicals**
- **diseases**
- **immunomodulators**
- **alkaloids**

TABLE 5.8 In vitro and in vivo Immunomodulatory Effects of Some Lectins.

Source	Isolated part	Phytochemical/ molecule name	Dose/day	Treatment case	Mechanism of action	References
Viscum album	Leaves	Lectin (VAA-I)	10 ng/ml	human PBMCs	Inducing the secretion of IL-2 and activating cytokine-induced NK	Hajto et al. (1998)
Cratylia mollis Mart	Seeds	Lectin (Cramoll 1,4)	25 µg/m	In vitro experimental cultures of mice lymphocytes		Melo et al. (2010)
Viscum album var. Coloratum	Leaves	Lectin (KML)	Dose-independent	Human dendritic cells	Induction of IL-2 secretion	Lyu and Park. (2010)
Alium sativum	Bulbs	Lectin (ASA-I)	0.5 mg/ml	Murine spleen cells	Inducing IL-12 production through of p38 mitogen-activated protein kinase and ERK activation in macrophages and stimulating IFN-γ production	Dong et al. (2011)

REFERENCES

Abd-Alla, H. I.; Moharram, F. A.; Gaara, A. H.; El-Safty, M. M.; Phytoconstituents of *Jatropha curcas* L. Leaves and Their Immunomodulatory Activity on Humoral and Cell-Mediated Immune Response in Chicks. *Z. Naturforsch. C.* **2009,** *64,* 495–501.

Ablise, M.; Leininger-Muller, B.; Wong, C. D.; Siest, G.; Loppinet, V.; Visvikis, S. Synthesis and *in Vitro* Antioxidant Activity of Glycyrrhetinic Acid Derivatives Tested with the Cytochrome P450/Nadph System. *Chem. Pharm. Bull.* **2004,** *52,* 1436–1439.

Agarwal, S.; Reynolds, M. A.; Pou, S.; Peterson, D. E.; Charon, J. A.; Suzuki, J. B. The Effect of Sanguinarine on Human Peripheral Blood Neutrophil Viability and Functions. *Oral Microbiol. Immunol.* **1991,** *6,* 51–61.

Aguilar, J. L.; Rojas, P.; Marcelo, A.; Plaza, A.; Bauer, R.; Reininger, E.; Klaas, C. A.; Merfort, I. Anti-inflammatory Activity of Two Different Extracts of *Uncaria tomentosa* (Rubiaceae). *J. Ethnopharmacol.* **2002,** *81,* 271–276.

Alarcón de la Lastra, C.; Villegas, I. Resveratrol as an Anti-Inflammatory and Anti-Aging Agent: Mechanisms and Clinical Implications. *Mol. Nutr. Food Res.* **2005,** *49,* 405–430.

Al-Sa'aidi, J. A. A.; Dawood, K. A.; Latif, A. D. Immunomodulatory Effect of *Nigella Sativa* Seed Extract in Male Rabbits Treated with Dexamethasone. *Iraqi J. Vet. Sci.* **2012,** *26,* 141–149.

Amirghofran, Z.; Azadmeh, A.; Javidnia, K. *Haussknechtia Elymatica*: a Plant with Immunomodulatory Effects. *Iran. J. Immunol.* **2007,** *4,* 26–31.

Anderson, J. W.; Smith, B. M.; Gustafson, N. J. Health Benefits and Practical Aspects of High-Fiber Diets. *Am. J. Clin. Nutr.* **1994,** *59,* 1242–1247.

Aniszewski, T. *Alkaloids—Secrets of Life, Alkaloid Chemistry, Biological Significance, Applications and Ecological Role,* 1st ed.; Elsevier: Amsterdam, The Netherlands, 2007.

Aslanipour, B.; Gülcemal, D.; Nalbantsoy, A.; Yusufoglu, H.; Bedir, E. Secondary Metabolites from *Astragalus karjaginii* BORISS and the Evaluation of Their Effects on Cytokine Release and Hemolysis. *Fitoterapia.* **2017a,** *122,* 26–33.

Aslanipour, B.; Gülcemal, D.; Nalbantsoy, A.; Yusufoglu, H.; Bedir, E.; Cycloartane-type Glycosides from *Astragalus brachycalyx* FISCHER and their Effects on Cytokine Release and Hemolysis. *Phytochem. Lett.* **2017b,** *21,* 66–73.

Awad, E.; Awaad, A. S.; Esteban, M. A. Effects of Dihydroquercetin Obtained from Deodar (Cedrus Deodara) on Immune Status of *Gilthead Seabream* (*Sparus Aurata* L.). *Fish Shellfish Immunol.* **2015,** *43,* 43–50.

Bagchi, D.; Sen, C. K.; Bagchi, M.; Atalay, M. Anti-Angiogenic, Antioxidant, and Anti-Carcinogenic Properties of a Novel Anthocyanin Rich Berry Extract Formula. *Biochem.* **2004,** *69,* 75–80.

Bindoli, A.; Cavallini, L.; Siliprandi, N. Inhibitory Action of Silymarin of Lipid Peroxide Formation in Rat Liver Mitochondria and Microsomes. *Biochem. Pharmacol.* **1977,** *26,* 2405–2409.

Bin-Hafeez, B.; Haque, R.; Parvez, S.; Pandey, S.; Sayeed, I.; Raisuddin, S Immunomodulatory Effects of Fenugreek (*Trigonella Foenum Graecum* L.) Extract in Mice. *Int. Immunopharmacol.* **2003,** *3,* 257–265.

Bonacorsi, C.; Raddi, M. S. G.; Carlos, I. Z.; Sannomiya, M.; Vilegas, W. Anti-Helicobacter Pylori Activity and Immunostimulatory Effect of Extracts from *Byrsonima crassa* Nied (Malpighiaceae). *BMC Complementary Altern. Med.* **2009,** *9,* 1–7.

Borgi, W.; Recio, M. C.; Ríos, J. L.; Chouchane, N. Anti-Inflammatory and Analgesic Activities of Flavonoid and Saponin Fractions from *Zizyphus Lotus* (L.) Lam *S. Afr. J. Bot.* **2008,** *74,* 320–324.

Bouic, P. J. Plant Sterols and Sterolins. *Altern. Med. Rev.* **2001,** *6,* 203–206.

Bravo, L. Polyphenols: Chemistry, Dietary Sources, Metabolism, and Nutritional Significance. *Nutr. Rev.* **1998,** *56,* 317–333.

Chan, G. C.; Chan, W. K.; Sze, D. M. The Effects of Beta-Glucan on Human Immune and Cancer Cells. *J. Hematol. Oncol.* **2009,** *10,* 2–25.

Chang, S. L.; Chiang, Y. M.; Chang, C. L.; Yeh, H. H.; Shyur, L. F.; Kuo, Y. H.; Wu, T. K.; Yang, W. C. Flavonoids, Centaurein and Centaureidin, from *Bidens pilosa,* Stimulate IFN-gamma Expression. *J. Ethnopharmacol.* **2007,** *112,* 232–236.

Chiang, L. C.; Ng, L. T.; Chiang, W.; Chang, M. Y.; Lin, C. C. Immunomodulatory Activities of Flavonoids, Monoterpenoids, Triterpenoids, Iridoid Glycosides and Phenolic Compounds of Plantago Species. *Planta Med.* **2003,** *69,* 600–604.

Chiou, W. F.; Chen, C. F.; Lin, J. J. Mechanisms of Suppression of Inducible Nitric Oxide Synthase (Inos) Expression in Raw 264.7 Cells by Andrographolide. *Br. J. Pharmacol.* **2000,** *129,* 1553–1560.

Choi, C. Y.; Kim, J. Y.; Kim, Y. S.; Chung, Y. S.; Seo, J. K. W.; Jeong, H. G. Aqueous Extract Isolated from *Platycodon Grandiflorum* Elicits the Release of Nitric Oxide and Tumor Necrosis Factor-α from Murine Macrophages. *Int. Immunopharmacol.* **2001,** *1,* 1141–1151.

Christybapita, D.; Divyagnaneswari, M.; Dinakaran Michael, R. Oral Administration of Eclipta Alba Leaf Aqueous Extract Enhances the Non-Specific Immune Responses and Disease Resistance of *Oreochromis Mossambicus. Fish Shellfish Immunol.* **2007,** *23,* 840–852.

Chuang, C. C.; Mcintosh, M. K. Potential Mechanisms by Which Polyphenol-Rich Grapes Prevent Obesity Mediated Inflammation and Metabolic Diseases. *Annu. Rev. Nutr.* **2011,** *31,* 155–176.

Clemetson, C. A. B. B. In *Vitamin C*; Clemetson, C. A. B. ed.; CRC Press, Inc.: Boca Raton, FL, **1989**; pp 101–128.

Cushnie, T. P. T.; Cushnie, B.; Lamb, A. J. Alkaloids: an Overview of Their Antibacterial, Antibiotic-Enhancing and Antivirulence Activities. *Int. J. Antimicrob. Agents.* **2014,** *44,* 377–386.

da Silva, N. A.; Rodrigues, E.; Mercadante, A. Z.; de Rosso, V. V. Phenolic Compounds and Carotenoids from Four Fruits Native from the Brazilian Atlantic Forest. *J. Agric. Food Chem.* **2014,** *62,* 5072–5084.

Dang, Y.; Xu, Y.; Wu, W.; Li, W.; Sun, Y.; Yang, J.; Zhu, Y.; Zhang, C. Tetrandrine Suppresses Lipopolysaccharide-Induced Microglial Activation by Inhibiting Nf-Kb and Erk Signaling Pathways in Bv2 Cells. *PLoS One.* **2014,** *9,* 102522.

DeFuria, J.; Bennett, G.; Strissel, K. J.; Perfield, J. W.; Milbury, P. E.; Greenberg, A. S.; Obin, M. S. Dietary Blueberry Attenuates Whole-Body Insulin Resistance in High Fat-Fed Mice by Reducing Adipocyte Death and Its Inflammatory Sequelae. *J. Nutr.* **2009,** *139,* 1510–1516.

Doligalska, M.; Joźwicka, K.; Laskowska, M.; Donskow-Łysoniewska, K.; Pączkowski,C.; Janiszowska, W. Changes in *Heligmosomoides Polygyrus* Glycoprotein Pattern by Saponins Impact the BALB/C Mice Immune Response. *Exp. Parasitol.* **2013,** *135,* 524–531.

Dong, Q.; Sugiura, T.; Toyohira, Y.; Yoshida, Y.; Yanagihara, N.; Karasaki, Y. Stimulation of IFN-Gamma Production by Garlic Lectin in Mouse Spleen Cells: Involvement of IL-12 Via Activation of and Erk in Macrophages. *Phytomed.* **2011,** *18,* 309–316.

Dragano, N. R.; Marques, A.; Cintra, D. E.; Solon, C.; Morari, J.; Leite-Legatti, A. V.; Velloso, L. A.; Marostica-Junior, M. R. Freeze-Dried Jaboticaba Peel Powder Improves Insulin Sensitivity in High-Fat-Fed Mice. *Br. J. Nutr.* **2013,** *110,* 447–455.

Erlund, I. Review of the Flavonoids Quercetin, Hesperetin, and naringenin. Dietary Sources, Bioactivities, Bioavailability, and Epidemiology. *Nutr. Res.* **2004**, *24*, 851–874.

Esposito, D.; Chen, A.; Grace, M. H.; Komarnytsky, S.; Lila, M. A. Inhibitory Effects of Wild Blueberry Anthocyanins and Other Flavonoids on Biomarkers of Acute and Chronic Inflammation *in Vitro*. *J. Agric. Food Chem.* **2014**, *62*, 7022–7028.

Ghosal, S.; Srivastava, R. S.; Bhattacharya, S. K.; Upadhyay, S. N.; Jaiswal, A. K.; Chattopadhyay, U. Immunomodulatory and CNS Effects of Sitoindosides IX and X, Two New Glycowithanolides Form *Withania Somnifera*. *Phytother. Res.* **1989**, *2*, 201–206.

Gupta, G. S. *Animal Lectins: Form, Function and Clinical Applications*; Springer: Vienna, 2012.

Hajto, T.; Hostanska, K.; Weber, K.; Zinke, H.; Fischer, J.; Mengs, U.; Lentzen, H.; Saller, R. Effect of a Recombinant Lectin, Viscum Album Agglutinin on the Secretion of Interleukin-12 in Cultured Human Eripheral Blood Mononuclear Cells and on NKcell-Mediated Cytotoxicity of Rat Splenocytes *in Vitro* and *in Vivo*. *Nat. Immun.* **1998**, *16*, 34–46.

Harborne, J. B. *Phytochemical Methods;* Chapman and Hall, Ltd.: London, 1973; pp 49–188.

Harborne, J. B. The Chemical Basis of Plant Defense. In *Plant Defenses against Mammalian Herbivory*; Palo, R. T., Robbins, C. T., Eds.; CRC Press: Boca Raton, Florida, 1991; pp 45–59.

Ho, L. J.; Juan, T. Y.; Chao, P.; Wu, W. L.; Chang, D. M.; Chang, S. Y.; Lai, J. H. Plant Alkaloid Tetrandrine Downregulates IκBα Kinases-IκBα-NF-κB Signaling Pathway in Human Peripheral Blood T Cell. *Br. J. Pharmacol.* **2004**, *143*, 919–927.

Hu, Z. Q.; Toda, M.; Okubo, S.; Hara, Y.; Shimamura, T. Mitogenic Activity of (−) Epigallocatechin Gallate on B-Cells and Investigation of Its Structure-Function Relationship. *Int. J. Immunopharmacol.* **1992**, *14*, 1399–1407.

Im, S. A.; Kim, K.; Lee, C. K. Immunomodulatory Activity of Polysaccharides Isolated from *Salicornia Herbacea*. *Int. Immunopharmacol.* **2006**, *6*, 1451–1458.

Ivanovska, N.; Philipov, S. Study on the Anti-Inflammatory Action of Berberis Vulgaris Root Extract, Alkaloid Fractions and Pure Alkaloids. *Int. J. Immunopharmacol.* **1996**, *18*, 553–561.

Jie, Y. H.; Cammisuli, S.; Baggiolini, M. Immunomodulatory Effects of Panax Ginseung C. Meyer in the Mouse. *Agents Actions* **1984**, *15*, 386–391.

Kandhare, A. D.; Raygude, K. S.; Ghosh, P.; Ghule, A. E.; Gosavi, T. P.; Badole, S. L.; Bodhankar, S. L. Effect of Hydroalcoholic Extract of Hibiscus Rosa Sinensis Linn. Leaves in Experimental Colitis in Rats. *Asian Pac. J. Trop. Biomed.* **2012**, *2*, 337–344.

Kensil, C. R. Saponins as Vaccine Adjuvants. *Crit. Rev. Ther. Drug Carrier Syst.* **1996**, *13*, 1–55.

Kim, S.H.; Hong, J.H.; Lee, Y.C.; Chelidonine, a principal isoquinoline alkaloid of Chelidonium *majus*, attenuates eosinophilic airway inflammation by suppressing IL-4 and eotaxin-2 expression in asthmatic mice. *Pharmacol Rep.* **2015**, *67*, 1168–1177.

Kong, J.M.; Chia, L.S.; Goh, N.K.; Chia, T.F.; Brouillard, R.; Analysis and biological activities of anthocyanins. *Phytochem.* **2003**, *64*, 923–33.

Kui, Z.; Wang, Q.; He, Y.; He, X.; Evaluation of radicals scavenging, immunity-modulatory and antitumor activities of longan polysaccharidesRadicals Scavenging, Immunity-Modulatory and Antitumor Activities of Longan Polysaccharides with Ultrasonic Extraction on in S180 Tumor Mice Models [J]. *Int. J. Biol. Macromol.* **2010**, *47*, 356–360.

Kulkarni, S.; Desai, S. Immunostimulant Activity of Inulin Isolated from *Saussurea Lappa* Roots. *Indian J. Pharm. Sci.* **2001**, *63*, 292–294.

Li, F.; Wang, H. D.; Lu, D. X.; Wang, Y. P.; Qi, R. B.; Fu, Y. M.; Li, C. J. Neutral Sulfate Berberine Modulates Cytokine Secretion and Increases Survival in Endotoxemic Mice. *Acta Pharmacol. Sin.* **2006,** *27,* 1199–1205.

Li, W.; Fan, T.; Zhang, Y.; Niu, X.; Xing, W. Effect of Chelerythrine Against Endotoxic Shock in Mice and Its Modulation of Inflammatory Mediators in Peritoneal Macrophages Through the Modulation of Mitogen-Activated Protein Kinase (Mapk) Pathway. *Inflammation* **2012,** *35,* 1814–1824.

Lin, X.; Yin, L.; Gao, R.; Liu, Q.; Xu, W.; Jiang, X.; Chong, B. H. The Effects of Panaxadiol Saponins on Megakaryocytic Maturation and Immune Function in a Mouse Model of Immune Thrombocytopenia. *Exp. Hematol.* **2015,** *43,* 364–373.

Lyu, S. Y.; Park, W. B. Mistletoe Lectin Transport by M-Cells in Follicle-Associated Epithelium (FAE) and IL-12 Secretion in Dendritic Cells Situated Below FAE in vitro. *Arch. Pharm. Res.* **2010,** *33,* 1433–1441.

Matheus, M. E.; Violante, F. D. A.; Garden, S. J.; Pinto, A. C.; Fernandes, P. D. Isatins Inhibit Cyclooxygenase-2 and Inducible Nitric Oxide Synthase in a Mouse Macrophage Cell Line. *Eur. J. Pharmacol.* **2007,** *556,* 200–206.

Mauray, A.; Felgines, C.; Morand, C.; Mazur, A.; Scalbert, A.; Milenkovic, D. Nutrigenomic Analysis of the Protective Effects of Bilberry Anthocyanin-Rich Extract in Apo E-Deficient Mice. *Genes Nutr.* **2010,** *5,* 343–353.

Melo, C. M. L. D.; De Castro, M. C. A. B. D.; Oliveira, A. P.; Gomes, F. O. S.; Pereira, V. R. A.; Correia, M. T. S.; Coelho, L. C. B. B.; Paiva, P. M. G. Immunomodulatory Response of Cramoll 1,4 Lectin on Experimental Lymphocytes. *Phytother. Res.* **2010,** *24,* 1631–1636.

Middleton, E.; Kandaswami, C. Effects of Flavonoids on Immune and Inflammatory Cell Function. *Biochem. Pharmacol.* **1992,** *43,* 1167–1179.

Mishra, K. P.; Padwad, Y. S.; Dutta, A.; Ganju, L.; Sairam, M.; Banerjee, P. K.; Sawhney, R. C. Aqueous Extract of Rhodiola Imbricata Rhizome Inhibits Proliferation of an Erythroleukemic Cell Line K-562 by Inducing Apoptosis and Cell Cycle Arrest At G2/M Phase. *Immunobiology.* **2008,** *213,* 125–131.

Mohamed, S. Functional Foods against Metabolic Syndrome (Obesity, Diabetes, Hypertension and Dyslipidemia) and Cardiovascular Disease. *Trends Food Sci. Technol.* **2014,** *35,* 114–128.

Myers, L.; Bouic, P. J. D. Flow Cytometric Analysis of the TH1-TH2 Shift in Allergic Individuals Using ModucareTM (sterols/sterolins). *26th Annual Congress of the Physiology Society of Southern Africa,* 1998.

Nalbantsoy, A.; Nesil, T.; Yılmaz-Dilsiz, O.; Aksu, G.; Khan, S.; Bedir, E. Evaluation of the Immunomodulatory Properties in Mice and in Vitro Anti-Inflammatory Activity of Cycloartane Type Saponins from Astragalus Species. *J. Ethnopharmacol.* **2012,** *139,* 574–581.

Neyrinck, A. M.; Van Hée, V. F.; Bindels, L. B.; De Backer, F.; Cani, P. D.; Delzenne, N. M. Polyphenol-Rich Extract of Pomegranate Peel Alleviates Tissue Inflammation and Hypercholesterolaemia in High-Fat Diet-Induced Obese Mice: Potential Implication of the Gut Microbiota. *Br. J. Nutr.* **2013,** *109,* 802–809.

Niu, X.; Fan, T.; Li, W.; Huang, H.; Zhang, Y.; Xing, W. Protective Effect of Sanguinarine against Acetic Acidinduced Ulcerative Colitis in Mice. *Toxicol. Appl. Pharmacol.* **2013,** *267,* 256–265.

Oda, K.; Matsuda, H.; Murakami, T.; Katayama, S.; Ohgitani, T.; Yoshikawa, M. Adjuvant and Haemolytic Activities of 47 Saponins Derived from Medicinal and Food Plants. *Biol. Chem.* **2000,** *381,* 67–74.

Oda, K.; Matsuda, H.; Murakami, T.; Katayama, S.; Ohgitani, T.; Yoshikawa, M. Relationship between Adjuvant Activity and Amphipathic Structure of Soya Saponins. *Vaccine.* **2003,** *21,* 2145–2151.

Okwu, D. E. Phytochemicals and Vitamin Content of Indigenous Spices of South Eastern Nigeria. *J. Sust. Agric. Environ.* **2004,** *6,* 30–37.

Park, J. E.; Cuong, T. D.; Hung, T. M.; Lee, I.; Na, M.; Kim, J. C.; Ryoo, S.; Lee, J. H.; Choi, J. S.; Woo, M. H.; Min, B. S. Alkaloids from *Chelidonium Majus* and Their Inhibitory Effects on LPS-Induced No Production in RAW264.7 Cells. *Bioorg. Med. Chem. Lett.* **2011,** *21,* 6960–6963.

Pegel, K. H. The Importance of Sitosterol and Sitosterolin in Human and Animal Nutrition. *SA J. Sci.* **1997,** *93,* 263–268.

Podder, B.; Jang, W. S.; Nam, K. W.; Lee, B. E.; Song, H. Y. Ursolic Acid Activates Intracellular Killing Effect of Macrophages During *Mycobacterium Tuberculosis* Infection. *J. Microbiol. Biotechnol.* **2015,** *25,* 738–744.

Punturee, K.; Wild, C. P.; Kasinrerk, W.; Vinitketkumnuen, U. Immunomodulatory Activities of *Centella Asiatica* and *Rhinacanthus Nasutus* Extracts. *Asian Pac. J. Cancer Prev.* **2005,** *6,* 396–400.

Puri, A.; Saxena, R.; Saxena, R. P.; Saxena, K. C.; Srivastava, V.; Tandon, J. S. Immunostimulant Activity of Nyctanthes Arbor-Tristis L. *J. Ethnopharmacol.* **1994,** *42,* 31–37.

Puri, A.; Saxena, R. P.; Guru, Y. P.; Kulshresta, D.; Saxena, K. C.; Dhawan, B. N. Immunostimulatant Activity of Picroliv, the Irioid Glycoside Fraction of *Picrorhiza Kurroa* and Its Protective Action Against *Leishmania Donovani* in Hamster. *Planta Med.* **1992,** *58,* 528–532.

Rabi, T.; Bishayee, A. Terpenoids and Breast Cancer Chemoprevention. *Breast Cancer Res. Treat.* **2009,** *115,* 223–239.

Rechner, A. R.; Kroner, C. Anthocyanins and Colonic Metabolites of Dietary Polyphenols Inhibit Platelet Function. *Thromb. Res.* **2005,** *116,* 327–334.

Sacchettini, J. C.; Poulter, C. D. Creating Isoprenoid Diversity. *Science* **1997,** *277,* 1788–1789.

Schepetkin, I. A.; Quinn, M. T. Botanical Polysaccharides: Macrophage Immunomodulation and Therapeutic Potential. *Int. Immunopharmacol.* **2006,** *6,* 317–333.

Seeram NP.; Adams LS.; Henning SM.; Niu Y.; Zhang Y.; Nair MG.; Heber D *In Vitro* Anti-Proliferative, Apoptotic and Antioxidant Activities of Punicalagin, Ellagic Acid and a Total Pomegranate Tannin Extract are Enhanced in Combination with Other Polyphenols as Found in Pomegranate Juice. *J. Nutr. Biochem.* **2005,** *16,* 360–367.

Senchina, D. S.; Hallam, J. E.; Thompson, N. M.; Nguyen, N. A.; Robinson, J. R.; Perera, M. A. Alkaloids and Endurance Athletes. *Track Cross Ctry. J.* **2012,** *2,* 2–18.

Senchina, D. S.; McCann, D. A.; Asp, J. M.; Johnson, J. A.; Cunnick, J. E.; Kaiser, M. S.; Kohut, M. L. Changes in Immunomodulatory Properties of *Echinacea* Spp Root Infusions and Tinctures Stored At 4 Degrees C for Four Days. *Clin. Chim. Acta.* **2005,** *355,* 67–82.

Sergent, T.; Piront, N.; Meurice, J.; Toussaint, O.; Schneider, Y. J. Anti-Inflammatory Effects of Dietary Phenolic Compounds in an *in Vitro* Model of Inflamed Human Intestinal Epithelium. *Chem. Biol. Interact.* **2010,** *188,* 659–667.

Singh, B.; Sharma, R. Plant Terpenes: Defense Responses, Phylogenetic Analysis, Regulation and Clinical Applications. *Biotech.* **2015,** *5,* 129–151.

Singh, S.; Khajuria, A.; Taneja, S. C.; Johri, R. K.; Singh, J.; Qazi, G. N. Boswellic Acids: a Leukotriene Inhibitor Also Effective Through Topical Application in Inflammatory Disorders. *Phytomed.* **2008,** *15,* 400–407.

Souto, A. L.; Tavares, J. F.; da Silva, M. S.; de Diniz, M. F. F. M.; de Athayde-Filho, P. F.; Barbosa Filho, J. M. Anti-Inflammatory Activity of Alkaloids: an Update from 2000 to 2010. *Molecules.* **2011,** *16,* 8515–8534.

Staniek, A.; Bouwmeester, H.; Fraser, P. D.; Kayser, O.; Martens, S.; Tissier, A.; Krol, S. V. D.; Wessjohann, L.; Warzec, D. H. Natural Products—Modifying Metabolite Pathways in Plants. *Biotechnol. J.* **2013,** *8,* 1159–1171.

Sun, H.; He, S.; Shi, M. Adjuvant-Active Fraction from Julibrissin Saponins Improves Immune Responses by Inducing Cytokine and Chemokine At the Site of Injection. *Int. Immunopharmacol.* **2014,** *22,* 346–355.

Torel, J.; Cillard, J.; Cillard, P. Antioxidant Activity of Flavonoids and Reactivity with Peroxy Radical. *Phytochemistry.* **1986,** *25,* 383–385.

Van Damme, E. J. M.; Peumans, W. J.; Barre, A.; Rougé, P. Plant Lectins: a Composite of Several Distinct Families of Structurally and Evolutionary Related Proteins with Diverse Biological Roles. *Crit. Rev. Plant. Sci.* **1998,** *17,* 575–692.

Veena, N.; Arora, S.; Kapila, S.; Singh, R. R. B.; Katara, A.; Pandey, M. M.; Rastogi, S.; Rawat, A. K. S. Immunomodulatory and Antioxidative Potential of Milk Fortified with *Asparagus Racemosus* (Shatavari). *J. Med. Plants Stud.* **2014,** *2,* 13–19.

Venkatalakshmi, P.; Vadivel, V.; Brindha, P. Role of Phytochemicals as Immunomodulatory Agents: a Review. *IJGP.* **2016,** *10,* 1–18.

Wu, P.; Gao, H.; Liu, J. X.; Liu, L.; Zhou, H.; Liu, Z. Q. Triterpenoid Saponins with Anti-Inflammatory Activities from *Ilex Pubescens* Roots. *Phytochemistry.* **2017,** *134,* 122–132.

Yadav, V. S.; Mishra, K. P.; Singh, D. P.; Mehrotra, S.; Singh, V. K. Immunomodulatory Effects of Curcumin. *Immunopharmacol. Immunotoxicol.* **2005,** *27,* 485–497.

Yang, C. W.; Chen, W. L.; Wu, P.-L.; Tseng, H. Y.; Lee, S. J. Anti-Inflammatory Mechanisms of Phenanthroindolizidine Alkaloids. *Mol. Pharmacol.* **2006,** *69,* 749–758.

Yendo, A. C.; de Costa, F.; Cibulski, S. P.; Teixeira, T. F.; Colling, L. C.; Mastrogiovanni, M.; Soulé, S.; Roehe, P. M.; Gosmann, G.; Ferreira, F. A.; Fett-Neto, A. G. A Rabies Vaccine Adjuvanted with Saponins from Leaves of the Soaptree (*Quillaja Brasiliensis*) Induces Specific Immune Responses Andprotects Against Lethal Challenge. *Vaccine.* **2016,** *34,* 2305–2311.

Yilma, A. N.; Singh, S. R.; Fairley, S. J.; Taha, M. A.; Dennis, V. A. The Anti-Inflammatory Cytokines, Interleukin-10 Inhibits Inflammatory Mediators in Human Epithelial Cells and Mouse Macrophages to Live and UV-Inactivated Chlamydia Trachomatis. *Mediators Inflammation.* **2012,** *10,* 1–10.

Yu, J.; Shi, F. S.; Hu, S. Improved Immune Responses to a Bivalent Vaccine of Newcastle Disease and Avian Influenza in Chickens by Ginseng Stem-Leaf Saponins. *Vet. Immunol. Immunopathol.* **2015,** *167,* 147–155.

Zelensky, A. N.; Gready, J. E. The C-Type Lectin-Like Domain Superfamily. *FEBS J.* **2005,** *272,* 6179–6217.

Zhao, Z.; Xiao, J.; Wang, J.; Dong, W.; Peng, Z.; An, D. Anti-Inflammatory Effects of Novel Sinomenine Derivatives. *Int. Immunopharmacol.* **2015,** *29,* 354–360.

Zhou, M.; Huang, L.; Li, L.; Wei, Y.; Shu, J.; Liu, X.; Huang, H. New Furostanol Saponins with Anti-Inflammatory and Cytotoxic Activities from the Rhizomes of Smilax Davidiana. *Steroids.* **2017,** *127,* 62–68.

CHAPTER 6

PHYTOCHEMICALS AS NUTRACEUTICALS AND PHARMAFOODS

ANYWAR GODWIN

Makerere University, Department of Plant Sciences, Microbiology and Biotechnology, P.O. Box 7062, Kampala, Uganda,
Tel: +256 702983410/+256782983410

Corresponding author. E-mail: godwinanywar@gmail.com;
ganywar@cns.mak.ac.ug; ganywar@cartafrica.org;
ORCID: https://orcid.org/0000-0003-0926-1832

ABSTRACT

Owing to changes in lifestyle, diet, and improvement in healthcare leading to longer life expectancy, mankind is faced with the ever-rising global threat of non-communicable diseases, carrying with them several morbidities and mortalities. There is a global shift in treatment modalities, with the proactive approach of using preventive medicine on the rise. This has largely taken the form of nutraceuticals, pharmafoods, functional, and designer foods. However, there is a lot of confusion in distinguishing these substances, based on what they are, what they do, and how they can be obtained inter alia. They have been shown to prevent and even treat various diseases such as cancers, cardiovascular diseases, and hypertension among others. This chapter focuses on nutraceuticals from plant sources, their classification, phytochemistry, as well as their biological and the therapeutic activities. A clear understanding of what these substances are, where they can be obtained from, and encouraging their regular consuming, can go a long way in mitigating disease and improving our quality of life.

6.1 INTRODUCTION

Nutraceuticals and other categories of medical or therapeutic foods have received substantial interest because of their potential nutritional and therapeutic effects as well as their apparent safety (Rajasekaran, 2017). The emergence of "pharmafoods" and "nutraceuticals" blurs the distinction between food and medicine (Etkin and Johns, 1998). There is no clear difference between the terms "pharmafoods" and "nutraceuticals" or even medical foods, functional foods, dietary supplements, and designer foods among others (Nasri et al., 2014). Schmitt and Ferro (2013) noted that the definitions of these terms may differ depending on where they are being used and are mainly used for marketing purposes. This causes a lot of confusion and results in different people using the terms interchangeably under different circumstances (Nasri et al., 2014).

Accordingly, the terms functional foods, nutraceuticals, pharmaconutrients, and dietary integrators are used erroneously and indiscriminately to mean nutrients or foods augmented with nutrients that can prevent or treat diseases (Hardy, 2000). However, the following distinctions are necessary

6.1.1 NUTRACEUTICALS

DeFelice of the Foundation for the Innovation of Medicine coined the term "nutraceutical" in 1989. He defined nutraceuticals as "any substance that may be considered a food or part of a food and provides medical or health benefits such as in the prevention and treatment of disease" (DeFelice, 1994). Nutraceuticals are therefore not drugs (Mueller, 1999), and are rarely legally classified as such, with some exceptions like coenzyme Q10 (CoQ10) in Japan and melatonin in the UK (Lockwood, 2009). Foods or food products can be considered as nutraceuticals if they have medical or health benefits (Mueller, 1999). Nutraceuticals are juxtaposed between medical foods and drugs (Singh, 2007), straddled beyond the diet but before drugs, since they combine both nutritional and health benefits of food extracts (Santini et al., 2017).

6.1.2 FUNCTIONAL FOODS

The concept of functional food was first used in Japan in 1984 to refer to food products fortified with special constituents with advantageous physiological effects (Hardy, 2000). Goldberg (1994) defined functional foods as any food or ingredient that in addition to having a nutritive value has a positive impact on an individual's health, physical performance, and state of mind. The regulatory authorities in Japan identified three conditions that must be met for foods to be qualified as functional foods namely (i) they should be naturally occurring ingredients, not capsules, tablets, or powders, (ii) they can be consumed as part of the daily diet and, (iii) when ingested, they should improve or regulate a particular biological process or mechanism to prevent or control a specific disease (Hardy, 2000).

6.1.3 MEDICAL FOODS

A medical food is a formulated food for consumption or administration through the enteral route, under the supervision of a physician. It is intended for the specific dietary management of a disease or condition, for which unique nutritional requirements based on standard scientific principles are determined by medical evaluation (Goldberg, 1994). Medical foods are the major source of nutrition for patients with metabolic disorders but do not provide total nutrition support (Singh, 2007).

6.1.4 DIETARY SUPPLEMENT

The US dietary supplement health and education act of 1994 defined a dietary supplement as a product (besides tobacco) that is meant to supplement the diet that contains one or more ingredients such as vitamins, mineral, a herb, an amino acid, or a concentrate, metabolite, constituent, extract, or combinations of these.

6.1.5 DESIGNER FOODS

"Designer foods" are foods that are fashioned to have some health benefits other than its traditional nutritional value. They are synonymous with "fortified food." Fortified foods are basically foods enriched with nutrient content already present in it or other complementary nutrient. The term was introduced in Japan in the 1980s to refer to processed food containing nutrients of some additional health benefits apart from its inherent nutritional value (Arai, 1996). Some well-known examples of a designer food include health drinks enriched with docosahexaenoic acid (DHA) to improve brain and visual development, the use of probiotics to enhance immune response and sports nutrition among others (Rajasekaran, 2017).

By the year 2000, nutraceuticals were the fastest growing segment of the food industry, with an estimated market value of $6–$60 billion (Hardy, 2000). Transparency Market Research (2015) reported that the global nutraceuticals market stood at $165.62 billion in 2014. They also indicated that the growth rate is rising at a compound annual growth rate (CAGR) of 7.3% from 2015 to 2021 with projections of the nutraceutical market value expected to reach $278.96 billion by the end of 2021.

Currently, there is an increasing consumer awareness of the health-promoting foods. Nutraceuticals can be used to improve general well-being, slow down the aging process, and prevent chronic diseases and so on. (Zhao, 2007). Nutraceuticals can be used effectively in preventive medicine by incorporating them into the daily diet (Santini et al., 2017).

6.2   SOURCES OF PHYTONUTRACEUTICALS

Nutraceuticals are typically components of food synthesized in plants during their natural development, and they can be consumed in their natural state or extracted and added to other foods (Lockwood, 2009; Marinangeli and Jones, 2013). Several plant species contain various compounds with known or proven nutraceutical properties. Other nutraceutical products include isolated nutrients, dietary supplements, genetically engineered designer foods, herbal products, and processed foods such as cereals, soups, and beverages (DeFelice, 1994). Plants are by far the greatest source of nutra-ceuticals. These nutraceuticals are often used as single purified compounds, for example, lycopene, lutein, zeathanin and γ-Linolenic acid (GLA), or multiple-component products such as grape seed proanthocyanidin extract, soy isoflavones, tea catechins, and pycnogenol or even whole plant foods such as soy, pomegranate, tea, olives, flaxseed, cranberry, and cocoa (Lock-wood, 2009).

6.3   CLASSIFICATION OF NUTRACEUTICALS AND THEIR THERAPEUTIC ACTIVITY

The classification of nutraceuticals can be premised on (i) their chemical nature, for example, flavonoids, carotenoids, terpenes, and so forth (ii) the type of food items from which they are derived such as vitamins, minerals, and dairy products (iii) whether they are traditional or not such as fruits and fortified juices (Dudeja and Gupta, 2017) and (iv) their pharmacological action such anticancer, antidiabetic, antioxidant, and so forth (Rajasekaran, 2017).

There are several compounds with nutraceutical properties that have been researched on to date. Some of the better-known sources of these nutraceuticals include the following

6.3.1 PHENOLICS

Plants and food contain large varieties of phenolic derivatives such as phenolic acids like gallic and caffeic acid, flavonoids, stilbenes, coumarins, tannins, lignans, and lignins. Phenolics are the most abundant antioxidants in the human diet, with over 4000 known polyphenols from various plant foods. They modulate the activity of numerous enzymes and cell receptors (Rajasekaran, 2017). Dietary fruits rich in polyphenolic compounds can lower the incidence of cancer by inhibiting certain enzymes that promote cell proliferation or enzymatic activity that results in cell death.

6.3.2 FLAVONOIDS

Flavonoids are classified as phenolic compounds. They occur as yellow and white plant pigments and are ubiquitous within the plant kingdom, with over 8000 known varieties (Pengelly, 2004). They are the most common plant pigments after chlorophyll and carotenoids. They belong to one of the largest classes of secondary metabolites from plants (Taiz and Zieger, 2006). Various plants studied contain a series of closely interrelated flavonoids with varying degrees of oxidation and or hydroxylation patterns (Pengely, 2004).

Generally, flavonoids differ in their substitution patterns at the functional groups. Specific classes and examples of well-known flavonoids are (i) flavones such as diosmin, luteolin, and apigenin; (ii) flavanols such as quercetin, kaempferol, myricetin (iii) flavanonol such as taxifolin; (iv) Isoflavones such as genistein, tectorigenin, and daidzein and (v) flavan-3-ols such as (+) catechin, (−) epicatechin, and (−) epigallocatechin (Tapas et al., 2008). However, the most commonly occurring flavonoids are flavones such as apigenin and flavonols such as quercetin (Fig. 6.1) (Pengely, 2004).

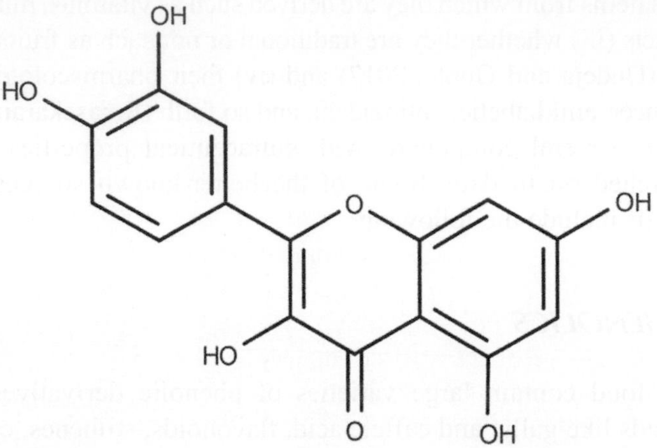

FIGURE 6.1   Quercetin.

Isoflavones are flavonoid isomers largely confined to the Fabaceae (legume) family. They rarely occur in glycosidic form and are structurally similar to estrogens. They have been classified among phytoestrogens, which are compounds, which bind to estrogen receptors but with relatively low estrogen activity (Pengely, 2004).

Flavonoids polymerize into large molecules called tannins. These include the proanthocyanidins or condensed tannins and the hydrolyzable tannins. They act as an antioxidant by accepting free radicals, but the antioxidant activity depends on their chemical structure (Pengely, 2004; Rajasekaran, 2017).

6.3.2.1   PHYTOCHEMISTRY OF FLAVONOIDS

Flavonoids occur both in a free state and as glycosides (Pengely, 2004). Flavonoid aglycones which are flavonoids without a sugar moiety attached exist in very diverse structural forms. All these forms contain 15 carbon atoms in their basic nucleus: two six-membered rings linked with a three-carbon unit, (C6–C3–C6) which may or may not be a part of a third ring (Middleton, 1984; Pengely, 2004). The three-carbon chain is generally closed to form a heterocyclic ring. Flavonoids are formed by the condensation of phenylpropanoid precursor with three malonyl coenzyme A units from both the shikimic acid and acetate pathways (Pengely, 2004).

6.3.2.2 BIOLOGICAL ACTIVITY OF FLAVONOIDS

Flavonoids play a very significant role in plants. They protect the plant tissues from the harmful ultraviolet radiation by acting as antioxidants, enzyme inhibitors, pigment, and light screens (Middleton, 1988). They are also involved in photosynthesis and energy transfer, the action of plant growth hormones and regulators, and defense against infection (Middleton, 1988).

They are key components of human diet with an estimated average consumption of 1 g per person daily. However, flavonoids are generally poorly absorbed, until they are hydrolyzed by bacterial enzymes in the intestine (Pengely, 2004). Because of their protection against environmental stress, flavonoids have been referred to as "environmental stress modifiers" (Middleton, 1988).

Flavonoids possess a very wide spectrum of biological activity (Robak and Gryglewski, 1996). Tapas et al. (2008) extensively reviewed the biological activity of flavonoids including their antimicrobial, antiulcer, hepatoprotective, anti-inflammatory, antidiabetic, antiatherosclerotic, cardioprotective, antiviral, and antineoplastic effects. Other well-documented therapeutic benefits of flavonoids include hepatoprotective, antihypertensive, and antiatheromatous (Pengely, 2004). For example, quercetin is an important inhibitor of the enzyme aldose reductase, which causes diabetic cataracts (Pathak et al., 1991). However, these effects depend on their degree of absorption. Genistein, an isoflavone from soymilk and other soy products, has been proven to relieve hot flushes and other menopausal-related symptoms as well as preventing tumors and other cancers (Albert et al., 2002). Rutin is widely acknowledged for its nutraceutical and several pharmacological effects (Ganeshpurkar and Saluja, 2017), such as antifatigue (Su et al., 2014) immunostimulatory (Lin et al., 2009).

6.3.3 CAROTENOIDS

Carotenoids are lipid-soluble yellow–orange–red pigments found in all higher plants and some animals. They belong to a class of compounds called isoprenoid polyenes (Tanaka et al., 2012). The carotenoids can be grouped into four main categories namely (i) vitamin A precursors that shows no pigmentation such as β-carotene; (ii) pigments with partial vitamin A activity such as cryptoxanthin; (iii) non-vitamin A precursors that do not pigment or pigment poorly, for example, violaxanthin and neoxanthin; and (iv) non-vitamin A precursors that pigment such as lutein, zeaxanthin, and canthaxanthin.

Carotenoids derive their name from carrots (*Daucus carota*) and xantho-phylls or phylloxanthins. Xanthos and phyllo are Greek words for yellow and leaf. Carotenoids and anthocyanins are the most complex class of natural food colorants with over 750 different structures identified. Carotenoids are selectively absorbed in the intestine (Tanaka et al., 2012). β-carotene is the most abundant dietary carotenoid (Heinonen and Albanes, 1994).

6.3.3.1 PHYTOCHEMISTRY OF CAROTENOIDS

Owing to their numerous conjugated double bonds and cyclic end groups, carotenoids present a diversity of stereoisomers with different chemical and physical properties (Tanaka et al., 2012). According to Hendry (1993), about 600 carotenoids have been described, and many of them are of animal origin, although they are derived from ingested plant carotenoids. An example is the plumage of birds (Tanaka et al., 2012). Carotenoids play a central role in photosynthesis and have little variation in their structure. Several plant-derived carotenoids are currently available as single compound nutraceuticals with multiple activities. They include lycopene (Fig. 6.2), lutein (Fig. 6.3), zeathanin (Fig. 6.4), and GLA among others (Lockwood, 2009). Like flavonoids, carotenoids protect the plant against photooxidative damage by absorbing light and transferring energy to chlorophyll during photosynthesis (Armstrong and Hearst, 1996).

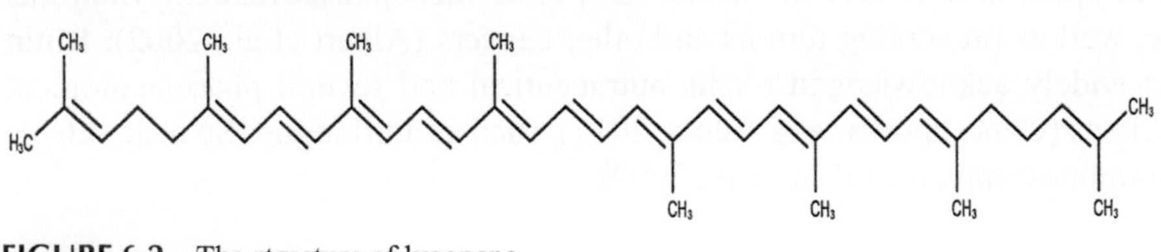

FIGURE 6.2   The structure of lycopene.

6.3.3.2 BIOLOGICAL ACTIVITY OF CAROTENOIDS

Several naturally occurring carotenoids, apart from β-carotene have demon-strated chemopreventive and or anticancer properties (Chew et al., 1999). The anticancer activity of carotenoids has been postulated to be mainly due to the presence of multiple conjugated double bonds that reduces the reactive oxygen species (Rajasekaran, 2017). Lycopene is a precursor in the biosynthesis of β-carotene (Tanaka et al., 2012) and is present in red fruits such as tomatoes, guavas, watermelon, and vegetables. The recommended daily intake of lycopene is 35 mg (Lockwood, 2009). Lycopene is a permitted food colorant in the European Union and as well as an approved food supplement in the USA (Tanaka et al., 2012).

6.3.4 LUTEIN AND ZEAXANTHIN

Lutein and zeaxanthin (Figs. 6.3 and 6.4) are the two major components of the macular pigments of the retina. The macula lutea "yellow spot" in the retina is responsible for central vision and visual activity. There are the only carotenoid pigments found in both the macula and lens of the human eye. They have dual functions in both tissues as powerful antioxidants and high-energy blue light filter (Landrum and Bone, 2001).

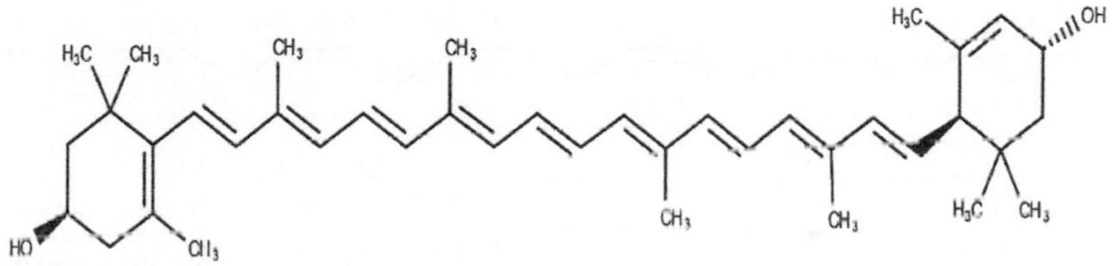

FIGURE 6.3 The structure of lutein.

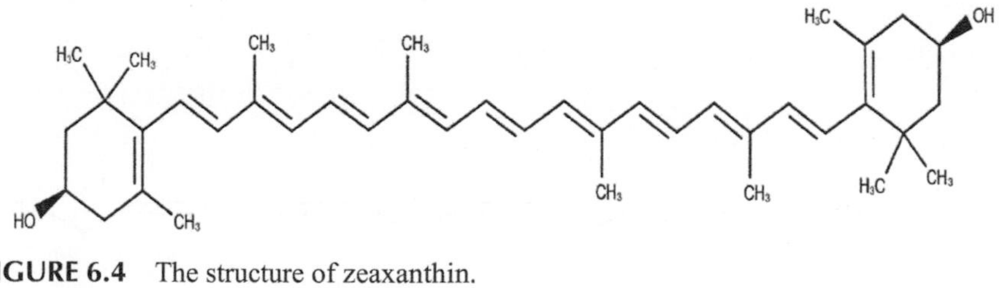

FIGURE 6.4 The structure of zeaxanthin.

Zeaxanthin is isomeric with lutein with the difference arising from a shift in a single double bond so that in zeaxanthin all double bonds are conjugated (Hadden et al., 1999). Zeaxanthin is the main pigment of yellow corn, *Zea mays* L. from which the name is derived but is also found in oranges and tangerines among others (Humphries and Khachik, 2003). Lutein is a very common carotenoid and one of the main xanthophylls present in dark green leafy vegetables but is also found in corn and egg yolks among others (Krinsky et al., 2003). Generally, foods that are yellow in color are good sources of lutein (Lockwood, 2009).

6.3.5   POLYUNSATURATED FATTY ACIDS

Polyunsaturated fatty acids (PUFA) contains multiple unsaturated double bonds found mostly in fish and plant oils. They include linoleic acid, eicosapentaenoic acid (EPA), DHA, α-linolenic acid (ALA), and GLA. EPA, DHA, and ALA are known as omega-3 fatty acids or n-3 PUFAs because their double bonds are located at the third carbon atom from the terminal end (Fig. 6.5). Linoleic and GLA are called as omega-6 or n-6 PUFAs because their first double bond is at the sixth carbon. Although the human body has the ability to synthesize fatty acids, it cannot synthesize these PUFA's since they are essential fatty acids. Therefore, they have to be obtained through the diet (Hargis and Van Elswyk, 1993; Sinclair et al., 2002; Kapoor and Nair, 2005).

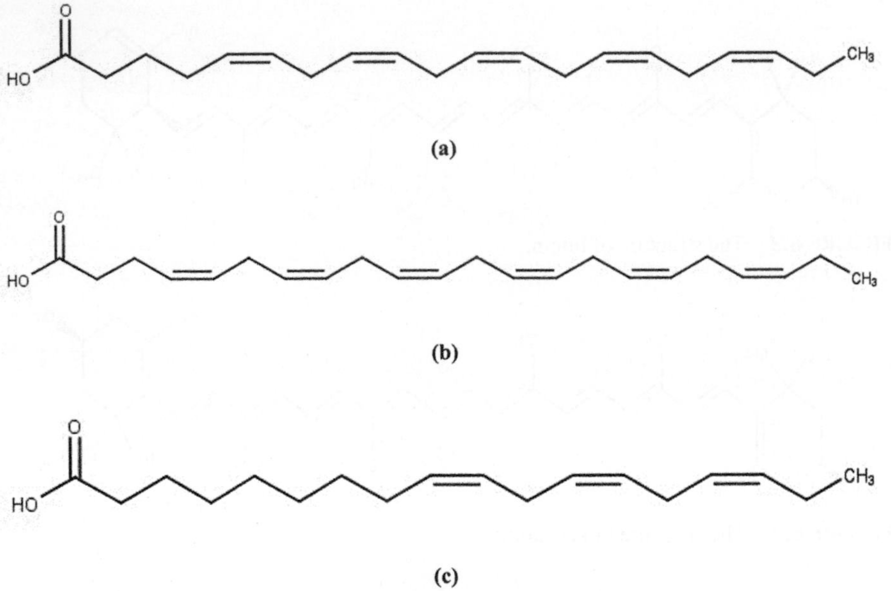

(a)

(b)

(c)

FIGURE 6.5   Omega 3-fatty acids; (a) eicosapentanoic acid; (b) docosahexaenoic acid; (c) α-Linolenic acid.

Long chain omega-3-PUFAs are of huge significance because of their effectiveness in prevention of coronary heart disease, diabetes, autoimmune disorders, hypertension, and cancer and are essential for maintenance and normal growth and development, especially for the brain (Rajasekaran, 2017).

6.3.5.1 γ-LINOLENIC ACID

GLA (Fig. 6.6) is an omega-6, 18 carbon (18C) PUFA not only found in human milk and several plant seed oils particularly borage, blackcurrant, and evening primrose (Sergeant et al., 2016) but also in several other plant sources (Lockwood, 2009). Unpurified GLA is usually used as a dietary supplement and is typically consumed as a part of a dietary supplement (Lockwood, 2009; Sergeant et al., 2016). It has been widely used for symptomatic relief of people suffering from atopic dermatitis or eczema (Simon, 2014; Sergeant et al., 2016), premenstrual syndrome as well as anti-inflammatory effects (Lockwood, 2009).

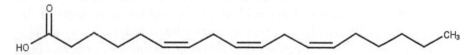

FIGURE 6.6 γ-linolenic acid, an omega 6 fatty acid.

GLA has selective tumoricidal action especially against malignant glioma cells both in vitro and in vivo (Das, 2004). Yoon et al. (2014) demonstrated that GLA in combination with omega-3 fatty acid could be used as a therapeutic adjuvant for acne patients.

6.3.5.2 ALPHA-LINOLENIC ACID

ALA can be obtained from several sources, although flaxseed oil (*Linum usitatissimum*) contains the most abundant source of ALA, with more than 50% ALA. Other sources of this essential fatty acid are the seeds of pumpkin, hemp, and walnut among others (Lockwood, 2009). ALA has antiatherosclerotic properties. In one study, it reduced the burden of plaques in carotid and femoral arteries in high cardiovascular risk patients (Sala-Vila et al., 2011). ALA also protects against depression (Kurotani et al., 2014). ALA supplementation in mouse models and human primary cell cultures was shown to impair arterial thrombus formation, vascular tissue factor expression, and plate activation making it a prospective nutritional intervention with direct dual antithrombotic effects (Holy et al., 2011).

6.3.6 COENZYME Q10

CoQ10 is a naturally occurring small hydrophobic substance and essential element of the mitochondrial electron transport chain. It freely moves throughout the inner mitochondrial membrane where it acts as an electron carrier (Rozen et al., 2002). CoQ10 is also known as a ubiquinone or ubidecarenone (Rajasekaran, 2017). CoQ10 can be found in vegetables, particularly spinach, where it is widely distributed (Lockwood, 2009).

CoQ10 has been the most comprehensively studied substance for the treatment of mitochondrial disorders. It has been shown to be safe with almost no detectable side effects in humans. CoQ10 prevents migraines (Rozen et al., 2002), and its deficiency has been associated with a variety of neurological disorders that respond to oral supplementation (Quinzii et al., 2007). CoQ10 has powerful antioxidant effects and has been used in the treatment of cardiovascular diseases including heart failure, hypertension, and angina among others (Lockwood, 2009) anti-inflammatory effects (Zhai et al., 2017).

6.3.7 ORGANOSULFUR COMPOUNDS

Glucosinolates are nitrogen and sulfur-containing compounds present in cruciferous vegetables, such as horseradish and mustards among others. Both garlic and onion belong to allium genus and contain high amount of sulfur compounds including thiosulfinates such as allicin, organosulfur volatiles such as diallyl disulfide, diallyl sulfide, and ajoene which help in preventing various diseases such as cancer, cardiovascular disease, obesity, hypertension, type 2 diabetes, and modulate the immune system (Traka and Meithein, 2009; Touloupakis and Ghanotakis, 2010; Santhosha et al., 2013).

Onions are also rich in the powerful antioxidant, quercetin which prevents DNA damage by free radicals decreases cancer tumor initiation, promotes healing of stomach ulcers, and inhibits the proliferation of breast, ovarian, and colon cancer (Potter, 1999), and irritable bowel disease (Hodge et al., 2002).

6.3.8 PLANT STEROLS

Plant sterols/phytosterols are naturally occurring compounds in plants. They are similar to cholesterol in structure (Shahzad et al., 2017).

Significant amounts of phytosterols are found in green and yellow vegetable nuts, seeds, legume, fruits, and grains (Rajasekaran, 2017). The most abundant plant sterols include sitosterol, campesterol, and stigmasterol with typical daily intakes ranging from 150 to 400 mg/day (Rajasekaran, 2017).

Phytosterols are minor but beneficial components of the human diet since they may inhibit the growth of tumors and help in the regulation of blood cholesterol (Pengely, 2004). They are also a useful starting material in the synthesis of steroidal drugs. Phytosterols possess various bioactive properties such as reducing intestinal cholesterol absorption, which alleviates blood low-density lipoproteins cholesterol and cardiovascular problems, lowers the risk of cancer, and enables antitumor responses by improving immune response recognition of cancer among others (Shahzad et al., 2017).

6.3.9 OTHER PHYTONUTRACEUTICALS

Vitamins and minerals have also been looked at as nutraceuticals (Rajasekaran, 2017). Additionally, various plant sources have been looked at as significant sources of specific nutraceutical compounds for example *Glycine max* (Soy and its isoflavones), *Punica granatum* (pomegranates) which are particularly rich in punicalagin, anthocyanins, and flavonoids with numerous therapeutic activities; Olives containing numerous phenolic compounds, cranberries (*Vaccinium oxycoccos*) with different flavonoids, *Camellia sinensis* (tea) and *Theobroma cacao* (cocoa) with various catechins, and *Vitis vinifera* (grapes) all with several therapeutic nutraceuticals (Lockwood, 2009; Rajasekaran, 2017).

6.4 CONCLUSION

In conclusion, plants are a rich source of nutraceuticals, which have proven therapeutic and prophylactic roles in many disease processes. Owing to our changing lifestyles and diet, we are living longer but are also suffering from various non-communicable diseases such as diabetes, hypertension, cancers, and cardiovascular diseases. By regularly consuming these nutraceuticals, we can significantly reduce the chances of suffering from these diseases and leave healthier lifestyles.

KEYWORDS

- **nutraceuticals**
- **pharmafoods**
- **functional**
- **designer foods**
- **phytochemicals**

REFERENCES

Albert, A.; Altabre, C.; Baro, F.; Buendia, E.; Cabero, A.; Cancelo, M. J.; Castelo-Branco, C.; Chantre, P.; Duran, M.; Haya, J.; Imbert, P.; Julia, D.; Lanchares, J. L.; Llaneza, P.; Manubens, M.; Minano, A.; Quereda, F.; Ribes, C.; Vazquez, F. Efficacy and Safety of a Phytoestrogen Preparation Derived from *Glycine max* (l.) Merr in Climacteric Symptomatology: A Multicentric, Open, Prospective and Non-Randomized Trial. *Phytomedicine* **2002**, *9*(2), 85–92 DOI: 10.1078/0944–7113–00107.

Arai, S. Studies on Functional Foods in Japan—State of the Art. *Biosci. Biotechnol. Biochem.* **1996**, *60*(1), 9–15. DOI: 10.1271/bbb.60.9.

Armstrong, G. A.; Hearst, J. E. Carotenoids 2: Genetics and Molecular Biology of Carotenoid Pigment Biosynthesis. *FASEB J.* **1996**, *10*, 228–237.

Chew, B. P.; Park, J. S.; Wong, M. W.; Wong, T. S. A Comparison of The Anticancer Activities of Dietary β-Carotene, Canthaxanthin and Astaxanthin in Mice in Vivo. *Anti-Cancer Res.* **1999**, *19*, 1849–1853.

Das, U. N. From Bench to the Clinic: γ-Linolenic Acid Therapy of Human Gliomas. *Prostaglandins, Leukotrienes Essent. Fatty Acids* **2004**, *70*(6), 539–552. DOI: https://doi.org/10.1016/j.plefa.2003.12.001.

DeFelice, S. L. What is a True Nutraceutical? And-What is the Nature and Size of the U.S. Nutraceutical Market? 1994, http://www.fimdefelice.org/p2462.html (accessed Dec 11, 2017).

Dudeja, P.; Gupta, R. K. Chapter 40—Nutraceuticals. In *Food Safety in the 21st Century;* Gupta, R. K., Dudeja, P., Singh M., Eds.; Academic Press: San Diego, 2017; pp 491–496.

Etkin, N. L.; Johns, T. "Pharmafoods" and "Nutraceuticals": Paradigm Shifts in Biotherapeutics. In *Plants for Food and Medicine*; Proceedings of the Joint Conference of the Society for Economic Botany and the International Society for Ethnopharmacology, London; Prendergast, H. D. V., Etkin, N. L., Harris, D. R., Houghton, P. J., Eds.; Royal Botanic Gardens, Kew: London, 1998.

Ganeshpurkar, A.; Saluja, A. K.; The Pharmacological Potential of Rutin. *Saudi Pharm. J.* **2017**, *25*(2), 149–164. DOI: 10.1016/j.jsps.2016.04.025.

Goldberg, I. In *Functional Foods, Designer Foods, Pharmafoods, Nutraceuticals;* Chapman & Hall: London, 1994.

Hadden, W. L.; Watkins, R. H.; Levy, L. W.; Regalado, E.; Rivadeneira, D. M.; van Breemen, R. B.; Schwartz, S. J. Carotenoid composition of marigold (*Tagetes erecta*) Flower Extract Used as Nutritional Supplement. *J. Agric. Food Chem.* **1999**, *47*, 4189–4194.

Hardy, G. Nutraceuticals and Functional Foods: Introduction and Meaning. *Nutrition* **2000,** *16*(7–8), 688–689. DOI: 10.1016/j.tox.2006.01.014.

Hargis, P. S.; Van Elswyk, M. E. Manipulating the Fatty Acid Composition of Poultry Meat and Eggs for the Health Conscious Consumer. *World's Poultry Sci. J.* **1993,** *49,* 251–264.

Heinonen, O. P.; Albanes, D. The Effect of Vitamin E and β Carotene on the Incidence of Lung Cancer and Other Cancers in Male Smokers. The α-Tocopherol, β-Carotene Cancer Prevention Study Group. *N. Engl. J. Med.* **1994,** *330,* 1029–1035.

Hodge, G.; Hodge, S.; Han, P. *Allium sativum* (garlic) Suppresses Leukocyte Inflammatory Cytokine Production in Vitro: Potential Therapeutic Use in the Treatment of Inflammatory Bowel Disease. *Cytometry* **2002,** *48*(4), 209–215. DOI: 10.1002/cyto.10133.

Holy, E. W.; Forestier, M.; Richter, E. K.; Akhmedov, A.; Leiber, F.; Camici, G. G.; Mocharla, P.; Lüscher, T. F.; Beer, J. H.; Tanner, F. C. Dietary α-Linolenic Acid Inhibits Arterial Thrombus Formation, Tissue Factor Expression, and Platelet Activation. *Arterioscler. Thromb. Vasc. Biol.* **2011,** *31*(8), 1772–1780. DOI: 10.1161/atvbaha.111.22611.

Humphries, J. M.; Khachik, F. Distribution of Lutein, Zeaxanthin, and Related Geometrical Isomers in Fruit, Vegetables, Wheat, and Pasta Products. *J. Agric. Food Chem.* **2003,** *51,* 1322–1327.

Kapoor, R.; Nair, H. *Gamma Linolenic Acid Oils Bailey's Industrial Oil and Fat Products;* John Wiley and Sons, Inc., 2005.

Krinsky, N. I.; Landrum, J. T.; Bone, R. A. Biologic Mechanisms of the Protective Role of Lutein and Zeaxanthin in the Eye. *Annu. Rev. Nutr.* **2003,** *23,* 171–201.

Kurotani, K.; Sato, M.; Ejima, Y.; Kashima, K.; Nanri, A.; Pham, N. M.; Kuwahara, K.; Mizoue, T. Serum Alpha-Linolenic and Linoleic Acids are Inversely Associated with Depressive Symptoms in Adults. *e-SPEN J.* **2014,** *9*(1), e7–e12. DOI: https://doi.org/10.1016/j.clnme.2013.12.003.

Landrum, J. T.; Bone, R. A. Lutein, Zeaxanthin, and the Macular Pigment. *Arch. Biochem. Biophys.* **2001,** *385,* 28–40.

Lin, J. P.; Yang, J. S.; Lu, C. C.; Chiang, J. H.; Wu, C. L.; Li, J. J.; Lin, H. L.; Yang, M. D.; Liu, K. C.; Chiu, T. H.; Chung, J. Rutin Inhibits the Proliferation of Murine Leukemia WEHI-3 Cells in Vivo and Promotes Immune Response in Vivo. *Leuk. Res.* **2009,** *33*(6), 823–828.

Lockwood,, B.G. B. G. The Plant Nutraceuticals. In *Pharmacognosy. ,* 15th ed.; Trease, E. C. W.; ., Evans,, D. Eds.; 15th ed. London: Elsevier Ltd., : London, 2009.

Marinangeli, C. P. F.; Jones, P. J. H. Gazing into the Crystal Ball: Future Considerations for Ensuring Sustained Growth of the Functional Food and Nutraceutical Marketplace. *Nutr. Res. Rev.* **2013,** *26,* 12–21.

Middleton, E. The Flavonoids. *Trends Pharmacol. Sci.* **1984,** *5,* 335–338.

Middleton, Jr. E. Plant Flavonoids Effects on Mammalian Cell Systems. In *Herbs, Spices and Medicinal Plants;* Cracker, L. E., Simon, J. E., Eds.; Oryx Press: Arizona, 1988; Vol. 3, *Trends Pharmacol. Sci. 5,* 335–338

Mueller, C. The Regulatory Status of Medical Foods and Dietary Supplements in the United States. *Nutrition* **1999,** *15*(3), 249–251. www.fimdefelice.org/p2410.html.

Nasri, H.; Baradaran, A.; Shirzad, H.; Rafieian-Kopaei, M. New Concepts in Nutraceuticals as Alternative for Pharmaceuticals. *Int. J. Prev. Med.* **2014,** *5*(12), 1487–1499.

Onel, S. Functional Foods, Nutraceuticals, Designer Foods. *Regulatory Affairs Focus.* 2001; April 17.

Pathak, D.; Pathak, K.; Gingla, A. K. Flavonoids as Medicinal Agents-Recent Advances. *Fitoterapia* **1991,** LXII, 371–389.

Pengelly, A. *The Constituents of Medicinal Plants: An Introduction to the Chemistry and Therapeutics of Medicinal Plants,* 2nd ed.; CABI Publishing: Cambridge, 2004.

Potter, J. D. Colorectal Cancer: Molecules and Populations. *J. Natl. Cancer Inst.* **1999,** *91,* 916–932.

Quinzii, C. M.; Di Mauro, S.; Hirano, M. Human Coenzyme Q10 Deficiency. *Neurochem. Res.* **2007,** *32*(4), 723–727. DOI: 10.1007/s11064–006–9190-z.

Rajasekaran, A. 1.05—Nutraceuticals. In *Comprehensive Medicinal Chemistry III;* Chackalamannil, S., Rotella, D., Ward, S. E., Eds.; Oxford: Elsevier. 2017; pp 107–134.

Robak, J.; Gryglewski, R. J. Bioactivity of Flavonoids. *Pol. J. Pharmacol.* **1996,** *48,* 555–564.

Rozen, T. D.; Oshinsky, M. L.; Gebeline, C. A.; Bradley, K. C.; Young, W. B.; Shechter, A. L.; Silberstein, S. D. Open Label Trial of Coenzyme Q10 as a Migraine Preventive. *Cephalalgia* **2002,** *22*(2), 137–141. DOI: 10.1046/j.1468–2982.2002.00335.x.

Sala-Vila, A.; Cofán, M.; Núñez, I.; Gilabert, R.; Junyent, M.; Ros, E. Carotid and Femoral Plaque Burden is Inversely Associated with the α-Linolenic Acid Proportion of Serum Phospholipids in Spanish Subjects with Primary Dyslipidemia. *Atherosclerosis* **2011,** *214*(1), 209–214. DOI: https://doi.org/10.1016/j.atherosclerosis.2010.10.026.

Santhosha, S. G.; Jamuna, P.; Prabhavathi, S. N. Bioactive Components of Garlic and Their Physiological Role in Health Maintenance: A Review. *Food Biosci.* **2013,** *3,* 59–74.

Santini, A.; Tenore, G. C.; Novellino, E. Nutraceuticals: A Paradigm of Proactive Medicine. *Eur. J. Pharm. Sci.* **2017,** *96,* 53–61. DOI: 10.1016/j.ejps.2016.09.003.

Schmitt, J.; Ferro, A. Nutraceuticals: Is There Good Science Behind the Hype? *Br. J. Clin. Pharmacol.* **2013,** *75*(3), 585–587. DOI: 10.1111/bcp.12061.

Sergeant, S.; Rahbar, E.; Chilton, F. H. Gamma-Linolenic Acid, Dihommogamma Linolenic, Eicosanoids and Inflammatory Processes. *Eur. J. Pharmacol.* **2016,** *785,* 77–86. DOI: 10.1016/j.ejphar.2016.04.020.

Shahzad, N.; Khan, W.; Md, S; Ali, A.; Saluja, S. S.; Sharma, S.; Al-Allaf, F. A.; Abduljaleel, Z.; Ibrahim, I. A. A.; Abdel-Wahab, A. F.; Afify, M. A.; Al-Ghamdi, S. S. Phytosterols as a Natural Anticancer Agent: Current Status and Future Perspective. *Biomed. Pharmacother.* **2017,** *88*(Suppl C), 786–794. DOI: https://doi.org/10.1016/j.biopha.2017.01.068.

Simon, D.; Eng, P. A.; Siegfried, B.; Kägi, R.; Zimmermann, C.; Zahner, C.; Jürgen, D.; Hess, H.; Ferrari, F.; Lautenschlager, S.; Wüthrich, B.; Schmid-Grendelmeier-Linolenic, P. Acid Levels Correlate with Clinical Efficacy of Evening Primrose Oil in Patients with Atopic Dermatitis. *Adv. Ther.* **2014,** *31*(2), 180–188. DOI: 10.1007/s12325–014–0093–0.

Sinclair, A. J.; Attar-Bashi, N. M.; Li, D. What is the Role of Alpha-Linolenic Acid for Mammals? *Lipids* **2002,** *37*(12), 1113–1123.

Singh, R. The Enigma of Medical Foods. *Mol. Genet. Metab.* **2007,** *92*(1), 3–5. DOI: https://doi.org/10.1016/j.ymgme.2007.07.002.

Su, K. Y.; Yu, C. Y.; Chen, Y. W.; Huang, Y. T.; Chen, C. T.; Wu, H. F.; Chen, Y. L. Rutin, a Flavonoid and Principal Component of *Saussurea involucrata,* Attenuates Physical Fatigue in a Forced Swimming Mouse Model. *Int. J. Med. Sci.* **2014,** *11*(5), 528–537.

Taiz, L. and Zeiger, Plant Physiology and Development, 4th ed.; Sinauer Associates: Sunderland, Massachusetts, USA, 2006.

Tanaka, T.; Shnimizu, M.; Moriwaki, H. Cancer Chemoprevention by Carotenoids. *Molecules* **2012,** *17*(3), 3202.

Tapas, A. R.; Sakarkar, D. M.; Kakde, R. B. Flavonoids as Nutraceuticals: A Review. *Trop. J. Pharm. Res.* **2008,** *7*(3), 1089–1099.

Touloupakis, E.; Ghanotakis, D. F. Nutraceutical Use of Garlic Sulfur-Containing Compounds. *Adv. Exp. Med. Biol.* **2010,** *698,* 110–121.

Traka, M.; Meithein, R. Glucosinolates Isothiocyantes and Human Health. *Phytochem. Rev.* **2009,** *8,* 269–282.

Transparency Market Research. Nutraceuticals Market—Global Industry Analysis, Size, Share, Growth, Trends, and Forecast 2015–2021. 2015, https://www.transparencymarketresearch. com/global-nutraceuticals-product-market.html (accessed Nov 21, 2017).

US Dietary Supplement Health and Education Act (DSHEA) of 1994. https://ods.od.nih.gov/ About/DSHEA_Wording.aspx#sec3.

Zhai, J.; Bo, Y.; Lu, Y.; Liu, C.; Zhang, L. Effects of Coenzyme Q10 on Markers of Inflammation: A Systematic Review and Meta-Analysis. *Plos One.* **2017,** *12*(1), e0170172. DOI: 10.1371/journal.pone.0170172.

Zhao, J. Nutraceuticals, Nutritional Therapy, Phytonutrients, and Phytotherapy for Improvement of Human Health: A Perspective on Plant Biotechnology Application. *Recent Pat. Biotechnol.* **2007,** *1*(1), 75–97.

CHAPTER 7

ROLE OF PHYTOCHEMISTRY IN PLANT CLASSIFICATION: PHYTOCHEMOTAXONOMY

FELIX IFEANYI NWAFOR[1,*]and IFEOMA CELESTINA ORABUEZE[2]

[1]Department of Pharmacognosy and Environmental Medicines, University of Nigeria, Nsukka, Enugu State, Nigeria, Tel.: +2348036062242

[2]Department of Pharmacognosy, University of Lagos, Lagos State, Nigeria

*Corresponding author. E-mail: felix.nwafor@unn.edu.ng; felixnucifera@gmail.com
ORCID: *https://orcid.org/0000-0003-1889-6311

ABSTRACT

The recognition and application of phytochemistry in plant taxonomy could be said to have started from the early man. Man began to classify plants as edible and nonedible, aromatic, colorful, tasty, and medicinal obviously based on their chemical constituents and such grouping of characters has been attributed to their differences in chemical diversity. Chemotaxonomy is a system of taxonomy that classifies organisms based on their chemical constituents. Phytochemical markers of taxonomic importance include the directly visible particles (including crystals, raphides, and starch granules), primary metabolites, and the secondary metabolites. In this chapter, the authors detailed the concept and origin of chemotaxonomy and the different classes of phytochemicals that have been successfully utilized in classification and delimitation of plants at all taxonomic levels. The challenges and limitations of this branch of science and suggestions of possible remedies were also highlighted. Researchers and students in the fields of plant taxonomy, phytochemistry, and natural products chemistry will find this chapter exceptionally relevant.

7.1 INTRODUCTION

Plant taxonomy is considered as one of the oldest branch of science that has been into practice from the beginning of human existence. Earlier documentaries show that man's dependence on plants for food and survival led to vernacular names given to plants in various cultures and in different forms. Different tribes and countries have given different names to a particular plant in different languages while different plants sometimes bear the same name given by different peoples. However, in order to overcome this problem of ambiguities in terms of naming of plants, professional botanists (taxonomists) have come up with a methodical system of identifying, classifying, and naming of plants for international communication. Plant taxonomy is, therefore, a scientific study of classification and naming of plants following certain rules or principles. It is a science that brings about lawful arrangement and orderliness to the plant kingdom, and before a scientific study can be initiated on any given plant species, there must be, first of all, proper identification of that plant species (Pandey and Misra, 2008; Inya-Agha et al., 2017).

Plant taxonomists employ evidence from different areas of study, including morphology, anatomy, palynology, cytology, molecular phylogeny, and phytochemistry in the delimitation and classification of taxa and in solving problems of misidentification of crude drugs (AbdulRahamanet al., 2014). Morphological and anatomical studies have remained the bedrock of plant classification but are supported by evidence from other areas of study (Agbagwa and Nduka, 2004). On this note, chemotaxonomy is simply the systematic study of the diversity of chemical constituents in the living organism and the use of such variations in the delimitation of taxa. Plants possess chemical substances especially the secondary metabolites that serve as diagnostic characters and chemical markers for taxonomy. The contribution of phytochemicals to plant taxonomy lies in the fact that chemotaxonomists believe that they are widely distributed in plants, stable, unambiguous, and not easily changeable. These properties suggest that they can provide information on the interrelationships amongst plants the same way as morphological and anatomical characters (Pandey and Misra, 2008; Bhargava et al., 2013; Singh, 2016).

Chemical characters have been used to delimit plants at all taxonomic levels. In the Euphorbiaceae, for instance, the members of the Tribe

Euphorbieae are distinguished by the presence of milky exudates (latex) (Hutchinson and Dalziel, 1963). Essential oils are characteristic of the Rutaceae (e.g., *Citrus*), Lamiaceae (e.g., mints, thyme, etc.) and Myrtaceae (e.g., *Eucalyptus*). Terpenoids and flavonoids have wide distributions in the members of Asteraceae, Lauraceae, Poaceae, Apiaceae, Lamiaceae, Rubiaceae, Cactaceae, and Cupressaceae (Bhargava et al., 2013). Alkaloids have been characterized and used in the delimitation of taxa in the members of Apocynaceae and Solanaceae. Nicotine is distributed in *Nicotiana* spp. and ephedrine in *Ephedra*. Their distribution is often specific and thus of taxonomic importance. Morphine is present only in *Papaver somniferum* (Solanaceae) (Pandey and Misra, 2008). Phenolics and caffeol extracted from *Erigeron bonariensis* validated its separation from the closely related genus *Conyza* (Bhargava et al., 2013). A number of nonprotein amino acids occur in high concentrations in certain groups of plants. For example, lathyrine is known only to occur in *Lathyrus* (Fabaceae) and on the basis of its distribution seven intrageneric groups have been recognized in the genus (Pandey and Misra, 2008). Pigments in living organisms are the basis of classification, from cyanobacteria, algae, fungi to lichens et al. classified based on their cell pigments (Delgado-Vargas et al., 2000; Nayaka, 2005). Even though most chemotaxonomists recognize three broad categories of chemical compounds – primary metabolites, secondary metabolites, and semantides as important taxonomic tools, directly visible particles, including calcium oxalate crystals, raphides, and starch granules that are ubiquitous in plants cells have also been found useful (Ekeke and Agbagwa, 2014). Calcium oxalate crystals and raphides have been used in the delimitation of toxic plants and varieties in the morphology and ornamentation of starch granules largely contribute to the chemotaxonomy of members of the Poaceae (grains) and tuberous species (Mathew, 1984; Gott et al., 2006; Singh, 2016).

7.2   ORIGIN AND CONCEPT OF CHEMOTAXONOMY

The recognition and application of phytochemistry in plant taxonomy could be said to have started from early man. Man began to classify plants as edible and nonedible, aromatic, colorful, tasty, and medicinal obviously based on their chemical constituents and such grouping of characters has been attributed to their differences in chemical constituents. We could easily tell the identity of a food plant when consumed by the flavor or taste and medicinal plants from their therapeutic activities because of the presence of bioactive molecules in them. It is not until recent times has chemotaxonomy been considered as an autonomous field of study. This has largely promoted the advent of advanced modern technology and research methodologies especially in the areas of bioprospecting novel chemical agents and drug discovery (Pandey and Misra, 2008).

A. P. de Candolle (1816) was the first to introduce the term chemotaxonomy when he postulated that (1) plant taxonomy will be the most useful guide to man in his research for new industrial and medicinal plants, and (2) that chemical characteristics of plants will be most valuable to plant taxonomy in the future. Both statements are evident in the present days as scientists explore every available technique of chemotaxonomy in research and discovery of novel drugs and other bioactive constituents of industrial applications. Depending on the study objectives, chemical diagnostic features can be used in the description and classification of plants and/or in tracing their phylogenetic relationships with others. On this note, biosystematics, or in this case chemosystematics tends to cover the knowledge of plant diversities, their classification, and evolutionary relationships. The definition of chemotaxonomy (interchangeably expressed as chemosystematics) could, therefore, be structured to fit into the definition of plant systematics by Stace (1980). Thus, chemotaxonomy is the study and description of variation in chemical constituents of organisms, the investigation of causes (including evolutionary changes), and consequences of this variation and the manipulation of the data obtained to produce a system of classification (Pandey and Misra, 2008; Singh, 2016).

7.3 RELEVANCE OF CHEMOTAXONOMY

The contribution of chemotaxonomy and comparative phytochemistry to modern scientific studies include but are not limited to the following:

1. It provides new taxonomic diagnostic characters to supplement the existing systems of plant classification.
2. It is used in solving problems of ambiguity in plant classification.
3. It helps to interpret and understand the ontogenetic and phylogenetic relationships among plant taxa.
4. It is used to interpret hybridization in plants.
5. Chemotaxonomy can serve as a starting point to bioprospecting, discovery of novel drugs and other bioactive compounds of industrial application, and their conservation (Misra and Srivasta, 2016).
6. Comparative phytochemistry also helps to analyze environmental influences and evolutionary changes in a particular taxon.

7.4   PHYTOCHEMICALS IN PLANT TAXONOMY

A wide range of chemical compounds are found in plants and to them are added various chemicals produced in various metabolic pathways (Harvey, 2000). Phytochemical markers of taxonomic importance include the directly visible particles (sometimes treated as morphological characters); macromolecules that include non-semantide (plant molecules that are not involved in information transfer such as starches, cellulose etc.) and semantides (information-carrying molecules such as DNA, RNA, and proteins); micromolecules (both primary and secondary metabolites). Primary metabolites are micromolecules that are involved in vital metabolic pathways, for example, citric acid, aconitic acid, protein, and amino acids, whereas secondary metabolites are phytocompounds which are the by-products of primary metabolism and often perform non-vital functions, for example, nonprotein amino acids, phenolic compounds, alkaloids, glucosinolates, terpenoids, cardiac glycosides among others (Pandey and Misra, 2008, Salim et al., 2008). In this context, emphasis will be focused on the directly visible particles and the micromolecules.

7.4.1   DIRECTLY VISIBLE PARTICLES

The most studied directly visible particles in chemotaxonomy are the calcium oxalates and starch granules.

7.4.1.1   CALCIUM OXALATE CRYSTALS

Among the directly visible particles utilized in chemotaxonomy are calcium oxalate (CaOx) crystals – the most distributed mineral deposits in plants. They are found in diverse forms and in over 215 plant families including algae, lichens, and fungi. Distributed in almost all plant organs or tissues such as stems, roots, leaves, flowers, and seeds, they vary in shapes and forms and the most common types are raphides, druses, styloids, and prisms. Crystals are majorly formed in special cell vacuoles called idioblasts and sometimes accumulate in other cell organelles including the cell walls of gymnosperms. Their contribution to plant development remains unclear but they have been found to be helpful in calcium regulation in plant cells, provide protection against herbivory, detoxify heavy metals or oxalic acid, and provide tissue strength to the plant (Prychid and Rudall, 1999; Ekeke and Agbagwa, 2014). The abundance and varieties in types and sizes of these crystals together with the belief that these morphological differences are controlled by the genes suggest their potential in taxonomic studies. Mathew (1984) earlier identified members of the family Verbenaceae based on their type and shapes of calcium oxalate crystals.

7.4.1.2 STARCH GRANULES

Plants store their food in form of starch. Starch granules occur in most tissues but are found more abundantly in storage organs such as tubers, seeds, roots, and fruits. The granules consist almost entirely of two glucose polymers, amylose, and amylopectin, with small amounts of lipids, minerals, and phosphorus. The variability in starch granule distribution, type, shape, size, and ornamentation as a result of the complexity of starch biosynthesis has made them useful taxonomic tools in the delimitation of plant groups and has been utilized properly by taxonomists and pharmacognosists in plant identification and standardization of crude drugs. Types of starch granules vary from simple, compound to semi-compound depending on how they are formed (compartments) in the amyloplasts. Their shapes may be oval, discs, spherical, elongated, rounded, kidney-shaped, or polyhedral, even though some intermediate/irregular forms have been documented in some plants while their sizes range from 1 to 100 μ, and sometimes up to 175 μ in rhizomes of some plants (Gott et al., 2006; Ekeke and Agbagwa, 2014).

7.4.2 MICROMOLECULES

7.4.2.1 PRIMARY METABOLITES

Naturally occurring compounds can be divided into three broad groups. The first group consists of compounds such as phytosterols, acryl lipids, nucleotides, amino acids, and organic acids, are found in every cell and are essential for fundamental metabolic pathways and production of the cells. They are known as the primary metabolites. Plants utilize primary metabolites for their growth and basic developmental functions such as respiration and cell differentiation. They are commonly distributed in large quantity in the plant kingdom. The general degradation of carbohydrates and sugars through glycolysis process, the oxidation of fatty acids from fat through β-oxidation process, interconversion or degradation of amino acids are undergone by all organisms via different metabolic processes for the release of energy. The various primary metabolic pathways for modifying, synthesizing, and degrading energy-rich organic compounds such as proteins, fats, carbohydrates, and nucleic acids are basically the same in all organisms. Thus, primary metabolites play a minor role in chemotaxonomic classification. The second group includes the cellular structures such as cellulose, lignins, and proteins (Muranaka and Saito, 2010), while the third is the secondary metabolites (see next section).

7.4.2.2 SECONDARY METABOLITES

The third group, known as the secondary metabolites, is limited in distribution but specific in functions. They are compounds produced from key intermediates of primary metabolism. They are found in only specific organisms, or groups of organisms, and expression of the individuality or species. Secondary metabolites are not produced all the time or under all conditions but at certain stages of growth or stress. They could be produced for defense against environmental threat (such as against herbivory, mechanical damage, and microbial infection), toxic material as a defense against predators, or as coloring agents to attract or warn other species (Osawa et al., 1994). In the past, they have been regarded as "waste products" because they are not particularly needed for growth and development of the plants. Studies have proven most secondary metabolites to be pharmacologically active natural products acting on other organisms. Over 40% of conventional human medicines have been directly or indirectly originated from these natural products. Secondary metabolites are also greatly utilized in manufacturing and food industries.

There is no clear-cut distinction between the primary and the secondary metabolites. Some groups of natural products can be grouped under both primary and the secondary metabolites. Good examples are sugars and fatty acids, which at best are regarded as primary metabolites but some rare types are found only in some species, unlike primary metabolites. On the basis of functionality, primary metabolites drive nutrition and essential metabolic processes inside the plant, while secondary metabolites (natural products) influence interactions with other organisms and environment (Irchhaiya et al., 2014).

Secondary metabolites are produced in plants in minute quantities by specialized cells at particular stages of the plant growth, thereby making their extraction and isolation processes difficult. Secondary metabolites that are "chemotaxonomically" close have a lot in common (Irchhaiya et al., 2014).

Secondary metabolites can be classified according to their biosynthetic pathway (e.g., phenylpropanoid); chemical structure (presence of ring, sugar, functional groups); composition of compounds (containing nitrogen or not), and their solubility in various solvents. They are generally divided into three groups based on their biosynthetic origins:

1. Phenolics (presence of hydroxyl functional group attached to aromatic rings, e.g., phenolic acids, tannins, flavonoids, and lignin).
2. Terpenes (contain five-carbon isoprenoid units, carbon and hydrogen molecule, e.g., monoterpenes, sesquiterpenes, diterpenes, triterpenes, and cardiac glycosides).
3. Nitrogen-containing compounds (greatly diverse and may also contain sulfur, e.g., alkaloids, glucosinolates, and cyanogenic glycosides).

1. Phenolic compounds

Phenolic compounds are formed either by shikimic acid or malonate/acetate pathways (Croteau et al., 2000; see Chapter 2). They consist of one or more "acidic" hydroxyl (–OH) functional group attached directly to an aromatic hydrocarbon group and the simplest member of this class is the phenol. Many naturally occurring phenolics are generated from phenylpropanoid and phenylpropanoid-acetate pathways. Plant phenolics are easily oxidized to brownish products on exposure to air. This reaction generates products that form complexes with proteins and inhibit enzyme activity. Phenolic compounds can be grouped into two broad classes, the non-flavonoids and the flavonoid (Irchhaiya et al., 2014).

(i) Non-flavonoids

This group of secondary metabolites includes the phenolic acids, hydroxy-cinnamic acid, and the polyphenolics stilbenes.

Phenolic acids are widespread throughout the plant kingdom and are essential for physiological development and defense of plants. They are also called hydroxybenzoates of which Gallic acid is the basic component. Gallic acids are intermediates in plant production of tannins, an important raw material in hide and skin tanning and food industries. Tannins are present in most plant species. It exhibits antimicrobial activities, thus aids in protecting the plant (Ramawat, 2007).

Stilbenes are polyphenols produced by plants as a defensive response to microbial attack. Salicylic acid, generated by some plant species in response to the fungal attack has been synthesized and modified in the laboratory to serve as anti-inflammatory, pain reliever, and fever-reducing agent (Irchhaiya et al., 2014).

(ii) Flavonoids

These are polyphenolic compounds that exist relatively in large quantities in almost all plant species. They are highly valuable to plant as they are involved in diverse functions for the survival of the plant. They protect the plant from ultraviolet (UV) radiation, stimulate nitrogen-fixing nodules, and protect the plant from disease infections. Subclasses of flavonoids include isoflavanones, flavones, flavonols, flavanones, isoflavonoids, anthocyanidins, and chalcones. Flavonoids are associated with the antioxidant properties of many classes of food and medicinal plants (Pandey and Rizvi,2009).

Isoflavanones are synthesized mostly by leguminous plants as a defensive agent when attacked by microbes among which soybean has been reported to have the highest concentration (Irchhaiya et al., 2014). They have been demonstrated to have antioxidant properties and are very useful in the control of degenerative and chronic diseases. Antioxidant activity of phenolic compounds is mainly due to their redox properties in adsorbing and neutralizing free radicals, quenching singlet and triplet oxygen, or decomposing peroxides. Food and beverage industries utilize plant phenolics to improve or impart fragrance/odor, flavor, and taste. Vanillin from the vanilla bean, capsaicin from red peppers, and cinnamate and gingerol derivatives from cinnamon and ginger, respectively, all impart delightful taste and flavor (Osawa, 1994).

The bright pigmentation of some plant flowers and fruits is as a result of the presence of phenolic pigments such as anthocyanidins and anthocyanins. They function as attractants, attracting insects and pollen grain carriers for both pollination and fruit dispersal (Pandey and Rizvi, 2009).

Phenolic lignins contained in cell walls of some plants act as protection shield and deterrents as they provide strength to plants.

2. Terpenes

This group is large and widely varied and is synthesized in almost all plants. When terpenes are modified by oxidation or rearrangement of the carbon skeleton, the resulting compounds are referred to as terpenoids which are also known as isoprenoids. Terpenes and terpenoids are important raw materials as natural flavors in food and as a fragrance in cosmetic industries, in traditional aromatherapy, insect attractants and antifeedants, and they are also good antibiotics (Irchhaiya et al., 2014).

Terpenes are hydrocarbons usually containing one or more primary C=C double bonds and they usually fall under five-carbon units (isoprene units) derived from isopentenyl (3-methylbut-3-en-1-yl) pyrophosphate. These C_5 molecules are joined to each other in a regular pattern of head to tail by fusion of two small terpene precursors of up to 40carbons (Xu et al., 2004). Classification of terpenes is based on the number of isoprene or isopentane units present in the basic molecular skeleton. Examples of terpene are essential oils from plants such as eucalyptus, clove, and cinnamon.

(a) Monoterpenes and Sesquiterpenes

Monoterpenes have $C_{10}H_{16}$ molecular structure and could be linear or cyclic. They are made up of two C_5 isoprene units while Sesquiterpenes consist of three isoprene units. They are the principles that gave plants their unique odor. Their compounds are lipophilic in nature and easily evaporate (volatile) even at room temperature because of their low-molecular weight. Menthol, cineole, and thymol are examples of monoterpenes (Fig. 7.1) and they possess antimicrobial activities (Gurib-Fakim, 2006).

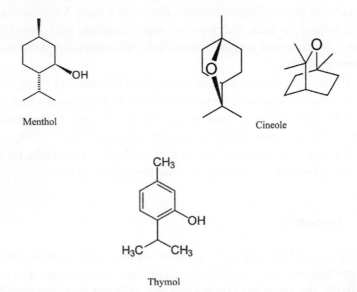

Menthol   Cineole

Thymol

FIGURE 7.1   Chemical structures of some monoterpenes.

Sesquiterpenes are also biologically active and have exhibited promising anti-infective potentials. The currently World Health Organization approved artemisinin, an antimalarial compound is of this group.

(b) Diterpenes and Sesterterpenes

Diterpene compounds are mostly polar compounds and are 20 carbon units skeletal structures, consisting of four isoprene units. Phytol, a diterpene, is found in most plants and has been reported to have pharmacological activities. The popular antitumor compound, paclitaxel (Fig. 7.2) belongs to this class of terpenes.

Sesterterpenes are 25 carbon compounds. They easily undergo cyclization and different oxidation level and possess many biological activities.

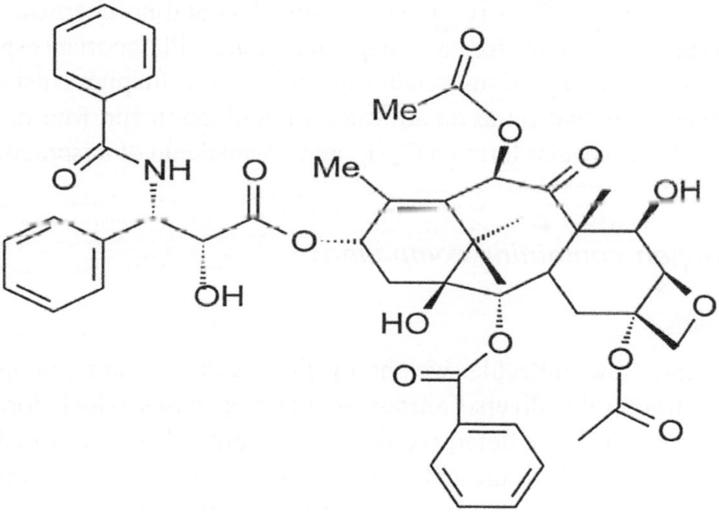

FIGURE 7.2 Chemical structures of paclitaxel (Taxol).

(c) Triterpenes

Triterpenes are greatly diverse and consist of a 30-carbon skeletal unit and 6 isoprene units. They can exist as acyclic or pentacyclic configuration. Squalenes at cyclization give rise to triterpene pentacyclic ring. Triterpenoids are triterpenes with one or more oxygen molecules and many of them are bioactive compounds with irritant properties, antiseptic and sedative potentials. Figure 7.3 is an example of two triterpenoidswith anticancer potentials, lupeol and ursolic acid (Dzubak et al., 2005; Tolstikova et al., 2006).

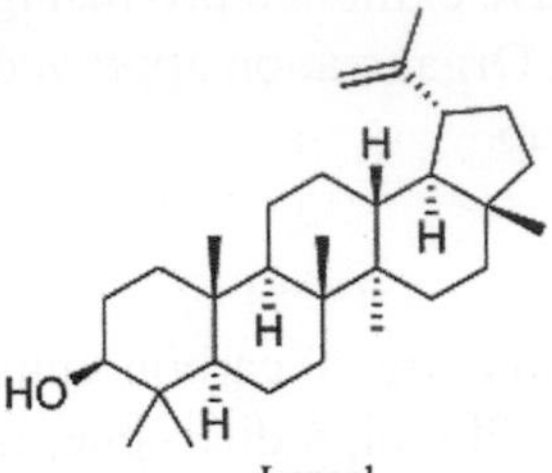

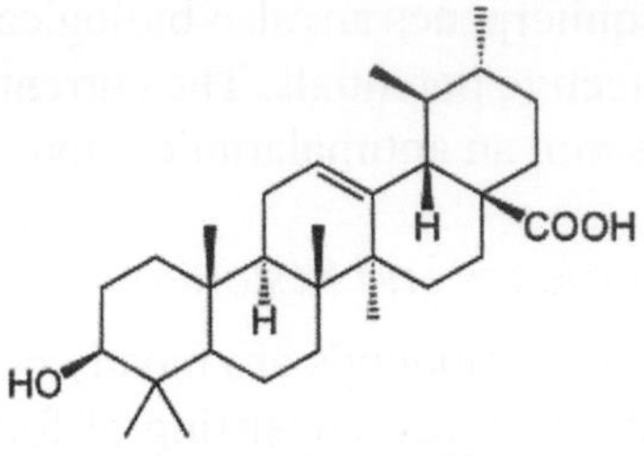

FIGURE 7.3   Chemical structures of lupeol and ursolic acid.

(d) Tetraterpenes

More than 650 carotenoids (C_{40}) exist in this class and no pharmacological potentials have been noted for this group but they are still important especially due to the role they play in human nutrition and the colorful pigmentation they give to plant parts that act as an attractant in pollination and fruit dispersal. They have the molecular formula $C_{40}H_{64}$ and are made up of 8 isoprene units.

3.   Nitrogen-containing compounds

(i) Alkaloids

Alkaloids are low-molecular-weight cyclic organic natural compounds. They are structurally diverse nitrogen-containing bases which form salts with acids and induce a defensive response to animal or insect herbivory. The structure of the molecule and the position of the functional groups determine the degree of basicity. The nitrogen part of alkaloids is derived from amino acids such as lysine, tyrosine, ornithine, and tryptophan. Alkaloids are limited in distribution and are found in plants, microbes, and animal species. They are widely distributed in plant families such as Solanaceae, Fabaceae, Berberidaceae, Rubiaceae, Papaveraceae, Apocynaceae, and Ranunculaceae. They are purified from crude extracts by acid–base extraction and used as recreational drugs, local anesthetic, and in the treatment of gastritis, typhoid, malaria, fever, and so forth (Pandey and Misra, 2008).

Alkaloids may be grouped based on the structure of the ring system containing the nitrogen atom and they include piperidine, isoquinoline, and indole alkaloids. This can reflect their biosynthetic origin from amino acid (which provides both the nitrogen atom and the fundamental portion of the alkaloidal skeleton). The indole alkaloids contain indole as the parent base. Indole alkaloids are formed from two building blocks secologanin and tryptamine or tryptophan through a single precursor, strictosidine. Examples of bioactive indole alkaloids include reserpine, an antihypertensive and tranquilizing agent found in *Rauvolfia* spp. Nicotine obtained from *Nicotiana tobaccum* (Solanaceae) is of pyridine alkaloid.

One of the best-known prescription alkaloids is the antitussive and analgesic codeine isolated from opium poppy. Plant alkaloids have also served as models for modern synthetic drugs such as morphine, vincristine, and vinblastine (anticancer), codeine (cough), atropine (used to dilate the pupil during eye examinations), scopolamine, hyoscyamine (anticholinergic), and quinine (indole-derived antimalarial and antipyretics).

(ii) Glycosides

Glycosides are produced by many plants and some species of toad as venom. They are stored in plant vacuoles as inactive constituents till needed for defense. Glycosides occur in fruit and flower pigments. They consist of two major parts – the sugar (glycone) and the non-sugar entity (aglycone) linked by four types of linkages namely, C-; O-; S-; and N-glycosidic bond. The aglycone entity may be a derivative of another metabolite (e.g., alcohol, glycogen, or starch).

Cardiac glycosides consist of a steroidal nucleus (aglycone) and a sugar molecule. The sugar moieties that are mostly attached are D-fructose, D-digitalose, D-digitoxose, L-rhamnose, D-digginose, D-glucose, D-sarmentose, and D-sarmentose. They are pharmacologically active in the treatment of heart diseases. They are found in *Digitalis* (Scrophulariaceae), *Strophanthus* (Apocynaceae), Squill bulb (Liliaceae) as digoxin, digitoxin, and digitonin.

(iii) Cyanogenic glycosides

Cyanogenic glycosides are bioactive toxins derived from amino acids found in over 2500 plant species. They are widely distributed in the members of Asteraceae, Fabaceae, Rosaceae, and Linaceae. Cyanogenic glycosides serve in defensive mechanism against herbivores and some fungal pathogens and they have been found useful as natural pesticides.

(iv) Saponins

Saponins are triterpenoids or steroids having one or more sugar molecule attached to it. They are high-molecular glycosides. They have hemolytic properties but are biological useful as anti-infective amongst others.

7.5 SUCCESSFUL APPLICATION OF CHEMOTAXONOMY IN DIFFERENT PLANT GROUPS

Review of available literature shows that chemotaxonomists have attempted the use of chemical markers in identification, classification, and study of evolutionary relationships in plants and recorded great success at all levels of taxonomic hierarchy. The distribution and complexity of phytochemicals vary in different plants groups and, therefore, in this section we will be discussing chemotaxonomic application based on particular plant groups.

7.5.1 CHEMOTAXONOMYINLOWERPLANTSCLASSIFICATION

Lower plants are one of the oldest organisms on earth together with bacteria. The fact they are nonvascular means they lack vascular systems and specialized organs – true leaves, stem, and roots. They include bryophytes (mosses and liverworts) and algae. Bryophytes and algae make use of light energy from the sun through the process of photosynthesis to manufacture their own food. Most bryophytes thrive in dark wet places, but some occur in dry places and can withstand desiccation. Algae need moisture to survive and occur in a wide range of habitats, from the freshwater to sea, and from freezing conditions to hot springs. They can also be found living as endophytes– within living tissues or epiphytic on living organisms and rocks. They also include microalgae and the seaweeds.

7.5.1.1 CHEMOTAXONOMY OF ALGAE

The chemical characters considered for classification of algae into different classes are the pigmentation and nature of their food reserves. These pigments are majorly chlorophylls, carotenoids (carotenes and xanthophylls), and phycobilins. While all photosynthetic algae contain chlorophyll a, chlorophyll b is dominant in division Chlorophyceae (green algae); chlorophyll d is found in Rhodophyceae (red algae) while chlorophyll c is dominant in Phaeophyceae (brown algae), many diatoms, and some dinoflagellates (Delgado-Vargas et al., 2000; Coupel et al., 2015).

Carotenoids are a group of yellow, orange, red, and brown protective pigments that act as a screen to light and as accessory pigments (Goodwin, 1992). They are grouped into carotenes (α, β, γ, ε, flavicine, and lycopene) and xanthophylls and are common pigments in Chlorophyceae, Phaeophyceae,

Rhodophyceae, and Cyanophyceae, and occur insignificantly in other algal groups. In most of algae β-carotene is present. In Bacillariophyceae (diatoms) and some members of Cryptophyceae, ε-carotene is present. In the case of xanthophylls, fucoxanthin is found in Chrysophyceae, Bacillariophyceae, and Phaeophyceae. Peridinin occurs only in Dinophyceae. Myxoxanthin and myxoxanthophyll are xanthophylls found in Cyanophyceae (blue–green algae). Taraxanthin is present in Rhodophyceae and antheraxanthin is found in Euglenophyceae. Violaxanthin is dominant in chlorophytes, prasinophytes, chrysophytes, and in some dinoflagellates while zcaxanthin dominates in cyanobacteria, pelagophytes, chrysophytes, and a few dinoflagellates (Jeffrey et al., 1997; Higgins et al., 2011; Coupel et al., 2015).

Phycobilins are water-soluble blue or red pigments that also serve as accessory pigments to chlorophylls. Tetrapyrrolic, a compound joined to globin proteins is present in Cyanophyceae, Rhodophyceae, and Cryptophyceae. On the basis of absorption spectra, we have three types of phycobilins: phycocyanin that is found in Cyanophyceae; phycoerythrin found in Rhodophyceae, and Allophycocyanin found both in Cyanophyceae and Rhodophyceae.

Reserved foods in algae are also of taxonomic importance. The first group consists of polysaccharides in which glucose subunits are joined with α-1, 4 linkages. They include starch for Chlorophyceae and Charophyceae, floridean starch for Rhodophyceae, and myxophycean starch for Cyanophyceae. Others are polysaccharides with β-1, 3 linkages. They are laminarin for Phaeophyceae, chrysolaminarin for Chrysophyceae and Bacillariophyceae, and paramylon for Euglinophyceae.

The next phytochemicals of chemotaxonomic values in algae are the fatty acids. Fatty acids have a more complex composition and greater variety in algae than in vascular plants (Dembitsky et al., 2003). This variety in composition at all hierarchical levels of algal taxonomy has proven them valuable taxonomic features in the delimitation of taxa. In green algae, for example, C_{16} and C_{18} polyunsaturated fatty acids (PUFAs) have generally been reported to be the most abundant (Khotimchenko, 1993; Gocke et al., 2010). In their study of the chemotaxonomic relevance of fatty acids, Xu et al. (1998) recorded 37 fatty acids, including palmitic acid, oleic acid, linolenic acid, myristic acid, and hexadecatrienoic acid, as useful diagnostic characters in six *Codium* spp.. In a similar study, Goecke et al. (2010) differentiated three species of *Codium* (*C. dimorphum*, *C. fernandezianum*, and *C. fragile*) based on their fatty acid composition.

Kenyon (1972) classified cyanobacteria (Cyanophyceae) into four groups based on their fatty acid composition. The first group comprised strains that lacked PUFA, containing only saturated and mono-unsaturated fatty acids. The second and third groups consisted of strains with linoleic or linolenic acids, respectively, and the last group consisted of strains containing octa-decatetraenoic acid (Kenyon, 1972). Borah et al. (2016) used the same fatty acid parameters to differentiate strain of *Cylindrospermum* and *Nostoc*. Tetradecanoic acid, pentadecanoic acid, and 12-hydroxy-9-octadecenoic acid were found to occur only in *Cylindrospermum* strains, whereas trideca-noic acid occurred in *Nostoc* strains but absent in *Cylindrospermum* (Borah et al., 2016). Similar reports have been given on cyanobacteria by Cohen and Vonshak (1991) and Gugger et al. (2002).

Amico (1995) studied the chemotaxonomy of brown algae and reported that species of *Cystoseira* generally synthesized tetraprenyltoluquinols while species of *Bifurcaria* and *Cystophora* and some *Cystoseira* produced linear diterpenoids. Tetraprenyltoluquinols have never been found in *Caulocystis* and *Acrocarpia,* instead, they accumulate acetogenins and *Landsburgia*is the only genus that produces naphthoquinone derivatives (Amico, 1995).

Moretti and Muchassio (2009) validated the inclusion of *Porphyridium* Näg. in*Rhodophyta* with the evidence of floridosides and γ-linolenic acid (compounds believed to occur only in red algae) isolated from *P. aerugineum* and *P. cruentum.*

7.5.1.2 CHEMOTAXONOMY OF BRYOPHYTES (MOSSES AND LIVERWORTS)

Mosses possess carbohydrates as their structural components, as well as, secondary metabolites that are responsible for their numerous biological activities (Maksimova et al., 2013). The specific groups that have been studied include fatty acids, lipids, essential oils among others (Klavina et al., 2015). Hu et al. (2011) classified five species of mosses (*Ptychomi-trium sinense, P. dentatum, P. polyphylloides, Macromibiuma ferriei,* and *M. syntrichophyllum*) based on their chemical components using Fourier transform infrared spectroscopy and chemometrics.

Caldicott and Eglinton (1976) had earlier reported the chemotaxonomic significance of cutin acids: 15-hydroxyhexadecanoic acid, 8, 16-, 9, 16- and 10, 16-dihydroxyhexadecanoic acids in species of *Sphagnum* moss and liverworts. Klavina et al. (2015) isolated and identified different phenolic compound in some species of mosses for the first time. They include

3'''-desoxydicranolomin, 5,6,7,8-tetrahydroxycoumarin-5-β-glucopyranoside, 7,8-dihydroxy-5-methoxycoumarin-7-β-sophoroside, and others while matairesinol, apigenin, atraric acid, abscisic acid were also recognized. Sphagnic acid, a substance previously supposed to occur only in *Sphagnum* was reported in other mosses species and in *Sphagnum rubellum*, some unique substances not characteristic for other tested mosses were found, such as hydroxyharmane and harmol propionic acid ester, which are derivatives of alkaloid harmol (Klavina et al., 2015).

Liverworts are known to produce unique sesquiterpenoids with carbon skeletons that otherwise are lacking in higher plants, and they play important roles in their delimitation. Examples include (-)-frullanolide and (-)-caryo-phyllene which are found in species of *Frullania* and *Scapania undulata* respectively (Andersen et al., 1977). The monoterpenes, camphene, β-pinene, limonene, linalool, α-thujene and β-phellandrene, previously isolated in higher plants have also been identified in liverworts (Asakawa, 1994).

7.5.1.3 CHEMOTAXONOMY OF LICHENS

It is important to consider the lichens in this context because of the symbiotic association between the photosynthetic algae (lower plant) and fungi. Although lichens are classified as part of the fungi kingdom, the algae are protected within the fungus and supply the fungus with energy from photosynthesis as the fungus cannot make its own food because they lack chlorophyll. The metabolites produced by algae could serve as a basis for chemoxanomical classifications. Lichens are found in a wide range of habitats throughout the world and dominate terrestrial ecosystems with about 20,000 species documented globally. They are economically important to man as a dye, food, medicine, source of industrial raw material, and their ability to detect changing climatic condition and air pollution has made them be considered good bioindicators. These properties can only be attributed to the phytochemicals found in them. They produce primary metabolites such as amino acids, polyols, carotenoids, polysaccharides, and vitamins. It is estimated that about 700 secondary metabolites have been isolated, of which 550 are unique to them and not available in any other plant group, including the much exploited usnic acid used as an antibiotic (Molnar and Farkas, 2010).

In addition to morphological and anatomical features, secondary metabolites (popularly referred to as lichen substances) have contributed to the identification and classification of lichens (especially lichenan and

isolichenan) through classic spot test, microcrystal test, thin layer chromatography, or high-performance liquid chromatography (Walker and James,
1995). Some lichen's thallus emits fluorescence (yellowish, bluish) when
observed under UV light due to the presence of the lichen substance called
lichexanthone, and it is an important taxonomical character for identification
of species in few cases (Nayaka, 2005) and carotenoid compounds have also
been intensely studied for insights to evolutionary relationships.

The first attempt to the chemotaxonomy of lichens was by William
Nylander in the 1980s when he separated C+ red *Cetrelia olivetorum* from
the identical C−*C. cetrarioides*. Ever since then, lichenologists have been
utilizing the pigments in the classification of lichens. The family Teloschis-
taceae is characterized by the orange anthraquinone pigment − parietin and
vulpinic acid which is a characteristic of the species of *Letharia*. The cortical
substance atranorin is found in *Physcia* spp. while it is lacking in the closely
related *Phaeophyscia* spp. In *Punctelia*, the cortex contains atranorin while
in *Flavopunctelia* the cortex produces usnic acid (Nayaka, 2005).

7.5.2   CHEMOTAXONOMY IN HIGHER PLANTS CLASSIFICATION

Higher plants, also known as vascular plants and botanically grouped as
tracheophytes, include most plants that are easily recognized around us. They
differ from lower plants in having specialized and more complex organs.
They range in structure and complexity from pteridophytes (including ferns
and club mosses) to gymnosperms (including conifers) and angiosperms
(flowering plants). Their complexity in structure and functions correlate with
the wide diversity and distribution of phytochemicals found in them. Among
those that have been applied in chemotaxonomic studies are the directly
visible particles, semantides, and primary and secondary metabolites.

Directly visible particles such as ergastic substances produced in plants
including tannins, crystals of calcium oxalates, starch granules have contributed immensely to chemotaxonomic studies of higher plants. Nwachukwu
and Edeoga (2006) confirmed the separation of species of *Indigofera* based
on the nature and distribution of starch grains and calcium oxalate crystals.
Konyar et al. (2014) highlighted their relationship and contribution to the
identification of poisonous plants.

Raphides, one of the most common types of oxalate crystals were
studied by previous researchers and their relevance as taxonomic tools
were recorded: Based on their morphology, they have been classified into

basically four types occurring in specific plant families (Saadi and Mondal, 2011). Saadi and Mondal (2011) recognized two types of raphides in the family Araceae and used their structures and distribution to differentiate 14 species in the family. Similar successes were recorded in Vitaceae (Web, 1999; Arnott and Webb, 2000), Typhaceae, Solanaceae (Horner et al., 1981), Agavaceae (Wattendorff, 1976), Dioscoreaceae (Prychid and Rudall, 1999), Malvaceae, Tiliaceae (Faheed et al., 2013), and Asteraceae (Meric, 2009).

Electrophoresis has made it possible for chemotaxonomists to utilize the variation in seed protein electrophoretic patterns in studying relationships in plants. Previous authors have used this technique to delimit species of *Vicia* (Sammour, 1989*), Sesbania* (Badr et al., 1998), *Zygophyllum* (El-Ghameryet al., 2003; Khafagi, 2003), and *Anagallis* (Aboel-Atta, 2004). Species of *Tribulus* have been separated based on proteins and isoenzymes isolated from their seeds through electrophoresis techniques.

Bhargava et al. (2013) reviewed the relevance of terpenoids and essential oils to the chemotaxonomy of eight plant families. Diterpenoids were used to successfully delimit species of Garryaceae, a family that is difficult to classify by their morphological characters and linearol, lineral, isolinearol, and siderol were terpenoids of taxonomic importance in species of *Sideritis* (Norgard, 1974). It was also important to note that the identity of *Erigeron bonariensis* that was traditionally mistaken for *Conyza* due to their morphological resemblance was successfully confirmed by the phenolic content and caffeol derivatives present in it (Ansari, 1992). Methylated, prenylated, and acetylated phloroglucinol derivatives present in the essential oils of the family Myrtaceae (c.g., *Eucalyptus* spp.) helps in their taxonomic delimitation. Similarly, the Rutaceae is another family rich in essential oils such as evodionol and aromatic compounds such as furano and dimethyl pyranocoumarins. Other families with characteristic essential oils of chemotaxonomic importance include Lamiaceae, Verbenaceae, Piperaceae, and Malvaceae (Bhargava et al., 2013). Mandal et al. (2016) separated eight members of the Lauraceae by thin-layer chromatography, based on their essential oil, anthraquinone, flavonoids, and phenolics compositions.

Riveria et al. (1997) confirmed the separation of *Populus* (Salicaceae) into four taxonomic sections by earlier researchers (Diaz-Gonzalez and Llamas, 1987; Crane, 1988; English et al., 1991; English et al., 1992; Blanco, 1993) based on the flavonoid contents. From their report, Sect. *Populus* and *Thuranga* lacked flavonoids with cinnamic acid derivatives and hydrocarbons, the major components in the former. Sect. *Tacamahaca* had dihydrochalcones and sesquiterpenols but lacked flavones, flavanones, flavanonols, and pinobanksin which were characteristic to Sect. *Aigeiros* (Rivera et al., 1997).

Suau et al. (2002) successful classified 10 *Fumaria* spp. into three groups based on the alkaloid contents. In their study through gas chromatography–massspectrometry technique, phthalideisoquinoline alkaloid was found to be peculiar to *F. macrosepala* and rare in others. Protopine was common in all species but in varying amounts (Suau et al., 2002). Hillig and Mahlberg (2004) grouped *Cannabis* spp. into three chemotypes based on their variations in cannabinoid contents.

An extensive chemotaxonomic study of some monocotyledons was conducted by Ankanna et al. (2012). They found wide distribution of flavonoids, phenols, tannins, and steroids in 40 species belonging to 16 families and emphasized their taxonomic importance (Ankanna et al., 2012). Míka et al. studied the chemotaxonomy of the Poaceae and used phenolic compounds as chemical markers in delimiting different species and cultivars of *Dactylis, Festuca rubra,* and *Bromus* (2005). The phenolic compound that showed interesting contrasts were caffeic acid, ferulic acid, *p*-coumaric acid, chlorogenic acid, rosmarinic acid, and flavonoid compounds such as quercetin, rhamnetin, isorhamnetin, and others (Mika et al., 2005). Another chemotaxonomic study in Monocots was that of Zafar et al. (2011) who reported the distribution of flavanols, phenolic acids, and aurone, and their taxonomic importance in four species of *Cyperus*.

7.6 CHALLENGES AND LIMITATIONS IN CHEMOTAXONOMY

Chemotaxonomy has been proved to be a promising area of study that could provide useful information that, when combined with pieces of evidence from morphological aspects, would help taxonomists create a reliable phylogenetic system of classification. However, it involves sophisticated techniques and is not void of challenges. The following challenges and limitations may be considered:

7.6.1 PARALLELISM AND CONVERGENCE

These phenomena have been contributing to difficulties in all approaches to taxonomy and chemotaxonomy. They are phenomena where a certain taxonomic character (in this case a chemical character) fails to diverge and runs parallel (parallelism) or converge (convergence) along the line of evolution (Pandey and Misra, 2008). Simply put, when similar chemical marker (or function) occurs separately in two or more species that share the same lineage (ancestor), it is said to be parallel evolution but when the same chemical character occurs in species that share entirely distinct lineages (ancestors), it is termed convergent evolution (Zhang and Kumar, 1997). Certain chemical compounds occur sporadically in plant families that are not even genetically related and synthesized by different biogenetic pathways. Therefore, adequate knowledge of the biosynthetic pathways (and whether they are reversible or not) of every chemical marker used in chemotaxonomy is needed in order to construct a valid phylogenetic classification system. The various biosynthetic pathways are detailed in Chapter 2 of this book.

7.6.2 CHEMICAL REDUCTION

This can be a problem to creating a valid phylogenetic classification system based on chemotaxonomic characters given that there are shreds of evidence that larger molecules or having a more complex molecular structure do not necessarily imply that the said chemical compound is more advanced than the other. This is because chemical reduction may occur at any point along the biosynthetic pathway of that molecule due to metabolic or environmental changes.

7.6.3 ENVIRONMENTAL INFLUENCE

Many chemical compounds and their biosynthesis can be affected by environmental factors and climatic changes such as temperature anomaly, nutrient availability/deficiency, and certain industrial and anthropogenic activities. It was earlier noted that certain secondary metabolites are secreted by plants as a response to stress, insect attack, or mechanical damage. This may cause a significant change in both quantitative and qualitative composition of the phytochemicals when compared with unaffected species.

7.6.4 CHEMICAL VARIABILITY

Chemical variability may occur in an individual plant over a geographic range, time of collection, and/or stage of development within the period of study. In other words, a certain plant organ may yield more phytochemicals at the earlier stages of development (e.g., at budding or early flowering stages than at maturity), and some chemical substances may be found to be more concentrated in a plant organ at sunrise than at sunset and vice versa.

7.6.5   INADEQUATE FUNDS AND RESOURCES

One of the causes of loss of interest in research in the developing and underdeveloped countries has been poor funding and research facilities. Some scientists who have the interest in the biological diversity provided by nature to carryout research may not have access to some of the modern equipment needed to accomplish the task. Advanced phytochemotaxonomy involves isolation, characterization, and structural elucidation of the isolated compounds in order to infer their biosynthetic pathway and possibly their phylogenetic relationships. This remains a dream to such scientists as they lack those sophisticated equipment (e.g., nuclear magnetic resonance spectroscopy, etc.) need for such study in their research institutions. Furthermore, human resources and funds to attend training programs (that involves long distance travels) are not easily available to young researchers.

7.7   CONCLUSION

Notwithstanding the criticisms thrown its way, comparative phytochemistry has over the years contributed immensely to plant taxonomy and systematics and will unarguably continue to be the bedrock of drug research and discovery in the future. With the advancement of analytical methods today, studies should be intensified to obtain more knowledge of the biosynthetic pathways of most phytochemicals used as taxonomic markers in order to provide a clearer understanding of their phylogenetic relationships and possibly create a classification system that will be based on taxonomic keys derived from chemical characters. This, however, should not be a replacement but rather a supplementary to the already existing taxonomic keys constructed from morphological characters for a better experience.

KEYWORDS

- **phytochemicals**
- **chemotaxonomy**
- **plant classification**
- **phytochemistry**
- **secondary metabolite**

REFERENCES

Abdul Rahaman, A. A.; Kolawole, O. S.; Oladele, F. A. Leaf Epidermal Features as Taxonomic Characters in Some *Lannea species* (Anacardiaceae) from Nigeria. *Phytol. Balcan.* **2014**, *20* (2–3), 227–231.

Aboel-Atta, A. I.I. On the Delimitation of *Anagallis arvensis* L. (Primulaceae) – Evidence Based on SEM of Leaf and Seed Coat and SDS-PAGE of Seed Protein Profile. *Egypt. J. Biotechnol.* **2004**, *16*, 61–74.

Agbagwa,I. O.;Ndukwu, B. C.The Value of Morpho-Anatomical Features in the Systematics of *Curcubita* L. Species in Nigeria. *Afr. J. Biotechnol.* **2004**, *3* (10), 541–546.

Amico, V.Marine Brown Algae of Family Cystoseiraceae: Chemistry and Chemotaxonomy. *Phytochemistry.* **1995**, *39* (6), 1257–1279.

Andersen,N. H.;Bissonette, P.;Liu,C. B.;Shunk, B.;Ohta, Y.;Tseng,C. W.;Moore, A.;Huneck, S.Sesquiterpenes ofNine Europeans Liverworts from the Genera *Anastrepta, Bazzania, Jungermannia, Lepidozia*, and *Scapania. Phytochemistry* **1977**, *16*, 1731–1751.

Ankanna, S.;Suhrulatha, D.;Savithramma, N.Chemotaxonomical Studies of Some Important Monocotyledons. *Bot. Res. Int.* **2012**, *5* (4), 90–96.

Ansari, S. H.*Essentials of Pharmacognosy,* 4th ed.; Birla Publishers: New Delhi,1992.

Arnott,H. J.;Webb, M. A.Twinned Raphides of Calcium Oxalate in Grape (Vitis): Implications for Crystal Stability and Function. *Int. J. Plant. Sci.* **2000**, *161*, 133–142.

Asakawa, Y.Highlights in Phytochemistry of Hepaticae – Biologically Active Terpenoids and Aromatic Compounds. *Pure Appl. Chem.* **1994**, *66*, 2193–2196.

Badr, A.;Abuo-Elanain,M. M.;El-Shazly, H. H.Variation in Seed Protein Electrophoretic Pattern and Species Relationships in *Sesbania.* In *Proceedings Sixth Egyptian Botanical Conference, Cairo University. Giza,* III:1998, 493 501.

Bhargava, V. V.; Patel, S. C.; Desai, K. S. Importance of Terpenoids and Essential Oils in Chemotaxonomic Approach. *Int. J. Herbal Med.* **2013**, *1*(2), 14–21.

Blanco, P.Salix. In *Flora Liberica 3;* Castroviejo, S., Eds.; Real Jardin Botanica: Madrid, 1993; pp 477–517.

Borah, I.;Vimala, N.;Thajuddin, N.Chemotaxonomy of Cyanobacteria Isolated from Assam, North-East India. *Phytochemistry.* **2016**, *46* (2), 33–45.

Caldicott, A. B.; Eglinton, A. B.Cutin Acids from Bryophytes: An ω-1 Hydroxy Alkanoic Acid in Two Liverwort Species. *Phytochemistry.* **1976**, *15*(7), 1139–1143.

Cohen, Z.; Vonshak, A. Fatty Acid Composition of *Spirulina* and *Spirulina*-Like Cyanobacteria in Relation to Their Chemotaxonomy. *Phytochemistry.* **1991**, *30*(1), 205–206.

Coupel, P.; Matsuoka, A.; Ruiz-Pino, D.; Gosselin, M.; Marie, D.; Tremblay, J. E.; Babin, M.Pigment Signatures of Phytoplankton Communities in the Beaufort Sea. *Biogeosciences.* **2015**, *12*, 991–1006.

Crane, E. *Beekeeping: Science, Practice and WorldResources;* Heinemann: London, 1988.

Croteau, R.; Kutchan, T. M.; Lewis, N. G. Natural Products (Secondary Metabolites). In *Biochemistry and Molecular Biology of Plants;* Buchanan, B., Gruissem, W., Jones, R., Eds.; John Wiley and Sons Ltd.: Rockville, MD, 2000; pp 1250–1318.

Delgado-Vargas, F.; Jiménez, A. R.; Paredes-López, O. Natural Pigments: Carotenoids, Anthocyanins and Betalains – Characteristics, Biosynthesis, Processing, and Stability. *Crit. Rev. Food Sci. Nutr.* **2000**, *40* (3), 173–289.

Dembitsky, V. M.; Rezankova, H.; Rezanka, T.; Hanus, L. O. Variability of the Fatty Acids of the Marine Green Algae Belonging to the Genus *Codium. Biochem.Syst. Ecol.* **2003**, *31*, 1125–1145.

Diaz-Gonzalez,T. E.; Llamas, F. Aportaciones Al Conocimiento Del Genero*Salix* L. (Salicaceae) En La Provincial De Leon (NW Espana). *Acta Bot. Malacitana.* **1987**, *12*, 111–150.

Dzubak, P.; Hajduch, M.; Vydra, D.; Hustova, A.; Kvasnica, M.; Biedermann, D.; Markova, L.; Urban, M.; Sarek, J. *Nat. Prod. Rep.* **2005**, *2*, 394–411.

Ekeke, C.; Agbagwa, I. O. Ergastic Substances (Calcium Oxalate Crystals) in the Leaf of *Combretum* Loefl. (Combretaceae) Species in Nigeria. *Am. J. Plant. Sci.* **2014**, *5*, 2389–2401.

El-Ghamery, A. A.; Abdel-Azeem, E. A.; Kasem, A. M. Electrophoretic Seed Protein, Isozyme Patterns and Nucleic Acids Content in Some Egyptian Taxa of the Genus *Zygophyllum*. *Egypt. J. Biotechnol.* **2003**, *13*, 268–283.

English, S.; Greenway, W.; Whatley, F. R. Analysis of Phenolics of *Populus trichocarpa* BudExudate by GC-MS. *Phytochemistry* **1991**, *30*, 531–533.

English, S.; Greenway, W.; Whatley, F. R. Analysis of Phenolics in the Bud Exudates of *Populus deltodes, P. fremontii, P. sargentii* and *P. wislizenii* by GC-MS. *Phytochemistry.* **1992**, *31*, 1255–1260.

Faheed, F.; Mazen, A.; Elmohsen, S. A. Physiological and Ultrastructural Studies on Calcium Oxalate Crystal Formation in Some Plants.*Turk. J. Bot.* **2013**, *37*, 139–152.

Goecke, F.; Hernández, V.; Bittner, M.; González, M.; Becerra, J.; Silva, M. Fatty Acid Composition of Three Species of *Codium* (Bryopsidales, Chlorophyta) in Chile. *Revista de Biología Marina y Oceanografía.* **2010**, *45*(2), 325–330.

Goodwin, T. W. Biosynthesis of Carotenoids: An Overview. *Method. Enzymol.* **1992**, *214*(B), 330–340.

Gott, B.; Barton, H.; Samuel, D.; Torrence, R. Biology of Starch. In *Ancient Starch Research;* Torrence, R., Barton, H., Eds.; Left Coast Press: California, 2006; pp35–45.

Gugger, M.; Lyra, C.; Suominen, I.; Tsitko, I.; Humbert, J. F.; Salkinoja-Salonen, M. S.; Sivonen, K. Cellular Fatty Acids as Chemotaxonomic Markers of the Genera Anabaena, Aphanizomenon, Microcystis, Nostoc and Planktothrix (Cyanobacteria). *Int. J. Syst. Evol. Microbiol.* **2002**, *52*, 1007–1015.

Gurib-Fakim, A. Medicinal Plants: Traditions of Yesterday and Drugs of Tomorrow. *Mol. Aspect. Med.* **2006**, *27*, 1–93.

Harvey, A. Strategies for Discovering Drugs from Previously Unexplored Natural Products. *Drug Discov. Today.* **2000**, *5*(7), 294–300.

Higgins, H. W.; Wright, S.W.; Schlüter, L. Quantitative Interpretation of Chemotaxonomic Pigment Data. In *Phytoplankton Pigments: Characterization, Chemotaxonomy and Applications in Oceanography;* Roy, S., Llewellyn, C.A., Egeland, E.S., Johnsen, G., Eds.; Cambridge University Press: United Kingdom, 2011; pp 257–313.

Hillig, K. W.; Mahlberg, P. G.A Chemotaxonomic Analysis of Cannabinoid Variation in *Cannabis* (Cannabaceae). *Am. J. Bot.* **2004**, *91*(6), 966–975.

Horner, H. T.; Kausch, A. P.; Wagner, B. L. Growth and Change in Shape of Raphide and Druse Calcium Oxalate Crystals as a Function of Intracellular Development in *Typha angustifolia* L. (Typhaceae) and *Capsicum annuum* L. (Solanaceae). *Scan. Electron. Microsc.* **1981**, *3*, 251–262.

Hu, T.; Jin, W.; Cheng, C. Classification of Five Kinds of Moss Plants with the Use of Fourier Transform Infrared Spectroscopy and Chemometrics. *J. Spectrosc.* **2011**, *25*, 271–285.

Hutchinson, J.; Dalziel, J. M. *Flora of West Tropical Africa;* Crown Agent for Overseas Governments and Administration: London, 1963; Vol. 2.

Inya-Agha, S. I.; Nwafor, F. I.; Ezugwu, C. O.; Ezejiofor, M. Herbarium Techniques. In *Phytoevaluation: Herbarium Techniques and Phytotherapeutics;* Inya-Agha, S.I., Ezea, S.C., Nwafor, F.I., Eds.; Paschal Communication: Enugu State, 2017; pp 8–22.

Irchhaiya, R.; Anurag, K.; Anumalik, Y.; Nitika, G.; Swadesh, K.; Nikhil, G.; Santosh, K.; Vinay, Y.; Anuj, P.; Himanshu, G. Metabolites in Plant and Classification. *World J. Pharm. Pharma. Sci.* **2014**, *4*(1), 286–305.

Jeffrey, S. W.; Mantoura, R. F. C.; Wright, S. W. *Phytoplankton Pigments in Oceanography: Monographs on Oceanographic Methods;* UNESCO: Paris,1997.

Kenyon, C. N. Fatty Acid Composition of Unicellular Strains of Blue-Green Algae. *J. Bacteriol.* **1972**, *109*, 827–834.

Khafagi, A. A. The Significance of Seed Proteins in *Zygophyllum* Species (Zygophyllaceae) in Egypt. *Egypt. J. Biotechnol.* **2003**, *15*, 186–194.

Khotimchenko, S. V. Fatty Acids of Green Macrophytic Algae from the Sea of Japan. *Phytochemistry.* **1993**, *32*, 1203–1207.

Klavina, L.; Springe, G.; Nikolajeva, V.; Martsinkevich, I.; Nakurte, I.; Dzabijeva, D.; Steinberga, I. Chemical Composition Analysis, Antimicrobial Activity and Cytotoxicity Screening of Moss Extracts (Moss Phytochemistry). *Molecules.* **2015**, *20*, 17221–17243.

Konyar, S. T.; Öztürk, N.; Dane, F.Occurrence, Types and Distribution of Calcium Oxalate Crystals in Leaves and Stems of Some Species of Poisonous Plants. *Bot. Stud.* **2014**, *55*, 32–40.

Maksimova, V.; Klavina, L.; Bikovens, O.; Zicmanis, A.; Purmalis, O. Structural Characterization and Chemical Classification of Some Bryophytes Found in Latvia. *Chem. Biodivers.* **2013**, *10*, 1284–1294.

Mandal, P.; Choudhury, D.; Ghosal, M.; Das, A.P. TLC Based Chemotaxonomic Approach of Some Laurels Present in Sub-Himalayan Terai and Duars Region of West Bengal, India. *Int. J. Pharm. Sci. Rev. Res.* **2016**, *41*(2), 193–196.

Mathew, L.Crystals and Their Taxonomic Significance in Some Verbenaceae.*Bot. J. Linnean Soc.* **1984**, *88*, 279–289.

Míka, V.; Kubáň, V.; Klejdus, B.; Odstrčilová, V.; Nerušil, P. Phenolic Compounds as Chemical Markers of Low Taxonomic Levels in the Family Poaceae. *Plant Soil Environ.* **2005**, *51*(11), 506–512.

Misra, A.; Srivastava, S. Chemotaxonomy: An Approach for Conservation and Exploration of Industrially Potential Medicinal Plants. *J. Pharmacogn. Nat. Prod.* **2016**, *2*, 108.

Molnar, K.; Farkas, E. Current Results on Biological Activities of Lichen Secondary Metabolites: A Review. *Z. Naturforsch.* **2010**, *65c*, 157–173.

Moretti, A.;Musacchio, A.Chemotaxonomic Notes on Porphyridiumnäg. (Rhodophyta, Porphyridiales). *G. Bot. Ital.* **2009**, *116*(5–6), 269–274.

Muranaka, T.; Saito, K. Production of Phytochemicals by Plant Tissue Cultures. In*Comprehensive Natural Products II: Chemistry and Biology;* Mander, L., Liu, H. W., Eds.; Elsevier: Oxford, 2010; Vol. 3, pp 615–628.

Nayaka, S. Studying Lichens. Sahyadri E-News, Western Ghats Biodiverstity Information System – Issue XVI, 2005. http://wgbis.ces.iisc.ernet.in/biodiversity/bio_iden/lichens.htm; (accessed Nov 24, 2017).

Norgard, S. Qualitative and Quantitative Examination of Four Algal Species for Carotenoids. *Biochem. Syst. Ecol.* **1974**, *2*, 7–9.

Nwachukwu, C. U.; Edeoga, H. O. Tannins, Starch Grains and Crystals in Some Species of *Indigofera* L. (Leguminosae – Papilionoideae). *Int. J. Bot.* **2006**, *2*(2), 159–162.

Osawa, K.; Yasuda, H.; Maruyama, T.; Morita, H.; Takeya, K.; Itokawa, H. Antibacterial Trichorabdal Diterpenes from *Rabdosia trichocarpa*. *Phytochemistry* **1994**, *36*, 1287–1291.

Pandey, K. B.; Rizvi, S. I. Plant Polyphenols as Dietary Antioxidants in Human Healthand Disease. *Oxid. Med. Cell. Longev.* **2009**, *2*(5), 270–278.

Pandey, S. N.; Misra, S.P. *Taxonomy of Angiosperms;* Ane Books Pvt. Ltd.: New Delhi, 2008.

Prychid, C. J.; Rudall, P. J. Calcium Oxalate Crystals in Monocotyledons: A Review of Their Structure and Systematics. *Ann. Bot.* **1999**, *84*, 725–739.

Ramawat, K. G. Secondary Plant Products in Nature. In *Biotechnology: Secondary Metabolites; Plants and Microbes,* Ramawat, K. G., Merillon, J. M., Eds.; Science Publishers: Enfield, NH. 2007; pp 21–57.

Riveria, D.; Obon, C.; Tomas-Barberan, F.; Arenas, M. J. Study of theFlavonoids as Chemotaxonomic Markers in *Populus* (Salicaceae) of Spain. *Lagascalia.* **1997**, *19*(1–2), 813–818.

Saadi, A. I.; Mondal, A. K. Studies on the Calcium Oxalate Crystals of Some Selected Aroids(Araceae) in Eastern India. *Adv. Biores.* **2011**, *2*(1), 134–143.

Salim, A. A.; Chin, Y. W.; Kinghorn, A.D. Drug Discovery from Plants. In *Bioactive Molecules and Medicinal Plants;* Ramawat, K.G., Merillon, J. M., Eds.; Springer: USA, 2008; pp10–25.

Sammour, R. H. Electrophoresis of Seed Proteins of *Vicia faba* L. and its Immediate Progenitors.*Pl. Breed.* **1989**, *104*, 196–201.

Singh, R. Chemotaxonomy: A Tool for Plant Classification. *J. Med. Plants Stud.* **2016**, *4*(2), 90–93.

Stace, C. A. The Significance of the Leaf Epidermis in the Taxonomy of the Combretaceae: Conclusion. *Bot. J. Linn. Soc.* **1980**, *81*, 327–339.

Suau, R.; Cabezudo, B.; Rico, R.; Nájera, F.; López-Romero, J. M. Direct Determination of Alkaloid Contents in *Fumaria* Species by GC-MS. *Phytochem. Anal.* **2002**, *13*, 363–367.

Tolstikova, T. G.; Sorokina, I. V.; Tolstikov, G. A.; Tolstikov, A. G.; Flekhter, O. B. Biological Activity and Pharmacological Prospects of Lupane Terpenoids: I. Natural Lupane Derivatives. *Bioorg. Khim.* **2006**, *32*(1), 42–55.

Wattendorff, J.A Third Type of Raphide Crystal in the Plant Kingdom: Six-Sided Raphides with Laminated Sheaths in *Agave americana* L. *Planta.* **1976**, *130*, 303–311.

Webb, M. A. Cell-Mediated Crystallization of Calcium Oxalate in Plants. *Plant Cell* **1999**, *11*, 751–761.

Xu, R.; Fazio, G. C.; Matsuda, S. P.T. Review on the Origins of Triterpenoid Skeletal Diversity. *Phytochemistry.* **2004**, *65*, 261–291.

Xu,X. Q.; Hung,V. T.; Kraft, G.; Beardall, J. Fatty Acids of Six *Codium* Species from Southeast Australia. *Phytochemistry.* **1998**, *48*, 1335–1339.

Zafar, M.; Ahmad, M.; Khan, M. A.; Sultana, S.; Jan, G.; Ahmad, F.; Jabeen, A.; Shah, G. M.; Shaheen, S.; Shah, A. Chemotaxonomic Clarification of Pharmaceutically Important Species of *Cyperus* L. *Afr. J. Pharm. Pharmacol.* **2011**, *5*(1), 67–75.

Zhang, J.; Kumar, S. Detection of Convergent and Parallel Evolution at the Amino Acid Sequence Level. *Mol. Biol. Evol.* **1997**, *14*, 527–536.

CHAPTER 8

PLANT METABOLOMICS

SAGAR SATISH DATIR[1,*] and RAKESH MOHAN JHA[1]

[1]*Department of Biotechnology, Savitribai Phule Pune University, Pune 411007, Maharashtra, India, Tel.: +918412013810*

*Corresponding author. E-mail: datirsagar2007@gmail.com
ORCID: *https://orcid.org/0000-0003-0065-498X.*

ABSTRACT

Plant metabolomics deals with the analytical characterization of the metabolites present in the cells at a specific time and under specific conditions. It detects metabolic pathways in plants which help to identify and alter the novel gene function using genetic engineering approaches. Metabolomics based on the high-throughput detection of metabolites will facilitate understanding and discovery of complex metabolic networks in plants. Metabolomics approaches have been targeted to understand plant–pathogen interactions, abiotic stresses, identification of novel plant-derived compounds, and phytoremediation. However, the identification of metabolites under stressful conditions have been mainly complicated by metabolite complexity and often subjected to the fluctuations in environmental conditions. Therefore, the development and progress are multidimensional and advanced chromatographic separations coupled with high-throughput technologies may allow for the deeper mining of plant metabolites. This chapter provides a comprehensive review of recent scientific developments in plant metabolomics.

8.1 INTRODUCTION

Plants are abundant in the universe and encompass almost every aspect of human life including food, agriculture, and medicine. They produce a very large number of structurally diverse metabolites or phytochemicals which play diverse roles in plant growth, development, and response to various stress conditions. Metabolites are classified as primary and secondary. Secondary metabolites are organic compounds that differ widely across the plant kingdom and are not directly involved in the normal growth and development but are very crucial in plant defense against various diseases as well as necessary for a plant to survive under stressful conditions (Scossa et al., 2016). However, the diversity of plant metabolites is complicated by a complex regulatory mechanism which highlights the necessity to explore the underlying physiological and biochemical nature (Hall et al., 2008). Due to the lack of complete knowledge and the immense metabolic diversity amongst plants, metabolomics has become a key analytical tool in plant analysis (Hall et al., 2002).

Metabolomics is based on modern omic's techniques (Fig. 8.1) for a comprehensive analysis of metabolite pool in an organism which provides a functional screen of the cellular state (Oliver et al., 1998). It achieves qualitative and quantitative metabolite data from biological samples grown under a specific set of experimental conditions. Metabolomics provides both quantitative and qualitative measurements of diverse cellular metabolites which gives a complete knowledge of the biochemical status of an organism that can be further used to understand the function of the gene (Fiehn et al., 2000; Bino et al., 2004). Both qualitative and quantitative identification of plant-derived metabolites is critical and necessary. For instance, plant responses to environmental stimuli involve altered gene expression, which result in qualitative changes in metabolite pools. Accurate and reproducible quantitative methods are also essential as some responses may result only in temporal or spatial changes in metabolite concentrations. Therefore, quantitative methods differentiate samples at a level that can be used to study the functional relationship between genes and metabolites (Sumner et al., 2003). Plant metabolomics, therefore, aims to study the plant system at the molecular level to provide a non-biased characterization of the total metabolite pool (the metabolome) from plants in response to various environmental conditions (Fiehn, 2002; Hall et al., 2002; Fernie et al., 2004; Hall, 2006).

The identification of plant metabolites using metabolomics approaches has become a center of research interest in many research laboratories and has been widely studied to investigate plant metabolite responses to various kinds of abiotic stresses (Degenkolbe et al., 2013; Dias et al., 2015), to study plant–pathogen interactions (Allwood et al., 2010; Rudd et al., 2015), identification of novel plant-derived compounds (Taamalli et al., 2015; Chen et al., 2017), plant development processes (Businge et al., 2012), and phytoremediation studies (Liu et al., 2013; Pidatala et al., 2016). Table 8.1 describes examples of metabolomics tools used in various plant processes. Metabolomics approaches which involve identification of plant-derived metabolites would be of interest for the production of novel compounds, for drug development, increasing plants resistance against biotic stress, introduction of health beneficial compounds in food plants (Ye et al., 2000) using genetic engineering approaches, and for identification of the specific genes/metabolites that are responsible for tolerance to various abiotic stresses (Genga et al., 2011).

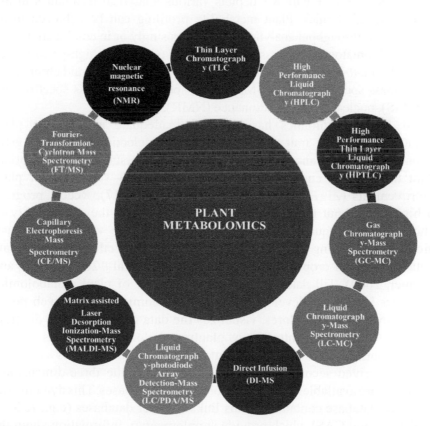

FIGURE 8.1   Different techniques in plant metabolomics.

Considering diverse applications, research on plant metabolomics has led to the development of multiple experimental and analytical platforms that collectively produce millions of metabolite profiles. Such experiments generate a vast amount of metabolomics data that leads to the development of public databases which provides the scientific community with comprehensive knowledge and information about metabolite data generation, annotation, and cross talk of various metabolic pathways (Bais et al., 2010). However, a single analytical technique cannot identify and quantify all the metabolites found in plants. Hence, a multiple qualitative and quantitative analytical and separation techniques or integrated approaches now found usefulness in the systematic characterization of various biological processes. Metabolite profiling using high-throughput operation provides in-depth analysis of metabolites economically, that is, low unit cost per sample (Schauer and Fernie, 2006). Figure 8.1 depicts various analytical techniques in use in plant metabolomics. Plant metabolite profiling can be achieved using various high-throughput analytical techniques singly or in combination such as gas chromatography–mass spectrometry (GC-MS), high-performance liquid chromatography (HPLC)–mass spectrometry (MS), liquid chromatography–mass spectrometry (LC-MS), mass spectrometry–mass spectrometry (MS-MS), nuclear magnetic resonance (NMR), and so forth.

So far, metabolomics has received inadequate attention in plant science, mainly for trait mapping and plant selections. It offers great potential in the advancement of the current understanding of important plant traits which enables the development of new strategies for plant improvements (Zivy et al., 2015; Kumar et al., 2017). Recent progress in high-throughput techniques in metabolomics and the accessibility of whole-genome sequence data, genome-wide genetic variants and cost-effective genotyping assays opens new avenues to effectively integrate metabolomics in crop breeding program (Hall et al., 2002; Fernie and Schauer, 2009). Till date, a very limited number of plant metabolomics databases have been developed. PlantMetabolomics.org is a web portal and database which explores, visualizes the data generated from different analytical platforms (http://www.plantmetabolomics.org; Bais et al., 2010). Another database such as Plant Metabolome Database is a database of plant-derived secondary metabolites in which the three-dimensional structures are available in the various biological databases. This dynamically compiled database contains various links to other databases (e.g., KEGG, PubChem, and CAS) which provide supplementary information about the metabolites (http://www.sastra.edu/scbt/pmdb; Udayakumar et al., 2012). Madison-Qingdao Metabolomics Consortium Database is a resource for metabolomics research using NMR spectroscopy and MS tools that provides the identification and characterization of metabolites present in biological samples (http://mmcd.nmrfam.wisc.edu/; Cui et al., 2008). Medicinal plants metabolomics resource provides a framework for generating

TABLE 8.1 Examples of Metabolomics Tools Used in Various Plant Processes.

Plant species	Analytical method	Remark	Reference
Mangifera indica	Proton transfer reaction-time of flight-mass spectrometry	Metabolite profiling of ripening Mangoes	White et al. (2016)
Zingiber officinale cv. Ogawa Umare	Liquid-chromatography mass spectrometry (LC-MS)	Chemical properties – medicinal and edible ginger cultivars	Tanaka et al. (2015)
Catharanthus roseus and *Vinca minor*	Gas chromatography (GC) and LC-MS	Metabolite profiling	Chen et al. (2017)
Hamelia patens	Nuclear magnetic resonance (NMR) spectrometry	Metabolite profiling	Flores-Sanchez et al. (2016)
Mentha pulegium and *Origanum majorana*	Reversed-phase ultra-high-performance liquid chromatography coupled to electrospray ionization quadrupole time-of-flight mass spectrometry	Metabolite profiling	Taamalli et al. (2015)
Boerhaavia diffusa	Gas chromatography-mass spectrometry (GC-MS)	Metabolite profiling	Pereira et al. (2009)
Arabidopsis thaliana and the bacterial disease caused by *Pseudomonas syringae*	Fourier transform infrared spectroscopy	Plant–pathogenic interaction	Allwood et al. (2010)
Oryza sativa and sheath blight – causal organism – *Rhizoctonia solani*	Flight mass spectrophotometry Capillary Electrophoresis Time-of-Flight Mass Spectrometry (CE-TOF-MS)	Plant–pathogen interaction	Suharti et al. (2016)
Triticum aestivum and fungal disease caused by *Zymoseptoria tritici*	Ultra performance liquid chromatography-tandem mass spectrometry	Plant–pathogen interaction	Rudd et al. (2015)
Lotus japonicus	Gas chromatography coupled to electron impact ionization–time of flight–mass spectrometry (GC/EI-TOF-MS)	Drought stress	Sanchez et al. (2012)

TABLE 8.1 *(Continued)*

Plant species	Analytical method	Remark	Reference
O. sativa	GC	Drought stress	Degenkolbe et al. (2013)
O. sativa	NMR Spectroscopy	Salinity stress	Nam et al. (2015)
Lens culinaris	GC/EI-TOF-MS	Drought stress and salinity stress	Muscolo et al. (2015)
Cicer arietinum	Liquid chromatography coupled to triple quadrupole–mass spectroscopy and gas chromatography coupled to triple quadrupole–mass spectroscopy	Salinity stress	Dias et al. (2015)
Suaeda salsa	NMR Spectroscopy	Phytoremediation	Liu et al. (2013)
Chrysopogon zizanioides	Liquid chromatography-mass spectrometry-mass spectrometry	Phytoremediation	Pidatala et al. (2016)
Raphanus sativus	GC-MS	Phytoremediation	Wang et al. (2015)
Sedum alfredii	GC-MS	Phytoremediation	Luo et al (2016)
Fragaria X ananassa	GC and high-performance liquid chromatography	Fruit development and maturation	Zhang et al. (2011)
Picea abies	Gas chromatography coupled to time-of-flight–mass spectrometry	Plant development	Businge et al. (2012)

experimentally testable hypotheses about the metabolomics network with specialized compounds, identifying genes that control the biosynthesis of these generated compounds, and establishing a basis for modeling metabolism in less studied species (Wurtele et al., 2012). An economical development of herbal medicine using NMR-based metabolomics provides a valuable tool for identifying potential biomolecule from medicinal plants (Heyman and Meyer, 2012; Mukherjee et al., 2016). These software tools were developed to generate metabolomics databases containing enormous data; henceforth, it will become important to map novel findings into metabolic pathways and fully illustrate the function of genes and its products such as encoded proteins and metabolites (Roessner, 2007).

8.2 MECHANISMS UNDERLYING PLANT SECONDARY METABOLISM

Since prehistoric times, plants have been extensively used in the treatment of various human diseases. Plants are the major producers of natural compounds which are biologically active molecules rich in health beneficial metabolites (Liu et al., 2017). However, metabolomics data is still not known for many medicinally important plants. Moreover, the characterization of the metabolic pathway which leads to the generation of medicinally important compounds is not well known. Metabolite analysis of plant-derived products is a first step towards the understanding of associated gene function and enzymatic regulatory pathway associated with it (Wurtele et al., 2012). Characterization of metabolites using high-throughput technologies is becoming an indispensable tool in the move towards the vision of personalized medicine (Frédérich et al., 2016) and personalized nutrition (German et al., 2011). There is major public health concern about dreadful diseases such as cancer, diabetes, dengue, HIV, and so forth. Therefore, there is an increasing demand to develop alternative methods to treat these diseases. Plant-derived natural compounds are currently gaining momentum in scientific research for the well-being of the community (Greenwell and Rahman, 2015). Current research in medicinal plants makes extensive use of metabolomics in the identification of the molecular targets of natural products which is an important aspect of current drug discovery, as knowledge of the molecular targets will greatly aid drug development (Akiyama et al., 2008; Wang et al., 2012). Therefore, in the understanding of drug action, it is crucial to have knowledge about the protein targets of natural products (Wang et al., 2008).

Metabolomics characterization of medicinal plants such as *Catharanthus roseus* (Apocynaceae) and *Vinca minor* (Apocynaceae) reveals the presence of terpenoid indole alkaloid (TIA). These metabolites are crucial in the treatment of various human diseases (Belal et al., 2009). GC-MS and LC-MS metabolite profiling of these two plants revealed the presence of 58 compounds comprised of 16 sugars, eight amino acids, nine alcohols, and 18 organic acids. Both plants showed the presence of nine typical alkaloids with the abundance of TIA intermediates of loganin, serpentine, and tabersonine. Metabolomics approaches for comparison between *C. roseus* and *V. minor* revealed the metabolite annotation for their divergence (Chen et al., 2017).

Comprehensive understanding of various secondary metabolites in traditional herbal medicine is important to study its medicinal properties. Traditionally, ginger (Zingiberaceae) has been considered medicinally important and global consumption of ginger has been increasing rapidly. Ginger is an ideal natural candidate chiefly used as an additive for food and beverages (Tanaka et al., 2015). Their metabolomics studies using LC-MS revealed that apart from gingerol and shogaol, there is the presence of several acetoxy derivatives in rhizome.

Hamelia patens (Rubiaceae), is a medicinal shrub known for the treatment of chronic wound and tumor (Leonti et al., 2002; Mena-Rejon et al., 2009). The biosynthesis and production of biologically active monoterpenoid indole alkaloids (MIAs) and monoterpenoid oxindole alkaloids (MOAs) in *H. patens* were studied using NMR-based metabolic profiles when treated with the stress hormone jasmonic acid (JA). Metabolomics approaches of *H. patens* plants showed that JA activates significant changes in the expression of MIAs and MOAs. These alkaloids are found to be associated with ethnomedical use (Sanchez et al., 2016). Due to its antioxidant and healthy properties in plants, researchers are actively engaging in the identification of phenolic compounds from plants. In view of this, metabolite profiling of *Mentha pulegium* (Lamiaceae) and *Origanum majorana* (Lamiaceae) were performed using reversed-phase ultra-HPLC coupled to electrospray ionization quadrupole time-of-flight mass spectrometry. The result revealed the presence of 85 metabolites such as nucleosides, phenolic compounds, amino acids, organic acids, and its derivatives as well as other polar metabolites. Further results revealed that gallocatechin is the main compound in *M. pulegium* extract, whereas quercetin dimethyl ether, jaceidin, and dihydrokaempferide were the chief ones in *O. majorana*. Such metabolomics approaches provide comprehensive information for the quality evaluation and pharmacokinetic studies of the plants (Taamalli et al., 2015).

These studies suggested that metabolomics can be an effective method for the complete assessment of the qualities of medicinal plants and also for advancing our understanding of their efficacy and mode of action of traditional medicines. However, metabolomics is complicated due to intricate data, which frequently include many experimental artifacts. Therefore, to overcome metabolite complexity, there is an urgent need to develop a combination of multidimensional chromatographic separations with multidimensional MS analysis so as to achieve maximum output of existing technologies (Shyur and Yang, 2008; Bowen and Northen 2010).

8.3 METABOLIC ANALYSIS OF PLANT–PATHOGEN INTERACTIONS

Plants are continually under attack by various pathogens such as viruses, fungi, protozoa, nematodes, and pests which causes a constant threat to agricultural production and thus to food security generating economic losses around the world (Heil and Baldwin, 2002; Pais et al., 2013; Bigeard et al., 2015). For instance, the fungus *Puccinia striiformis* is a causative agent of yellow rust disease which affects wheat production worldwide, leading to complete crop loss when left untreated (Beddow et al., 2015). The understanding of how plants respond and develop the defense mechanisms is crucial for developing a sustainable crop enhancement program. Plants synthesize a variety of compounds and these secondary metabolites play a major role in the resistance of plants against various pathogens (Schafer et al., 2009). These secondary metabolites which are involved in defense are synthesized from various metabolic pathways which are categorized into three major groups namely; terpenes, phenolics, and nitrogen-containing compounds (Großkinsky et al., 2012). Extensive metabolic profiles have been generated using advances in analytical techniques during plant–pathogen and plant–pest interactions. Metabolomics also plays a significant role in understanding plant–pathogen interactions (Allwood et al., 2010). However, metabolomics approaches in studying plant–pathogen interactions are very restricted and have been performed in a limited number of crops.

So far, metabolomics studies have been mainly conducted in understanding plant–fungal interactions. For instance, high-throughput metabolomics/bioinformatics protocol was developed for soybean (Leguminosae) against its soil-borne fungal pathogen *Rhizoctonia solani*. Metabolite detection and identification were accomplished using Orbitrap MS and GC-MS. In response to *Rhizoctonia* infection, the mobilization of carbohydrates, disturbance of the amino acid pool, and activation of isoflavonoid, a-linolenate, and phenylpro-panoid biosynthetic pathways of the soybean plants were observed. Several metabolites with antioxidant properties and bioactivity such as phytoalexins, coumarins, flavonoids, signaling molecules, and hormones were identified in response to pathogen's invasion. The metabolomics strategy reported in this research provides soybean's metabolism during fungal infection and these results could be further exploited in marker-assisted crop breeding, agrochemical, food, and pharmaceutical industries (Aliferis et al., 2014).

Cultivated rice (Poaceae) is severely affected by fungal pathogens such as *Magnaporthe grisea* and its capable of infecting many related cereals like barley, wheat, rye, and millet (Talbot, 2003). Jones et al. (2011) used NMR and GC-LC–MS-MS approaches to study the infection of the rice with compatible and incompatible strains of the rice blast fungal pathogen *M. grisea*. However, NMR identified 56 metabolites, GC-MS detected 67 metabolites with some overlap with the NMR in both the compatible and incompatible interactions. Studies revealed a good correlation between time of fungal penetration into the leaf and the divergence of metabolites such as alanine together with malate glutamine, proline, cinnamate, and an unknown sugar in each interaction. Therefore, metabolomics approaches used to iden-tify various types of metabolites in rice leaves can provide valuable informa-tion about the mechanisms of infection and plant/pathogen interaction of this disease. Likewise, bacterial leaf blight disease caused by *Xanthomonas oryzae* causes severe crop losses in rice. Metabolomics was applied to inves-tigate responses of rice plants when infected with *X. oryzae*. Many different metabolic responses were revealed between wild-type and genetically modi-fied rice with disease resistance. Moreover, various biosynthetic pathways such as acetophenone, xanthophylls, fatty acids, alkaloids, glutathione, carbohydrate, and lipid synthesis were affected (Sana et al., 2010). Such studies will help to understand a complexity of infection in response to a pathogen (Tarpley et al., 2005). NMR-based metabolite response of tomato leaves revealed that the identification of metabolites responsible for the differences between control and infected samples can provide information about the chemical diversity of the signaling compounds involved in the defense response in plant–pathogen interaction (López-Gresa et al., 2010).

Plant parasitic nematodes cause crop yield loss worldwide. Diseases caused by nematode are extremely difficult to control mainly due to their hidden nature and hence, generally overlooked (Singh et al., 2015c). Root-knot nematodes (RKNs) are widely distributed determining a significant impact on agriculture (Pierre et al., 2003). A GC-MS untargeted analysis was performed to identify important metabolites and biomarkers that occur in tomato plants after 2 months of infestation with *Meloidogyne incognita*. Tomato (Solanaceae) leaves showed induction in β-alanine, phenylalanine, and melibiose, while the reduction in ribose, glycerol, myristic acid, and palmitic acid was noted in response to RKN stimuli. Sugars such as ribose, sucrose, fructose, and glucose were upregulated, whereas glycine and fumaric acid were downregulated in tomato stems. These studies provided a powerful and reliable approach to study-level changes of plant metabolites after RKN infestation with adequate sensitivity and specificity to distinguish an infested plant from controls (Eloh et al., 2016).

Metabolomics approaches using various high-throughput techniques such as NMR and GC-MS not only help to understand changes in metabolites during plant–pathogen interactions but also open up new opportunities to evaluate the dynamic biochemical networks of plant–pathogen interactions.

8.4 METABOLOMICS AND PLANT RESPONSES TO ABIOTIC STRESSES

Adverse environmental conditions such as temperature, drought, and salinity are considered as major abiotic factors which limit agriculture crop productivity worldwide. Responses of plants to abiotic stresses include not only at the transcriptional level and post-translational levels but also in the identification of specific metabolites which leads to the generation of specific physiological response or phenotype (Verslues et al., 2006). Abiotic stresses activate several genes which result in the accumulation of various primary and secondary metabolites as well as proteins which are important in understanding the basics of plant stress physiology and biochemistry (Rodziewicz et al., 2014). For improvement of crop species to abiotic stresses, the information about the role played by low-molecular-weight primary and secondary metabolites in the stress tolerance process is essential. However, the function of these metabolites in the process of various abiotic stress tolerance of plants is comparatively least understood (Rodziewicz et al., 2014). Metabolomics has become an indispensable tool in the selection process of plants which are resistant to changing climatic conditions (Obata and Fernie, 2012). For instance, it has been applied to study the metabolic responses of *Arabidopsis* to abiotic stresses, such as heat, freezing, drought, and salinity (Kaplan et al., 2004; Qi and Zhang, 2014).

Plant responses to drought and salinity stresses involves the production of certain metabolites such as proline, soluble carbohydrates, glycine betaine, and γ-aminobutyric acid (Renault et al., 2013; Singh et al., 2015a). These metabolites not only help to maintain the osmotic compatibility within the cell but also to decrease the entropy levels, and to also provide support to proteins in the folded native tertiary structure (Muscolo et al., 2015). Effects of salinity and drought on two developmental stages such as germination and early growth followed by identification of particular changes in metabolite profile of lentil (Fabaceae) plants were performed. Responses of lentil culti-vars to these stresses were evaluated with respect to changes in polyamines, organic acids, sugars and polyols, amino acids, and other metabolites using GC/EI-TOF-MS. Metabolite indicators such as ornithine and asparagine can be used as biomarkers of drought stress, while stress indicators such as alanine and homoserine act as important biomarkers of salinity stress . Therefore, for identification of suitable physiological traits at an early stage would help plant breeders in specific selection programs (Muscolo et al., 2015). Metabolomics if combined with transcriptomics approaches can be useful in identification of secondary metabolites/key candidates associated with abiotic stress tolerance.

Rice is susceptible to salinity and the sensitivity to salt stress mainly depends on three factors such as growth stages, organ types, and cultivars which further limit plant growth. In view of this, metabolic markers were iden-tified using ^{1}H-NMR spectroscopy in 38 rice genotypes subjected to salinity stress using metabolite profiling. A total of five conserved salt-responsive metabolic markers of rice roots were identified, that is, sucrose, allantoin, glutamate, glutamine, and alanine. Further results revealed that sucrose, allantoin, and glutamate were accumulated in response to salinity stress, however, the levels of both glutamine and alanine found to be decreased. These studies identified a positive correlation between metabolite variations with growth potential and salinity tolerance of different rice genotypes for allantoin and glutamine, suggesting that metabolomics approaches help in the identification of conserved metabolic markers in response to long-term mild salinity stress in rice (Nam et al., 2015). Metabolomics approaches provide a deeper knowledge and understanding of biochemical pathways and molecular mechanisms. Therefore, the knowledge of genes, transcripts, and proteins involved cannot alone help to understand the biological process but essential to have a complete information of various metabolites that are engaged in abiotic stress mechanism (Deshmukh et al., 2014).

More than 200,000 plant secondary metabolites found to display huge chemical diversity in specific organs, tissues, and cells (Hartmann et al., 2007). These secondary metabolites found to contribute wine quality in grapes (Vitaceae). In grapes, the flavonoid accumulation was governed by water deficit, which further leads to quantitative and compositional varia-tions in anthocyanin pigments. However, in case of white grapes, the effect of water deficit on metabolite accumulation is largely unknown. Effects of water deficit in grapes from early stages of berry development to berry harvest using chromatography techniques revealed that in response to water deficit several secondary metabolic pathways lead to the production of phenylpropanoids, the carotenoid zeaxanthin, and of volatile organic compounds like monoterpenes. Moreover, water deficit condition also altered grape and wine antioxidant potential, composition, as well as sensory features. When transcriptome analysis was performed, it identified 18 phenylpropanoids, 16 flavonoids, nine carotenoids, and 16 terpenoid structural genes were found to be modulated in response to water deficit. These results demonstrated the transcriptional regulation of various secondary metabolic pathways in grape berries when exposed to water deficit. Identification of candidates through metabolomics approaches will provide a deeper understanding of the role and regulation of various secondary metabolites during water deficit condition in grapes (Savoi et al., 2016). These studies demonstrated that metabolomics is helpful to elucidate how the plant's metabolic process respond to stressful conditions (Obata et al., 2012). However, due to the complexity of metabolic pathways, it is challenging to identify the key regulatory metabolites involved in abiotic stress responses (Jain, 2013).

Although the function of several metabolites induced by abiotic stress in vivo is largely unknown, integrated metabolomics is an important powerful approach to reveal their function (Nakabayashi and Saito, 2015). Therefore, to improve the plant's tolerance to abiotic stress, there is an urgent need to identify novel genes/secondary metabolite pathways (Jain, 2013). Such metabolites can be further utilized to create stress tolerance crops using genetic engineering approaches.

8.5 METABOLITE PROFILING FOR HEAVY METAL TOLERANCE

Environmental pollution due to global mechanization, urbanization, rapid industrialization, modern agricultural practices, and increased anthropogenic activities results into the release of toxic compounds such as heavy metals (HMs) into the biosphere (Eapen and D'Souza, 2005; Kavamura and Esposito, 2010; Miransari, 2011; Mosa et al., 2016). The contamination of water and soil due to HMs like lead (Pb) and cadmium (Cd) represents a major environmental hazard to human health (Gupta et al., 2012; Liu et al., 2013; Mosa et al., 2016). Hence, it is important to develop suitable approaches and mechanisms for remediation of contaminated soil and water. The development of environment friendly and sustainable methods such as bioremediation, phytoremediation, and rhizoremediation for the cleanup of contaminated sites are widely preferred over physical remediation strategies which are not economical, nonspecific, and often renders the soil infertile for farming and other uses by altering the soil ecosystem (Mosa et al., 2016). Studies suggested that many important physiological and biochemical alterations have been induced in plants upon exposure to HMs. Hence, to cope with the undesirable effects of HM toxicity, plants need to adopt strategies (Singh et al., 2015b). However, identifying the biochemical and cellular targets by which plants respond to HM toxicity are very complex and challenging (Wang et al., 2015). It has been reported that Pb and Cd are the most common HM contaminants, which can be first absorbed by plants through HM contaminated water and soil which further enters into the food chain (Pourrut et al., 2013; Seregin and Ivanov, 2001). However, there is little knowledge and information available about the biochemical mechanisms responsible for HM tolerance in plants. It has been predicted that upon HM stress, plants might synthesize various metabolites and signaling molecules to acclimatize and cope with the presence of HM in their tissue. Moreover, in extreme metal toxicity, antioxidants, osmoprotectants, plant growth regulators, organic acids, phenolic compounds, and signal transduction molecules are known to be produced (Le Lay et al., 2006; Zoghlami et al., 2011). Some metabolites are known to be involved in HM stress tolerance, and therefore, recent advances in metabolomics have assisted in the study of various metabolites involved in HM tolerance, which in turn can be utilized for generating HM-tolerant crops (Singh et al., 2015b).

Remediation of soils that are highly contaminated with HM has been performed using plant root system. For instance, the radish (*Raphanus sativus,* Brassicaceae), an important root vegetable crop was found to be vulnerable to HM such as Cd and Pb (Uraguchi et al., 2009; Kapourchal et al., 2009). Therefore, to explore the HM-response mechanisms, the regulatory network at molecular levels of tolerance and homeostasis, metabolomic analysis was performed to find out novel metabolites and specific biological pathways involved in Pb and Cd stress in radish roots. GC-MS analysis revealed various metabolites such as sugars, amino acids, organic acids, inorganic acids, and others were altered in response to Pb or Cd stress in radish roots. Furthermore, various biochemical changes in carbohydrate metabolism, energy metabolism, and glutathione metabolism were observed when radish roots were exposed to Pb stress. While, in response to Cd stress, significant variations in energy production, amino acid metabolism, and oxidative phosphorylation-related pathways were noted. These findings suggested that metabolomic analysis can facilitate further dissection of the processes involved in HM accumulation tolerance in plants and that may provide the effective strategy to manage the HM contamination in vegetable crop plants by genetic engineering (Wang et al., 2015).

The contamination of residential soils due to Pb is a major problem in urban areas. Although phytoremediation is inexpensive and effective remediation strategy, it is still a promising approach to remove Pb from residential soils (Saminathan et al., 2010). The plant cultivar, Vetiver (*Chrysopogon zizanioides*), which belongs to the family Poaceae is an ideal plant for phytoremediation due to its noninvasive nature, fast-growing ability with high biomass. It can also tolerate high amount of Pb in its tissues. The identification of secondary metabolite pathways associated with Pb tolerance and detoxification in Vetiver by metabolic profiling was performed using LC/MS/MS. It was observed that when Vetiver plants were exposed to various concentrations of Pb in a hydroponic culture, higher amounts of Pb were accumulated in root tissue compared to shoot tissue. Metabolomics profiling of both root and shoot tissue exhibited remarkable induction in important metabolic pathways such as amino acid metabolism, sugar metabolism, and an increase in synthesis of osmoprotectants, such as betaine and polyols as well as metal-chelating organic acids. Although these studies provided a comprehensive insight into the overall HM response mechanisms in Vetiver, a further comparison with an HM non-accumulating plant would illustrate the differential response of Vetiver with susceptible plants.

Recently, Luo et al. (2016) performed comparative metabolic profiling of root exudates from two different ecotypes such as Pb-accumulating and non-accumulating of *Sedum alfredii* (Crassulaceae) using GC-MS. A total of 56 compounds were detected and out of which 15 compounds were identified and assumed to be potential biomarkers associated with Pb accumulation or tolerance. Further leaching experiments indicated that metabolites such as l-alanine, l-proline, and oxalic acid have a positive effect to activate Pb in soil while glyceric acid and 2-hydroxyacetic acid have a common effect to stimulate Pb in the soil. Both 4-Methylphenol and 2-methoxyphenol somehow may activate Pb in the soil, whereas glycerol and diethyleneglycol might stabilize Pb in the soil, however, the activation effect and stabilization effect were all not obvious. Further studies are warranted to study the interaction between HM and metabolite accumulation. Therefore, such methods will help to produce plants that are more suitable for phytoremediation of HM-contaminated soils (Gill et al., 2011).

These studies suggest that metabolomics approaches in the identification of specific metabolites playing a very significant role in HM tolerance may provide clean, efficient, inexpensive, and environment-friendly technology for the removal of contaminants from soil and water (Weis and Weis, 2004).

There has been the implication of using such hyperaccumulators in HM tolerance studies mainly because such plants possess the greater capability of HM uptake, root-to-shoot translocation of HM, and detoxification and sequestration of HM (Singh et al., 2015b).

8.6   CONCLUSION

Plants synthesizes a variety of secondary metabolites during their life span. These metabolites play a very crucial role not only during growth and development but also to withstand during various biotic as well as abiotic stresses. Apart from this, plant-derived metabolites have special significance in human diseases. To identify and functionally characterize such metabolites, a high-throughput metabolomics is needed. Metabolomics provides a qualitative and quantitative analysis of metabolites which can be utilized in the understanding of plant–pathogen interactions, abiotic stress tolerance, phytoremediation, and identification of important drug candidates. It may also help to understand the biochemical basis of seed germination, plant growth, development and physiology, fruit ripening, and post-harvest shelf life. Metabolomics if combined with other omic's approaches like transcriptomics and proteomics may help to engineer bioactive secondary metabolites which can be further utilized in system biology and in the improvement of human health.

ACKNOWLEDGMENT

The authors are thankful to Prof. Ameeta Ravikumar, HOD, Department of Biotechnology, Savitribai Phule Pune University for her kind support during the writing of the book chapter.

KEYWORDS

- abiotic stress
- chromatography
- mass spectrometry
- metabolomics
- nuclear magnetic resonance

REFERENCES

Akiyama, K.; Chikayama, E.; Yuasa, H.; et al. PRIMe: A Website that Assembles Tools for Metabolomics and Transcriptomics. *In Silico Biol.* **2008**, *8*, 339–345.

Aliferis, K. A.; Faubert, D.; Jabaji, S. A Metabolic Profiling Strategy for the Dissection of Plant Defense Against Fungal Pathogens. *PLoS One.* **2014**, *9*, e111930. DOI: 10.1371/journal.pone.0111930.

Allwood, J. W.; Clarke, A.; Goodacre, R.; Mur, L. A. J. Dual Metabolomics: A Novel Approach to Understanding Plant-Pathogen Interaction. *Phytochemistry* **2010**, *71*, 590–597.

Bais, P.; Moon, S. M.; He, K.; et al. PlantMetabolomics.org: A Web Portal for Plant Metabolomics Experiments. *Plant Physiol.* **2010**, *152*, 1807–1816.

Beddow, J. M.; Pardey, P. G.; Chai, Y.; Hurley, T. M.; Kritico, D. J.; Braun, H. J.; Park, R. F.; Cuddy W. S.; Yonow, T. Research Investment Implications of Shifts in the Global Geography of Wheat Stripe Rust. Nat. Plants. **2015**, *1, 1–5.*

Belal, T. S.; Barary, M. H.; Sabry, S. M.; Elsayed, M.; Ibrahim, A. L. Kinetic Spectrophotometric Analysis of Naftidrofuryl Oxalate and Vincamine in Pharmaceutical Preparations Using Alkaline Potassium Permanganate. *J. Food Drug Anal.* **2009**, *17*, 415–423.

Bigeard, J.; Colcombet, J.; Hirt, H. Signalling Mechanisms in Pattern-Triggered Immunity (PTI). *Mol. Plant.* **2015**, *8*, 521–539.

Bino, R.; Hall, R.; Fiehn, O.; Kopka, J.; Saito, K.; Draper, J.; Nikolau, B.; Mendes, P.; Roessner-Tunali, U.; Beale, M.; Trethewey, R.; Lange, B.; Wurtele, E.; Sumner, L. Potential of Metabolomics as a Functional Genomics Tool. *Trends Plant Sci.* **2004**, *9*, 418–425.

Bowen, B. P.; Northen, T. R. Dealing with the Unknown: Metabolomics and Metabolite Atlases. *J. Am. Soc. Mass Spectrom.* **2010**, *21*, 1471–1476.

Businge, E.; Brackmann, K.; Moritz, T.; Egertsdotter, U. Metabolite Profiling Reveals Clear Metabolic Changes During Somatic Embryo Development of *Norway spruce* (*Picea abies*). *Tree Physiol.* **2012**, *32*, 232–244.

Chen, Q.; Lu, X.; Guo, X.; Guo, Q.; Li, D. Metabolomics Characterization of Two Apocynaceae plants, *Catharanthus roseus* and *Vinca minor*, Using GC-MS and LC-MS Methods in Combination. *Molecules* **2017**, *22*, 997. DOI: 10.3390/molecules22060997.

Cui, Q.; Lewis, I. A.; Hegeman, A. D.; Anderson, M. E.; Li J.; Schulte, C. F.; Westler, W. M.; Eghbalnia, H. R.; Sussman, M. R.; Markley, J. L. Metabolite Identification Via the Madison Metabolomics Consortium Database. *Nat. Biotechnol.* **2008**, *26*, 162.

Degenkolbe, T.; Do, P. T.; Kopka, J.; Zuther, E.; Hincha, D. K.; Köhl, K. I. Identification of Drought Tolerance Markers in a Diverse Population of Rice Cultivars by Expression and Metabolite Profiling. *PLoS One.* **2013**, *8*(5), e63637.

Deshmukh, R.; Sonah, H.; Patil, G.; Chen, W.; Prince, S.; Mutava, R.; Vuong, T.; Valliyodan, B.; Nguyen, H. T. Integrating Omic Approaches for Abiotic Stress Tolerance in Soybean. *Front Plant Sci.* **2014**, *5*, 244. DOI: 10.3389/fpls.2014.00244.

Dias, D. A.; Camilla Beate Hill, C. B.; Jayasinghe, N. S.; Atieno, J.; Sutton, T., Roessner, U. Quantitative Profiling of Polar Primary Metabolites of Two Chickpea Cultivars with Contrasting Responses to Salinity. *J. Chromatogr. B.* **2015**, *1000*, 1–13.

Eapen, S.; D'Souza, S. F. Prospects of Genetic Engineering of Plants for Phytoremediation 1423 of Toxic Metal. *Biotechnol. Adv.* **2005**, *23*, 97–114.

Eloh, K.; Sasanelli, N.; Maxia, A.; Caboni, P. Untargeted Metabolomics of Tomato Plants After Root-Knot Nematode Infestation. *J. Agric. Food Chem.* **2016**, *64*, 5963–5968.

Fernie, A. R.; Schauer, N. Metabolomics-Assisted Breeding: A Viable Option for Crop Improvement? *Trends Genet.* **2009**, *25*, 39–48.

Fernie, A. R.; Trethewey, R. N.; Krotzky, A. J.; Willmitzer, L. Metabolite Profiling: From Diagnostics to Systems Biology. *Nat. Rev. Mol. Cell. Biol.* **2004**, *5*, 763–769.

Fiehn, O. Metabolomics: The Link Between Genotypes and Phenotypes. *Plant Mol. Biol.* **2002**, *48*, 155–171.

Fiehn, O.; Kopka, J.; Dörmann, P.; Altmann, T.; Trethewey, R. N.; Willmitzer, L. Metabolite Profiling for Plant Functional Genomics. *Nat. Biotechnol.* **2000**, *18*, 1157–1161.

Flores-Sanchez, I. J.; Vega, D. P.; Reyes, I. V.; Cerda-García-Rojas, C. M.; Valdivia, A. C. Alkaloid Biosynthesis and Metabolic Profiling Responses to Jasmonic Acid Elicitation in *Hamelia patens* Plants by NMR-Based Metabolomics. *Metabolomics* **2016**, *12*, 66, DOI: 10.1007/s11306-016-0999-4.

Frédérich, M.; Pirotte, B.; Fillet, M.; de Tullio, P. Metabolomics as a Challenging Approach for Medicinal Chemistry and Personalized Medicine. J. Med. Chem. **2016**, *59*, 8649–8666.

Genga, A.; Mattana, M.; Coraggio, I.; Locatelli, F.; Piffanelli, P.; Consonni, R. Plant Metabolomics: A Characterization of Plant Responses to Abiotic Stresses. In *Abiotic Stress in Plants – Mechanisms and Adaptations;* Shanker, A., Ed.; InTech, 2011; DOI: 10.5772/23844. https://www.intechopen.com/books/abiotic-stress-in-plants-mechanisms-and-adaptations/plant-metabolomics-a-characterisation-of-plant-responses-to-abiotic-stresses (accessed Dec 7, 2017).

German, J. B.; Zivkovic, A. M.; Dallas, D. C.; Smilowitz, J. T. Nutrigenomics and Personalized Diets: What will they Mean for Food? *Annu. Rev. Food Sci.* Technol. **2011**, *2*, 97–123.

Gill, S. S.; Khan, N. A.; Anjum, N. K.; Tuteja, N. Amelioration of Cadmium Stress in Crop Plants by Nutrients Management: Morphological, Physiological and Biochemical Aspects. *Plant Stress.* **2011**, *5*, 1–23.

Greenwell, M., Rahman, P. K. S. M. Medicinal Plants: Their use in Anticancer Treatment. *Int. J. Pharm. Sci. Res.* **2015**, *1*, 4103–4112.

Großkinsky, D. K.; Vander Graaff, E.; Roitsch, T. Phytoalexin Transgenics Inc Rop Protection—Fairy Tale with a Happy End? *Plant Sci.* **2012**, *195*, 54–70.

Gupta, N.; Khan, D.; Santra, S. Heavy Metal Accumulation in Vegetables Grown in a Long-Term Wastewater-Irrigated Agricultural Land of Tropical India. *Environ. Monit. Assess.* **2012**, *184*, 6673–6682.

Hall, R. D. Plant Metabolomics: From Holistic Hope, to Hype, to Hot Topic. *New Phytol.* **2006**, *169*, 453–468.

Hall, R.; Beale, M.; Fiehn, O.; Hardy, N.; Sumner, L.; Bino, R. Plant Metabolomics: The Missing Link In Functional Genomics Strategies. *Plant. Cell.* **2002**, *14*, 1437–1440.

Hall, R. D.; Brouwer, I. D.; Fitzgerald, M. A. Plant Metabolomics and its Potential Application for Human Nutrition. *Physiol. Plant.* **2008**, *132*, 162–175.Hartmann, T. From Waste Products to Ecochemicals: Fifty Years Research of Plant Secondary Metabolism. *Phytochemistry* **2007**, *28*, 2831–2846.

Heil, M.; Baldwin, I. T. Fitness Costs of Induced Resistance: Emerging Experimental Support for a Slippery Concept. *Trends Plant Sci.* **2002**, *7*, 61–67.

Heyman, H. M.; Meyer, J. J. M. NMR-Based Metabolomics as a Quality Control Tool for Herbal Products. *South Afr. J. Bot.* **2012**, *82*, 21–32.

Jain, M. Emerging Role of Metabolic Pathways in Abiotic Stress Tolerance. *J. Plant Biochem. Physiol.* 2013, 1, 108. DOI: 10.4172/2329-9029.1000108.

Jones, O. A. H.; Maguire, M. L.; Griffin, J. L.; Jung, Y.-H.; Shibato, J.; Rakwal, R.; Agrawal, G. L.; Jwa, N.-S. Using Metabolic Profiling to Assess Plant-Pathogen Interactions: An Example Using Rice (*Oryza sativa*) and the Blast Pathogen *Magnaporthe grisea*. *Eur. J. Plant. Pathol.* **2011**, *129*, 539–554.

Kaplan, F.; Kopka, J.; Haskell, D. W.; Zhao, W.; Schiller, K. C.; Gatzke, N.; Sung, D. Y.; Guy, C. L. Exploring the Temperature-Stress Metabolome of *Arabidopsis*. *Plant Physiol.* **2004**, *136*, 4159–4168.

Kapourchal, S. A.; Kapourchal, S. A.; Pazira, E.; Homaee, M. Assessing Radish (*Raphanus sativus* L.) Potential for Phytoremediation of Lead-Polluted Soils Resulting from Air Pollution. *Plant Soil Environ.* **2009**, *55*, 202–206.

Kavamura, V. N.; Esposito, E. Biotechnological Strategies Applied to the Decontamination of 1690 Soils Polluted with Heavy Metal. *Biotechnol. Adv.* **2010**, *28*, 61–69.

Kumar, R.; Bohra, A.; Pandey, K.; Pandey, M. K.; Jumar, A. Metabolomics for Plant Improvement: Status and Prospects. *Front. Plant Sci.* **2017**, *8*, 1302. DOI: 10.3389/fpls.2017.01302.

Le Lay, P.; Isaure, M. P.; Sarry, J. E.; Kuhn, L.; Fayard, B.; Le Bail, J. L.; Bastien, O.; Garin, J.; Roby, C.; Bourguignon, J. Metabolomic, Proteomic and Biophysical Analyses of *Arabidopsis thaliana* Cells Exposed to a Caesium Stress. Influence of Potassium Supply. *Biochimie* **2006**, *88*, 1533–1547.

Leonti, M.; Sticher, O.; Heinrich, M. Medicinal Plants of the Popoluca, Mexico: Organoleptic Properties as Indigenous Selection Criteria. *J. Ethnopharmacol.* **2002**, *81*, 307–315.

Liu, X.; Song, Q.; Tang, Y.; Li, W.; Xu, J.; Wu, J.; Wang, F.; Brookes, P. C. Human Health Risk Assessment of Heavy Metals in Soil-Vegetable System: A Multi-Medium Analysis. *Sci. Total Environ.* **2013**, *463*, 530–540.

Liu, K.; Abdullah, A. A.; Huang, M.; Nishioka, T.; Md. Altaf-Ul-Amin; Kanaya, S. Novel Approach to Classify Plants Based on Metabolite-Content Similarity. *BioMed. Res. Int.* **2017**, Article ID 5296729, https://doi.org/10.1155/2017/5296729.

López-Gresa, M. P.; Maltese, F.; Bellés, J. M.; Conejero, V.; Kim, H. K.; Choi, Y. H.; Verpoorte, R. Metabolic Response of Tomato Leaves upon Different Plant Pathogen Interactions. *Phytochem. Anal.* **2010**, *21*, 89–94.

Luo, Q.; Wang, S.; Sun, Li-na.; Wang, H. Metabolic Profiling of Root Exudates from Two Ecotypes of *Sedum alfredii* Treated with Pb Based on GC-MS. *Sci. Rep.* **2016**, *7*, 39878. DOI: 10.1038/srep39878.

Mena-Rejon, G.; Caamal-Fuentes, E.; Cantillo-Ciau, Z.; Cedillo-Rivera, R.; Flores-Guido, J.; Moo-Puc, R. In Vitro Cytotoxic Activity of Nine Plants used in Mayan Traditional Medicine. *J. Ethnopharmacol.* **2009**, *121*, 462–465.

Miransari, M. Hyperaccumulators, Arbuscular Mycorrhizal Fungi and Stress of Heavy Metal. *Biotechnol. Adv.* **2011**, *29*, 645–653.

Mosa, K. A.; Saadoun, I.; Kumar, K.; Helmy, M.; Dhankher, O. P. Potential Biotechnological Strategies for the Cleanup of Heavy Metals and Metalloids. *Front. Plant Sci.* **2016**, *7*, 303. DOI: 10.3389/fpls.2016.00303.

Mukherjee, P. K.; Harwansh, R. K.; Bahadur, S.; Biswas, S.; Kuchibhatla, L. N.; Tetali, S. D.; Raghavendra, A. S. Metabolomics of Medicinal Plants – A Versatile Tool for Standardization of Herbal Products and Quality Evaluation of Ayurvedic Formulations. *Curr. Sci.* **2016**, *111*, 1624–1630.

Muscolo, A.; Junker, A.; Klukas, C.; Weigelt-Fischer, K.; Riewe, D.; Altmann, T. Phenotypic and Metabolic Responses to Drought and Salinity of Four Contrasting Lentil Accessions. *J. Expt. Bot.* **2015**, *66*, 5467–5480.

Nakabayashi, R.; Saito, K. Integrated Metabolomics for Abiotic Stress Responses in Plants. *Curr. Opin. Plant Biol.* **2015**, *24*, 10–16.

Nam, M. H.; Bang, E.; Kwon, T. Y.; Kim, Y.; Kim, E. H.; Cho, K.; Park, W. J.; Kim, B.-G.; Yoon, I. S. Metabolite Profiling of Diverse Rice Germplasm and Identification of Conserved

Metabolic Markers of Rice Roots in Response to Long-Term Mild Salinity Stress. *Int. J. Mol. Sci.* **2015**, *16*, 21959–21974.

Obata, T.; Fernie, A. R. The use of Metabolomics to Dissect Plant Responses to Abiotic Stresses. *Cell Mol. Life Sci.* **2012**, *69*, 3225–3243.

Oliver, S. G.; Winson, M. K.; Kell, D. B.; Baganz, F. Systematic Functional Analysis of the Yeast Genome. *Trends Biotechnol.* **1998**, *16*, 373–378.

Pais, M.; Win, J.; Yoshida, K.; Etherington, G. J.; Cano, L. M.; Raffaele, S.; Banseld, M. J.; Jones, A.; Kamoun, S.; Saunders, D. G. From Pathogen Genomes to Host Plant Processes: The Power of Plant Parasitic Oomycetes. *Genome Biol.* **2013**, *14*, 211. DOI: 10.1186/gb-2013-14-6-211.

Pereira, D. M.; Faria, J.; Gaspar, L.; Valentão, P.; Andrade, P. B. *Boerhaavia diffusa*: Metabolite Profiling of a Medicinal Plant from Nyctaginaceae. *Food Chem. Toxicol.* **2009**, *47*, 2142–2149.

Pidatala, V. R.; Li, K.; Sarkar, D.; Ramakrishna, W.; Datta, R. Identification of Biochemical Pathways Associated with Lead Tolerance and Detoxification in *Chrysopogon zizanioides* L. Nash (Vetiver) by Metabolic Profiling. *Environ. Sci. Technol.* **2016**, *50*, 2530–2537.

Pierre, A.; Bruno, F.; Marie-Noelle, R.; Philippe, C.-S. Root-Knot Nematode Parasitism and Host Response: Molecular Basis of a Sophisticated Interaction. *Mol. Plant Pathol.* **2003**, *4*, 217–224.

Pourrut, B.; Shahid, M.; Douay, F.; Dumat, C.; Pinelli, E. Molecular Mechanisms Involved in Lead Uptake, Toxicity and Detoxification in Higher Plants. In *Heavy Metal Stress in Plants;* Dharmendra, K. G., Francisco, J. C., José, M. P., Ed.; Springer: Heidelberg, Germany, 2013; pp 121–147.

Qi, X.; Zhang, D. Plant Metabolomics and Metabolic Biology. *J. Integr. Plant Biol.* **2014**, *56*, 814–815.

Renault, H. E.; Amrani, A.; Berger, A.; Mouille, G.; Soubigou-Taconnat, L.; Bouchereau, A.; Deleu, C. γ-Aminobutyric Acid Transaminase Deficiency Impairs Central Carbon Metabolism and Leads to Cell Wall Defects During Salt Stress in *Arabidopsis* Roots. *Plant Cell Environ.* **2013**, *36*, 1009–1018.

Rodziewicz, P.; Swarcewicz, B.; Chmielewska, K.; Wojakowska, A.; Stobiecki, M. Influence of Abiotic Stresses on Plant Proteome and Metabolome Changes. *Acta. Physiol. Plant.* **2014**, *36*, 1–19.

Roessner, U. Uncovering the Plant Metabolome: Current and Future Challenges. In *Concepts in Plant Metabolomics;* Nikolau, B. J., Wurtele, S. E., Eds.; Springer: Heidelberg, Germany, 2007; pp 71–85.

Rudd, J. J.; Kanyuka, K.; Hassani-Pak, K. Transcriptome and Metabolite Profiling of the Infection Cycle of *Zymoseptoria tritici* on Wheat Reveals a Biphasic Interaction with Plant Immunity Involving Differential Pathogen Chromosomal Contributions and a Variation on the Hemibiotrophic Lifestyle Definition. *Plant Physiol.* **2015**, *167*, 1158–1185.

Saminathan, S. K.; Sarkar, D.; Andra, S. S.; Datta, R. Lead Fractionation and Bioaccessibility in Contaminated Soils with Variable Chemical Properties. *Chem. Spec. Bioavailab.* **2010**, *22*, 215–225.

Sana, T. R.; Fischer, S.; Wohlgemuth, G.; Katrekar, A.; Jung, K.-H.; Ronald, P. C.; Fiehn, O. Metabolomic and Transcriptomic Analysis of the Rice Response to the Bacterial Blight Pathogen *Xanthomonas oryzae* pv. *Oryzae. Metabolomics.* **2010**, *6*, 451–465.

Sanchez, D. H.; Schwabe, F.; Erban, A.; Udvardi, M. K.; Kopka, J. Comparative Metabolomics of Drought Acclimation in Model and Forage Legumes. *Plant Cell Environ.* **2012**, *35*, 136–149.

Savoi, S.; Wong, D. C. J.; Arapitsas, P.; Miculan, M.; Bucchetti, B.; Peterlunger, E.; Fait, A.; Mattivi, F.; Castellarin, S. D. Transcriptome and Metabolite Profiling Reveals that Prolonged Drought Modulates the Phenylpropanoid and Terpenoid Pathway in White Grapes (*Vitis vinifera* L.). *BMC Plant Biol.* **2016**, *16*, 67. DOI: 10.1186/s12870-016-0760-1.

Schafer, H.; Wink, M. Medicinally Important Secondary Metabolites in Recombinant Microorganisms or Plants: Progress in Alkaloid Biosynthesis. *Biotechnol. J.* **2009**, *4*, 1684–1703.

Schauer, N.; Fernie, A. E. Plant Metabolomics: Towards Biological Function and Mechanism. *Trends Plant Sci.* **2006**, *11*, 508–516.

Scossa, F.; Brotman, Y.; de Abreu e Lima, F.; Willmitzer, L.; Nikoloski, Z.; Tonga, T.; Fernie, A. R. Genomics-Based Strategies for the use of Natural Variation in the Improvement of Crop Metabolism. *Plant Sci.* **2016**, *242*, 47–64.

Seregin, I.; Ivanov, V. Physiological Aspects of Cadmium and Lead Toxic Effects on Higher Plants. *Russ. J. Plant Physiol.* **2001**, *48*, 523–544.

Shyur, L.-F.; Yang, N.-S. Metabolomics for Phytomedicine Research and Drug Development. *Curr. Opin. Chem. Biol.* **2008**, *12*, 66–71.

Singh, M.; Kumar, J.; Singh, S.; Singh, V. P.; Prasad, S. M. Roles of Osmoprotectants in Improving Salinity and Drought Tolerance in Plants: A Review. *Rev. Environ. Sci. Biotechnol.* **2015a**. DOI: 10.1007/s11157-015-9372-8.

Singh, S.; Parihar, P.; Singh, R.; Singh, V. P.; Prasad, S. M. Heavy Metal Tolerance in Plants: Role of Transcriptomics, Proteomics, Metabolomics, and Ionomics. *Front. Plant Sci.* **2015b**. https://doi.org/10.3389/fpls.2015.01143.

Singh, S.; Singh, B.; Singh A. P. Nematodes: A Threat to Sustainability of Agriculture. *Procedia Environ. Sci.* **2015c**, *29*, 215–216.

Suharti, W. S.; Nose, A.; Zheng, S.-H. Metabolite Profiling of Sheath Blight Disease Resistance in Rice: In the Case of Positive Ion Mode Analysis by CE/TOF-MS. *Plant Prod. Sci.* **2016**, *19*, 279–290.

Sumner, L. W.; Mendes, P.; Dixon, R. A. Plant metabolomics: Large-scale Phytochemistry in the Functional Genomics Era. *Phytochemistry.* **2003**, *62*, 817–836.

Taamalli, A.; Arráez-Román, D.; Abaza, L.; Iswaldi, I.; Fernández-Gutiérrez, A.; Zarrouka, M.; Segura-Carretero, A. LC-MS-Basedmetabolite Profiling of Methanolic Extracts from the Medicinal and Aromatic Species *Mentha pulegium* and *Origanum majorana*. *Phytochem. Anal.* **2015**, *26*, 320–330.

Talbot, N. J. On the Trail of a Cereal Killer: Exploring the Biology of *Magnaporthe grisea*. *Annu. Rev. Microbiol.* **2003**, *57*, 177–202.

Tanaka, K.; Arita, M.; Sakurai, H.; Ono, N.; Tezuka, Y. Analysis of Chemical Properties of Edible and Medicinal Ginger by Metabolomics Approach. *Biomed. Res. Int.* **2015**, 671058. DOI: 10.1155/2015/671058.

Tarpley, L.; Duran, A. L.; et al. Biomarker Metabolites Capturing the Metabolite Variance Present in a Rice Plant Developmental Period. *BMC Plant Biol.* **2005**, *5*, 8. https://doi.org/10.1186/1471-2229-5-8.

Udayakumar, M.; Chandar, D. P.; Mathangi, A. J.; Hemavathi, K.; Seenivasagam, R. PMDB: Plant Metabolome Database-A Metabolomic Approach. *Med. Chem. Res.* **2012**, *21*, 47–52.

Uraguchi, S.; Mori, S.; Kuramata, M.; Kawasaki, A.; Arao, T.; Ishikawa, S. Root-to-Shoot Cd Translocation Via the Xylem is the Major Process Determining Shoot and Grain Cadmium Accumulation in Rice. *J. Exp. Bot.* **2009**, *60*, 2677–2688.

Verslues, P. E.; Agarwal, M.; Katiyar-Agarwal, S.; Zhu, J. Zhu, J.-K. Methods and Concepts in Quantifying Resistance to Drought, Salt and Freezing, Abiotic Stresses that Affect Plant Water Status. *Plant J.* **2006**, *45*, 523–539.

Wang, L.; Zhou, G. B.; Liu, P.; Song, J. H.; Liang, Y. Dissection of Mechanisms of Chinese Medicinal Formula Realgar-Indigo Naturalis as an Effective Treatment for Promyelocytic Leukemia. *Proc. Natl. Acad. Sci. USA.* **2008**, *105*, 4826–4831.

Wang, X.; Zhang, A.; Sun, H. Future Perspectives of Chinese Medical Formulae: Chinmedomics as an Effector. *OMICS* **2012**, *16*, 414–421.

Wang, Y., Xu, L.; Shen, H.; Wang, J.; Liu, W.; Zhu, X.; Sun, R. W. X.; Liu, L. Metabolomic Analysis with GC-MS to Reveal Potential Metabolites and Biological Pathways Involved in Pb & Cd Stress Response of Radish Roots. *Sci. Rep.* **2015**, *5*, 18296.

Weis, J. S.; Weis, P. Metal Uptake, Transport and Release by Wetland Plants: Implications for Phytoremediation and Restoration. *Environ. Intl.* **2004**, *30*, 685–700.

White, I. R.; Blake, R. S.; Taylor, A. J.; Monks, P. S. Metabolite Profiling of the Ripening of Mangoes *Mangifera indica* L. cv. 'Tommy Atkins' by Real-Time Measurement of Volatile Organic Compounds. *Metabolomics* **2016**, *12*, 57. DOI: 10.1007/s11306-016-0973-1.

Wurtele, E. S.; Chappell, J.; Jones, A. D.; Celiz, M. W. et al. Medicinal Plants: A Public Resource for Metabolomics and Hypothesis Development. *Metabolites* **2012**, *2*, 1031–1059.

Ye, X.; Al-Babili, S.; Klöti, A.; Zhang, J.; Lucca, P.; Beyer, P.; Potrykus, I. Engineering the Provitamin A (β-Carotene) Biosynthetic Pathway into (Carotenoid Free) Rice Endosperm. *Science* **2000**, *287*, 303–305.

Zhang, J.; Wang, X.; Yu, Q.; Tang, J.; Gu, X.; Wan, X.; Fang, C. Metabolic Profiling of Strawberry (*Fragaria X ananassa* Duch.) During Fruit Development and Maturation. *J. Exper. Botany.* **2011**, *62*, 1103–1118.

Zivy, M.; Wienkoop, S.; Renaut, J.; Pinheiro, C.; Goulas, E.; Carpentier, S. The Quest for Tolerant Varieties: The Importance of Integrating "Omics" Techniques to Phenotyping. *Front. Plant Sci.* **2015**, *6*, 448. DOI: 10.3389/fpls.2015.00448.

Zoghlami, L. B.; Djebali, W.; Abbes, Z.; Hediji, H.; Maucourt, M.; Moing, A.; Brouquisse, R.; Chaibi, W. Metabolite Modifications in *Solanum lycopersicum* Roots and Leaves Under Cadmium Stress. *Afr. J. Biotechnol.* **2011**, *10*, 567–579.

PART II
Methods and Techniques

PHYTOCHEMICAL EXTRACTION, ISOLATION, AND DETECTION TECHNIQUES

TEMITOPE TEMITAYO BANJO[1,*], PAUL AKINNIYI AKINDUTI[2], TEMITOPE OLUWABUNMI BANJO[3], and VINESH KUMAR[4]

[1]*Department of Biological Sciences, Wellspring University, Irhirhi Road, PMB 1230, Benin, Edo, Nigeria, Tel.: +2347030121326*

[2]*Department of Biological Sciences, Covenant University, Ota, Ogun, Nigeria*

[3]*Institute for Human Resources Development, University of Agriculture, Alabata Road, PMB 2240, Abeokuta, Ogun, Nigeria*

[4]*Department of Sciences, Kids' Science Academy, Roorkee, Uttarakhand, India*

*Corresponding author. E-mail: topebanjo4rever@gmail.com
ORCID: http://orcid.org/0000-0002-5836-1752.

ABSTRACT

Phytochemicals are bioactive compounds present in different parts of plants (leaves, flowers, seeds, barks, roots, and pulps). The growing popularity of phytochemicals is because of their therapeutic importance in the control and treatment of diverse infections or diseases. Owing to the diverse bioactive molecules present in plants, this chapter details the various extraction methods, techniques involved in isolation, and those for the identification of bioactive compounds. The extraction methods include cold extraction method, solvent extraction method, serial exhaustive method, supercritical fluid extraction, microwave-assisted extraction and so forth. Similarly, the techniques involved in the isolation of phytochemicals include the thin-layer chromatography, column chromatography, gas chromatography, high-performance liquid chromatography, and so forth. This chapter also discusses the various spectroscopic techniques involved in the identification of isolated compounds such as ultraviolet spectroscopy, infrared spectroscopy, Fourier-transform infrared spectroscopy, nuclear magnetic resonance spectroscopy, and mass spectroscopy.

9.1 INTRODUCTION

The increasing demand and applications of plant products have led to an increased study and search for new medicinal plants with therapeutic properties (Cosa et al., 2006). There is increasing reliance on the use of medicinal plants for therapeutic purposes in most developing countries and the world at large (Ameh, 2010). Plants have many constituents which are of therapeutic importance in the control and treatment of diseases (Duraipandiyan et al., 2006). Moreover, the resistance of microorganisms to the conventional drugs employed in the treatment of diseases has increased the growing popularity and acceptance of medicinal plants (Van de Bogaard et al., 2000). The prices of synthetic drugs are very high compared to herbal medicine (Uzoekwe and Hamilton-Amachree, 2016). The increasing reliance on the use of medicinal plants and the prevalence of multiple-drug-resistant strains of a number of pathogenic bacteria has stimulated more research work in the use of medicinal plants for the treatment of diseases. Plants are the rich sources of biologically active constituents. This chapter focuses on the methods of extraction, analysis, and identification of the active components present in medicinal plants.

9.2 FACTORS TO CONSIDER DURING EXTRACTION

There are some factors to consider during phytochemical extraction. They include the nature of the plant material, choice of solvent, amount of the material, heating temperature, extraction methods, and duration of extraction. These factors may affect the quality and the quantity of the extract.

The choice of solvent is crucial during phytochemical extraction and some important factors to consider are its volatility, toxicity, cost, corrosivity, viscosity, and chemical stability, and so forth. The solvent used for extraction process, for instance, should have high volatility so that it can be easily removed from the extract. The solvent should be non-toxic or have a very low toxicity. The solvent should not be too expensive and have low corrosivity. The desired compound to be extracted should be soluble in the selective solvent. It should have a less boiling point in comparing to solute, that is, easy to separate out.

Some solvents used for the extraction of different classes of compounds are:

1. Water is used for the extraction of anthocyanins, starches, tannins, saponins, terpenoids, polypeptides, and lectin.
2. Ethanol is used for the extraction of tannins, polyphenols, polyacetylenes, flavonols, terpenoids, sterols, and alkaloids.
3. Methanol is used for the extraction of anthocyanins, terpenoids, saponins, tannins, xanthoxylene, totarol, quassinoids, lactones, flavones, phenones, and polyphenols.
4. Chloroform is used for the extraction of terpenoids and flavonoids.
5. Ether is used for the extraction of alkaloids, terpenoids, coumarins, and fatty acids.
6. Acetone is used for the extraction of phenol and flavonols.

9.3 EXTRACTION METHODS

The methodologies employed in the extraction depend upon the nature of the active compounds present in the plant materials. On the other way round, extraction methods have a significant effect on the quality of the phytochemical extracted. The extraction of bioactive compound is a tedious process because of the presence of different compounds in plants. Moreover, different conditions must be maintained during the extraction process. There may be a need for further separation of the biologically active components from other components present in the plant material. The commonly used methods for extraction are cold extraction, solvent extraction, serial exhaustive extraction, microwave-assisted extraction, ultrasound-assisted extraction (UAE), accelerated solvent extraction, supercritical fluid extraction (SFE), and hydrodistillation.

9.3.1 COLD EXTRACTION

As the name implies, plant extracts are obtained without the application of heat. But first, the plant parts may be dried at a temperature range of 50–60°C and ground into fine powder. The dried powder can be taken in specific amount into a glass container containing appropriate solvent and allowed to stand for 48 h or more. In the process, the solution should be shaken intermittently or by the use of mechanical or orbital shakers. Thereafter, the extract can be filtered using filter paper under vacuum and dried using an evaporating dish. The differences in weight of each dish prior to drying of the extracts and after drying will be useful for the calculation of percentage yield (Krishnananda et al., 2017).

$$\text{Percent of extracts} = \frac{\textit{Weight of extract obtained}}{\textit{Weight of plant sample taken}} \times 100$$

9.3.2 SOLVENT EXTRACTION METHOD (SOXHLET EXTRACTION METHOD)

Depending upon the nature of material or compounds to be isolated, the solvent may be either hexane, ethyl acetate, acetone, ethanol or water, and so forth. In this method, the dried powder of various plant parts is placed in glass thimble for extraction purpose using appropriate solvent. The temperature of the setup is to be kept below the boiling point of the solvent. The extract can be concentrated in a vacuum concentrator to obtain the crude extract.

9.3.2.1 PROCEDURE

The plant material to be extracted is placed inside the thimble and loaded into the main chamber of the extractor. The distillation flask is filled with the extraction solvent. The distillation flask is then placed on the heating element. The Soxhlet extractor should be properly placed on top of flask after which the extractor, a reflux condenser, is placed to condense the evaporated solvent.

On heating, the solvent inside the distillation flask starts to change into the vapor state and travel up to the reflux condenser. The reflux condenser cools down the vapor which drips into the chamber having the thimble of material in the form of droplets. In the warm solvent, some desired compounds may dissolve and when the chamber fills with solvent, the siphon empties it and the solvent is returned back to the distillation flask. This cycle may be allowed to repeat many times for some hours. After these cycles, the desired compounds are concentrated in the distillation flask of the extractor by rotary evaporator, yielding the extract. After drying, the respective extracts are weighed and the percentage extractive values (w/w) can be determined using following the formula.

$$\text{Percent of extracts} = \frac{\textit{Weight of extract obtained}}{\textit{Weight of plant sample taken}} \times 100$$

9.3.3 SERIAL EXHAUSTIVE EXTRACTION

Serial exhaustive extraction is an extraction method aimed at fractionating a crude extract from plant materials. This method is usually employed because different solvents are capable of extracting different phytochemical groups. This involves the use of solvents of varying polarities in combination or differently. Depending on the phytochemical of interest, the setup could start from the stepwise use of non-polar solvents down to very polar solvents. By this process, there is an enhanced isolation of compounds from the complex crude extracts. Sometimes, this process could be coupled to solvent extraction method from which the residue remains in the thimble is weighed and used for next successive extraction using another solvent as given in Figure 9.1.

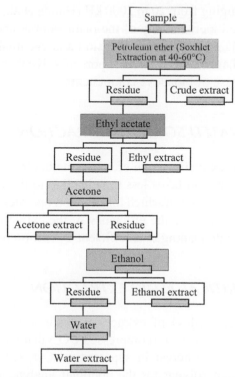

FIGURE 9.1   A typical serial exhaustive extraction procedure.

9.3.4   MICROWAVE-ASSISTED EXTRACTION

In this method, microwave energy is used to facilitate the elution of the bioactive compounds from the plant sample into the solvent (Trusheva et al., 2007). This extraction method combines microwave and the traditional solvent extraction. In this extraction method, the plant material is heated by microwave. The water present in plant cells by changing into vapor state exerts pressure on plant cell walls and results in the rupturing of plant cell walls. There is a subsequent release or discharge of bioactive compounds from the cell, hence increasing the yield of phytoconstituents (Mittleman, 2013).

9.3.5   ULTRASOUND-ASSISTEDEXTRACTIONORSONICATION

UAE or sonication extraction is a simple and relatively low-cost technology which can be applied in both small and large scale phytochemical extraction. The principle of operation of this extraction method is the use of ultrasound with frequencies ranging from 20 to 2000 kH (Handa et al., 2008). The ultrasound increases the kinetic energy of the plant sample and the appropriate solvent, thus increasing their rate of collision and eventual rupturing of the cell walls. This enhances the mass transport of solvent into the plant cells resulting in the release of bioactive components.

9.3.6   ACCELERATED SOLVENT EXTRACTION

Accelerated solvent extraction is an effective method of extraction because it requires less solvent and takes less time leading to the better recovery of the extract. The principle upon which this method operates is the use of high temperature, which increases the efficiency of the extraction and keeps the solvent in a liquid state leading to an efficient extraction process.

9.3.7   SUPERCRITICAL FLUID EXTRACTION

The SFE is another method of extraction which uses supercritical fluid (SF). An example of SF is CO_2 (compressed CO_2) that become SF at above 31.1°C and 7380 kPa. Interest in supercritical-CO_2 (SC-CO_2) extraction is due to its excellent solvent for the nonpolar analyte. In this extraction process, pumping of the SF is done through a cylinder packed with the plant material to be extracted. The separation of the extract from the SF occurred in a chamber. This method allows for the reuse of the SF over and over again. Patil et al. (2014) reported an optimum yield of extract from *Wadelia calendulacea* with the use of SFE methodology.

9.3.8 HYDRODISTILLATION

In this method, plant tissues are directly submerged in a boiling water for the extraction of volatile constituents especially essential oils. Plant materials are usually hydrodistilled for 4 h using a clevenger type apparatus. The extracted oil can then be dried over anhydrous sodium sulfate (Na_2SO_4) and then kept in a sealed vial in a refrigerator until analysis (Kumar and Sharma, 2016).

9.4 ISOLATION OF PHYTOCHEMICALS

Plant extracts contain various types of bioactive compounds having different polarities. Therefore, separation, identification, and characterization become a challenge. Some common techniques employed in the separation and identification of bioactive compounds are thin-layer chromatography (TLC), column chromatography, high-performance liquid chromatography (HPLC), high-performance TLC (HPTLC), gas chromatography (GC), and optimum performance laminar chromatography (OPLC).

9.4.1 THIN-LAYER CHROMATOGRAPHY

TLC is a simple chromatographic technique employed for quick observation of compounds present in the extract, hence its application in phytochemical studies. TLC is being used in phytochemical studies due to the following reasons:

1. It enables rapid analysis of herbal extracts with minimum sample clean-up requirement.
2. It allows for rapid analysis of plant extracts of medical importance.
3. Enables the quantification of chemical constituents.

The basis of separation of constituents is by adsorption. The constituents with a higher affinity toward the adsorbent move slower while the one with a low affinity toward the adsorbent moves faster thus ensuring the separation of the constituents.

TLC is detailed further in Chapter 11 of this book.

9.4.2   COLUMN CHROMATOGRAPHY

This method of chromatography is also known as liquid chromatography. It is a type of adsorption chromatography because the separation of components depends on the extent of adsorption to stationary phase. The principle of operation of this method of chromatography is the affinity and adsorption of compounds to be separated to the stationary phase mostly fine sand. The compounds with lower adsorption to the stationary phase move faster and are separated out first while those with higher adsorption are separated out last.

9.4.3   GAS CHROMATOGRAPHY

GC is another method of chromatographic used for the separation of volatile compounds (Littlewood, 2013). In other words, it is used in separating compounds that can be vaporized without decomposition. In this method, extracts distribute between gas and a liquid phase. However, while the gas phase is flowing, the liquid phase remains stationary in GC. The level and speed at which constituents separated, depends on their distribution in the gas phase. Constituents of the plant extract flow through the column with the gas as mobile phase at different rates. This movement is dependent on their properties and interactions with the stationary phase (Ardrey, 2003). Moreover, the distribution of the constituents in the mobile phase (gas) determines their migration and eventual separation.

9.4.4   HIGH-PERFORMANCE LIQUID CHROMATOGRAPHY

HPLC or high-pressure liquid chromatography is an analytical technique for the separation and determination of phytochemicals (Krishnananda et al., 2017). It involves the separation of constituents of a plant extract based on the interaction of the sample and the chromatography column. In this method of chromatography, high pressure up to 400 bars is required to elute the analyte through column before they pass through a diode array detector.

It measures the absorption spectra of the analyte to aid in their identification. The time at which the different constituents come out of the column (retention time) is characteristic of each constituent and is a basis for identification of each constituent of the extract. This chromatographic method also provides a good complement to GC (Katz, 2009). HPLC is further detailed in Chapter 12 and 13.

9.4.5 HIGH-PERFORMANCE THIN-LAYER CHROMATOGRAPHY

HPTLC is an efficient, simple, and rapid method of resolution of plant extracts into its different components. It is an enhanced form of TLC with better resolution of constituents. The principle of operation of HPTLC is similar to TLC. The basis of separation of constituents is by adsorption. The constituents with higher affinity toward the adsorbent move slower while the one with low affinity toward the adsorbent moves faster thus ensuring the separation of the constituents. Detailed information with pictorial representation of a typical HPTLC can be accessed in Chapter 13.

9.4.6 OPTIMUM PERFORMANCE LAMINAR CHROMATOGRAPHY

OPLC is formerly referred to as overpressure layer chromatography is a powerful liquid chromatography separation technique that combines two or more features of other chromatographic techniques. It is a tool suitable for research and quality control laboratories. The mode of operation of OPLC is like that of other methods of chromatography, in which the mobile phase (liquid) is forced through a stationary phase, such as silica or a bonded phase medium. What makes OPLC unique from other chromatographic method is the optimum laminar flow of mobile phase over the adsorbent layer in an automated controlled system.

9.5 DETECTION AND IDENTIFICATION OF PHYTOCHEMICALS

The different bioactive components present in plant extracts have been identified through different methods of detection such as The Fourier-transform infrared spectroscopy (FTIR). The nuclear magnetic resonance (NMR) spectroscopy, mass spectrometry (MS), ultraviolet (UV) Spectroscopy, infrared (IR) spectroscopy, and X-ray crystallography.

9.5.1   ULTRAVIOLET-VISIBLE SPECTROSCOPY

It involves the measurement of absorbance of a beam of light after reflection from a sample surface. The absorbance of the analyte solution can be measured using Beer–Lambert's law to determine its concentration (Beer–Lambert's law is the linear relationship between absorbance and concentration of a solution). Hence, UV spectroscopy can be used to determine the concentration and characterize the absorption of bioactive compounds from plants. This is used for the detection of unsaturation in the compounds. A comprehensive overview of UV/Vis spectroscopy is detailed in Chapter 12 of this book.

9.5.2   INFRARED SPECTROSCOPY (IR)

IR spectroscopy measures the interaction between molecules and radiation from the infrared region of the electromagnetic spectrum. In IR spectroscopy, infrared radiation is passed through a sample and a detector is used to plot the percentage transmission of the radiation through the sample against the wavenumber of the radiation. This technique is also employed in the identification of a particular compound and as a tool to determine the newly synthesized or novel molecule.

9.5.3   FOURIER-TRANSFORM IR

FTIR is one of the most preferred methods of spectroscopy because of its speed and sensitivity. This method analyzes frequency simultaneously unlike some other methods where the frequency is analyzed in sequence. The type of sample to be analyzed determines how the sample will be prepared. In liquid samples, a thin film is formed by placing a drop of the sample between two plates of sodium chloride, whereas solid samples are mixed with potassium bromide substrate. The solution is then placed onto a single high-attenuated total reflectance plates and spectra were recorded in terms of percentage transmittance. The peaks at specific wave number were assigned by bonding and the functional group as per the reference is given in Varian FTIR instrument manual (Koparde, 2017).

9.5.4   NUCLEAR MAGNETIC RESONANCE SPECTROSCOPY

The NMR spectroscopy is a spectroscopic method which utilizes the magnetic properties of the nuclei of atoms. It is a convenient method for determining the presence of known biomolecules and for assigning the chemical structure of novel ones. One dimensional technique is routinely used but the complicated structure of the molecules could be achieved through two-dimensional NMR techniques. The principle of operation of this technique is based on the electric charge on the nuclei. A transfer of energy takes place from the base energy to a higher energy level with the application of an external magnetic field. The nucleus releases energy at the frequency of the radio wave applied. The signal that matches this energy transfer is processed to yield a spectrum for the particular nucleus (Krishnananda et al., 2017)

9.5.5 MASS SPECTROMETRY

MS is used in the determination and identification of the structure and properties of phytochemicals. This technique is used for the identification of isolated compounds by determining its molecular weight. This method is used in the structural elucidation of organic compounds and phytochemicals. It is used in monitoring the existence of previously characterized compounds in complex mixtures with a high specificity by defining both the molecular weight and a diagnostic fragment of the molecule simultaneously.

9.5.6 X-RAY CRYSTALLOGRAPHY

X-ray crystallography is a spectroscopic technique used to determine the electronic structure of compounds with the use of X-ray excitation. The electron cloud of atoms leads to the scattering of incident X-rays in many directions. From this, a three-dimensional shape of the electron density which reflects their chemical bonds and other critical information about the compound is constructed, that is, a model is progressively built into the experimental electron density, refined against the data and the result is a quite accurate molecular structure.

9.6 CONCLUSION

Bioactive compounds occurring in plant materials consist of multi-component mixtures, thus making their extraction, identification, and determination challenging. Their separation may involve a combination of methods to extract and isolate the bioactive constituents of the plant materials. The characterization of the isolated compound is also the critical but important part of the phytochemical analysis. For this purpose, different spectroscopic methods have been used. Each method describes the special characteristics of the isolated molecule. The application of some of this techniques for the test of phytochemicals was presented in Chapter 15.

KEYWORDS

- **phytochemicals**
- **bioactive molecules**
- **solvent extraction method**
- **cold extraction method**
- **infrared spectroscopy**

REFERENCES

Ameh, G. I. Evaluation of the Phytochemical Composition and Antimicrobial Properties of Crude Methanolic Extract of Leaves of *Ocimum gratissimum* L. *J. Nat. Sci. Eng. Tech.* **2010,** *9*(1), 147–152.

Ardrey, R. E. *Liquid Chromatography-Mass Spectrometry: An Introduction;* John Wiley and Sons: New Jersey, 2003.

Cosa, P.; Vlietinck, A. J.; Berghe, D. V.; Maes, L. Anti-Infective Potential of Natural Products: How to Develop a Stronger In Vitro Proof-of-Concept. *J Ethnopharmacol.* **2006,** *106,* 290–302.

Duraipandiyan, V.; Ayyanar .M; Ignacimuthu. S. Antimicrobial Activity of Some Ethno Medicinal Plants Used by Paliyar Tribe from Tamil Nadu, India. *BMC Complement Altern. Med.* **2006,** *6,* 35–41.

Handa, S. S.; Khanuja, S. P. S.; Longo, G.; Rakesh, D. D. *Extraction Technologies for Medicinal and Aromatic Plants;* United Nations Industrial Development Organization and the International Centre for Science and High Technology: Italy, 2008.

Katz, E. D. *High Performance Liquid Chromatography: Principle and Methods in Biotechnology;* John Wiley & Sons: New Jersey, India, 2009.

Koparde, A. A.; Magdum, C. S.; Doijad, R. C. Phyto Active Compounds from Herbal Plants Extracts: Its Extraction, Isolation and Characterization. *World J. Pharm. Res.* **2017,** *6*(8), 1186–1205.

Krishnananda, P. I.; Amit, G. D.; Dipika, A. P.; Mahendra, S. D.; Mangesh, P. M.; Vaibhav,C. K. Phytochemicals: Extraction Methods, Identification and Detection of Bioactive Compounds from Plant Extracts. *J. Pharmacogn. Phytochem.* **2017,** *6*(1), 32–36.

Kumar, V.; Sharma, S. Chemical Composition and Antibacterial Activity of Essential Oils of *Tanacetum longifolium. Int. J. Curr. Microbiol. App. Sci.* **2016,** *5*(10), 836–841.Littlewood, A. B. *Gas Chromatography Principle, Techniques and Applications;* Academic Press: London, U.K., 2013.

Mittleman, D. *Sensing with Terahertz Radiation;* Springer: New York, 2013.

Patil, A. A.; Sachin, B. S.; Wakte, P. S.; Shinde, D. B. Optimization of Supercritical Fluid Extraction and HPLC Identification of Wedelolactone from *Wedeliaca lendulacea* by Orthogonal Array Design. *J. Adv. Res.* **2014,** *5,* 629–635.

Trusheva, B.; Trunkova, D.; Bankova, V. Different Extraction Methods of Biologically Active Components from Propolis: A Preliminary Study. *Chem. Cent. J.* **2007,** *1*, 13. DOI:10.1186/1752s-153X-1-13.

Uzoekwe, N. M.; Hamilton-Amachree, A. Phytochemicals and Nutritional Characteristics of Ethanol Extract of the Leaf and Bark of Njangsa (*Ricinodendron Heudelotii*) Plant. *J. Appl. Sci. Environ. Manage.* **2016,** *20*(3), 522–527.

Van den Bogaard, A. E.; Stobberingh, E. E. Epidemiology of Resistance to Antibiotics: Links between Animals and Humans. *Int. J. Antimicrob. Agents.* **2000,** *14,* 327–335.

Voravuthikunchai, S. P.; Kitpipit, L. Activities of Crude Extracts of Thai Medicinal Plants on Methicillin-Resistant *Staphylococcus aureus. J. Clin. Microbiol. Infect.* **2003,** *9,* 236.

CHAPTER 10

TECHNIQUES IN PHYTOCHEMOTAXONOMY

IFEOMA CELESTINA ORABUEZE[1] and FELIX IFEANYI NWAFOR[2,*]

[1]Department of Pharmacognosy, University of Lagos, Akoka, Lagos, Nigeria

[2]Department of Pharmacognosy and Environmental Medicines, University of Nigeria, Nsukka, Enugu, Nigeria, Tel.: +2348036062242

*Corresponding author. E-mail: felix.nwafor@unn.edu.ng; felixnucifera@gmail.com
ORCID: *https://orcid.org/0000-0003-1889-6311

ABSTRACT

Chemotaxonomic studies begin with the collection of plant samples and extraction of their phytoconstituents before they can be characterized and analyzed. Techniques may vary depending on the nature and the physical characteristics of the phytochemicals to be studied. Common extraction techniques include maceration, infusion, percolation, and hot continuous extraction (Soxhlet) and sometimes a combination of two or more techniques is desired for optimum result. Modern techniques employed in advanced chemotaxonomic studies for the isolation and characterization of the phytochemicals include electrophoresis, thin-layer chromatography, column chromatography, gas chromatography, high-performance liquid chromatography, spectroscopy (nuclear magnetic resonance, etc.), Fourier-transform infrared among others. These techniques have been successfully applied in the delimitation of taxa both at the lower and higher levels of taxonomic hierarchy and even though some challenges and limitations exist, when harnessed, chemotaxonomy will remain the bedrock of phytochemical studies and drug discovery.

10.1　INTRODUCTION

Chemotaxonomic study begins with the collection of plant sample and extraction of its phytoconstituents. An important preparatory step towards good extraction result is grinding or breaking down to smaller particles in an effort to increase surface area and to rupture the cell membranes of the plant material. This can be done by dry grinding in a mechanized blender or homogenizing using the extraction solvent. Another important step is bringing the ground material in contact with the extraction solvent, undisturbed for predetermined time at a temperature that will not allow degradation of desired active compound(s) to be isolated. Enough time with intermediate shaking or vibration is observed to ensure as much extraction of plant constituents into extraction solvent. The resulting slurry is filtered to obtain a filtrate free of particulate matters. The filtrate can be used directly for some assays or concentrated by removing the extraction solvent before storage. In advanced chemotaxonomic study, the crude extract can be further fractionated and subjected to high-tech separation techniques to obtain semi-purified fractions or pure compounds. Modern techniques employed in chemotaxonomic studies include chemomicroscopy, electrophoresis, thin-layer chromatography (TLC), column chromatography (CC), gas chromatography (GC), high-performance liquid chromatography (HPLC), spectroscopy (nuclear magnetic resonance [NMR], etc.), Fourier-transform infrared among others. In this chapter, the science, significance, techniques, and applications of chemotaxonomy in plant classification have been highlighted.

10.2　CHEMOMICROSCOPY

Chemomicroscopy is performed in order to study the distribution of directly visible particles in plant tissues. This may be achieved by clearing and sectioning of a fresh plant part with a microtome and stained with standard biological stains to create contrast within the plant tissues before observing under a microscope. Alternatively, chemomicroscopy may be conducted on dried powdered plant material– a method frequently adopted by pharmacognosists in standardization and identification of powdered crude drugs. In this method, a clearing agent, usually, chloral hydrate solution is dropped on a glass slide containing a judicious amount of the powder and passed through a Bunsen burner until bubbles are formed. This signifies successful clearing of tissues. Standard stains and reagents are now dropped and the preparation is observed under a microscope usually with an attached microscope camera for photomicrography. Different kinds of stains and reagents are chosen depending on the nature of plant material to be studied.

10.3 ELECTROPHORESIS

Electrophoresis is a technique employed by modern chemotaxonomists to study the origin and relationship of proteins and nucleic acids in plants. This separation technique of proteins has now become popular in chemotaxonomic study of closely related taxa, both at the population level or in comparison to sympatric species within the same genus. This separation method is based on the differential rate of migration of charged species in an applied direct current electric field. The rate of such migration depends on the charge, size, efficiency, and resolution. Common in application is the gel electrophoresis using polyacrylamide gel which is preferred to paper and cellulose acetate in taxonomy of higher plants and considered the best medium supports for resolving larger number of protein bands with desirable clarity. The percentage of polyacrylamide in the electrophoresis medium is usually 7%, in a Tris-glycine buffer at pH 8.1, but may be varied in some cases for optimum result. The source of protein is usually seeds of plants as they are believed to be less affected by environmental factors. Other sources for successful taxonomic study include pollen grains, leaves, and other protein-containing plant organs. This technique without doubts has attracted modern plant taxonomists who are interested in protein studies and feasibility of chemotaxonomic approaches through electrophoresis in higher plants (Suranto, 2002; Mohamed, 2006).

10.4 EXTRACTION PROCEDURES

Extraction is an important step taken by phytoscientists attempting to isolate and identify phytoconstituents or chemical groups from natural products using selected extraction technique(s) and solvents. The resulting crude extract contains many active and non-active plant metabolites, such as alkaloids, glycosides, phenolics, terpenoids, and flavonoids (Azwanida, 2015). Selecting suitable method and solvent to be used is crucial in extracting the desired compounds.

Traditional methods of medicinal plant extraction involve relatively simple extraction procedures with a wide range of organic solvents, water, and their mixtures. Solvent system used in extraction is known as menstruum. The solvent employed in extraction to a large extent determines the constituents to be extracted. Only substances that can be dissolved in a solvent can be extracted by it. Single or combination of solvents can be used for extraction depending on the desired component target. Commonly used traditional methods of extraction include: maceration, infusion, percolation, and hot continuous extraction (Soxhlet). Recent extraction methods exhibit significant advanced procedures such as limited solvent use, elimination of additional sample cleanup, improvement in extraction efficiency (extraction yield), selectivity, and kinetics of extraction (Huie, 2002). Such modified or improved techniques require cost-oriented, sophisticated, and specific equipment. Modern extraction methods include; microwave-assisted extraction (MAE), ultrasound-assisted extraction (UAE), and supercritical-fluid extraction (SFE), solid-phase microextraction, pressurized-liquid extraction, surfactant-mediated techniques, and phytonic extraction (with hydrofluorocarbon solvents) (Azwanida, 2015). For volatile or essential oil material, steam distillation, hydrolytic maceration followed by distillation, expression, effleurage (cold fat extraction), headspace trapping, solid-phase microextraction, protoplast extraction, microdistillation may be employed (Handa, 2008).

Grinding extraction sample breaks the particles into smaller sizes and increases the surface area for easy and fast and high-yield extraction. Next is bringing the grounded sample in contact with an extraction solvent, undisturbed under predetermined conditions. These are two initiating steps towards good extraction. The resulting slurry is filtered to obtain a filtrate free of particulates, which may be used directly or concentrated to dryness for further use. Gradient extraction is possible by drying of filtrate and re-extraction with different solvents of increasing polarity (Vvedenskaya et al., 2004).

10.4.1 MACERATION

Maceration is a simple extraction procedure performed at room temperature. It involves the act of soaking whole or coarsely powdered sample material with a solvent of choice for a defined period with constant stirring or agitation for a period of time, 2–3 days after which it is filtered (Handa, 2008). This method has the setback of long extraction periods, use of the large volume of solvent, low-extraction yield, and the ease of compound decomposition for a solvent unstable compound but suitable for thermolabile drugs.

10.4.2   PERCOLATION

A general extracting percolation percolator has two openings, a wide-mouthed at the top and a valve-fixed draining outlet at the base for out flow. The sample material is tightly packed in the percolator and extracting solvent is filled to cover the packed plant material. The plant material is allowed to stand for several hours or overnight to allow sample constituents to seep into the extraction solvent. The base outlet is then opened a little and solvent saturated with solute is slowly collected via the base valve while an additional solvent is added at the top of the percolator to replace losses from the bottom.

10.4.3   INFUSION

An infusion is prepared by soaking sample materials in boiled or cold solvent or water for a short period and drained. It gives a low concentrated or dilute solution. Soft and high water content plant tissues such as the leaves, flowers, fleshy fruits, and so forth can easily be extracted using this infusion method, especially when the components of the sample are very soluble in the solvent of extraction.

10.4.4   DECOCTION

This extraction method is suitable for strong and difficult-to-penetrate plant parts (such as roots, twigs, dry and hard fruits, and barks) and usually resulted in more oil-soluble compounds compared to simple maceration and infusion. The sample is boiled, strained, cooled, and taken within 24 h. It is recommended only for extractions of phytochemicals that are heat stable and soluble in water. The duration of boiling depends on how hard the sample is and desired concentration.

10.4.5   DIGESTION

This process is a modified form of maceration. It involves slight heating of the sample in a solvent preheated to the desired temperature. The heating period could vary from 30 min to 24 h with constant agitation. This method of extraction is recommended for very hard plant parts that contain insoluble but heat-stable constituents.

10.4.6   PLANT TISSUE HOMOGENIZATION

This is a simple and fast way of extracting phytochemicals from plant materials. The plant sample to be extracted is blended in a solvent to fine particles. More solvent is added, shaken continuously for about 15 min or allowed to stand for 24 h after which the extract is filtered and centrifuged if clear solution if desired.

10.4.7   HOT CONTINUOUS EXTRACTION (SOXHLET)

The most commonly used extractor is Soxhlet device. It is a modified percolation procedure. Extraction takes place in an enclosed system with continuous heating at a controlled temperature. The advantage of this system is its reduced solvent consumption; it allows a large amount of sample to be extracted with a minimal amount of solvent. Extraction solvent is continuously heated in a round bottom flask, vaporizes, passes through packed sample material in the thimble chamber, condenses back into the round bottom flask, and the solvent recycling continues till exhausted. The solvent is only changed when it is spent. Gradient extraction using varying polar solvents (serial exhaustive extraction) makes this method popular when exhausted extraction is needed. Continuous heating facilitates the extraction process, but easily causes degradation of thermolabile compounds.

10.4.8   ULTRASOUND-ASSISTED EXTRACTION/SONICATION

UAE has the advantages of high extract yield, simple equipment and fast extraction rate, and lower extraction temperature (Soria and Villamiel, 2010; Ingle, 2017). The procedure involves the use of high-frequency sound (ultrasound) wave ranging between 20 and 2000 kHz to induce vibration (Handa, 2008). The procedure weakens and breaks down the intermolecular forces holding the plant material intact, due to the application of high-intensity vibration, which is known as acoustic cavitation (Tiwari, 2015). The resulting collapse of molecular structures of the plant material increases the permeability of cell walls and liberation of extractable phytochemicals from the plant materials. UAE could cause possible degradation of heat-labile compounds due to heat created during high-intensity vibration, formation of free radicals, and consequently undesirable changes in the plant molecules at high frequencies (Tiwari, 2015).

Plant material extraction using UAE method involves placing finely powdered plant material to be extracted in a glass container, covered by the extraction solvent and placed in temperature-controlled ultrasonic bath. Natural product extracts containing low-molecular-weight organic molecules such as alkaloids, phenolic, volatile oils have been reported to be extracted successfully using UAE with a recorded reduction in extraction time and improved yield (Toma et al., 2001; Palma and Barroso, 2002; Vilkhu et al., 2008).

10.4.9 MICROWAVE-ASSISTED EXTRACTION

MAE technology utilizes electromagnetic radiation from microwave energy to facilitate extraction of bioactive components of plant materials into a solvent system (Trusheva et al., 2007). Plant material to be extracted absorbs applied microwave energy, which it converts to heat energy. The level of microwave energy adsorption is dependent on the dielectric constants of plant material and solvent of extraction. Microwaves induce dipolar rotation of polar and polarizable molecules due to the electric field these molecules possess, causing dipole collisions between surrounding molecules. Thermal energy is released due to the collisions and the heating facilitates extraction process.

MAE method is a selective extraction procedure for polar molecules and solvents with high dielectric constants and capable of absorbing strongly microwave energy. Nonpolar solvents are not suitable for MAE as the energy transferred is only by dielectric absorption.

In general, this MAE technique reduced extraction time, solvent volume, improved analytes recovery, and reproducibility as compared to conventional methods. Efficacy of MAE is influenced by changes in factors like the solvent composition, temperature, and extraction time. Compounds that degrade at hightemperature such as tannin and antho-cyanins are not recommended for MAE. In such case, irradiation can be applied for short intervals with intervals of cooling time to avoid super boil of sample material. For instance, limonoids from neem seed kernel (*Azadirachta indica*) can be extracted by first defatting 2 g in petroleum ether, then extracted with 15 ml dichloromethane at 150 W, 30 s on, 30 s off cycle (Dai et al., 1999).

Other types of MAE are: ultrasonic MAE, vacuum MAE, nitrogen-protected MAE, or Dynamic MAE.

10.4.10 SUPERCRITICAL FLUID EXTRACTION

This extraction procedure resembles Soxhlet extraction except that supercritical fluids are used in place of organic solvents. Commonly used supercritical fluid is carbon dioxide (CO_2). Supercritical fluids such as CO_2 when compressed and heated above their critical temperatures and pressure exhibit both the physical characters of liquid and gas. At this critical point, the density of a supercritical fluid is extremely sensitive to minor changes in temperature and pressure. Above a bar pressure of 200 and 31.7°C, CO_2 has the solvating/dissolution power of a liquid and the diffusivity of a gas. At near liquid densities, the probability of CO_2 interacting with the substrate increases, behaving similarly but higher in degree to a liquid solvent (Abbas et al., 2008). The gas-like diffusivities of supercritical fluids allow exceptional mass flow or extraction of constituents than liquid solvents. Exhibiting gaseous properties such as, near zero surface tension and low viscosities, supercritical fluids easily penetrate microporous matrix of plant material to extract desired phytoconstituents. Thus, supercritical fluid has the ability to diffuse faster in a solid matrix than a liquid and solvent strength to extract phytoconstituents from the plant material (Brunner, 2005).

The ability to precisely control which component(s) in a complex plant material is extracted and which ones are left behind can easily be achieved with SFE (Fig. 10.1) through systemic control of several key parameters such as temperature, pressure, flow rates, and processing time. The properties of SFE makes it suitable for extracting, thermally labile and nonpolar bioactive compounds but the addition of small quantity of co-solvent or modifier, such as ethanol or methanol to the extracting fluid can increase the extractability of polar compounds using SFE.

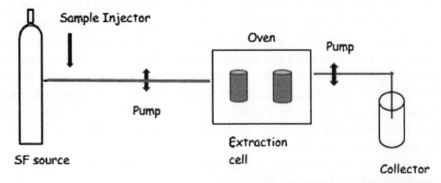

FIGURE 10.1   A simplified drawing of an idealized supercritical fluid extractor.

Removal of solvent from extracted phytoconstituents is easy to accomplish since CO_2 returns to its gaseous state upon exiting the extractor.

Natural products such as essential oils, gallic acid, quercetin, and essential oil from the flowers of *Achyrocline satureioides*; phenolics from grape peels (*Vitis labrusca*) have been extracted using SFE method of extraction (Ghafoor et al., 2010).

10.4.11 ACCELERATED(PRESSURIZED)SOLVENTEXTRACTION

Accelerated solvent extraction (ASE) is a liquid solvent extraction procedure and has the advantage of the minimal use of solvent and rapid extraction process. Online filtration device (cellulose filter paper) is fitted within the automatized extraction process of ASE. A moderate quantity of solid and semisolid plant sample can be extracted using this method.

Extraction is achieved using commonly available solvents and at an adjustable temperature and pressure. Sequential extraction with solvents of different polarity (from nonpolar to polar solvents) and a mixture of solvents at different ration is possible (Cicek et al., 2010). This allows possible gradient extraction and isolation of a wide range of plant constituents.

Plant material to be extracted is packed with an inert material such as sand (diatomaceous earth or sea sand) in the stainless steel extraction cell. Packing with a layer of sand is to prevent the sample from aggregating and blocking of the system tubing (Rahmalia et al., 2015). A simplified packing of ASE stainless steel extraction cell can be performed as described by Rahmalia et al. (2015), by placing a cellulose filter and sand layers at both capped ends, and sample-sand mixture in between. The ASE cell is then placed into ASE carousel for the extraction process. The temperature and pressure are adjustable for optimal extraction efficacy. Extracted products can be collected in small fixed volumes in vials. Extraction process on the sample material can be repeated to ensure exhausted extraction.

ASE is usually used as a sample preparation method for analytical purposes and many samples can be extracted automatically at once

10.4.12 DISTILLATION METHODS

Distillation is an extraction process applied in obtaining aromatic compounds from plant sources. Distillation occurs because different compounds vaporize at different temperatures due to their different boiling points.

This method, compared to other extraction techniques is not dependent on the solubility of a compound in either water or oil to initiate component separation. However, essential oils with high solubility in water and which is thermal sensitive cannot be extracted by this distillation method. Some variation of distillation exists.

10.4.12.1   STEAM DISTILLATION

Steam distillation method is recommended for extraction and isolation of water-insoluble and temperature-sensitive essential oils and other aromatic hydrocarbons from plants source. The principle of this technique is that at about 100°C, the combined vapor pressure of all contained essential oils in the sample is equal to the ambient pressure. This means that all volatile compounds in the sample can evaporate at a temperature lower than that of their individual boiling points or at a temperature close to that of water (100°C). The isolation works at atmospheric pressure and a temperature below 100°C even for essential oil of boiling point range of 150–300°C.

In this procedure, steam is generated from boiling water. The plant material is subjected to the generated water steam without direct contact with water. Steam is passed under pressure, from the base of the extractor through the packed sample material to the top. The steam on passing through the plant material, break up the pores and cell walls of the raw material and releases the essential oil/volatile compounds in vapor form. In the condensation chamber, the mixture of steam and the essential oil is cooled and forms two phases: the essential oil and the water. With a separating funnel, the two phases can be separated, essential oil floats on top, having a lower density than water. The aqueous phase may contain some residual soluble fragrant compounds and oils, which arecalled hydrosols. Most starting raw materials are fresh plant materials.

10.4.12.2   HYDRODISTILLATION

Hydrodistillation, also called water distillation is a type of steam distillation. However, in contrast to steam distillation, sample plant material is in contact with water and heat is applied, followed by liquefaction of the resulting steam in a condenser, giving two phases. The two phases can then be separated, the essential oil from the aqueous phase.

10.5   ISOLATION AND PURIFICATION

Plant crude extracts occur as complex, multicomponent mixture of phytoconstituents with different polarities. Isolation or separation of individual phytoconstituents for purpose of identification, fingerprinting or characterization is challenging and may require the use of different separation methods. The work or investigation in this area of science, natural products chemistry began with the work of Serturner, who first isolated morphine from opium and separation technology has improved greatly. Isolated and purified pure compounds are used for structure elucidation (identification) and bioassays (Handa, 2008).

Chromatographic techniques are separation methods based on differential distribution/partitioning of different constituents of a plant extract mixture between a mobile phase and stationary phase. Differential distribution of a compound between mobile and stationary phases is determined by its affinity to each of the phases and it is a key characteristic in chromatographic separations. For the qualitative purpose, evaluation factors such as retention, which is expressed as retention time or retention factor (R_f) depending on the elution method can be recorded. It measures the speed or time taken from point of injection of a sample to point of each component elution. This allows unknown compounds to be compared to known compounds since R_f is constant for any compound at the same operating conditions.

10.5.1   *LIQUID–LIQUID PARTITION/FRACTIONATION*

Some preliminary isolation techniques involve partition of the sample between two immiscible liquids and selective distribution of individual components of the sample between the two immiscible liquids. This separation or distribution is independent of percentage concentration of individual compounds or concentration of the solute but governed strictly by the principle of "partition coefficient" (affinity between the sample components/compounds and the two liquids involved). A single partitioning of extract between butanol and water often concentrates the saponins in the butanol fraction, thereby providing a preliminary clean-up step (Hostettman and Marston, 1995). This method has been reportedly used in the isolation of triterpene glycoside from *tetrapleura tetraptera*, a plant from Nigeria with molluscicidal activity (Hostettmann and Marston, 1995).

Paper chromatography is the oldest known method of liquid–liquid partition chromatography and mostly used for analytical separation. Recent implementations of partition chromatography are various types of countercurrent chromatography (CCC) (Hostettmann and Marston, 1995).

10.5.2 LIQUID–SOLID/ADSORPTIONCHROMATOGRAPHIC TECHNIQUES

Liquid–solid or adsorption chromatography are chromatographic separation methods with solid stationary phases either as planar or CC. Here, the sample components are adsorbed on the surface of the adsorbent (solid phase), displacing the initially loosely adsorbed solvent molecules. Separation of a mixture is achieved by differences in polarity of the individual components.

Adsorption chromatography is subdivided into normal-phase chromatography and reversed-phase chromatography. Normal-phase chromatography involves the use of polar (hydrophilic) stationary phase, usually on a silica or alumina support. Thus, the hydrophilic molecules in the solvent of elution (mobile phase) are held or adsorb to the silica gel in the column, while the hydrophobic molecules move through the column and are eluted first. The term reversed phase describes the chromatography that consists of modified silica surfaces, such that nonpolar (hydrophobic) materials are used for the stationary phase and mobile phase is a polar solvent. The polar solvent includes water-methanol mixtures or water-acetonitrile mixtures.

Some conventionally used adsorption chromatography are: TLC (planar method), vacuum liquid chromatography (VLC), flash chromatography (FC), HPLC, low-pressure liquid chromatography, medium-pressure liquid chromatography.

10.5.2.1 THIN-LAYER CHROMATOGRAPHY

TLC (Fig. 10.2) is a fast but simple, and relatively low-cost isolation procedure that can be used for both qualitative and semi-quantitative analysis of an unknown sample (Kim et al., 2013). The degree of purity of the compounds can be evaluated based on TLC generated information. The stationary phase is a thin layer of adsorbent (usually silica gel or alumina) coated on one side of a plate of glass or a strip of plastic or aluminum. The sample to be analyzed is spotted onto the plate as a single small dot near one end of the plate using a microcapillary tube. The plate is developed by allowing the spot to dry and placing of the spotted plate in a jar or developing chamber that contains a small volume of solvent (mobile phase). The chamber should have a lid that closes tightly enough to keep the chamber saturated. Mobile phase moves up the stationary phase by capillary action carrying along the resolving components of the test sample. Individual bands or components separate at different length of the TLC depending on the affinity of the components to the stationary phase. The color of the separated bands with different detecting reagents and R_f helps create TLC profile of resolved compounds and aid in their identification and authentication. The separated bands can be scrapped from the TLC plates for further purification and analysis.

The advantage of TLC is that the samples need little or no clean-up preloading process, very little quantity of the test sample is required and a wide range of detecting agents and mechanisms are available. The separated band can be scraped off the plate and be analyzed by other techniques (Sarkeret al., 2006; Pyka, 2014).

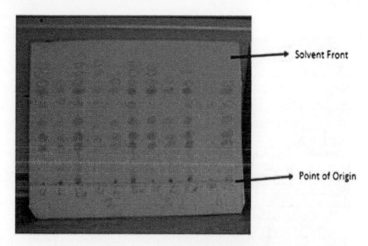

FIGURE 10.2 Separation on thin-layer chromatography plate.
Source: Pictures taken by the authors at the Department of Organic Chemistry, Natural Product Unit, University of Free State, Bloemfontein, South Africa.

10.5.2.2 COLUMN CHROMATOGRAPHY

CC is mostly used for preparative scale separation of components from crude plant extracts. CC consists of a vertical column, usually glass packed with particulate material (stationary phase), such as silica gel, aluminum oxide, or magnesium silicate and a selected solvent system (mobile phase) running through it at atmospheric, low, medium, or high pressure. The principle driving the separation could be liquid–solid (adsorption) or liquid–liquid (partition). Conventional systems rely on gravity to push the solvent through, but medium-pressure pumps are commonly used in modified systems such as flash CC. The sample can be preload either as wet or dry packing/slurry.

Care is taken not to overload the column with the sample to avoid over-running of separating bands (bleeding). Method of elution could be either gradient (gradual increase of mobile phase polarity) or isocratic (fixed solvent system) *elution and the collected* fractions are usually monitored by TLC (Guiochon, 2001; Schellinger and Carr, 2006).

In general, it has a poor resolution result, materials are lost due to irrevers-ible adsorption on the silica gel and the long length of time needed to perform the separation. Open CC (Fig. 10.3) was reported to be used at various stages in the separation process of dammarane glycosides actinostemmosides A–D from *Actinostemmalobatum* (Cucurbitaceae) (Asada et al., 1989; Hostett-mann and Marston, 1995).

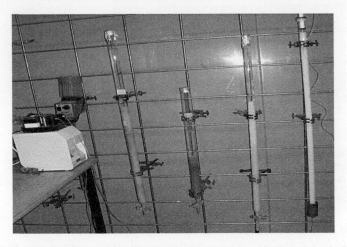

FIGURE 10.3   Open column chromatography showing the stationary phase (solid packing material).

Source: Pictures taken by the authors at the Department of Organic Chemistry, Natural Prod-uct Unit, University of Free State, Bloemfontein, South Africa.

10.5.2.3   *VACUUM LIQUID CHROMATOGRAPHY*

The technique used in VLC is force-flow CC to increase the rate of flow of the solvent system (mobile phase) through a short packed bed of adsorbent (stationary phase). Fractions are collected batch after batch. Each batch of mobile phase introduced is allowed to run dry before the introduction of another batch or run of the mobile phase. This is different from open CC where the mobile phase is a continuous run of the solvent system but comparable to preparative TLC where a plate can be dried and redeveloped (Hostettmann et al., 1998). Stationary phases available include silica gel (both normal and reversed phase), aluminum oxide (Al_2O_3), acetonitrile (CN), diol (polyols), and polyamide. VLC is mainly used for preliminary fractionation of crude extract into semi-purified fractions (Hostettmann et al., 1998; Reid and Sarker, 2006; Otto, 2008). Researchers have reported a successful use of VLC towards isolation of compounds (Joshi et al., 1992).

10.5.2.4 FLASH CHROMATOGRAPHY

Flash Chromatography (FC) (Fig. 10.4) and HPLC uses the same mechanism of applied pressure to drive the mobile phase through the column. The difference is in the level of pressure applied. FC uses medium pressure, while HPLC uses high pressure. The applied pressure improves the flow rate and reduces the separation runtime. Pressure is applied to the solvent through vacuum line attached to the bottom of a conventional separating column or pressurized gas/compressed air/air pumps fixed on top of conventional separating column in order to achieve a quicker result (Roge et al., 2011). A small particle size of FC stationary phase (silica gel 200–400 mesh) aids high-resolution separation (Swathi et al., 2015). Operating systems such as gradient pump, sample injection ports, fraction collector for the eluent, and online peak detection usually by coupling to a ultraviolet (UV) detector are all applicable in FC.

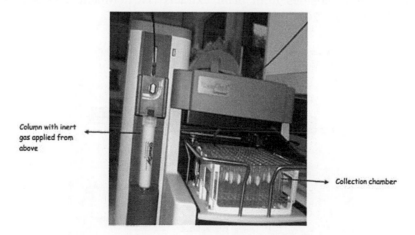

Column with inert gas applied from above

Collection chamber

FIGURE 10.4 Flash chromatograph column.

Source: Pictures taken by the authors at the Department of Organic Chemistry, Natural Product Unit, University of Free State, Bloemfontein, South Africa.

10.5.2.5   HIGH-PERFORMANCE LIQUID CHROMATOGRAPHY (HPLC)

HPLC (Fig. 10.5) is a popular chromatographic analytical technique that is used in the separation of multicomponent plant extract samples and purification of isolated compounds (Fan et al., 2006; Piana et al., 2013; Boligon and Athayde, 2014).The basic principle of HPLC is the use of small-sized particles (to increase surface area and resolution performance) and the application of high pressure at the inlet of a liquid chromatographic column to increase the rate of movement of the mobile phase through the stationary phase, thereby reducing the time of separation. Separation occurs due to different rates by which the separating compounds are being carried in the moving liquid phase, due to their differing interactions with the stationary and mobile phases (Hostellmann et al., 1998). Detectors are employed to aid in the identification of isolated compounds. Many detectors are available and may be coupled with structure elucidation spectrometer (SM) (Sasidharan et al., 2011).

In addition to the normal-phase columns (nonpolar solvent and a polar surface such as silica), there are reverse phase (RP) columns. RP HPLC is the method of choice for larger nonvolatile molecules (Prathap et al., 2013). The HPLC is usually linked to a SM (e.g., UV or mass spectrometry [MS]) evaporative light-scattering detector (Guiochon, 2001).

Analytical and preparative HPLC has been used in resolving mixtures of closely related compounds. A lot of researchers have reported successful separation of glycosides from plant extracts (Hostettmann and Marston, 1995; Gökay et al., 2010).

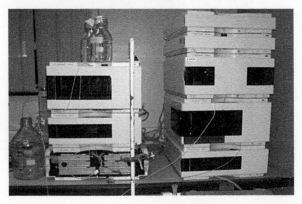

FIGURE 10.5   High performance liquidchromatography.
Source: Pictures taken by the authors at the Department of Organic Chemistry, Natural Product Unit, University of Free State, Bloemfontein, South Africa.

10.5.2.6 GEL PERMEATION CHROMATOGRAPHY (SIZE EXCLUSION CHROMATOGRAPHY)

This is a low-resolution chromatography technique and mostly reserved for last step "cleanup" of an isolated compound purification process. Gel chromatography, also known as size-exclusion chromatography because separation is according to the size of molecules involved. High molecules and low-molecular-weight particles are selectively separated and eluted based on their sizes. Dextran gels, which are used as stationary phases well up to form gel matrix of different pore sizes when in suitable solvents and these pores restrict movement of sample solutes according to their sizes and shape as the mobile phase moves along the column. The larger molecules which cannot enter the matrix pores move faster through the column and are eluted first, while the smaller-sized solutes are held in the pores and elute last.

It is a method commonly used in the separation of proteins, polypeptides carbohydrates, and chlorophyll elutes first (Guiochon, 2001; Reid and Sarker, 2006; Bucar et al., 2013). Commonly available gel permeation chromatography is Sephadex (Sephadex LH-20) and agarose.

10.5.2.7 GAS CHROMATOGRAPHY (GC)

GC is a chromatographic technique in which the mobile phase is a gas and stationary phase which could be either solid (gas–solid chromatography) or liquid (gas–[GLC]). The stationary phase for GLC is immobilized on a supporting inert solid. A carrier gas is usually an inert gas, such as hydrogen, helium, nitrogen, argon, or carbon dioxide which is applied under pressure to transport the sample for separation through the column till the components are eluted. The principle of separation here is based on differences in boiling point (volatility) and affinity for the stationary phase. GC is restricted to sample containing molecules (or derivatives) that are thermally stable and volatile to pass through the GC system intact at the operating temperatures (Niessen, 2001; König and Hochmuth, 2004).

The length of the column affects the time it takes for the separated compounds to elute (Cseke et al., 2006). Slowly increasing the temperature of the column increases the rate of separation and widens the range of compounds that can be separated. The number of peaks indicates the number of components. Quantitatively the area under the peaks determines the amount of each peak (Hostettmann and Marston, 1995).

Available GC detectors include: flames (flame ionization detector, nitrogen phosphorous detector–flame photometric detector); by changes in properties of the carrier (thermal conductivity detector, electron capture detector–argon ionization detector–helium ionization detector); or by MS coupled with GC (Meshram and Srivastava, 2014; Meshram et al., 2015).

10.5.2.8   COUNTERCURRENT CHROMATOGRAPHY

Countercurrent chromatography (CCC) is a general term for liquid–liquid chromatography, where one of the liquids serves as support-free stationary phase and held in the spinning coil by centrifugal force (Berthod et al., 2009). The second immiscible liquid being the mobile phase contains the sample to be separated. Samples are fed into the separating column using injectors. This method can be used to separate, qualify, and quantify phytochemical components of natural products. There is total elution (recovery) of injected sample. During separation process in the column, the two immiscible phases mix, settle, and separate allowing components of the sample to separate based on their solubility/partition coefficient in the two liquid phases involved.

Modified CCC include high-speed CCC, droplet countercurrent chromatography, rotation locular countercurrent chromatography, and high-performance CCC (Reid and Sarker, 2006; Otto, 2008).

10.5.3   FRACTIONAL CRYSTALLIZATION

Crystallization is an old method of purification or production of crystals for determination of chemical structure by X-ray diffraction. Crystallization mostly depends upon the inherent character of the compound which forms crystals at the point of supersaturationin solvent in which it is soluble. A common method of crystallization is forming a supersaturated solution of the compound in a solvent that it is very soluble in. Then a second solvent in which it is not soluble is introduced in a larger volume. The resultant mixture is allowed to stand undisturbed till the crystals are grown. Controlling the temperature by placing in a cool place, improves the rate of crystal growth but smaller crystals are generated. Slowing the rate of crystal growth gives bigger crystals. Crystals can be removed from the mother liquor by filtering with sintered glass at the pump and perhaps air-drying by suction or oven dried for heat-stable compounds (Florence et al., 2006). Crystallization and recrystallization repeatedly in several different solvents gives a greater degree of purity.

10.6   OTHER SEPARATION AND PURIFICATION METHODS

Other separation methods include; overpressure layer chromatography, centrifugal TLC, centrifugal partition chromatography (CPC), high-performance CPC.

In spite of improved technology and high resolution obtainable on these techniques, a one-step separation step is not always possible. A pre-fractionation step may be needed and also a clean-up step may also be needed.

10.7   CHARACTERIZATION AND STRUCTURE ELUCIDATION

Structure elucidation involves the use of various spectroscopic techniques in determining the chemical structure of a compound. Commonly used technology are one-dimensional NMR (1-DNMR) and two-dimensional (2-D) proton NMR as well as C-13 NMR, infrared (IR), MS, and X-ray analysis.

10.7.1   NUCLEAR MAGNETIC RESONANCE SPECTROSCOPY (NMR)

NMR spectroscopy is analytical process concerned with the study of magnetic properties of some atomic nuclei, especially the nucleus of the hydrogen atom and that of carbon-13 isotope (^{13}CNMR). It is a very informative tool for identification and structural elucidation of an isolated pure compound. Analytical information for structure determination of compounds is based on the information obtained by absorption of electromagnetic energy in the radio-frequency region (Ogundani et al., 2000). The magnetic field is provided by an external magnet and atomic nuclei such as ^{1}H, ^{13}C, ^{15}N, ^{19}F are studied. NMR informs on the type of environment and how many such nuclei (^{1}H, ^{13}C and any other) are present in a molecule under study.

Information from 1-DNMR experiments only or in combination with 2-DNMR experiments, for more complicated molecular structures are used for structure elucidation (Hostettmann and Wolfender, 2001). Both protons (^{1}H) and carbons (^{13}C) are involved in 1-D and 2-D NMR.

10.7.1.1   ONE-DIMENSIONAL NMR
(^{1}H-NMR and ^{13}C-NMR)

Proton NMR is a plot of signals arising from absorption of radio frequency during an NMR experiment by the different protons in a compound under study as a function of frequency (chemical shift). In NMR spectrum, area under the plots indicates the number of hydrogen atom present in the molecule, signal intensity indicates the number of protons of that type, the position of the signals (the chemical shift) reveals information on how shielded or de-shielded (chemical and electronic environment) the proton is, and the splitting pattern shows the number of protons on adjacent/neighboring atoms.

Carbon NMR is a plot of signals arising from the different carbons as a function of chemical shift. The signals in ^{13}C NMR experiments normally appear as singlets because of the decoupling of the attached protons. The number of types of carbon present is shown by the number of peaks, which is seen as single lines. Different ^{13}C NMR experiments are available that can differentiate the types of carbons (primary, secondary, tertiary, and quaternary) present in a molecule. The range of the chemical shift values differs between the ^{1}H (normally 0–10) and ^{13}C NMR (normally 0–230 ppm) that arises from the two nuclei having different numbers of electrons around their corresponding nuclei as well as different electronic configurations (Kwan and Huang, 2008; Breton and Reynolds, 2013).

10.7.1.2   TWO-DIMENSIONAL TECHNIQUES (2D-NMR)

These experiments indicate relationships between the same type of nuclei, homonuclear ^{1}H-^{1}H (correlation spectroscopy [COSY], nuclear overhauser effect spectroscopy [NOESY], rotating frame nuclear overhauser effect spectroscopy, total COSY) and heteronuclear ^{1}H-^{13}C (heteronuclear multiple-quantum correlation [HMQC] and heteronuclear multiple-bond correlation [HMBC], heteronuclear single-quantum COSY), those that indicate relationships between different types of nuclei, often between proton and carbon.

COSY is a plot that shows coupling among neighboring protons. It provides information on the connectivity, in which H atoms are coupling with each other, within the molecule (Kwan and Huang, 2008; Breton and Reynolds, 2013). A line across the dark spots (on spectra) to each axis in a spectrum will show which protons couple with one another and which are, therefore, attached to neighboring carbons.

¹H-¹HNOESY is a homonuclear correlation via dipolar coupling; which correlates nuclei that are spatially close to each other and enables the assignment of relative configuration of substituents at chiral centers (Hostettmann and Wolfender, 2001; Kwan and Huang, 2008; Breton and Reynolds, 2013).

The HMQC spectroscopy correlates protons and a different nuclei (mostly carbon) signals separated by one bond. The spots in the spectrum indicate which proton signal is attached to which carbon.

The HMBC spectroscopy detects long-range coupling, 2–4 bonds away between ¹H and ¹³C (Hostettmann and Wolfender, 2001).

10.7.2 INFRARED AND ULTRAVIOLET SPECTROSCOPY

IR spectroscopy offers information relating to the functional groups present in a molecule, based on the spectra interpretation compared to reference values of different functional group wavenumbers and absorption bands. Individual functional groups have a characteristic absorption in the IR region.

UV-visible spectroscopy reveals information relating to the presence of sites of unsaturation in the structure. It indicates the chromophores present in the isolated compound.

10.7.3 MASS SPECTROMETRY (MS)

MS is an analytical instrument that involves generating charged particles (ions) from molecules of the analyte. The generated ions are analyzed to provide information on fragmentation, molecular mass, the formula of the compound, and its chemical structure.

10.7.4 GC–MS

GC equipment can be directly coupled to mass SM for the molecular mass analysis of volatile compounds of herbal medicines. The hyphenated equipment is sensitive with high efficiency in providing information for structural elucidation. GC vaporizes injected sample and moves it into the separating chamber. Separated compounds from the GC are immediately moved to the mass SM that generates the mass spectrum of the individual compounds (Hostettmann et al., 2001; Guo et al., 2006; Teo et al., 2008).

10.7.5 X-RAY CRYSTALLOGRAPHY

X-ray diffraction is an experimental technique for determining the finger-print and structure of crystalline compounds. This is achievable due to the ability of the crystalline atoms to diffract the beam of X-rays into several specific directions. Three-dimensional pictures of the density electrons, atom placement in the crystalline state, interatomic distance, and angles can be determined by measuring the intensities and angles of the diffracted beams.

The X-ray characteristic profile of each crystalline compound is unique to it and can be used as future identification fingerprint. The size of atoms, type, and lengths of chemical bonds in a structure can easily be determined using X-ray diffraction.

KEYWORDS

- **chemotaxonomy techniques**
- **chemomicroscopy**
- **electrophoresis**
- **extraction**
- **isolation and characterization**

REFERENCES

Abbas, K.A.; Mohamed, A.; Abdulamir, A.S.; Abas, H.A. A Review on Supercritical Fluid Extraction as New Analytical Method. *Am. J. Biochem. Biotechnol.* **2008,** *4*(4), 345–353.

Asada, Y.; Ueoka, T.; Furuya, T. Novel Acylated Saponins from Montbretia (*Crocosmiacrocosmiiflora*). Isolation of Saponins and the Structures of Crocosmiosides A, B and H. *Chem. Pharm. Bull.* **1989,** *37*, 2139–2146.

Azwanida, N.N. A Review on the Extraction Methods Use in Medicinal Plants, Principle, Strength and Limitation. *Med. Aromat. Plants.* **2015,** *4*, 196.

Berthod, A.; Maryutina, T.; Spivakov, B.; Shpigun, O.; Sutherland, I.A. Countercurrent Chromatography in Analytical Chemistry (IUPAC Technical Report). *Pure Appl. Chem.* **2009,** *81*, 355–387.

Boligon, A.A.; Athayde, M.I. Importance of HPLC in Analysis of Plant Extracts. *Austin Chromatogr.* **2014,** *1*(3), 2379–7975.

Breton, R.C.; Reynolds, W.F. Using NMR to Identify and Characterize Natural Products. *Nat. Prod. Rep.* **2013,** *30*, 501–505.

Brunner, G. Supercritical Fluids: Technology and Application to Food Processing. *J. Food Eng.* **2005**, *67*, 21–33.

Bucar, F.; Wube, A.; Schmid, N. Natural Product Isolation–How to Get from Biological Material to Pure Compounds. *Nat. Prod. Rep.* **2013**, *30*, 525–545.

Cicek, S.S.; Schwaiger, S.; Ellmerer, E. P.; Stuppner, H. Development of a Fast and Convenient Method for the Isolation of Triterpene Saponins from Actaearacemose by High-Speed Countercurrent Chromatography Coupled with Evaporative Light Scattering Detection. *Planta Med.* **2010**, *76*(5), 467–473.

Cseke, L.J.;Setzer, W.N.; Vogler, B.; Kirakosyan, A.; Kaufman, B. Traditional, Analytical, and Preparative Separations of Natural Products. In *Natural Products from Plants;* Cseke, L.J., Kirakosyan, A., Kaufman, P.B.,Warber, S.L., Duke, J.A.,Brieelmann, L., Eds.; Taylor and Francis: Boca Raton, 2006; pp 264–313.

Dai, J.; Yaylayan, V.A.; Raghavan, G.S.V.; Pare, J.R. Extraction and Colorimetric Determination of Azadirachtin-Related Limonoids in Neem Seed Kernel. *J. Agric. Food Chem.* **1999**, *47*, 3738–3742.

Fan, X.H.; Cheng, Y.Y.; Ye, Z.L.; Lin, R.C.; Qian, Z.Z. Multiple Chromatographic Fingerprinting and Its Application to the Quality Control of Herbal Medicines. *Anal. Chem. Acta.* **2006**, *555*, 217–224.

Florence, A.J.; Johnson, A.; Fernandes, P.; Shankland, N.; Shankland, K. An Automated Platform forParallei Crystallization of Small Organic Molecules. *J. Appl. Cryst.* **2006**, *39*, 922–924.

Ghafoor, K.; Park, J.; Choi, Y.H. Optimization of Supercritical Fluid Extraction of Bioactive Compounds from Grape Peel by Using Response Surface Methodology. *Innov. Food Sci. Emerg. Technol.* **2010**,*11*, 485–490.

Gökay, N.; Kühner, D.; Los, M.; Götz, F.; Bertsche, U.; Albert, K. An Efficient Approach for the Isolation, Identification and Evaluation of Antimicrobial Plant Components on an Analytical Scale, Demonstrated by the Example of Radix Imperatoriae. *Anal. Bioanal. Chem.* **2010**, *10*, 210–216.

Guiochon, G. Basic Principles of Chromatography. In *Handbook of Analytical Technology;* Günzler, H., Williams, A., Eds.; Wiley-VCH Verlag GmbH, Weinheim: Germany, 2001; pp 173–198.

Guo, F.Q.; Huang, L.F.; Zhou, S.Y.; Zhang, T.M.; Liang, Y.Z. Comparison of the Volatile Compounds ofAtractylodes Medicinal Plants by Headspace Solid-Phase Microextraction-Gas Chromatography-Mass Spectrometry. *Anal. Chim. Acta.* **2006**, *570*, 73–78.

Handa, S. S. An Overview of Extraction Techniques for Medicinal and Aromatic Plants. In *Extraction Technologies for Medicinal and Aromatic Plants*, Handa, S. S., Khanuja, S. P. S., Longo, G.,Rakesh, D. D., Eds.; United Nations Industrial Development Organization and the International Centre for Science and High Technology: Italy, 2008; pp 21–54.

Hostettmann, K.; Marston, A. *Chemistry and Pharmacology of Natural Products: Saponins;* Cambridge University Press: Cambridge, 1995.

Hostettmann, K.; Marston, A.; Hostettmann, M. *Preparative Chromatography Techniques: Applications in Natural Product Isolation*, 2nd ed.; Springer: Berlin/Heidelberg, 1998; pp 45–98.

Hostettman, K.; Wolfender, J.L.; Terreaux, C. Modern Screening Techniques for Plant Extracts. *Pharm. Biol.* **2001**, *39*(1), 18–32.

Huie, C.W. A Review of Modern Sample-Preparation Techniques for the Extraction and Analysis of Medicinal Plants. *Anal. Bioanal. Chem.* 2002, *373*, 23–30.

Ingle, K.P.; Deshmukh, A.G.; Padole, D. A.; Dudhare, M.S.; Moharil, M.; Khelurkar, V.C. Phytochemicals: Extraction Methods, Identification and Detection of Bioactive Compounds from Plant Extracts. *J. Pharmacogn. Phytochem.* **2017**, *6*(1), 32–36.

Joshi, B.S.; Moore, K.M.; Pelletier, S.W., Puar, M.S.; Pramanik, B. N.Saponins from *Collinsoniacanadensis*. *J. Nat. Prod.* **1992**, *55(10)*, 1468–1476.

Kim, B.S.; Song, M.; Kim, S.; Jang, D.; Kim, J.; Ha, B.; Kim, S.; Lee, K.J.; Kang, S.; Jeong, I.Y. The Improvement of Ginsenoside Accumulation in *Panax ginseng* as a Result of γ-Irradiation. *J. Ginseng Res.* **2013**, *37*(3), 332–340.

König, W.A.; Hochmuth, D.H. Enantioselective Gas Chromatography in Flavour and Fragrance Analysis. *J. Chromatogr. Sci.* **2004**, *42,* 423–439.

Kwan, E.E.; Huang, S.G. Structural Elucidation with NMR Spectroscopy: Practical Strategies for Organic Chemists. *Eur. J. Org. Chem.* **2008**, *16*, 2671–2688.

Meshram, A.; Srivastava, N. Molecular and Physiological Role of Epipremnum aureum. *Int. J. Green Pharm.* **2014**, *8,* 73–76.

Meshram, A.; Kumar, A.; Srivastava, N. Gas Chromatography-Mass Spectrometry (GC-MS) Analysis of Alkaloids Isolated from *Epipremnum aureum* (Linden and Andre) Bunting. *Int. J. Pharm. Sci. Res.* **2015**, *6,* 337–342.

Mohamed, A.H. Taxonomic Significance of Seed Proteins and Iso-Enzymes in *Tribulus* (*Zygophyllaceae*). *Int. J. Agric. Biol.* **2006**, *8*(5), 573–575.

Niessen, W.M.A. Principles and Instrumentation of Gas Chromatography-Mass Spectrometry. In *Current Practice of Gas Chromatography-Mass Spectrometry;* Niessen, W. M. A., Ed.; Marcel Dekker, Inc.: New York, USA, 2001; pp 1–29.

Ogundaini, A.A.; Ayim, J.S.K.; Ogungbamila, O.; Olugbade, T.O.; Olaniyi, A.A. Spectroscopic Methods II. In *The Principles of Drug Quality Assurance and Pharmaceutical Analysis;* Olaniyi, A.A., Eds.; Mosuro Publishers: Ibadan, 2000; pp 273–337.

Otto, S. Natural Product Isolation. *Nat. Prod. Rep.* **2008**, *25,* 517–554.

Palma, M.; Barroso, C.G. Ultrasound-Assisted Extraction and Determination of Tartaric and Malic Acids from Grapes and Winemaking By-Products. *Anal. Chem. Acta.* **2002**, *458,* 119–130.

Piana, M.; Zadra, M.; De Brum, T.F.; Boligon, A.A.; Gonçalves, A.F.; Da Cruz, R.C. Analysis of Rutin in the Extract and Gel of *Viola tricolor*. *J. Chromatogr. Sci.* **2013**, *51,* 406–411.

Prathap, B.; Dey, A.; Srinivasarao, G.H.; Johnson, P.; Arthanariswaran, P. Importance of RP-HPLC in Analytical Method Development. *Int. J. Novel Trends Pharma. Sci.* **2013**, *3,* 15–23.

Pyka, A. Detection Progress of Selected Drugs in TLC:A Review.*Biomed. Res. Int.* **2014**, *2014,* 1–19.

Rahmalia, W.; Fabre, J.F.; Mouloungui, Z. Effects of Cyclohexane/Acetone Ratio on Bixin Extraction Yield by Accelerated Solvent Extraction Method. *Procedia Chem.* **2015**, *14,* 455–464

Reid, R.; Sarker, S. Isolation of Natural Products by Low-Pressure Column Chromatography. In *Methods in Biotechnology, Natural Products Isolation;* Sarker, S.D., Latif, Z., Gray, A. I., Eds.; Humana Press Inc.: Totowa, NJ, 2006; Vol. 20, pp 120–140.

Roge, A.B.;Firke, S.N.;Kawade, R.M.; Sarje, S.K.; Vadvalkar, S.M. Brief Review on Flash Chromatography. *Int. J. Pharm. Sci. Res.* **2011**, *2*(8), 1930–1937.

Sarker, S.D.; Latif, Z.; Gray, A.I. *Methods in Biotechnology, Natural Products Isolation,* 2nd ed.; Humana Press Inc.: Totowa, NJ, 2006; Vol. 20.

Sasidharan, S.; Chen, Y.; Saravanan, D.; Sundram, K.M.; Yoga Latha, L. Extraction, Isolation and Characterization of Bioactive Compounds from Plants' Extracts. *Afr. J. Tradit. Complementary Altern. Med.* **2011**, *8,* 1–10.

Schellinger, A.P.; Carr, P.W. Isocratic and Gradient Elution Chromatography: A Comparison in Terms of Speed Retention Reproducibility and Quantitation. *J. Chromatogr. A.* **2006**, *1109,* 253–266.

Soria, A.C.; Villamiel, M. Effect of Ultrasound on the Technological Properties and Bioactivity of Food: A Review. *Trends Food Sci. Technol.* **2010**, *21,* 323–331.

Suranto, S. The Early Application of Electrophoresis of Protein in Higher Plant Taxonomy. *Biodiversitas* **2002**, *3*(2), 257–262.

Swathi G.; Srividya, A.; Ajitha, A.; Rao, V.U. Review on Flash Chromatography. *World J. Pharm. Sci.* **2015**, *4*(8), 281–296

Teo, C.C.; Tan, S.N.; Yong, J.W.H.; Hewb, C.S.; Ong, E.S. Evaluation of the Extraction Efficiency of Thermally Labile Bioactive Compounds in *Gastrodiaelata*Blume by Pressurized Hot Water Extraction and Microwave-Assisted Extraction. *J. Chromatogr. A.* **2008**, *1182,* 34–40.

Tiwari, B.K. Ultrasound: A Clean, Green Extraction Technology. *TrAC Trends Anal. Chem.* **2015**, *71,* 100–109.

Toma, M.; Vinatoru, M.; Paniwnyk, L.; Mason, T.J. Investigation of the Effects of Ultrasound on Vegetal Tissues during Solvent Extraction. *Ultrason. Sonochem.* **2001**, *8*(2), 137–142.

Trusheva, B.; Trunkova, D.; Bankova, V. Different Extraction Methods of Biologically Active Components from Propolis: A Preliminary Study. *Chem. Cent. J.* **2007**, *1* (13), 11–19.

Vilkhu, K.; Mawson, R.; Simons, L.; Bates, D. Applications and Opportunities for Ultrasound Assisted Extraction in the Food Industry – A Review. *Innov. Food Sci. Emerg. Technol,* **2008**, *9*(2), 161–169.

Vvedenskaya, I.O.; Rosen, R.T.; Guido, J.E.; Russell, D.J.; Mills, K.A.; Vorsa, N. Characterization of Flavonolsin Cranberry (*Vacciniummacrocarpon*) Powder. *J. Agric. Food Chem.* **2004**, *52,* 188–195.

CHAPTER 11

CHROMATOGRAPHICAL TECHNIQUES IN PHYTOCHEMICAL RESEARCH

SUMERA JAVAD[1,*] and SHAGUFTA NAZ[2]

[1]*Department of Botany, Lahore College for Women University, Lahore, Pakistan*

[2]*Department of Biotechnology, Lahore College for Women University, Lahore, Pakistan*

*Corresponding author. E-mail: zif_4 zif_4 <zif_4@yahoo.com
ORCID: *https://orcid.org/0000-0002-4703-9610*

ABSTRACT

There are different techniques which are being used for the isolation of plant metabolites, but the most common and reliable method for isolation is chromatography. Chromatography is a technique of separation of a mixture based on differential partitioning between the mobile and stationary phases. There are different types of chromatographical techniques. In phytochemical research, these techniques are selected based on the type of analysis, the target compound, and the nature of plant product involved. The world's flora is a rich treasure of phytochemicals which can be used in many industries. These photosynthetic machines can be said to be a gift from God because of their usefulness in the treatment and management of diseases. In this chapter, different chromatographic techniques used for the isolation and identification of phytochemicals are summarized.

11.1 INTRODUCTION

It is estimated that there are over 400,000 different species of plants. The reason for this diversity is mainly because of the bioadaptability of plants. This means that plants have a great potential to change their habits depending on their habitat. This is another reason why each day a new variety of plants are being added to the list.

11.1.1 PLANT METABOLITES

Plants produce phytochemicals which are being used in the fragrance industry, medicines, paints, cosmetics, textile, flavors, and food industries. There are two main types of plant metabolites, that is, primary and secondary plant metabolites. The primary metabolites are the amino acids, sugars, and fats, and so forth, which are part of primary metabolism and essential for plant survival. The secondary metabolites are the compounds which are plant specific. They are produced as a part of secondary metabolism which may be part of plant defense system but not required for ultimate survival. These include phenolics, flavonoids, tannins and glycosides, and so forth (Liu et al., 2002). These have equally important applications in the industry.

11.1.2 ISOLATION OF PLANT METABOLITES

Phytochemistry is a developing field of research. It is a combination of plant sciences, organic chemistry, and biochemistry. Phytochemistry focuses on the study of the chemicals produced by plants through the study of their natural biosynthetic pathways, its chemical natures, commercial importance, and methods to separate and purify them from plants.

In phytochemistry, there are quite a number of techniques utilized in the study of phytochemicals. The most important are the methods of extraction and isolation. Some methods involved are maceration (Sasidharan et al., 2011), soxhlet extraction (Huie, 2002), microwave-assisted extraction (Javad et al., 2014), supercritical fluid extraction (Herrero et al., 2006), and so forth.

11.2 CHROMATOGRAPHY

Chromatography is the combination of two words, "chrom" meaning color and "graphy" meaning to write. It was named so because at first, it was the separation of different colors from a mixture.

In this procedure, two phases are involved, one is known as the stationary phase while the other is known as the mobile phase. The mixture of interest (plant extract) comprises different components. These components are separated by chromatography on the basis of their solubility in the mobile or stationary phase. The mobile phase is a moving phase like a solvent or a carrier gas while the stationary phase is a fixed immobile phase like some solid or a liquid adsorbed on the surface of a solid. When the mobile phase enters the system containing stationary phase, it is known as the "eluent" and when it comes out it is known as the "eluate" (Fig. 11.1).

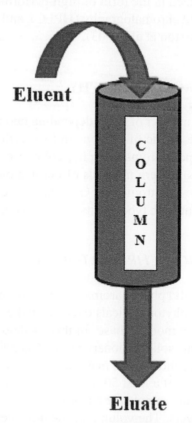

FIGURE 11.1 Eluent and eluate during elution in chromatography.

Elution is the process of removing the analytes from a mixture in a stepwise manner, based on their ability to flow out of the system with the eluent. This ability is based on their chemical nature or polarity. It follows the principle of "like dissolves like." Components which is more soluble in the mobile phase will be eluted first while least soluble will remain behind. Similarly, an analyte having more attraction for stationary phase tend to stay behind during elution (Ingle et al., 2017).

Historically, chromatography started from the work of Tsvet in 1903 on column chromatography. In a series of research and discoveries, it was found in 1941 that mobile phase cannot be a liquid only it can also be a vapor too. Martin and Synge in 1941 gave the idea of liquid–liquid chromatography. In 1952, paper chromatography was explained which was soon replaced by thin-layer chromatography (TLC) which was the first method for which a photograph was easily possible. Thereafter, research made these methods more modernized in the form of high-performance TLC (HPTLC), high-performance liquid chromatography (HPLC), and gas chromatography (GC), and so forth (Marston et al., 2003).

11.3   TYPES OF CHROMATOGRAPHY

Chromatography has a number of types depending upon the nature of mobile phase, stationary phase, mode of elution, and so forth. Some are primitive techniques such as paper chromatography, column chromatography while some are considered as modern methods of chromatography such as liquid chromatography–mass spectrometry, GC–mass spectrometry (GCMS), HPLC, and HPTLC. But each type has its own importance and applications.

11.3.1   ADSORPTION CHROMATOGRAPHY

This is also known as solid phase chromatography. It involves the interaction of functional groups of phytochemicals either with the solid stationary phase or with the liquid or gas mobile phase. In this method, part of loaded plant sample is adsorbed by the solid stationary phase depending upon the nature of sample and surface area and surface material of the stationary phase. Adsorbents with a surface area of a least 50 m^2/g are considered to be good adsorbents. Molecules from the sample are adsorbed, not absorbed, on the surface in the form of monolayers. The volume of the adsorbed surface is basically the product of thickness and surface area of column beds of the adsorbent surface. The sample size is also very important for the proper separation of the components, as very high sample size increases the retention volume of the sample components, which can cause their elution instead of adsorption.

11.3.2 ION-EXCHANGE CHROMATOGRAPHY

It is very important for plant protein separation. It consists of a charged surface to be used as a stationary phase which may be anionic as well as cationic. Ions or charged particles of the plant extract are then separated according to their charges. This process has moved from speed of 2 to 500 cm/h and has emerged as a fast pace process for identification of biological molecules. Even now it is possible to complete the process in 5 min for isolation of a protein of known weight. The limitation of this process is its incompatibility with mass spectrometry as its ions interfere with the ionic field of the mass spectrometer (Jungbauer and Hahn, 2004).

11.3.3 SIZE EXCLUSION CHROMATOGRAPHY

It is a type of chromatography which usually does not need any energy as it relies on the gravitational energy or gravitational movements of solute particles according to their sizes and pore sizes of stationary phase. In this type of chromatography, the stationary phase is made up of the inert material of different sizes because it does not chemically interact with the solution in contact (Wu, 2001). Beads of silica with different sizes may be used for the purpose. There are layers of different pore sizes so the components of plant sample are separated according to their molecular size.

11.3.4 GAS CHROMATOGRAPHY

GC is a powerful tool when equipped with a mass spectrometer as a detector. Moreover, it can be used just for the analysis of volatile components of an extract. In this type of chromatography, the mobile phase is a gas which is usually helium gas or in some cases a nitrogen gas.

GC has a number of applications in the field of volatile components of plant extract. It is used to identify, separate, and quantify different components. Compounds with very low boiling points are vaporized in the column by increasing the temperature of the column where it is carried by the gas mobile phase.

11.3.5   COUNTERCURRENT CHROMATOGRAPHY

It is a modern form of liquid–liquid chromatography. In this process, two immiscible liquids are used. The stationary phase is a solvent which is held in the column by centrifugal force. It is without a solid support and very effective in separating and isolating a mixture of different components such as plant extract (Guitele et al., 2013). In some types of countercurrent chromatography, both solvents enter from opposite sides of column and exit from opposite sides. But in some types, one liquid phase acts as the stationary phase. Functionally, it is almost similar to HPLC attached with a detector, and so forth.

11.3.6   THIN-LAYER CHROMATOGRAPHY (TLC)

In TLC, thin glass plates are coated with a stationary phase. The stationary phase may consist of silica gel or aluminum oxide. In TLC, the selection of the mobile phase is tactical which largely depends on the nature of the targeted analyte. The mobile phase may be a single solvent or a mixture of solvents. It may be polar, nonpolar, or intermediate in polarity according to the properties of the components in the mixture. The principle of TLC is based on the distribution of a compound between a solid fixed phase applied to a glass or aluminum plate and a liquid mobile phase, which is moving over the solid phase (Fig. 11.2). A small amount of a compound or mixture is applied to a starting point just above the bottom of TLC plate. The plate is then developed in the developing chamber that has a shallow pool of solvent just below the level at which the sample was applied. The solvent is drawn up through the particles on the plate through the capillary action, and as the solvent moves over the mixture, each component will either remain with the solid phase or will be dissolved in the solvent and will move up on the plate. Whether the compound moves up the plate or stays behind depend on the physical properties of that individual compound and thus depend on its molecular structure, especially functional groups. The solubility rule "like dissolves like" is followed. The more similar the physical properties of the compound to the mobile phase, the longer it will stay in the mobile phase. The mobile phase will carry the most soluble compounds the furthest up the TLC plate. The compounds that are less soluble in the mobile phase and have a higher affinity to the particles on the TLC plate will stay behind (Kumar et al., 2013). TLC is usually used as a precursor to select the mobile phase to be used on the HPLC for the separation of the target compound from the plant extract.

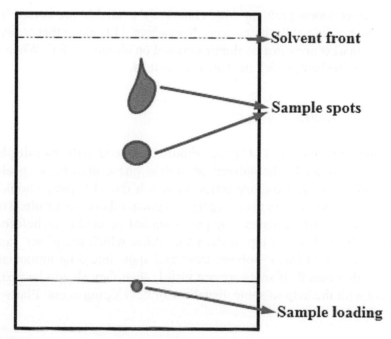

FIGURE 11.2 A thin-layer chromatography chromatogram after developing

11.3.6.1 LOADING OF SAMPLE

Putting the sample on TLC plate is known as loading of the sample. The sample can be loaded with some capillary tube, with a micropipette, or just with the help of a tip of the micropipette. The sample should be small and should not flow on the TLC plate. It is preferable to prepare the sample in some volatile liquid rather than water so that the solvent is evaporated as early as possible.

The sample should be loaded very carefully on one side of the plate, a few centimeters above the edge. If there is a need for repetition, a second drop can be applied just above the first drop.

Before sample loading, it is a good practice to ensure that the stationary phase that is over glass plate is smooth, not cracked, and completely dry. This is because if a TLC plate has any moisture, it will alter the polarity of the stationary phase, thus altering the final results. If problem arises, one can place the TLC plates for some time in the hot air dry oven to get rid of adsorbed solvents on the surface of TLC plates.

Another common problem with commonly available pre-coated TLC plates is the bending of the base sheets. Nowadays, TLC plates that are available in the market are silica or alumina coated on aluminum foil. When one cuts it, it may be bent, which may alter the results.

11.3.6.2   RUNNING OF TLC

After sample loading, the TLC plates should be placed in the mobile phase solution and covered. The solvent or mobile phase then rises up along the TLC plate due to capillary action in which the TLC plate should be kept straight as possible to make separation good, otherwise, results would not be clear with tilted plates. The plates should be held back before the solvent front reached the top of the plate. After which the plates can be removed from the beaker. Solvent front and spot should be immediately marked with a pencil. If spots are not visible then they should be marked afterward with the help of some visualizer or developing agent. Plates can then be dried.

11.3.6.3   DEVELOPING AGENTS

After plates are dried, they should be analyzed with different visualizing agents according to the nature of target compounds (Table 11.1). Some compounds are colored and are easily visible in a visible spectrum of light as colored spots such as chlorophyll, curcumin, and so forth. Some spots become visible when exposed to ultraviolet (UV) light. Therefore, when they are found, the spots should be encircled because once they are again in the visible light, they will be invisible again. Some spots can only be seen when in contact with some chemical reagents. These reagents are known as the developing agents.

Developing agents usually have one or more reactive group which reacts with the functional groups of target plant metabolites and they are specific in their reactions. Their reaction products are usually colored which we can see on TLC plate. Moreover, these spots when visible should be marked because these may not be long-lasting compounds and may be degenerate after a few hours or days. A list of few of the available developing agents is given in the form of Table 11.1. It shows specificity of the reagent for the functional group.

TABLE 11.1 Some Common Developing Agents for TLC and Recipes.

Developing agent	Target compound	Recipe
Aniline phthalate	Reducing sugars	Dissolve 0.93 g aniline and 1.66 g o-phthalic acid in 100 mL n-butanol
Antimony chloride	Flavonoids	10% solution in chloroform
Antimony chloride	Vitamin A, D, carotenoids, steroids, steroidal glycosides	25% solution in chloroform. Heat the plate after developing
Aluminium chloride	Flavonoids	1% solution in ethanol
Ceric ammonium sulfate	For alkaloids	1% ceric (IV) ammonium sulfate in 50% phosphoric acid
Ceric sulfate	For alkaloids	10% cerium sulfate in 15% sulfuric acid
Chloranil agent	Phenols	1% tetrachloro-p-benzoquinone in toluene
Dichlorodicyanobenzoquinone	Phenols	2% solution in toluene
Dinitrophenylhydrazine (DNP)	Aldehydes and ketones	12 g of DNP+ 60 mL of sulfuric acid+ 200 mL of 95% ethanol
Diphenyl amine	Glycosides	10 ml of 10% diphenylamine with ethanol+ 100 ml HCl+ 80 ml glacial acetic acid
Ferric chloride	Phenols	1% $FeCl_3$ in 50% aqueous methanol
Formaldehyde	alkaloids	37% solution in sulfuric acid
Iodine	For organic compounds, particularly sugars	
Ninhydrin	amino acids	1.5 g of ninhydrin+100 mL of nbutanol+ 3 mL of acetic acid
Paraanasaldehyde staine 2	Terpenes, Cineoles, acronecyne, steroids	anisaldehyde: $HClO_4$: acetone: water (1:10:20:80)
Potassium hexacyanoferrate	Phenols and aryl amines	Spray 1:1 g aminoantipyrine in 100 mL of 80% ethanol Spray 2:4 g potassium hexacyanoferrate in 20 mL water and make total vole 100 mL with ethanol Heat in warm air
Potassium permanganate	For oxidizing agents like alkenes, alkynes, amines	5 g of Potassium permanganate+ 10 g K_2CO_3, and 1.25 mL 10% NaOH in 200 mL water. Immerse in 1% solution then heat the plate after that
Ultraviolet (UV) light	For UV active compounds like with conjugation (alternative double bonds) or aromatic rings	

11.3.6.4 R_f VALUE

An R_f value (retardation factor or ratio to front) is usually calculated by using the formula.

$$R_f = \frac{Distance\ covered\ by\ sample\ spot}{Distance\ covered\ by\ solvent\ front}$$

A compound having more affinity for the mobile phase will be having higher R_f values. But these values vary with the mobile phase.

11.3.6.5   RESOLUTION

Resolution is the ability of the chromatographic system to separate two components or spots. It is the same definition for all the other types of chromatographical techniques.

11.3.7   HIGH-PERFORMANCE LIQUID CHROMATOGRAPHY

HPLC is one of the most accepted analytical tools for plant secondary metabolites. It is easy to handle and very much feasible to be connected to a number of detectors such as UV-visible spectrophotometer, mass spectrometer, infrared spectrometer, refractive index detector, evaporative light scattering detector, conductivity detector, fluorescent detector and diode array, and so forth. It was introduced in 1967 and since then, it has helped a lot to plant scientists (Spackman et al., 1958). Open column chromatography was used before but requires more solvents and is not cost effective and contributes hazards to the environment. Another main technique in use was TLC which is pretty much helpful in identification sometimes but not in measuring the concentration.

HPLC is a method which can be used to analyze a wide range of constituents of plant extracts with precision and accuracy. In this method, the stationary phase is once again attached to a column coated with very fine sized silica particles. These stationary phases may contain nonpolar or polar components according to the nature of separation to be carried out. They are small enough to bear the pressure of pumps associated with the mobile phase (60 MPa) which is the characteristic of the HPLC making it superior to other forms. Now ultra HPLC systems have also been developed in which column can bear a pressure up to 120 MPa.

11.3.7.1   SAMPLE PREPARATION AND LOADING

A very small amount of extract is enough to make analysis by HPLC, which makes it a powerful tool for the purpose. A 20 μl sample is usually used. The extract is filtered first by some fine HPLC grade filters such as filters with 0.45-μ pore size. Filtrates are then loaded to the HPLC column by a syringe which is usually made up of glass.

11.3.7.2   MOBILE PHASE SELECTION

Usually, when working with HPLC of plant products or metabolites, it is good to run TLC earlier to select a mobile phase for the target compound. Selection of mobile phase basically depends upon the target of research. Whether one is interested in isolation of a single compound like a single phenolic, or a group of compounds like all phenolics possible. Therefore, he/she selects the type of mobile phase accordingly. The solubility of a targeted analyte in the solvent system is also important. Moreover, it is important to note that before running the solvent on the HPLC system, it should be filtered and degassed by ultrasonics. This is necessary to avoid the chocking of the fine columns of the HPLC.

However, if the composition of the mobile phase remains same throughout the experiment, then it is known as the isocratic elution (same composition elution). The system in which the composition of mobile phase changes with the time is known as gradient elution. For example, if at the start of an experiment, the mobile phase is acetonitrile: water in a ratio of 1:9 and concentration gradually changed to 9:1 up to the end of the experiment. If isocratic elution is suitable, then it should not be replaced by the gradient. Gradient elution is sometimes preferred as it gives more sharp peaks for the eluents with more retention times (Adam and Carr, 2006).

11.3.7.3   COLUMNS

Larger columns are usually used for the industrial purposes where larger amounts of analytes are involved, while for research purposes where the targets are narrowed down, small columns with short diameters can be used. This increases the efficiencies of the columns as well as decrease the run time of the sample.

11.3.7.4   DETECTORS

When the sample is separated by HPLC column, they are passed through some particular detector attached. The software for that detector is usually loaded with HPLC software. One gets the results in the form of peaks (Fig. 11.3). In the chromatogram, the x-axis shows the retention time while the y-axis is related to the signal of the detector attached. Usually, a UV-visible spectrophotometer is a good universal detector, but some other detectors are also used according to the nature of target compound and the type of work. For example, Zhang et al. (2013) reported the detection of 14 phenolic compounds at a time by using UV diode array detector from grapes. While earlier Jandik et al. (2009) reported the isolation of phenolics by using disposable carbon electrodes coupled with HPLC.

11.3.7.5   CHROMATOGRAM

A result obtained in the form of a graph for different peaks is known as a chromatogram (Fig. 11.3).

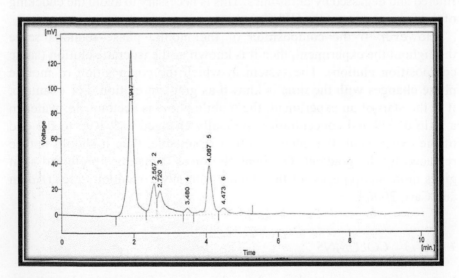

FIGURE 11.3   A typical high-performance liquid chromatoghraphy chromatogram showing peaks of analytes at different retention times.

The retention time along the x-axis (Fig. 11.3) indicates the time in which a compound is retained by the column. Sometimes to ensure the peak identity, one can do the spiking. In this process, a calculated amount of standard compound is added to the analyte, due to which that particular peak is spiked to confirm the results. Then by comparing the area of sample peak with the area of the standard peak, one can find out the concentration of the compound of interest. Samples are eluted at different retention times, where they are collected and labeled according to the relative peaks. Resolution is the ability of the system to differentiate two signals or two peaks.

11.4 APPLICATION OF CHROMATOGRAPHIC TECHNIQUES

Chromatographic techniques have been widely applied in the screening of the phytochemical composition of plants (Tables 11.2 and 11.3). Different techniques with different solvent systems have been developed for effective detection and quantification of plant phytochemicals. Plants secondary metabolites are very important in terms of applied fields. The chemodiversity of plant natural compounds can be exploited at every level to make new products such as food, medicines, cosmetics, perfumery, detergents, paints, and so forth. An important factor to consider is the experimental design. It should be one designed to get a maximum product with cost-effective setup in lesser time and little or no harm to the environment. Techniques selected at each step should be precise and accurate.

Chromatography is used for identification, isolation as well as purification of the plant components. TLCs and GC methods are identified to be the most appropriate for low-molecular-weight terpenoids. Basically, all classes of terpenoids such as mono, di, tri, sesquiterpenes, and so forth, can be detected and analyzed by TLC and GCMS. For TLC, H_2SO_4 is usually used as a developer. Sometimes additional heating is also required (Citoglu and Ozlem, 2012). Some of the researchers have also preferred column chromatography for the terpenoids and got good results (Abdelgaleil et al., 2008; Brown et al., 2003). TLC and HPLC methods are also strongly recommended for the isolation and quantification of alkaloids in the plant samples. Capillary GC is also suggested for a number of alkaloids (Talita et al., 2012). Alkaloids have also been identified from fungi by using column chromatography (Ishiuchi et al., 2011).

Lipopeptides have been separated from plants samples by using TLC, reverse phase HPLC, and Ion exchange chromatography (Symmank et al., 2002). A number of chromatographic methods have been modified and developed de novo to study the plant proteins such as diagonal chromatography (Walton et al., 2016), high-performance size exclusion chromatography (Barth 1982), and so forth.

TABLE 11.2 Applications of Chromatographic Techniques in the Isolation of Phenolics.

S/No.	Plant or source	Chromatography method	Mobile phase	References
1.	Grape wine	High-performance liquid chromatography (HPLC)	Water: methanol	Helene et al. (1984)
2.	Echinacea spp.	Reverse phase HPLC	Methanol: water: acetic acid	Glowniak et al. (1996)
3.	Apple and pear	HPLC	2% acetic acid in water: 0.5% acetic acid in acetonitrile	Schieber et al. (2001)
4.	Dimocarpus longan	HPLC-EIMS (HPLC coupled with electron ionization mass spectrometery)	Water: acetic acid: methanol	Soong and Barlow (2005)
5.	Prunella sp.	HPLC	Methanol	Sahin et al. (2013)
6.	Rice bran	Column chromatography	Petroleum ether, acetone	Wang et al. (2015)
7.	Olive oil	Gas chromatoghrpahy–mass spectrometry (GCMS)	Nitrogen gas	Bajoub et al. (2016)
8.	Arachis hypogaea	HPLC	Acetonitrile: water	Oldoni et al. (2016)
9.	Euphorbia lathyris	GCMS	Helium gas	Sosa et al. (2016)
10	Saccharum officinarum	Countercurrent chromatography	Methylated butyl ether: acetonitrile: water	Fang et al. (2017)
11.	Ormocarpum kirkii	High-speed countercurrent chromatography	Hexane: ethanol: water	Kamto et al. (2017)
12.	Sea algae	Liquid chromatography–mass spectrometry	Acetonitrile	Klejdus et al. (2017)
13.	Mangifera indica	Counter current chromatography	Hexane: ethyl acetate: methanol: water 4:6:4:6	Shaheen et al. (2017)

TABLE 11.3 Applications of Chromatographic Techniques in the Isolation of Alkaloids.

S/No.	Plant/resource	Chromatography technique	Mobile phase	Reference
1.	*Peganum harmala*	Thin-layer chromatography (TLC)	Chloroform:methanol	Pozzi et al. (2012)
2.	*Carica papaya*	HPLC	Methanol	Julianti et al. (2014)
3.	*Mahonia manipurensis*	TLC+ reverse phase HPLC	Methanol and formic acid	Pfoze et al. (2014)
4.	*Tea*	HPLC	Water:acetonitrile:methanol	Rahim et al. (2014)
5.	*Coptis chinensis*	Reverse phase HPLC	Acetonitrile:potassium dihydrogen phosphate 25%	Teng and Choi (2014)
6.	*Stephania sinica*	HPLC	Triethylamine with phosphoric acid:acetonitrile	Xie et al. (2014)
7.	*Rauvolfia nukuhivensis*	HPLC	Methanol:dichloromethane	Martin et al. (2015)
8.	*Chelidonium majus*	TLC	Chloroform:methanol	Moricz et al. (2015)
9.	*Berberis amurensis*	Ultra-performance liquid chromatography	Acetonitrile:water	Wu et al. (2015)
10.	*Sophora flavescens*	HPLC	Ethanol	Zhang et al. (2015)
11.	*Erythroxylum subsessile*	Countercurrent chromatography	Ethyl acetate:water	Cruz et al. (2016)
12.	*Achnatherum robustum*	HPLC	Formic acid	Jarmusch et al. (2016)

Chromatographic techniques are also used to test for the adulteration of herbal products with some synthetic chemical agents (Gokar et al., 2012). HPLC has been in continuous use in pharmaceutical industry as a quality control tool (Li et al., 2011).

KEYWORDS

- **chromatographic techniques**
- **thin-layer chromatography**
- **phytochemical screening**
- **high-performance liquid chromatography**
- **chromatogram**

REFERENCES

Abdelgaleil, S. A. M.; Abbassy, M. A.; Belal, A. H.; AbdelRasoul, M. A. A. Bioactivity of Two Major Constituents Isolated from the Essential Oil of *Artemisia judaica* L. *Bioresour. Technol.* **2008**, *99*, 5947–5950.

Adam, *P. S.;* Carr, *P. W.* Isocratic and Gradient Elution Chromatography: A Comparison in Terms of Speed, Retention Reproducibility and Quantitation. *J. Chromatogr. A* **2006**, *1109*, 253–266.

Bajoub, A.; Tiziana, P.; Elena, H.; Lucia, O.; Rocio, G.; Alberto, F.; Oleg, A. M.; Alegra, C. Comparing Two Metabolic Profiling Approaches (Liquid Chromatography and Gas Chromatography Coupled to Mass Spectrometry) for Extra-Virgin Olive Oil Phenolic Compounds Analysis: A Botanical Classification Perspective. *J. Chromatogr. A* **2016**, *1428*, 267–279.

Barth, H. G. High-Performance Size-Exclusion Chromatography of Hydrolyzed Plant Proteins. *Ann. Biochem.* **1982**, *124*(1), 191–200.

Brown, G. D.; Liang, G. Y.; Sy, L. K. Terpenoids from the Seeds of Artemisia Annua. *Phytochemistry* **2003**, *64*, 303–323.

Citoglu, G. S.; Ozlem, B. A. Column Chromatography for Terpenoids and Flavonoids. In *Chromatography and its Applications;* In-Tech Publishers: Croatia, 2012; pp 13–50.

Cruz, R. A. S.; Almeida, H.; Fernandes, C. P.; Pedro, J. N.; Rocha, L.; Gilda, G. L. A New Tropane Alkaloid from the Leaves of *Erythroxylum subsessile* Isolated by pH-Zone-Refining Counter-Current Chromatography. *J. Sep. Sci.* **2016**, *39*(7), 1273–1277.

Fang, Y. T.; Li, Q.; Cao, A. C.; Yuan, L.; Yun, W. Isolation and Purification of Phenolics Acids from Sugarcane (*Saccharum officinarum* L.) Rinds by pH-Zone Refining Counter Current Chromatography and Their Antioxidant Evaluation. *Food Anal. Meth.* **2017**, *10*(7), 2576–2584.

Glowniak, K.; Grazyna, Z.; Kozyra, M. Solid-Phase Extraction and Reversed-Phase High-Performance Liquid Chromatography of Free Phenolic Acids in Some Echinaceaspecies. *J. Chromatogr. A* **1996**, *730*(1–2), 25–29.

Goker, H.; Maksut, C.; Gulgun, A. K. Chromatographic Separation and Identification of Sildenafil and Yohimbine Analogues Illegally Added in Herbal Supplements. In *Chromatography and its Applications;* Dhanarasu, S., Ed.; In-Tech Publishers: Croatia, 2012; pp 51–68.

Guitele, D. G.; Pasillas, Y. H.; Choi, R. V. Chapter Nine—New Methods of Analysis and Investigation of Terpenoid Indole Alkaloids. *Adv. Bot. Res.* **2013**, *68*, 233–272.

Helene, M.; Auguste, S.; Bertrand, A. Wine Phenolics—Analysis of Low Molecular Weight Components by High Performance Liquid Chromatography. *J. Sci. Food Agric.* **1984**, *35*(11), 1241–1247.

Herrero, M.; Alejandro, C.; ELinel, B. Sub- and Supercritical Fluid Extraction of Functional Ingredients from Different Natural Sources: Plants, Food-By-Products, Algae and Microalgae: A Review. *Food Chem.* **2006**, *98*(1), 136–148.

Huie, C. W. A Review of Modern Sample-Preparation Techniques for the Extraction and Analysis of Medicinal Plants. *Anal. Bioanal. Chem.* **2002**, *373*(1–2), 23–30.

Ishiuchi, K.; Kubota, T.; Ishiyama, H.; Hayashi, S.; Shibata, T.; Mori, K.; Obara, Y.; Nakanhata, N.; Kobayashi, J. Lyconadins D and E, and Complanadine E, New *Lycopodium alkaloids* from *Lycopodium complanatum*. *Bioorg. Med. Chem.* **2011**, *19*, 749–753.

Jandik, P.; Pohl, C.; Cher, J. Determination of Phenolic Compounds Using HPLC and Electrochemical Detection with Disposable Carbon Electrodes, 2009. Available: http://www.chromatographyonline.com/determination-phenolic-compounds-using-hplc-and-electrochemical-detection-disposable-carbon-electrod (accessed Jan 20, 2018).

Jarmusch, A. K.; Musso, A. M.; Tatsiana, S.; Scott, A. J.; Miranda, J. W.; Mary, E. L.; Brandie, M. E.; Susana, S.; David, E. N.; Stanely, H. F.; Nadja, B. C. Comparison of Electrospray Ionization and Atmospheric Pressure Photoionization Liquid Chromatography Mass Spectrometry Methods for Analysis of Ergot Alkaloids from Endophyte-Infected Sleepygrass (*Achnatherum robustum*). *J. Pharm. Biomed. Anal.* **2016**, *117*, 11–17.

Javad, S.; Shagufta, N.; Saiqa, I.; Amna, T.; Farah, A. Optimization of the Microwave Assisted Extraction and its Comparison with Different Conventional Extraction Methods for Isolation of Stevioside from Stevia Rebaudiana. *Asian J. Chem.* **2014**, *26*(23), 8043–8048.

Julianti, T.; Maria, D. M.; Stefanie, Z.; Samad, N.; Marcel, K.; Markus, N.; Melani, R.; Reto, B.; Matthias, H. HPLC-Based Activity Profiling for Antiplasmodial Compounds in the Traditional Indonesian Medicinal Plant *Carica papaya* L. *J. Ethnopharmacol.* **2014**, *155*(1), 426–434.

Jungbauer, A.; Hahn, R. Monoliths for Fast Bioseperation and Bioconversion and Their Applications in Biotechnology. *J. Sep. Sci.* **2004**, *27*, 767–778.

Kamto, E. L. D.; Carvalho, T. S. C.; Josephine, N. M.; Marie, C. N. M.; Dieudonne, E. P.; Gilda, G. L. Alternating Isocratic and Step Gradient Elution High-Speed Counter-Current Chromatography for the Isolation of Minor Phenolics from *Ormocarpum kirkii* Bark. *J. Chromatogr. A* **2017**, *1480*, 50–61.

Klejdus, B.; Plaza, M.; Marie, S.; Lea, L. Development of New Efficient Method for Isolation of Phenolics from Sea Algae Prior to Their Rapid Resolution Liquid Chromatographic—Tandem Mass Spectrometric Determination. *J. Pharm. Biomed. Anal.* **2017**, *135*(20), 87–96.

Li, Y.; Zhao, J.; Yang, B. Strategies for Quality of Chinese Medicines. *J. Pharm. Biomed. Anal.* **2011**, *55*, 802–809.

Liu, J. R.; Choi, D. W.; Chung, H. J.; Woo, S. S. Production of Useful Secondary Metabolites in Plants: Functional Genomics Approaches. *J. Plant Biol.* **2002,** *45*(1), 1–6.

Martin, N. J.; Mael, N.; Gael, L.; Phila, R. Isolation and Characterization Procedure for Indole Alkaloids from the Marquesan Plant *Rauvolfia nukuhivensis. Bioprotocol* **2015,** *5*(20), 1–8.

Moricz, A. M.; Fornal, E.; Jesionek, W.; Barbaraa, M. D.; Choma, I. M. Effect Directed Isolation and Identification of Antibacterial *Chelidonium majus* L. Alkaloids. *Chromatographia* **2015,** *78*(9–10), 707–716.

Oldoni, T. L. C.; Melo, P. S.; Massarioli, A. P.; Moreno, A. M.; Bezerra, R. M. N.; Pedro, L. R.; Gil, V. J. S.; Andrea, M. N.; Severino, M. A. Bioassay-Guided Isolation of Proanthocyanidins with Antioxidant Activity from Peanut (*Arachis hypogaea*) Skin by Combination of Chromatography Techniques. *Food Chem.* **2016,** *192*(1), 306–312.

Pfoze, N. L.; Myrboh, B.; Kumar, Y.; Rohman, M. R. Isolation of Protoberberine Alkaloids from Stem Bark of *Mahonia manipurensis* Takeda Using RP-HPLC. *J. Med. Plant Stud.* **2014,** *2*(2), 48–57s.

Pozzi, F.; Nobuko, S.; Leona, M.; Lombardi, J. R. TLC-SERS Study of *Syrian rue* (*Peganum harmala*) and its Main Alkaloid Constituents. *J. Raman Spectrosc.* **2012,** *44*(1), 102–107.

Rahim, A. A.; Nofrizal, S.; Saad, B. Rapid Tea Catechins and Caffeine Determination by HPLC Using Microwave-Assisted Extraction and Silica Monolithic Column. *Food Chem.* **2014,** *147*, 262–268.

Sahin, S.; Ari, F.; Demir, C.; Ulukava, E. Isolation of Major Phenolic Compounds from the Extracts of *Prunella* L. Species Grown in Turkey and Their Antioxidant and Cytotoxic Activities. *J. Food Biochem.* **2013,** *38*(2), 248–257.

Sasidharan, S.; Chen, Y.; Saravanan, D.; Sundram, K. M.; Yoqa, L. L. Extraction, Isolation and Characterization of Bioactive Compounds from Plants' Extracts. *Afr. J. Tradit. Complementary Altern. Med.* **2011,** *8*(1), 1–10.

Schieber, A.; Petra, K.; Carle, R. Determination of Phenolic Acids and Flavonoids of Apple and Pear by High-Performance Liquid Chromatography. *J. Chromatogr. A* **2001,** *910*(2), 265–273.

Shaheen, N.; Yanzhen, L.; Ping, G.; Qian, S.; Yun, W. Isolation of Four Phenolic Compounds from *Mangifera indica* L. Flowers by Using Normal Phase Combined with Elution Extrusion Two-Step High Speed Countercurrent Chromatography. *J. Chromatogr. B* **2017,** *1046*(1), 211–217.

Soong, Y. Y.; Barlow, P. J. Isolation and Structure Elucidation of Phenolic Compounds from Longan (*Dimocarpus longan* Lour.) Seed by High-Performance Liquid Chromatography— Electrospray Ionization Mass Spectrometry. *J. Chromatogr. A* **2005,** *1085*(2), 270–277.

Sosa, A. A.; Bagi, S. H.; Imad, H. H. Analysis of Bioactive Chemical Compounds of Euphorbia Lathyrus Using Gas Chromatography-Mass Spectrometry and Fourier-Transform Infrared Spectroscopy. *J. Pharmacogn. Phytother.* **2016,** *8*(5), 109–126.

Spackman, D. H.; Stein, W. H.; Moore, S. Automatic Recording Apparatus for use in Chromatography of Aminoacids. *Anals Chem.* **1958,** *30*, 1190–1206.

Symmank, H.; Frank, P.; Saenger, W.; Bernhard, F. Modification of Biologically Active Peptides: Production of a Novel Lipohexapeptide After Engineering of *Bacillus subtilis* Surfactin Synthetase. *Protein Eng.* **2002,** *15*, 913–921.

Talita, P. C. C.; Ananda, C. C.; Luzia, K.; Regina, A. C. G.; Arildo, J. B. O. Use of Associated Chromatographic Techniques in Bio-Monitored isolation of Bioactive Monoterpenoid Indole Alkaloids from in *Aspidosperma ramiflorum*. In *Chromatography and its Applications;* Dhanarasu, S., Ed.; In-Tech Publishers: Croatia, 2012; pp 119–130.

Teng, H.; Choi, Y. H. Optimization of Ultrasonic-Assisted Extraction of Bioactive Alkaloid Compounds from Rhizoma Coptidis (*Coptis chinensis* Franch.) Using Response Surface Methodology. *Food Chem.* **2014,** *142,* 299–305.

Walton, A.; Liana, T.; Silke, J.; Stes, E.; Jorris, M.; Frank, V. B.; Sofie, G.; Kris, G. Diagonal Chromatography to Study Plant Protein Modifications. *Biochim. Biophys. Acta* **2016,** *1864,* 945–951.

Wang, W.; Jia, G.; Junnan, Z.; Jie, P.; Tianxing, L.; Zhihong, X. Isolation, Identification and Antioxidant Activity of Bound Phenolic Compounds Present in Rice Bran. *Food Chem.* **2015,** *171,* 40–49.

Wu, C. *Hand Book of Size Exclusion Chromatography and Related Techniques;* Chromatographic Science Series; Marcel Dekker Inc., 2001; Vol. 91.

Wu, J. K.; Sun, H.; Zhang, Y.; Zhang, W.; Meng, F.; Du, X. Optimizing the Extraction of Anti-Tumor Alkaloids from the Stem of *Berberis amurensis* by Response Surface Methodology. Ind Crops Prod **2015,** *69,* 68–75.

Xie, D. T.; Wang, Y. Q.; Yun, K.; Hu, Q. F.; Su, N. Y.; Huang, J. M.; Che, C. T.; Guo, J. X. Microwave-Assisted Extraction of Bioactive Alkaloids from *Stephania sinica. Sep. Purif. Technol.* **2014,** *130,* 173–181.

Zhang, A.; Wan, L.; Wu, C.; Fang, Y.; Han, G.; Li, H.; Zhang, Z.; Wang, H. Simultaneous Determination of 14 Phenolic Compounds in Grape Canes by HPLC-DAD-UV Using Wavelength Switching Detection. *Molecules* **2013,** *18,* 14241–14257.

Zhang, W.; Fan, H.; Liu, X.; Wan, Q.; Wu, X.; Liu, P.; Tang, J. Z. Simultaneous Extraction and Purification of Alkaloids from *Sophora flavescens* Ait. by Microwave-Assisted Aqueous Two-Phase Extraction with Ethanol/Ammonia Sulfate System. *Sep. Purif. Technol.* **2015,** *141,* 113–123.

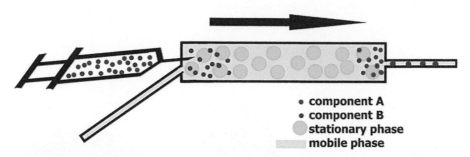

FIGURE 12.13   Distribution of analytes and liquid in an HPLC column.

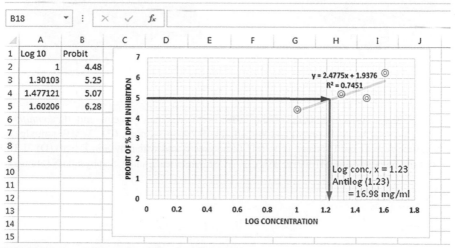

FIGURE 15.1   Illustration of IC_{50} determination.

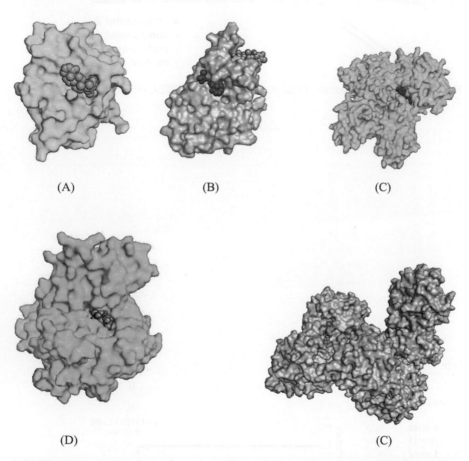

FIGURE 20.4 Surface structure of the different DNA repair proteins and *W. somnifera* phytochemicals; (A) 1EH8 (cyan) and withanolide B (deep salmon), (B) 2WMW (smudge)-withanolide A (red) and D (slate), (C) 3I6U (lime green) and withaphysalin F (red),(D) 3L3L (green) and withaphysalin M (marine blue), (E) 3U8U (light teal), and withaphysalin N (orange).

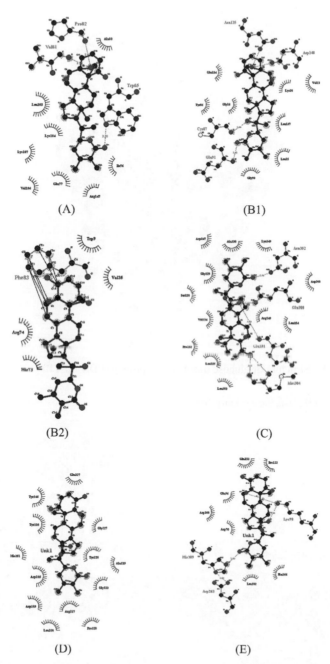

FIGURE 20.5 Interaction of various amino acids of target proteins with *W. somnifera* phytochemicals and type of interaction; (A) withanolide B_1EH8, (B1) withanolide A_2 WMW, (B2) withanolide D_2WMW, (C) withphysalin F_3I6U, (D) withaphysalin M_3L3L, (E) withaphysalin N_3U8U.

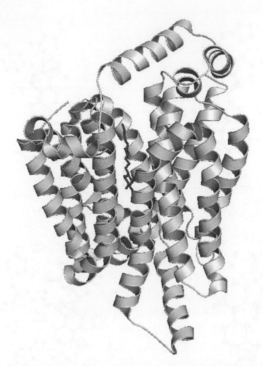

FIGURE 21.1   Structure of glucose transporter 1 protein (PDB=4PYP)[1].

_____

[1]PDB=4PYP (Protein Data Bank = Entry 4PYP).

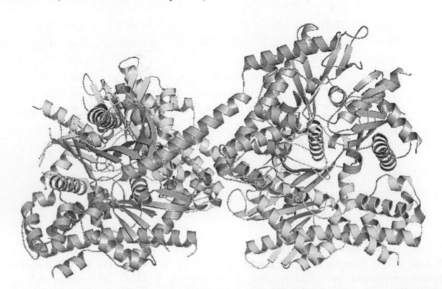

FIGURE 21.2   Structure of hexokinase 2 protein (PDB=2NZT).

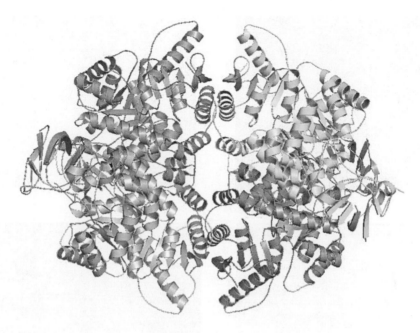

FIGURE 21.4   Structure of pyruvate kinase M2 protein (PDB=3GQY).

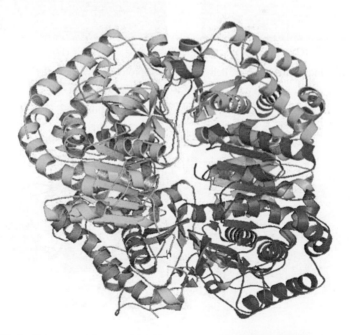

FIGURE 21.5   Structure of lactate dehydrogenase A protein (PDB=4AJP).

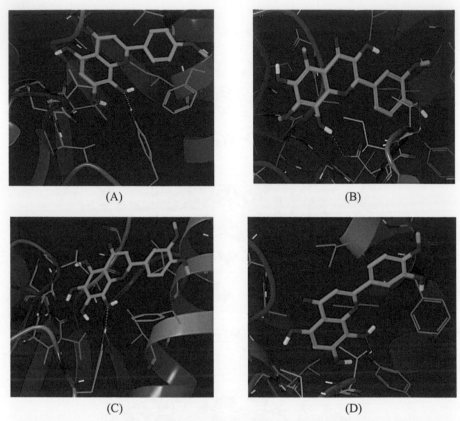

FIGURE 21.7   Interaction of lactate dehydrogenase A protein with lead methylated flavonoids.

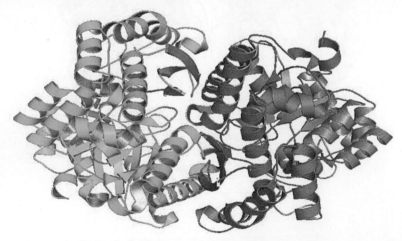

FIGURE 21.9   Structure of enolase 2 protein (PDB=5IDZ).

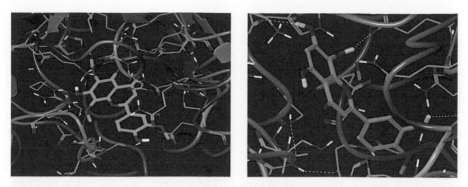

FIGURE 21.10　Interaction of enolase two protein with lead methylated flavonoids.

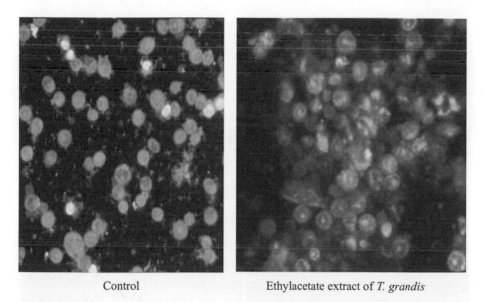

Control　　　　　　　　　　Ethylacetate extract of *T. grandis*

FIGURE 23.3　Morphological changes observed for control ethylacetate extract of *T. grandis*-treated MCF-7 cells stained with acridine orange and ethidium bromide. (1) viable cells have uniform bright green nuclei with organized structure; (2) early apoptotic cells have green nuclei, but perinuclear chromatin condensation is visible as bright green patches or fragments; (3) late apoptotic cells have orange to red nuclei with condensed or fragmented chromatin.

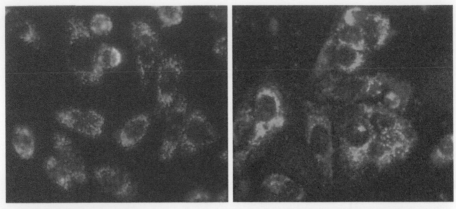

Control   Ethylacetate extract of *T. grandis*

FIGURE 23.4   Photomicrographs of MCF-7 breast cancer cells, JC-1 dye accumulated in the mitochondria of healthy cells as aggregates (red–orange fluorescing); in cells treated with ethyl acetate extract of *T. grandis*, due to collapse of mitochondrial membrane potential, the JC-1 dye remained in the cytoplasm its monomeric form, which fluoresced green.

Control   Ethylacetate extract of *T. grandis*

FIGURE 23.5   Deoxyribonucleic acid damage in ethylacetate extract of *T. grandis* treated MCF-7 cells is revealed in the comet assay. Comet images of DNA strand breaks at 12 h treatment of the ethylacetate extract of *T. grandis*.

CHAPTER 12

ULTRAVIOLET/VISIBLE SPECTROSCOPY AND HPLC IN PHYTOCHEMICAL ANALYSIS: AN INTRODUCTION

ADE KUJORE

Cecil Instruments, Milton Technical Centre, CB24 6AZ Cambridge, UK, Tel.:+44 (0) 1223 420821

E-mail: ade.kujore@cecilinstruments.com
ORCID: https://orcid.org/0000-0002-4588-5362

ABSTRACT

Ultraviolet (UV)/visible spectrophotometers are relatively inexpensive instruments that are quite simple to use in the detection and quantification of many compounds. The principle is based on the fact that some molecules have the capacity to absorb at particular wavelengths of UV or visible light. This follows that the quantity of light absorbed by a sample can be used to estimate its concentration. This obeys Beer–Lambert's law. This principle is also applicable to high-performance liquid chromatography (HPLC) only because it is a more complex technique which combines chromatography. HPLC offers wider advantages in the detection, identification, and quantification of a wider range of phytochemical compounds. This chapter is intended to be an in-depth discussion of UV/visible spectrophotometer and HPLC instrumentations and analysis. It focuses on the principles and its method of operations with some practical illustrations. It also provided tips on the calibration and qualifications of the equipment.

12.1   INTRODUCTION

Phytochemicals can be defined as those chemicals produced by plants, which are not essential nutrients to humans, but which may have effects on health.

Consequently, the analysis of phytochemicals is required for many reasons, including:

1. Ascertaining the purity and yield of phytochemical extracts.
2. Some phytochemicals may occur as chiral isomers, extraction of the required chiral type may be required. Examples include D-limonene in orange-flavored extracts; the pentacyclic triterpene acid, β-boswellic acid from frankincense, and S-(+)-Carvone from caraway seeds.
3. Checking the stated content of formulations containing phytochemical extracts.
4. Production checks during phytochemical elimination processing of final products. Such as checking for cannabinoid levels of hemp, or checking for cyanogenic glycosides in cassava and almonds.
5. Contamination and adulteration of phytochemical extracts, with, for example, pesticides and other environmental contaminants, synthetic analogs, mycotoxins, cheaper simulants, and so forth.
6. Identification of phytochemicals during discovery research.

During analysis, the analyst should be aware that many phytochemicals are naturally present in complex mixtures of a range of similar natural analogs. These mixtures can be difficult to effectively separate or extract. Hence, markers for the phytochemical of interest are sometimes used for identification and quantification purposes.

12.2   ULTRAVIOLET (UV)/VISIBLE SPECTROPHOTOMETRY

Ultraviolet (UV)/visible spectrophotometry is an established technique, with a flexibility to detect and measure many phytochemicals (compounds/analytes) within a wide variety of sample matrices. Figure 12.1 is an example of a typical Aquarius UV/visible spectrophotometer.

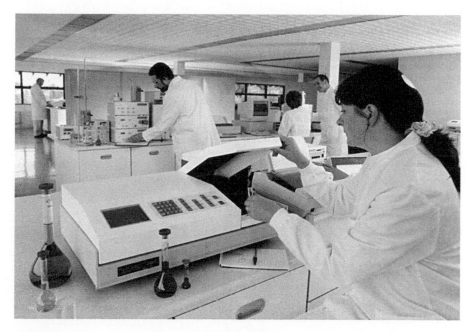

FIGURE 12.1 A typical aquarius ultraviolet/visible spectrophotometer being used within a laboratory.

Source: Courtesy to Cecil Instruments, Milton Technical Centre, Cambridge, CB24 6AZ, United Kingdom.

12.2.1 THEORY

Some molecules have the capacity to absorb particular wavelengths of UV or visible light. Compounds containing those molecules have a UV/**visible** chromophore.

At those particular wavelengths, the quantity of a UV/visible chromophore in a sample may be measured. In general, the higher the amount of UV/visible chromophore detected, the larger the concentration of that compound.

Light generated by some lamps, such as deuterium, tungsten, or xenon, is separated into discrete bands of wavelengths of light by a monochromator, which is then is passed through a sample after emerging from a slit. The sample with the UV/visible chromophore absorbs some light and the remaining light is detected by a detector.

Liquid samples are contained within cuvettes or cells (Fig. 12.2), which are placed inside a UV/visible spectrophotometer. The width of the cell, into which light passes through the sample is the path length, a standard path length used by many users is 10 mm.

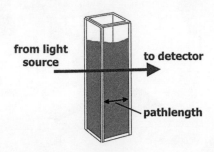

FIGURE 12.2   Light passing through a cuvette.

The Beer–Lambert law is then used to calculate the concentration of a specific analyte (compound) in a transparent liquid sample at a specific wavelength.

$$A = \epsilon \times l \times c,$$

where at a specific wavelength,

A   = the measured absorbance,
ϵ = the molar absorbtivity or extinction coefficient ($M^{-1}\cdot cm^{-1}$),
l = the pathlength (cm),
c = the analyte concentration (M).

The Beer–Lambert law provides for a linear relationship. There are a few restrictions on the law, and the linearity of the Beer–Lambert law is limited by instrumental and chemical factors.

Provided a concentration is measured in the linear portion of the calibration curve for each specific analyte, the law will apply in practice.

If transmittance measurements are required, then there is the following relationship:

$$A = - \log T.$$

Cuvettes are made of thin, uniform glass or plastic that is highly transparent to light at the wavelengths used. Wavelengths of the ultraviolet region (190–300 nm), require cuvettes which are made of other materials such as quartz or silica.

Two opposing sides of each cuvette will be rib textured, blackened, rough, or sintered (Fig. 12.3).

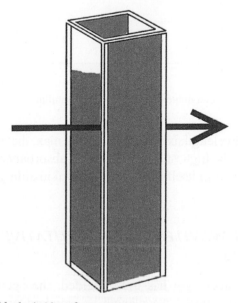

FIGURE 12.3 The blacked sides of a cuvette.

The surfaces of the cuvette through which light passes should be clean, clear, and free of fingerprints and grease. Handle cuvettes by touching the ribbed, blackened, rough, or sintered sides.

For very low analyte concentrations, cells of path lengths longer than 10 mm may be used. For very high analyte concentrations, cells of path length shorter than 10 mm may be used.

High analyte concentration solutions may be diluted so their absorbances are within the absorbance range of the spectrophotometer. And vice versa for solutions which have low analyte concentrations.

12.2.2 WAVELENGTH SCANNING

To determine the specific wavelength at which a user wishes to make a measurement, a wavelength scan is performed.

A wavelength scan is a plot involving absorbance on the y-axis and wavelength on the x-axis, for a particular analyte. This plot is termed a spectrum (Fig. 12.4).

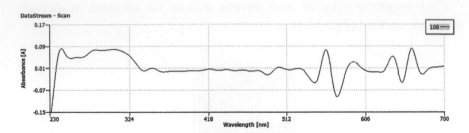

FIGURE 12.4   Spectrum of a dilute solution of methyl vanillin.

This specific wavelength is often the Lambda max, that is, the wavelength which gives rise to the highest clearly resolved absorbance value.

The scan or spectrum itself may also be useful in aiding in the identification of the analyte.

12.2.3   SINGLE WAVELENGTH QUANTITATIVE MEASUREMENTS

Once a specific wavelength has been decided, the spectrophotometer is programmed to that chosen wavelength. A standard or calibration curve of absorbance or transmittance, against concentration, needs to be plotted, (the various levels of concentration of a known standard and the resulting absorbance/transmittance readings are plotted) (Figs. 12.4 and 12.5). The amount of the unknown analyte in the sample is read off against the curve because a factor is derived from a calibration curve.

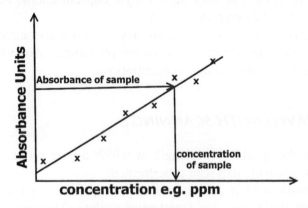

FIGURE 12.5   A typical absorbance calibration curve.

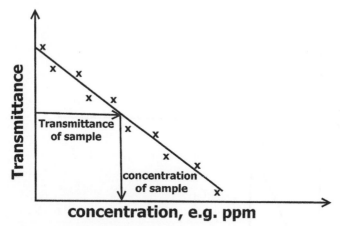

FIGURE 12.6 A typical transmittance calibration curve.

In general, concentration = factor × absorbance.

Often the factor is the gradient of a calibration curve and its intercept on the y-axis.

A factor is unique to an individual spectrophotometer, for a particular analyte, using a specific blank, after a specific type of sample pretreatment, for readings at a specific wavelength.

Before standard or sample readings are taken, a reference or blank (this is a material similar to the standard/sample, but does not contain the analyte of interest) should be placed into the spectrophotometer and the instrument zeroed for that blank at that the chosen wavelength.

The measured absorbance/transmittance of the standards and samples should not extend beyond the spectrophotometer's measuring range. Depending on the of the spectrophotometer's stray light, the best absorbances to aim for are 0.6–0.7 absorbance units.

Stray light is the detected light of any wavelength which is outside the selected wavelength's bandwidth. The larger the stray light, the greater the degree of inaccuracy of absorbance readings which are larger than around 1.5 absorbance units.

Be aware, many analytes exhibit the types of calibration curves shown below:

An analytical scientist cannot, therefore, use the whole of the calibration curves shown in Figures 12.7 and 12.8. They should only use the linear portions, where a clear single gradient (p to q) is seen. Consequently standard and sample concentrations are valid within the concentration range R.

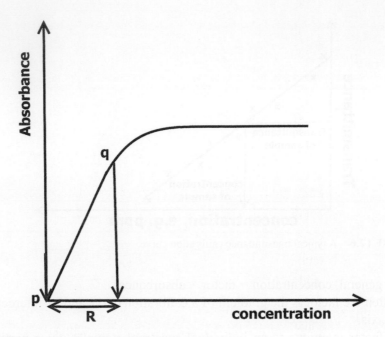

FIGURE 12.7   A typical whole calibration curve.

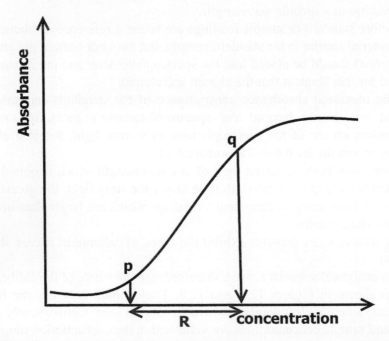

FIGURE 12.8   A sigmoid type of whole calibration curve.

12.2.4 SAMPLE TYPES

Most UV/visible spectrophotometer phytochemical samples are in a liquid form, but sometimes solid samples are used, especially in the determination of transmittance and for reflected color analyses, such as sometimes used for chlorophyll a.

The cuvette/cell or sample container should be appropriate to the type of sample present and the measurement to be determined.

If an analyte does not naturally contain a UV/visible chromophore, a chosen UV/visible chromophore may be added to it chemically, so that the resultant chemically modified or derivatized analyte, may be detected in a UV/visible spectrophotometer.

Additionally, samples may need to be pretreated, to isolate the analyte of interest from the remainder of the sample, or to reduce the levels of interference from other analytes within the sample.

12.2.5 SINGLE-BEAM SPECTROPHOTOMETERS

Here a single beam of light travels through a single sample container and the non-absorbed light is detected by a detector (Fig. 12.9). Many single-beam spectrophotometers, use A filter and a monochromator with a slit, divide the light to the chosen wavelength.

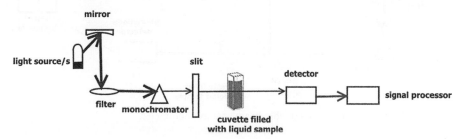

FIGURE 12.9 Schematic of a single-beam spectrophotometer.

The bandwidth (bandpass) of a spectrophotometer, relates to the size of the monochromator's slit, for example, 2 nm.

A narrow bandwidth will produce wavelength scans of higher resolution than scans at higher bandwidths. However, less light energy will reach the detector, so there can be a loss of sensitivity at narrow bandwidths.

When solely a filter is used to split the light, a very wide bandwidth results. In addition, it is not possible to perform wavelength scanning, as discrete filters need to be physically inserted for each wavelength range used.

Single-beam spectrophotometers are of the simplest in design, hence have lower capital and maintenance costs than other spectrophotometer types.

12.2.6   DOUBLE-BEAM SPECTROPHOTOMETERS

In the double-beam spectrophotometer (Fig. 12.10), the light leaving the monochromator is split, using a beam splitter, into a sample beam and a reference beam. After each beam of light is passed through its respective sample/reference (blank) container, each resulting beam is then detected by its own detector. The sample and reference are measured/scanned at the same time, thus saving time and helping to optimize accuracy.

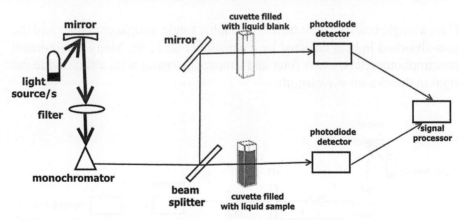

FIGURE 12.10   Schematic of a double-beam spectrophotometer.

Hence, the double-beam spectrophotometer has two detectors. Most detectors are silicon diodes. Double-beam spectrophotometers ensure that any fluctuations in the light emitted from the lamp are applied equally to both the sample and the reference beams. So double-beam spectrophotometers offer around 10 times better stability and two to five times lower baseline noise than single-beam spectrophotometers of the same brand.

For greater sensitivity, a single photomultiplier detector can replace the two silicon diode detectors. Photomultiplier detectors are used in the more expensive spectrophotometers and have a maximum wavelength range of 900 nm. In practice, most UV/visible measurements occur within the 190–750-nm wavelength range.

End-window photomultipliers will collect up to 100 times more light. Consequently, it is possible to measure highly light-scattering (LS) samples. A single photomultiplier detector simultaneously measuring both sample and reference beams is more precise than a two-detector system. Good accuracy and performance occur even at narrow optical bandwidths.

12.2.7 SPLIT-BEAM SPECTROPHOTOMETERS

Here light is divided into two beams, one beam passes through the sample and the other acts as a reference at the detector/s. Hence, a smaller amount of lamp energy is available for use in measurement; consequently, there is a lowering of sensitivity.

12.2.8 DIODE ARRAY SPECTROPHOTOMETERS

Some spectrophotometers have a "bank" of a thousand or so mini detectors or diodes, which are arranged as an array. Each diode will detect the band of wavelength of light which has been focused upon it.

With diode array spectrophotometers (Fig. 12.11), light from the lamp is passed through a polychromator after passing through the sample. The polychromator disperses the light onto the array of diodes so that each diode will measure a discrete band of wavelengths.

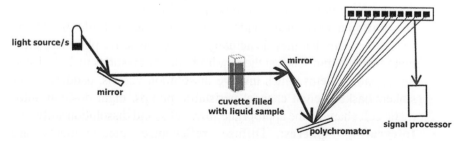

FIGURE 12.11 Schematic of a diode array spectrophotometer.

These diode array spectrophotometers can, therefore, produce a wavelength scan almost instantly, however, the sensitivity of measurements is compromised. No sample compartment lid is necessary and no moving parts are used.

12.2.9 COMMON ACCESSORIES AND CONSUMABLES

Individual spectrophotometers may be used with optional software and optional accessory hardware configurations, defined by an analytical scientist's individual requirements. Examples include:

- **Autosamplers:** These are useful when large numbers of samples require unattended measurement.
- **Calibration standards:** As part of the instrument validation process, these are used to check the wavelength accuracy, absorbance accuracy, stray light, and bandwidth of spectrophotometers. They can be solid filters or solutions.
- **Cells (cuvettes):** A wide variety of rectangular or circular cells are available. Typical path lengths range from 1 to 100 mm. Working volumes can start from 1 µl, especially if nano cell holders are used. Flow cells are used if liquids are to be continuously passed through a single cell. Fiber optic cells may be used if the sample is at some distance from the spectrophotometer.
- **Cell stirring:** There are occasions where the sample should be stirred while the measurements are taken, magnetic flea, cell stirrers are available.
- **Deuterium lamps:** These are used to create wavelengths within the 190–365-nm wavelength range. They are relatively expensive and consumable so that their life is often guaranteed. Many lamps will deteriorate over time, even if they are not used.
- **Dissolution accessories:** Controlled release tablets/capsules need to be tested to ensure that they do actually release the active pharmaceutical ingredient/s or nutrient/s at the required rate. Accessories include dissolution bath systems which involve dissolution vessels, paddles, tester sinkers/baskets, eight channel peristaltic pumps, eight position automatic cell changer, the appropriate flow cells, and dissolution software.
- **Integrating spheres:** Diffuse reflectance measurements are performed by means of an integrating sphere. An integrating sphere consists of a completely spherical chamber. The inner wall of the chamber is made of a material that provides the maximum possible reflectance over the entire visible wavelength range.

- **Multicell changers:** These can be useful, especially when more than one sample is to be measured within a short time space, or over a given period of time, and the process is to be repeated. These changers may be incorporated with temperature-controller devices.
- **PC use and control:** Programs are available to control spectrophotometers and to export spectrophotometer data to a PC/laptop.
- **Sipettes:** These are systems where a sample is aspirated into a flow cell, a reading taken, and the sample returned to its original container or to waste. This is useful for hazardous samples, as less user contact with the sample is achieved. Sipettes are also useful for continuous monitoring of processes.
- **Specular reflectance accessory:** Specular reflectance is normally used for the measurement of samples which reflect surface light but show very little scatter. For example, the reflecting properties of a coated optical mirror may be measured.
- **Temperature controllers:** Sometimes samples need to be measured at specific temperatures. Thermoelectric Peltier devices offer a fast and temperature programmable means. Circulating laboratory water baths may also be coupled to spectrophotometer cell holders to achieve a specific cell temperature.
- **Tungsten halogen lamps:** These are used to create wavelengths within the 320–1100-nm wavelength range.
- **Xenon lamps:** These are used to create wavelengths within the 190–1100-nm wavelength range. They are relatively expensive and consumable, so they often use "press to read" technology, to automatically switch on, when a measurement needs to be made. However, they do not emit good energy levels within the whole of the 190–1100-nm wavelength range, and they can emit an irritating high-pitched noise.

12.2.10   AN EXAMPLE OF A PRACTICAL PROCEDURE

Here is a typical procedure for the use of a double-beam spectrophotometer, in the determination of nicotine from a tobacco plant leaf sample:

1. Within a fume cupboard, use an accepted method to pretreat and derivatize nicotine standards of different concentrations from 0.5 to 5 µg/mL with potassium permanganate in the presence of sodium hydroxide to form a water-soluble green product. Also, treat a liquid blank in the same manner.

2. Within a fume cupboard, extract the nicotine from a dry finely ground leaf sample, by solubilization, precipitation, filtration, and centrifugation, using an accepted method. Derivatize the extract with potassium permanganate in the presence of sodium hydroxide.

3. Switch on the spectrophotometer and wait for any warm-up calibration checks to finish.

4. Fill to near the top, two 10-mm path length glass or silica cells with aliquots of the treated bank solution. Position each filled cuvette, into a cell holder of the spectrophotometer's sample compartment. Close the compartment cover.

5. Program the spectrophotometer to perform a baseline wavelength scan of the 400–750-nm wavelength range.

6. Remove the cell of the sample position, empty, rinse then fill with an aliquot of a treated standard.

7. Position the standard filled cuvette, into the sample position cell holder, of the spectrophotometer's sample compartment. Close the compartment cover.

8. Program the spectrophotometer to perform a wavelength scan of the 400–750-nm wavelength range.

9. Make a note of the Lambda max, this should be at around 610 nm.

10. Program the spectrophotometer to take absorbance readings at the Lambda max or 610 nm.

11. Remove the cell holder from the sample position, empty, rinse then fill with an aliquot of the treated blank.

12. Position the blank filled cuvette, into the sample position cell holder, of the spectrophotometer's sample compartment. Close the compartment cover.

13. Press the spectrophotometer's "zero" function and wait for the absorbance reading to show 0.000 absorbance units.

14. Remove the cell holder from the sample position, empty, rinse then fill with an aliquot of the lowest concentration treated standard.

15. Position the standard filled cuvette, into the sample position cell holder, of the spectrophotometer's sample compartment. Close the compartment cover. Note the absorbance reading.

16. Remove the cell holder from the sample position, empty, rinse then fill with an aliquot of the next lowest concentration treated standard.

17. Position the standard filled cuvette, into the sample position cell holder, of the spectrophotometer's sample compartment. Close the compartment cover. Note the absorbance reading.

18. Repeat steps 14 to 15 until readings have been taken of each standard. If any standards are too concentrated for an absorbance reading to be given, dilute with blank solution and make a note of the dilution.
19. Construct a calibration curve (see Section 2.3) and make a note of the factor obtained from the curve.
20. Remove the cell holder from the sample position, empty, rinse then fill with an aliquot of the treated sample.
21. Position the sample filled cuvette, into the sample position cell holder, of the spectrophotometer's sample compartment. Close the compartment cover. Note the absorbance reading.
22. Use this absorbance reading and the factor, to calculate the concentration of nicotine in the sample. If any dilutions of the treated sample were made, take this dilution into account for the final concentration of nicotine in the sample.

In practice, once a full calibration curve of some five to seven standards has been obtained, everyday analysis, using the same spectrophotometer, is often performed using just one or two standards.

12.2.11 CHECKS ON SPECTROPHOTOMETERS

Checks should be made that the spectrophotometer is functioning correctly, to the manufacturer's specifications.

When the spectrophotometer is first used, installation qualification (IQ) checks may be performed to ensure that the instrument has been adequately installed and configured.

Operating qualification (OQ) checks are used to ensure that the spectrophotometer is functioning correctly, to the manufacturer's specifications. These checks often involve verification of the wavelength accuracy, absorbance accuracy, stray light, and bandwidth.

Performance qualification (PQ) involves procedures when laboratory personnel regularly check to verify that the spectrophotometer is performing for its intended application.

As part of the above instrument validation process, certified solid filters and/or reagent solutions are used.

In addition to the above, when an analyte in an untried sample matrix is presented, and no established method is known of, analytical scientists may have to perform method development. This is where accurate, robust, reliable, and scientifically valid methods, to determine a particular analyte in the presence of a particular sample matrix is created and tested.

This developed method may then be validated, where checks on the accuracy, detection and quantitation limits, linearity, precision, repeatability, range, recovery, robustness, sample solution stability, and specificity/selectivity are performed. A validated method may then be sent (transferred) to other laboratories for use in the detection of that particular analyte in that particular sample matrix.

12.3   HIGH-PERFORMANCE LIQUID CHROMATOGRAPHY (HPLC)

High-performance liquid chromatography (HPLC) is an established technique, with inbuilt flexibilities to isolate, detect, and measure billions of phytochemical and impurity analytes within a wide variety of sample matrices. Figure 12.12 is a typical Q-Adept HPLC system.

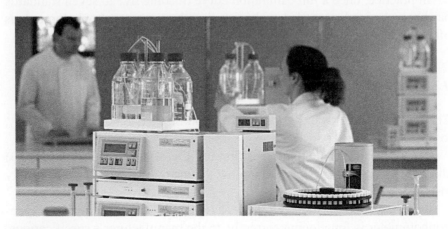

FIGURE 12.12   A typical Q-Adept high-performance liquid chromatography (HPLC) system.

Source: Courtesy to Cecil Instruments, Milton Technical Centre, Cambridge, CB24 6AZ, United Kingdom.

12.3.1   THEORY

HPLC is performed by the injection of a small amount of a sample liquid mixture into the flow of another liquid (called the mobile phase), which travels through a column packed with particles of stationary phase, under high pressure.

In a basic example (Fig. 12.13), component A has the same interaction with the stationary phase as the mobile phase. Component B has a stronger interaction with the stationary phase than it has with the mobile phase. After a mixture of both A and B has been injected into the column, these components will be forced through the column by the flow of the mobile phase. Molecules of component A will interact with the stationary phase and adsorb to it in the same way that the mobile phase does. Hence, component A will travel through or elute through the column with the same speed as the mobile phase.

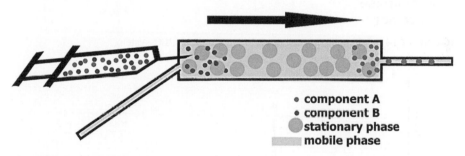

FIGURE 12.13 **(See color insert.)** Distribution of analytes and liquid in an HPLC column.

Because molecules of component B are more strongly adsorbed onto the stationary phase they will interact with the stationary phase for much longer than component A does. Hence, component B will move through the column at a slower rate than the mobile phase.

The presence of each component is detected by a signal within a detector (Fig. 12.14), after they have passed through the column. A detector is a device that senses the presence of components different from the liquid mobile phase and converts that information into an electrical signal. Different types of detectors can be used in HPLC, the type depends on which physical/chemical property of the analytes may be taken advantage of.

Hence, compounds A and B will exit the column at different times, that is, they have different retention times. The retention time is the time between injection and detection.

The detector will transmit this signal information to PC or Mac chromatography software, or to a printer plotter or to an integrator.

A plot of the analyte signal detected against retention time is a chromatogram (Fig 12.15).

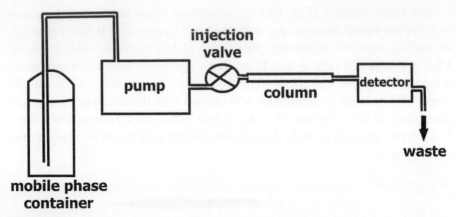

FIGURE 12.14 Schematic of the liquid flow within an HPLC system.

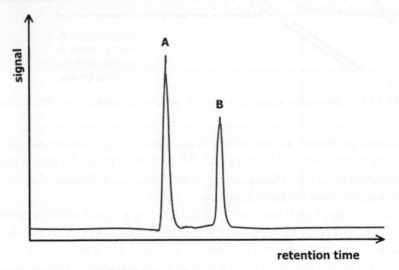

FIGURE 12.15 A general HPLC chromatogram.

The figure below represents the general shape of the chromatogram for the mixture of A and B, showing the effective separation of components A and B, within the mixture. The peaks of components A and B are adequately resolved from each other.

Within chromatograms, once all the expected analyte peaks are seen, the separation efficiency of peaks may be quantified by means of parameters such as resolution (Fig. 12.16), peak asymmetry, tailing factor, capacity factor, and theoretical plates. The degree of acceptability will vary within different laboratory environment types.

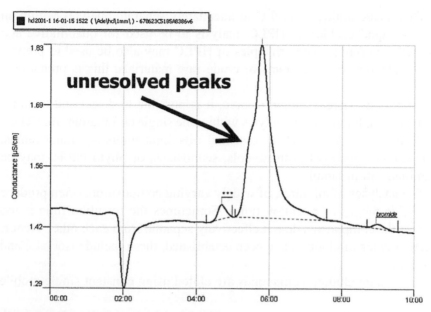

FIGURE 12.16 An unresolved chromatographic peak.

The figure below (Fig. 12.17) is a chromatogram for a mixture of artemisiten and artemisinin.

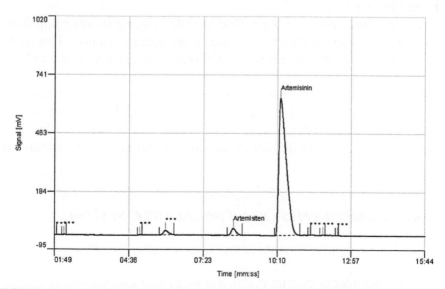

FIGURE 12.17 A chromatogram for a mixture of artemisiten and artemisinin.

This innate ability of HPLC to adequately separate analytes within an injected liquid enables an HPLC analysis to be used for quantitative and qualitative purposes. The principles of HPLC may also be used to prepare refined phytochemical extracts of crude raw materials, this is preparative HPLC.

Within one injected liquid sample, it is possible to detect and quantify one to several hundreds of analytes within one single chromatogram. Hence, whole analyte groups such as essential oils, cannabinoids, anthocyanins, capsaicinoids, tetrahydrocannabinols, sennosides, or phytosterols, may be examined within samples.

The analyses of mixtures, of widely varying composition, often produce very wide ranges of retention times. Sometimes the retention time is too long, or the components do not effectively separate from each other. Hence, different types of elution have been established, these include isocratic and gradient.

In isocratic elution, compounds are eluted using constant single mobile phase.

In gradient elution, components are eluted by increasing the strength of the mobile phase. Two different mobile phases (binary gradient), three different mobile phases (ternary gradient), or four different mobile phases (quaternary gradient) can be used. In practice most HPLC methods use a maximum of two different mobile phases, a few, use three, and only a very rare number use four.

With gradient elution, it is possible to elute compounds emerging from a column, more rapidly than they would, in an isocratic elution. This lends itself well in the case of complex mixtures of analyte groups, such as cannabinoids.

The interaction of the analyte with mobile and stationary phases can be manipulated through different choices of both mobile and stationary phases. As a result, HPLC incorporates a high degree of versatility and selectivity and thus has the ability to easily separate a wide variety of chemical mixtures.

12.3.2   COMPONENTS OF A TYPICAL HPLC SYSTEM

A typical HPLC system consists of the following (Fig. 12.18).

- Sample inlet or injector (valve and loop) instrumentation.
- An optional degasser instrument.

- A mobile phase system including mobile phase reservoir/s and pump/s instrumentation for delivering mobile phase.
- A column.
- Detector instrumentation.
- Instrumentation which will transfer data from the detector to a PC, integrator, printer, or chart recorder.

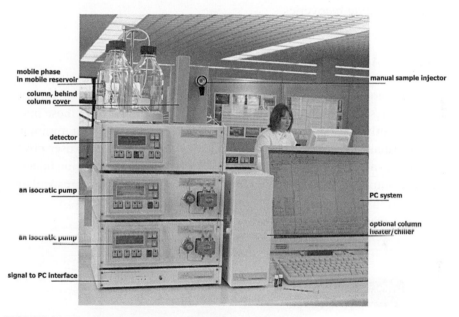

FIGURE 12.18 HPLC system components.

Some HPLC systems are supplied as modular instrumentation, so that analytical scientists may choose to mix and match the modular instrumentation components. Others are integrated as one single item of instrumentation.

12.3.2.1 SAMPLES

Representative homogenous samples introduced to HPLC systems must be in a liquid form. So solids may need to be dissolved, combusted, or melted, and gas samples need to be condensed or solubilized into liquid states.

In addition, samples may need to be pretreated by a variety of techniques such as grinding, homogenization, maceration, filtration, centrifugation, liquid/liquid extraction, and solid-phase extraction (SPE), in order to isolate the analyte/s of interest from the remainder of the sample (sample matrix), or to reduce the levels of interference from other analytes. Derivatization may also be required to render the analyte of interest detectable to the required detector. The pretreated sample may then diluted/concentrated as appropriate.

Storage of pretreated samples within certain temperature ranges and within nominated time periods may be specified.

Whatever sample treatment is used, it must be reproducible and produce acceptable analyte recoveries.

12.3.2.2   SAMPLE INLET OR INJECTORS

Physically, liquid solutions are injected into moving streams of pumped mobile phase/s at high pressures (Fig. 12.19). In order to perform these injections efficiently and safely, special injection valves are used. As a minimum, six-port manual injection valves may be used, where the HPLC user physically turns a valve for each injected liquid. The volume of the solution injected onto the column/s is limited by an injection loop. Injection loops are available in a wide variety of sizes, ranging from around 1 µl to several mL.

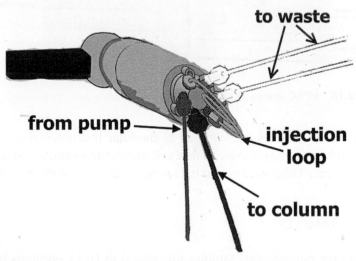

FIGURE 12.19   Typical manual injection valve and loop.

Large numbers of samples can be analyzed by HPLC without a user having to perform manual injections, by virtue of automatic sample injectors or autosamplers. Autosamplers are also very useful as their injection volume and technique is exactly the same for each required injection, hence they provide a large degree of injection volume precision.

12.3.2.3   DEGASSING

Mobile phase needs to be free of air before it reaches the pump/column. Scientists have three main options for degassing the mobile phase:

Sonication, by placing containers of mobile phase into ultrasonic water baths and sonicating until the air is deemed to have escaped the container. This method is off-line and time-consuming.

Sparging with an inert gas, here the mobile phase is sparged with an inert gas such as helium. This off-line method is very time-consuming.

Online degassers, these are machines which will remove gases by vacuum, from the mobile phase just before the mobile phase enters the pump. They are very efficient. The mobile phase is degassed as and when it is required.

12.3.2.4   MOBILE PHASE

The composition and polarity of the mobile phase have a great influence on retention time. Alteration of the mobile phase is one of the simplest means of improving chromatographic resolution of two overlapping analytes. However, the selection of mobile phase can be tricky, and this is part of the science of HPLC.

Depending on the analyte, column, and detector types, mobile phases can include an array of different solvents, used with different modifiers and/or buffers, at different pHs and concentrations.

A good starting point is a mixture of water and a polar organic solvent (methanol or acetonitrile).

If greater selectivity is required, a mobile phase composed of three or four different constituents may be used.

Anion/cation exchange columns involve a smaller choice of a choice of solvents, modifiers, buffers, and pHs.

12.3.2.5   PUMPS

In HPLC, the pump which is used to deliver the mobile phase at a uniform rate operates at very high pressures to around 40 MPa. Different pumps will operate at different ranges of flow rate capabilities, of a few microliters per minute at the nanoscale, to the preparative scale of liters per minute.

Gradient elutions may be achieved by use of high-pressure mixing systems, where individual isocratic high-pressure pumps are used to provide the proportions of each mobile phase. All the mobile phases are then blended under high pressure, into a homogenous mixture, before being introduced to the column.

As an alternative, low-pressure mixing systems may be used, where a single pump, with up to four channels, will blend proportions of up to four different mobile phases under low pressure and then pump at high pressures that homogenizes mixture onto a column.

The main advantage of low-pressure mixing is that it offers the ability to blend two or more mobile phases with one pump, hence a lower purchase price than for high-pressure mixing.

However, high-pressure mixing does offer a rapid proportioning response and a more precise creation and control of gradients.

12.3.2.6   COLUMNS

There is a bewildering array of different HPLC columns available, but it is helpful to remember that most columns fall into the following main category types:

- Reversed phase, for use where the analytes of interest are fairly polar. C8 and C18 columns being the most popular.
- Normal phase, for use where the analytes of interest are nonpolar.
- Size exclusion/gel permeation, for use where the analytes of interest have fairly large molecular weights.
- Chiral, for use where the analytes of interest are found in stable isomeric forms.
- Anion/cation exchange, for use where analytes are ions or can be converted to ions.
- Affinity, where ligand binding may be exploited.
- Specialist, for use with analytes with special functional groups such as glycoproteins.
- There are some column categories which will use a combination of separation modes, such as hydrophilic interaction liquid chromatography, for use with highly hydrophilic analytes.

The column on which the intended separation is performed is the analytical column. In order to preserve the life of the relatively expensive analytical column, a smaller and cheaper guard column is often used, so that the injected sample may first pass through the guard column, which will filter out extraneous material before the sample reaches the analytical column.

Generally, the analytical column can vary in size from around 70 μm in internal diameter (nano-HPLC) to around 50 mm in internal diameter (preparative HPLC). The length can vary from around 50 to some 300 mm.

12.3.2.7   COLUMN HEATER/CHILLERS

Maintaining analytical columns at constant temperatures helps to ensure that retention times are reproducible. Constant temperatures cannot usually be maintained if the column is kept at the ambient temperatures of the laboratory atmosphere. Column heater/chillers or ovens are housings, which provide constant and reproducible temperature control. In addition, in general, faster separations will occur when the temperature of the analytical column is increased, and vice versa at lower temperatures. There are some HPLC analyses, where temperature programming over the course of each elution is desirable.

12.3.2.8   DETECTORS

There are many types of detectors that can be used with HPLC. The more common detectors include:

12.3.2.8.1   UV/Visible Detectors

If the analytes have a UV/visible chromophore such as ergosterol, artemisinin, lanosterol, and campesterol or if a chromophore can be added, as in the case of some mycotoxins, a UV/visible detector may be of enormous value as UV/ visible detectors measure the ability of an analyte or its derivative, to absorb light. This can be accomplished at one or several wavelengths.

1.   Fixed wavelength detectors measure at only one wavelength, usually 254 nm.
2.   Variable wavelength detectors measure at one wavelength at a time, but can be used over a wide range of wavelengths.

3. Dual wavelength detectors can simultaneously measure at more than one wavelength.

4. Scanning detectors can simultaneously measure at more than one wavelength and can also perform spectral scanning over a range of wavelengths.

5. Diode Array detectors can measure at more than one wavelength and can also perform spectral scanning over a range of wavelengths.

UV/visible detectors usually have a maximum sensitivity of 1×10^{-8} or 1×10^{-9} g/mL.

12.3.2.8.2 Conductivity Detectors

These detectors focus on the electrical conductivity of ions, so will detect an analyte, such as oxalic acid, histamine, and malic acid, on the basis of ionic charge. Users can expect sensitivities of around 6×10^{-9} g/mL.

12.3.2.8.3 Fluorescence Detectors

These detectors measure the ability of analytes or treated analytes, such as lysergic acid and aflatoxins, to absorb then reemit light at given wavelengths. The typical maximum sensitivity is around 1×10^{-9}–1×10^{-11} g/mL.

12.3.2.8.4 Refractive Index Detectors

These detectors measure the ability of sample molecules such as sugars and alcohols, to bend or refract light. They are also particularly useful for large analyte molecules, such as long-chain oligosaccharides, some polyalcohols, tannins, and triglycerides. The typical maximum sensitivity limit is around 1×10^{-5} g/mL.

12.3.2.8.5 Radiochemical Detectors

Detection involves the use of radiolabelled material, usually tritium or carbon[14]. They operate by detection of fluorescence associated with β-particle ionization.

A typical maximum sensitivity limit is around 1×10^{-9}–1×10^{-10} g/mL.

12.3.2.8.6 Electrochemical Detectors

These detectors measure analytes such as flavonoids, capsaicins, and ergosines that undergo oxidation or reduction reactions within an electrical current. The typical maximum sensitivity limit is 1×10^{-12}–1×10^{-13} g/mL.

12.3.2.8.7 Mass Spectroscopy Detectors

There are various types of mass spectroscopy (MS) detectors. Here the analyte is ionized, then passed through a mass analyzer, and the ion current is detected. A wide range of analytes, particularly numerous analytes within a group, may be detected in this manner. The maximum sensitivity limit is around 1×10^{-8}–1×10^{-10} g/mL.

Other detectors include charged aerosol for nonvolatile analytes, nuclear magnetic resonance (NMR) detectors, LS detectors for large analyte molecules and near-infrared detectors.

12.3.2.9 SOFTWARE

In order to humanly visualize a chromatogram, data needs to be transferred from the detector, during the passage of time of a chromatogram, to a form which may be viewed by a human. Chart plotters, printers, and integrators were commonly used in the past to view chromatograms. Integrators, and/or rulers were used to take measurements of the chromatogram.

Nowadays, chromatographic software is mainly used. As a minimum, this should be able to acquire, manipulate, and process chromatograms. Most chromatography data systems will also control instrumentation, such as pumps, detectors, autosamplers, column heater/chillers, and so forth.

From the data, retention times, peak heights, and peak areas are viewed. After peak integration, calibration curves and automatic calculation of unknown quantities in samples should be possible.

Often users require traceability of the chromatogram acquisition and any modification to a chromatogram. The US Food and Drug Administration's codicil 21 CFR part 11 compliance of the software is used to this end.

Sometimes, automatic transfer of the reported chromatographic data to a laboratory information management system is required.

12.3.3 HPLC AS AN AID TO ANALYTE IDENTIFICATION

An analytical scientist must be certain that each resolved chromatographic peak seen, represents a single identified analyte. One must be sure that co-elution has not occurred. Co-elution is where two or more analytes elute within the same chromatographic peak.

Providing that each analyte has its own discernible profile/spectrum, there are some HPLC detectors which lend themselves very well to providing spectral scans of chromatographic peaks as they elute, in the determination of co-elution detection. These scanning detectors include mass spectrometers, ultrafast scanning UV/visible HPLC detectors, diode array, and some scanning fluorescence detectors.

In order to achieve a reasonable separation of all of the expected analytes within a reasonable time, the HPLC method may need to be tweaked, by attempting changes in column type, column dimensions, column temperatures mobile phase/s, flow rates, and detection wavelength/s (in the case of UV/visible and fluorescence detectors).

In addition, the identity of each peak must also be verified. So during the development of an HPLC method, it is common to check the identity of the eluted peak, using another analytical confirmatory technique, such as a MS technique, X-ray absorption fluorescence, X-ray diffraction, and NMR.

Once the identity of each fully resolved chromatographic peak has been established, qualitative HPLC analysis may be achieved, by comparing the retention time of eluted peaks in a sample, to those of a known standard (Fig. 12.20).

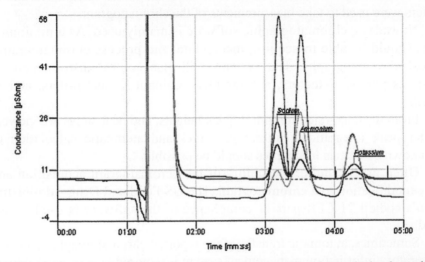

FIGURE 12.20   Overlaid chromatograms showing analyte peaks of a standard and samples.

12.3.4 HPLC AS AN AID TO ANALYTE QUANTITATION

Quantitative HPLC analysis is achieved by measurement of the areas or heights of the peaks in the chromatogram.

Before the area or height of a peak can be measured, the user must decide upon the location of the baseline of the chromatographic peak. This is termed peak integration, where the baselines of peaks in chromatograms, and the start and end of peaks are identified and drawn (Fig. 12.21).

If a chart recorder or printer is used, a user may manually draw the baseline with a ruler. If chromatography software or an integrator is used, parameters may be set to automatically or manually draw a baseline. The setting of automatic parameters can sometimes require a little trial and error, but it is worthwhile, as then all subsequent peaks of that type of chromatogram, will be automatically integrated.

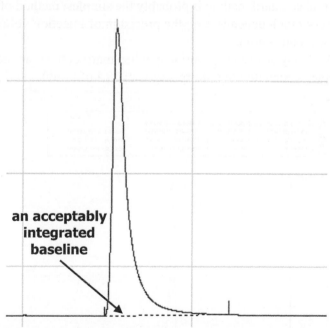

an acceptably integrated baseline

FIGURE 12.21   A chromatographic peak displaying its integrated baseline.

Once an analytical peak of interest has been successfully integrated, there are then four main modes of analyte calibration which an analytical scientist may use, for the quantification of analytes within their sample(s).

When each analyte has its own specific quantitative response to a detector, external standard, internal standard, and standard addition methods may be used. With each of these methods, initial determinations of the linear/proportional range of the concentrations are normally required. The analytical scientist must make up separate analytical standard solutions, using a high-purity chemical.

Normalization may be used for groups of analytes which do not have their own specific quantitative responses to a detector.

12.3.5 EXTERNAL STANDARD

Aliquots of an analyte standard of known concentrations, are injected separately from actual samples, and the acquired response factor, is used to calculate the concentration of that same analyte within a sample(s) (Figs. 12.22 and 12.23).

The external standard method is probably the simplest method of calibration and is very much dependent on the precision of injection volume, so it is good to use an autosampler.

The method may be used appropriately when matrix effects are negligible and for samples which do not require large degrees of sample pretreatment.

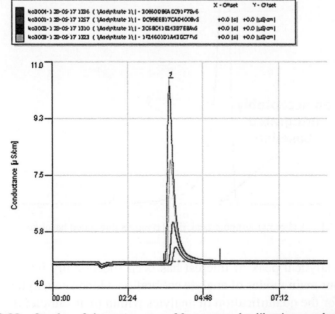

FIGURE 12.22 Overlay of chromatograms of four external calibration standards.

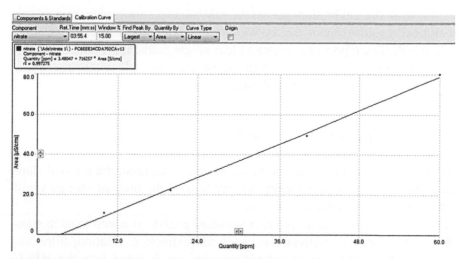

FIGURE 12.23 The calibration curve made using the four external standards.

A direct plot of the detector responses of each appropriate analyte standard peak, to its concentration, is used to create a calibration curve (Fig. 12.24).

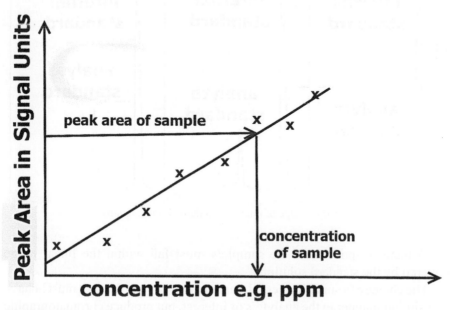

FIGURE 12.24 Individual chromatographic peak areas, of each standard, may be plotted onto a calibration curve.

As with the calibration curves of UV/visible spectrophotometers, an analytical scientist cannot use the whole of a calibration curve, they should only use the linear portions, where a clear single gradient is seen.

So the detector response/s of the sample/s must fall within the linear range covered by the standard solutions.

12.3.6   INTERNAL STANDARD

When a large amount of sample pretreatment is required, the internal standard method may be appropriate, as any loss of the internal standard will correlate to losses of the analyte/s of interest.

The same amount of an internal standard analyte is added to each standard/sample prior to pretreatment, such as (extraction, dilution, filtration, centrifugation, etc.). The standards/samples are injected into the HPLC system. The ratio of the detector response of the standard peak, to the internal standard peak, is used to create a calibration curve (Figs. 12.25 and 12.26).

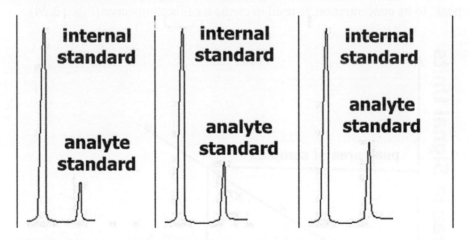

FIGURE 12.25   Composite image of internal standard chromatograms.

Detector response/s of the sample/s must fall within the linear range covered by the standard solutions.

The choice of a suitable internal standard can be complex as it must behave in a similar manner to the analyte/s of interest, but produce chromatographic peaks which are well resolved from the analyte/s of interest. The internal standard should also have a similar linear response as the sample.

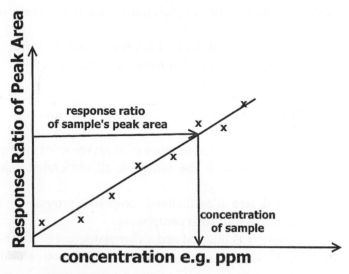

FIGURE 12.26 Individual chromatographic peak area ratios, of each standard, may be plotted onto a calibration curve.

12.3.7 STANDARD ADDITIONS

If sample matrix effects are problematic to resolve, the standard addition method may be used as a means of calibration. The standard additions calibration method is often used when working with complex sample matrices, such as clinical, biological, or food samples.

To negate interference from components within the sample matrix, a known amount of pure standard is added as a sample (spiking). This spiked sample then becomes a standard. The technique is also useful when a blank sample matrix is not available.

As an example, equal volumes of the same sample are added to say seven volumetric flasks. The same volume, but differing concentrations of the analytical standard, is then added to each of seven flasks. So each of the seven flasks represents an analyte concentration of say 0, 10, 20, 30, 40, 50, and 60 concentration units. Make up each flask to volume using a suitable solvent. Then pretreat (extract/dilute, centrifuge, filter etc.) each sample and inject on the HPLC system.

A direct plot of the detector response of each standard peak, to standard concentrations, is used to create a calibration curve. There will be an intercept on the detector response axis.

The detector response/s of the sample/s must fall within the range covered by the standard solutions.

Spiking may also be used to quickly check the identity, by virtue of retention time, of an analyte/s of interest's chromatographic peak.

12.3.8   NORMALIZATION

This applies to only a very limited number of analyses where the quantitative response of the detector is the same for all the eluted analytes of interest.

The percentage peak area of each eluted component provides an estimate of the relative concentration of each component.

Here, an actual sample is injected and a chromatogram is obtained.

For each peak of interest, a normalization calculation, based on the formula, is created:

$$percentage\ peak\ area\ of\ analyte\ A = \left(\frac{peak\ area\ of\ analyte\ A}{\sum of\ other\ relevant\ peak\ areas} \right) x100.$$

A one-off response factor must be obtained for one peak. The calculation is:

$$response\ factor = \frac{peak\ area\ of\ analyte\ A}{concentration\ of\ analyte\ A}.$$

To correlate the normalized quantity of peak B in a sample, the calculation would be:

$$\frac{percentage\ peak\ area\ of\ analyte\ B}{response\ factor}.$$

12.3.9   CHECKS ON AN HPLC SYSTEM

Checks should be made that an HPLC system is functioning correctly, to the manufacturer's specifications.

When the HPLC system is first used, IQ checks may be performed to ensure that the instrumentation has been adequately installed and configured.

OQ checks are used to ensure that the HPLC system is functioning correctly, to the manufacturer's specifications. These checks often involve verification of a UV/visible detector's wavelength accuracy, absorbance accuracy, absorbance linearity, stray light, and bandwidth; detector noise; pump flow rate accuracy, flow rate precision, proportioning accuracy, proportioning precision; column oven temperature accuracy and temperature precision; and autosampler sample volume reproducibility and carry over.

PQ is where laboratory personnel regularly check to verify that the HPLC is performing for its intended method. These checks are often included within system suitability checks. They include checks on retention time, theoretical plates, peak resolution, peak asymmetry (tailing factor), detection limits, precision, and recovery.

In addition to the above, when an analyte in an untried sample matrix is presented, and no established method is known of, analytical scientists may have to perform method development. This is where accurate, robust, reliable, and scientifically valid methods, to determine a particular analyte in the presence of a particular sample matrix is created and tested. This developed method may then be validated, where checks on the accuracy, detection and quantitation limits, linearity, precision, repeatability, range, recovery, robustness, sample solution stability, and specificity/selectivity are performed. A validated method may then be sent (transferred) to other laboratories for use in the detection of that particular analyte in the particular sample matrix.

12.3.10 TRENDS IN HPLC INSTRUMENTATION

Despite HPLC being a mature technique, enhancements on the basic concept, continuously arise. This is fuelled partly by the desire for increased speed, the reduction in the use of solvents and other required materials, simplification and space saving.

Developments such as online sample preparation, particularly in the form of SPE, sample filtration, pre-column derivatization and post-column derivatization; multidimensional hyphenated systems; nano-flow chip integrated circuit miniaturization (lab-on-a-chip); multidetector sequential analysis; high-throughput analysis, and fast and ultra-high pressure HPLC, are already occurring.

KEYWORDS

- UV/visible spectrophotometer
- HPLC
- identification
- quantification
- phytochemicals

REFERENCES

Kujore, A. Cecil Instruments. *Introduction to UV/Visible Spectrophotometers*. http://www. cecilinstruments.com/introduction-to-uv-visible-spectrophotometers.html (accessed Sep 5, 2017).

Kujore, A. Cecil Instruments. *Introduction to HPLC and Ion Chromatography*. http://www. cecilinstruments.com/introduction-to-HPLC-and-ion-chromatography.html (accessed Sep 12, 2017).

Kujore, A. Cecil Instruments. *HPLC and Ion Chromatography Calibration Primer*. http:// www.cecilinstruments.com/hplc-and-ion-chromatography-calibration-primer.html (accessed Oct 2, 2017.

Kujore, A. Cecil Instruments. *Response to a question on Research Gate*. https://www. researchgate.net/post/Is_it_necessary_to_use_istd_while_performing_HPLC_What_if_ istd_is_not_used (accessed Oct 8, 2017.

Kujore, A. Cecil Instruments. *Response to a question on Research Gate*. https://www. researchgate.net/post/How_to_determine_purity_of_an_isolated_unknown_compound_ without_using_standard (accessed Aug 8, 2017.

CHAPTER 13

HIGH-PERFORMANCE LIQUID CHROMATOGRAPHY AND HIGH-PERFORMANCE THIN-LAYER CHROMATOGRAPHY AS SOPHISTICATED TOOLS IN PHYTOCHEMICAL ANALYSIS

DEEPA R. VERMA[1],[*] and ROHAN V. GAVANKAR[2]

[1]*Department of Botany, VIVA College of Arts, Commerce and Science, Virar, Maharashtra, India, Mob.: +91-9766663740*

[2]*Department of Biotechnology, VIVA College of Arts, Commerce and Science, Virar, Maharashtra, India*

[*]*Corresponding author. E-mail: deepaverma@vivacollege.org*

ABSTRACT

Plants are rich in naturally occurring chemical compounds which are the end products of several metabolic pathways. These compounds are referred as phytochemicals (from Greek *phyto*, meaning plant). Phytochemicals are primarily synthesized to carry out the physiological functions of plants. Qualitative profiling and quantitative estimation of plant metabolites have become an area of interest for several researchers as these metabolites can be tapped for their therapeutic properties. However, the major challenge is separation and estimation of these phytoconstituents. The traditional screening methods with modern analytical tools can be a solution to this problem. The chapter highlights the significance of high-performance liquid chromatography and high-performance thin-layer chromatography as analytical tools to generate chemoprofiles of plants. The chapter illustrates the basic steps such as sample preparation, selection of mobile phase, the significance of derivatization, and data interpretation.

13.1   INTRODUCTION

Phytochemicals are naturally occurring chemical compounds which are the end products of several metabolic pathways. They are primarily synthesized to carry out the physiological functions of plants. These compounds give plant their color, flavor, and aroma. For example, the beautiful variegated foliage of *Coleus* is due to the anthocyanin, the flavor and aroma of *Mentha* are due to menthol and pulegone. These metabolites also protect the plant against pathogenic attack.

Ecologically, plants are referred to as "producers" which is the source of food and energy; physiologically, plants are nature's "chemical production units" which provide us with various chemical compounds which are explored for varied uses. Man's prime interest in the plant is to fulfill his basic need of food, clothing, and shelter. Plants have been traditionally used as a primary source in the cure of several diseases and have been mentioned in folklore and well scripted in Ayurveda. Today, several tribes depend on the plants not only for food but also for the cure of various diseases.

Natural vegetation has been a potential source of flavoring agents, food additives, preservatives in the manufacture of various industrial products, but considering the richness of the plant world, the knowledge and potential of plants acquired by man are still insufficient. The number of species about which men have reasonably detailed knowledge is probably less than 1% (Sivarajan, 1991). Several researchers are working in the fields of taxonomy, ethnobotany, and assessment of the plant genetic resources so as to explore and document the plant wealth which will serve as new resources of herbal drugs used by the aborigines. The World Health Organization describes a medicinal plant as any plant in which one or more of its organs contain substances that can be used for therapeutic purposes or which are precursors for the synthesis of useful drugs.

The medicinal values of these plants are direct function of the phytochemical constituents which are synthesized naturally by the various plant parts through metabolic pathways. These phytoconstituents can be used as therapeutic agents as they have a definite physiological effect on the microorganisms (antimicrobial properties) as well as on human body (pharmacological effect). The man has consumed plants or plant parts as a source of carbohydrates, protein, and lipids through the food. In addition to it, he has also consumed a multitude of compounds such as glycosides, alkaloids, flavonoids, and so forth in various Ayurvedic formulations.

On the basis of the physiological functions, phytochemicals can be divided into two groups

    i.   Primary metabolites: It comprises of common sugars, amino acid, proteins, and chlorophyll.

    ii.   Secondary metabolites: It comprises of alkaloids, terpenoids, saponins, phenolic compounds, flavonoids, tannins, and so on.

The qualitative and quantitative estimation of the phytochemical constituents of a medicinal plant (Fig. 13.1) is considered to be an important step in medicinal plant research (Kokate, 1994).

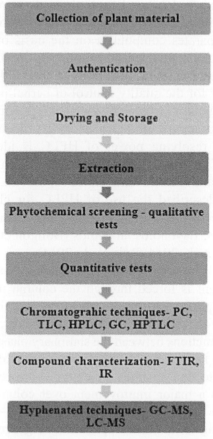

FIGURE 13.1   Steps involved in phytochemical analysis.

Qualitative profiling and quantitative estimation of plant metabolites have become an area of interest for several researchers as these metabolites can be tapped for their therapeutic properties. However, the major challenge is separation and estimation of these phytoconstituents. Traditional screening methods with modern analytical tools can be a solution to this problem.

13.2   HIGH-PERFORMANCE LIQUID CHROMATOGRAPHY (HPLC) – OVERVIEW

High-performance liquid chromatography (HPLC) is a widely used analytical technique and is versatile and robust. It is used for the separation as well as the determination of organic and inorganic solutes from the majority of samples (industrial, pharmaceutical, food, environment samples) and is being widely used for biological samples as well and for the isolation of natural products. HPLC also known as high-pressure liquid chromatography separates compounds on the basis of their interactions with solid particles of a tightly packed column and the solvent of the mobile phase. This technique is gaining popularity as one of the major choice for fingerprinting study for the quality control of herbal products (Fan et al., 2006). Natural products are frequently isolated following the evaluation of a relatively crude extract in a biological assay in order to fully characterize its properties. The resolving power of HPLC is ideally suited to the rapid processing of such multicomponent samples on both an analytical and preparative scale (Martin and Guichon, 2005). Many researchers and authors have described the use of HPLC for characterization and quantification of secondary metabolites in plant extracts, mainly phenol compounds, steroids, flavonoids, alkaloids (Boligon et al., 2013; Barbosa et al., 2014; Colpo et al., 2014; Reis et al., 2014).

HPLC is a highly improved form of column chromatography. In this technique, the solvent is forced through the column under high pressure of up to 400 atmospheres instead of solvent to drip through the column. Smaller particle size for the column packing material gives it a much greater surface area for interactions between the stationary phase and the molecules flowing past it. This facilitates much better separation of the components of the mixture. The detection methods are extremely sensitive and are highly automated which is a major improvement over column chromatography. There are two most commonly used mode of HPLC – normal phase and reverse phase. Owing to its broad application range, reversed-phase chromatography (Fig. 13.2) is the most commonly used separation technique in

HPLC. Over 65% of all HPLC separations are carried out in the reversed phase mode because of the simplicity, versatility, and scope of this method as it is able to handle compounds of a diverse polarity and molecular mass (Prathap et al., 2013); for example, to identify secondary plant metabolites (Boligon et al., 2012, 2013; Colpo et al., 2014).

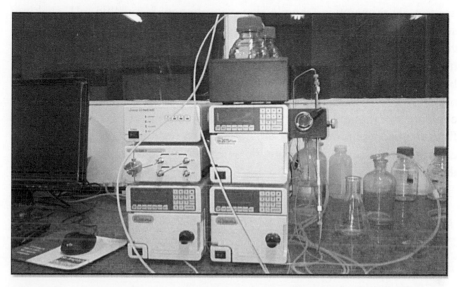

FIGURE 13.2 Representation of high-performance liquid chromatography (HPLC) instrument.
Source: (Courtesy to VCARD, VIVA College, Virar, Maharashtra, India).

13.3 SAMPLE PREPARATION AND METHOD DEVELOPMENT

The choice of solvent for sample reconstitution as well as the processing of a crude source material to provide a sample suitable for HPLC analysis can have a significant effect on the overall success of natural product isolation (Barbosa et al., 2014). The treatment of the source material, for example, the dried powdered plant will have to be done in such a way as to ensure that the compound of interest is efficiently extracted into solution. In the case of dried plant material, an organic solvent (e.g., methanol and chloroform) may be used following a period of maceration in which the solid material is then removed by decanting off the extract by filtration (Sasidharan et al., 2011; Janovik et al., 2012). The concentrated filtrate is then injected into HPLC for separation. The use of guard columns is necessary for the analysis of crude extract as many natural product materials contain a significant level of strongly binding components such as chlorophyll and so forth that may in the long-term, compromise the performance of analytical columns. Therefore, the guard columns will significantly protect the lifespan of the analytical columns (Ye et al., 2007; Goparaju and Kaushal, 2014).

HPLC analysis method is developed to identify, quantify, or purifying compounds of interest. The three critical components for a HPLC method are sample preparation (sample size, sample age, % organic, pH, shaking/sonication), analysis conditions (pH, flow rate, temperature, wavelength, and column age), and standardization (integration, wavelength, standard concentration, and response factor correction). All individual components should be investigated before the final method optimization during the preliminary method development stage. This gives the scientist a chance to critically evaluate the method performance in each component and streamline the final method optimization (FDA, 2000). The percentage of time spent on each stage is proposed to ensure the scientist will allocate sufficient time to different steps.

13.3.1   STEPS FOR HPLC METHOD DEVELOPMENT

The steps for HPLC method development are:
1. Sample Information
2. Defining of separation goals
3. Sample pretreatment (if any), special procedure requirement
4. Detector selection and setting
5. Optimization of separation conditions
6. Checking for problems or special procedure requirements
7. Recovery of purified material
8. Quantitative calibration/Qualitative method
9. Method validation for release to laboratories

13.3.2   REQUIREMENTS FOR GOOD METHOD DEVELOPMENT

13.3.2.1   CHOOSING THE APPROPRIATE HPLC COLUMN

C18 columns are the commonly used columns in HPLC method analysis. C8 or octyl bonded phases are also used occasionally. Like C18, they are nonpolar, but not as hydrophobic. Therefore, retention times for hydrophobic compounds are typically shorter.

13.3.2.2   COLUMN DIMENSIONS

This refers to the length and internal diameter of the packing media bed within the column tube. Short columns (30–50 mm) offer short run times, fast equilibration, low back pressure, and high sensitivity, whereas long columns (250–300 mm) provided higher resolving power but create more backpressure, lengthen analysis times, and use more solvent. Narrow column (2.1 mm and smaller) beds inhibit sample diffusion and produce narrower, taller peaks, and a lower limit of detection (LOD). They may require instrument modification to minimize distortion of the chromatography. Wider columns (10–22 mm) offer the ability to load more sample.

13.3.2.3   PARTICLE SHAPE

Most modern chromatographic packing has spherical particles, but few of them are irregular in shape. Spherical particles offer reduced back pressures and longer column life when using viscous mobile phases, for example, 50:50 McOH:H_2O.

13.3.2.4   PARTICLE SIZE

Particle size refers to the average diameter of the packing media particles. Standard particle sizes range from 3 μm (high efficiency) to 15–20 μm (preparative). A 5 μm particle size offers a good compromise between efficiency and back pressure. Smaller particles pack into columns with a higher density, allowing less diffusion of sample bands between particles and causing narrower, sharper peaks. However, smaller particles also cause higher solvent back pressures. As a rule of thumb, 1.5 or 3-μm particle sizes are to be chosen for resolving complex, multicomponent samples. Otherwise, 5 or 10-μm packings should be considered.

13.3.2.5   SURFACE AREA

It is expressed in m^2/g and the total surface area of a particle is the sum of the outer particle surface and the interior pore surface. High surface areas generally provide longer retention, greater capacity, and higher resolution and hence solute retention is greater on packings that have a high surface area. As a rule of thumb, a base material with a maximum surface area is to be used for resolving complex and multicomponent samples.

13.3.2.6   PORE SIZE

This refers to the average size of the pores or cavities present in porous packing particles. Pore sizes range from 60 Å on the low end to greater than 10,000 Å on the high end. A pore size of 150 Å or less is chosen for samples having MW ≤2000 and for samples with the molecular weight greater than 2000, columns with a pore size of 300 Å or greater are to be used. Larger pores allow larger solute molecules to be retained longer through maximum exposure to the surface area of the particles.

13.3.2.7   BONDING TYPE

The attachment of bonded phase to the base material is referred to as bonding type. Single-point attachment of each bonded phase molecule to the base material is seen in monomeric bonding, whereas polymeric bonding uses multipoint attachment of each bonded phase molecule to the base material. Polymeric bonding offers increased column stability, particularly when highly aqueous mobile phases are used. Polymeric bonding also enables the column to accept higher sample loading.

13.3.2.8   CARBON LOAD

Carbon load refers to the amount of bonded phase attached to the base material. The carbon load is a good indicator of hydrophobic retention for C18, C8, and phenyl packings. Higher carbon loads generally give higher column capacities, greater resolution, and longer run times; on the contrary, low carbon loads may show different selectivity because of greater exposure of the base material and also shorten run times. For complex samples that require the maximum degree of separation, it is good to choose high carbon loads. Suitable carbon loads must be selected to give shorter analysis times for simple sample mixtures and for samples which require high water content for solubility or stability.

13.3.2.9   ENDCAPPING

Endcapping applies only to reversed phase chromatography and is the process of bonding short hydrocarbon chains to free silanols remaining after the primary bonded phase has been added to the silica base. It reduces peak-tailing of polar solutes that interact excessively. Non-end capped packings provide a different selectivity than do the end-capped packings, especially for polar samples.

13.3.2.10 DETECTORS

Various detectors used in HPLC instrument include ultraviolet (UV)-visible detector, photodiode array detector, fluorescence detector, conductivity detector, refractive index detector, electrochemical detector, mass spectrometer detector, and evaporative light scattering detector. UV-visible detectors are typically used in many laboratories as they can detect a wide array of compounds.

13.3.2.11 pH RANGE

Method development within the different pH (ranges from 1 to 12 for better chromatographic resolution) depends upon three main factors, column efficiency, selectivity, and retention time. Column efficiency can improve by change in the mobile phase pH because it alters both the ionization of the analyte and the residual silanols and it also minimizes secondary interactions between analytes and the silica surface that lead to poor peak shape. To achieve optimum resolution, it requires change in the pH of the mobile phase. Method development can proceed by investigating parameters of chromatographic separations first at low pH and then at higher pH until optimum results are achieved (Dolan, 2002).

13.3.2.12 MOBILE PHASE COMPOSITION

Mobile phase composition also is known as solvent strength plays an important role in reversed phase high performance chromatography (RP-HPLC) separation. Acetonitrile (ACN), methanol (MeOH), and tetrahydrofuran (THF) are commonly used solvents in RP-HPLC having low UV cutoff of 190, 205, and 212 nm, respectively. These solvents are miscible with water. Mixture of acetonitrile and water is the best initial choice for the mobile phase during method development.

13.3.2.13   COLUMN TEMPERATURE

Selection of the right column temperature can enhance the separation of many samples. Higher column temperature reduces system backpressure by decreasing mobile phase viscosity, which in turn allows the use of longer columns with higher separation efficiency. However, an overall loss of resolution between mixture components in many samples occurs by increasing column temperature. The nature of the mixture components is also a deciding factor for the optimum temperature. The overall separation can be improved by the simultaneous changes in column temperature and mobile phase composition (Deng et al., 2009; Nguyen et al., 2010; Fu et al., 2010).

13.4   HPLC METHOD VALIDATION

The validation of an analytical method demonstrates the scientific soundness of the measurement or characterization. It is required to provide validation data throughout the regulatory submission process. The validation processes indicate that an analytical method measures the correct substance, in the correct amount, and in the appropriate range for the intended samples. It allows the analyst to understand the behavior of the method and to establish the performance limits of the method (Julia et al., 2011; Khan et al., 2012). The main goal is to identify the critical parameters and to establish acceptance criteria for method system suitability. The method can be validated for use as a screening (qualitative), semiquantitative (5–10 ppm), or quantitative method. It can also be validated for use on single equipment, different equipment in the laboratory, different laboratories or even for international use at different climatic and environmental conditions. The criteria for each type of validation will, of course, be different with the validation level required (Hill and Reynolds, 1999). The various validation parameters include linearity, accuracy, precision, ruggedness, robustness, LOD, limit of quantitation (LOQ), and selectivity or specificity

13.4.1   LINEARITY

The linearity of an analytical procedure is its ability (within a given range) to obtain test results that are directly proportional to the concentration of the analyte in the sample (Krier et al., 2011; Chan et al., 2004). For determination of the useful range at which the instrumental response is proportional to the analyte concentration, linearity is extremely important. Generally, a value of correlation coefficient (r) > 0.998 is considered as the evidence of an acceptable fit of the data to the regression line (Chitturi et al., 2008). The significance of deviation of intercept of calibration line from the origin can be evaluated statistically by determining confidence limits for the intercept, generally at 95% level (Shabir et al., 2007; Miller and Miller, 2005).

13.4.2 ACCURACY

Accuracy is defined by International Organization for Standardization (ISO) as "closeness of agreement between a measured quantity value and a true quantity value." It is a qualitative characteristic that cannot be expressed as a numerical value. It has an inverse relation to both random and systematic errors, where higher accuracy means lower errors (Mowafy, 2012). Accuracy is evaluated by analyzing test drug at different concentration levels. Samples are prepared in triplicate and relatively known amounts of related substances and the drug substance in placebo are spiked to prepare an accurate sample of known concentration of the related substance.

13.4.3 PRECISION

It expresses closeness of agreement (degree of scatter) between a series of measurements obtained from multiple sampling of the same homogeneous sample under the prescribed conditions. Precision may be considered at three levels: repeatability, intermediate precision, and reproducibility (ICH, 2005). Repeatability is also known as intra-assay precision. It is a measure of the precision of analysis in one laboratory wherein one operator uses one piece of equipment over a relatively short time span. It is degree of agreement of results when experimental conditions are maintained as constant as possible, and expressed as relative standard deviations of replicate values. The objective is to verify that the method will provide the same results despite differences in room temperature and humidity, variedly experienced operators, different characteristics of equipments (e.g., delay volume of an HPLC system), variations in material and instrument conditions (e.g., mobile phase composition, pH, flow rate of mobile phase in HPLC), equipment and consumables of different ages, columns from different suppliers or different batches and solvents, reagents, and other material with different quality (Staes et al., 2010).

13.4.4   SELECTIVITY AND SPECIFICITY

Selectivity and specificity are sometimes used interchangeably to describe the same concept in method validation. ISO defines selectivity of an analytical method as "property of a measuring system, used with a specified measurement procedure, in which it provides measured quantity values for one or more measures such that the values of each measure is independent of other measured or other quantities in the phenomenon, body, or substance being investigated." Specificity is the ability to assess unequivocally the analyte in the presence of components that may be expected to be present. By comparing test results from an analysis of samples containing impurities, degradation products, or placebo ingredients with those obtained from an analysis of samples without impurities, degradation products, or placebo ingredients specificity of a test method is determined. Specificity can best be demonstrated by the resolution between the analyte peak and the other closely eluting peak (Elbarbry et al., 2006).

13.4.5   LIMIT OF DETECTION AND LIMIT OF QUANTITATION

LOD of an analytical procedure is the lowest concentration of an analyte in a sample which can be detected but not necessarily quantitated as an exact value, whereas LOQ is the lowest amount of analyte in a sample that can be quantitatively determined with suitable precision and accuracy.

13.4.6   RANGE

The range of an analytical procedure is the interval between the upper and lower concentrations of analyte in the sample. It includes the concentrations for which it has been demonstrated that the analytical procedure has a suitable level of precision, accuracy and linearity (Chan et al., 1999). It is established by confirming that the analytical procedure provides an acceptable degree of linearity, accuracy, and precision when applied to samples containing amounts of analyte within or at the extremes of the specified range of the analytical procedure. The range of an analytical method can also vary with its intended purpose. It is generally 80–120% of the test concentration for the assay of a drug substance or a finished (drug) product, 70–130% of the test concentration for content uniformity, ±20% over the specified range for dissolution testing, reporting level of an impurity to 120% of the specification for the determination of an impurity. It should correspond with

LOD or LOQ (the control level of impurities), for impurities known to be unusually potent or to produce toxic or unexpected pharmacological effects.

13.4.7 ROBUSTNESS

The robustness of an analytical procedure is a measure of its capacity to remain unaffected by small, but deliberate variations in method parameters. It provides an indication of its reliability during normal usage. A number of chromatographic parameters, for example, flow rate, column temperature, injection volume, detection wavelength, and mobile phase composition are varied within a realistic range and quantitative influence of the variables is determined for the determination of method robustness. If the influence of the parameter is within a previously specified tolerance, the parameter is said to be within the method's robustness range. Obtaining data on these effects will allow to judge whether a method needs to be revalidated when one or more of parameters are changed, for example, to compensate for column performance over time (Hernández et al., 2011; Trani et al., 2012). Variation in method conditions for robustness should reflect typical day-to-day variation and also be small. Critical parameters are identified during the method development process. Only these critical method parameters should be investigated for robustness. Common critical method parameters can be divided into two categories. The HPLC conditions include HPLC column (brand, lot, and age), mobile phase composition (pH ±0.05 unit, organic content ±2%) and HPLC instrument (detection wavelength ±2 nm, column temperature ±5°C, flow rate, and dwell volume). The sample preparation variations include sample solvent (pH ±0.05 unit, organic content ±2%), sample preparation procedure (shaking time, different membrane filters), and HPLC solution stability.

13.5 HIGH-PERFORMANCE THIN-LAYER CHROMATOGRAPHY (HPTLC) – OVERVIEW

High-performance thin-layer chromatography (HPTLC) (Fig. 13.3) is the sophisticated form of thin-layer chromatography (TLC) which explores the use of chromatographic layers of utmost separation efficiency and the employment of state-of-the-art instrumentation facilities with sophistication and automation. HPTLC do not only mean performing TLC on pre-coated plates with modern equipment but it optimally combines technology with scientific theories and concepts to generate standardized methodology that is consistent and reproducible performance hence referred as HPTLC.

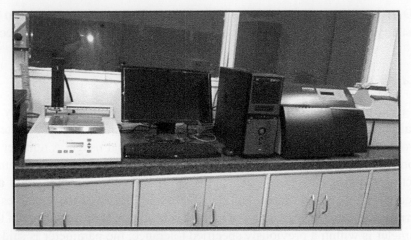

FIGURE 13.3   Representation of HPTLC instrumentation.

Source: (Courtesy to VCARD, VIVA College, Virar, Maharashtra, India).

The entire process of HPTLC (Fig. 13.4) is a concept-based standardized methodology which is based on scientific facts. It also utilizes validated methods for qualitative evaluation and quantitative estimation of the components. The validated methods have greater reproducibility and can be included in the various pharmacopeia. HPTLC is a user-friendly tool which meets all the quality requirements of today's analytical laboratories.

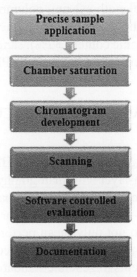

FIGURE 13.4   Schematic flow of various steps in HPTLC.

13.5.1 HPTLC METHOD DEVELOPMENT

Herbal industry is an upcoming industry gaining wider share in global markets. The shift of consumers from synthetic products to natural or plant-based products is mainly because of the safety associated with these products. There are enormous varieties of plant-based products on the market but have no comprehensive methods using HPTLC to assure its purity. HPTLC fingerprints are also lacking in pharmacopeia hence most of the pharmacopeias are in the process of revising and updating their monographs to include HPTLC methodology for botanicals.

13.5.1.1 SAMPLE PREPARATION

Sample preparation is a crucial step in HPTLC analysis as direct spotting of unprocessed samples may not generate an accurate fingerprint. Molecules such as proteins need to be hydrolyzed before spotting on the plate. Several compounds need pretreatment and washing prior to chromatographic separation.

13.5.1.2 SELECTION OF SUITABLE STATIONARY PHASE

Stationary phase selection is the most crucial step in the generation of a chromatographic fingerprint. The choice of the stationary phase is mainly dependent on the kind of major components in the plant material which are to be separated. Polar or an intermediately polar stationary phase can be preferably used. There is a great selection of ready-to-use pre-coated plates in the market. Almost all stationary phases used in columns can also be found as plates. Silica gel used for TLC is a porous material with a regular tetrahedron structure wherein each silica atom is surrounded by four oxygen atoms. The chemically bonded silica is slightly acidic in nature and retains molecules in accordance to the polarity hence the separation of compounds or the analytes is dependent on the migration rate and polarity (Fried and Sherma, 1994).

13.5.1.3 PREWASHING AND ACTIVATION OF PLATES

Cleaning of plates is recommended prior to the quantitative work as sorbent material with the larger surface area can adsorb air, water vapors, and other impurities from atmosphere also the condensation of volatile substances takes place after the opening of the packed plates (Sethi and Charegaonkar, 2008). This step of cleaning the plates to eliminate the interference of impurities is termed as prewashing of plates. The interaction of solutes to be separated using the stationary phase results in the tailing or leading peaks, this can be corrected by modification of the sorbent using a modifier. The modifier can be added to the mobile phase or HPTLC plate could be prewashed with the mobile phase containing modifier, or with methanol containing a modifier. It is necessary to wash the plates prior to separation; this can be done by migration of an appropriate solvent. The plates may also be impregnated by procedures such as development, immersion, or spraying. The plates may be activated, if necessary, by heating in an oven at 120°C for 20 min before use (British Pharmacopoeia, 2007). The better resolution that is sharper separations, significantly low signal to noise ratio and a straight baseline are the advantages of prewashing and activation of plate used for HPTLC (Sethi and Charegaonkar, 2008).

13.5.1.4   SAMPLE APPLICATION

The sample application is one of the important and critical steps in the entire process of method development using HPTLC. The selection of a sample application technique and the device to be used depends on factors such as nature of the work, qualitative or quantitative analysis of the raw material, workload, time constraints, type of separation, and sample volume to be applied. All these factors when observed yields a better-resolved chromatogram. The avoidance of manual sample application is one of the important characteristics of HPTLC as it hinders standardization of herbals. Automated sample application reduces the manpower consumption time and leads to high precision and accuracy. During automated sample application with the help of an applicator, a sample should be completely transferred from the applicator to the sorbent layer to form a compact zone and the application procedure should not damage the sorbent layer. Samples may be applied either spot wise with a device with controllable delivery speed, or they are sprayed on in the form of narrow bands (Sethi, 2001).

The advantages of the application of sample in form of a band instead of a spot were described by Sethi and Charegaonkar (2008):

- Better separation because of the rectangular area in which the components are present on the plate.

- Equal retention factor (R_f) values for the compounds from the sample and reference solutions.
- Matrix effects of extracted and applied excipients are significantly reduced as the solution is distributed over a larger area.
- Response of densitometer is higher than observed from an equal amount/equal volume of the same solution is applied to a spot. It appears that light may not gain access to all the sample material applied to a spot while scanning. Drugs are that detector linear response range is small for spot-wise application than for band-wise application.
- Spot broadening in the direction of development is smaller if band-wise application is practiced.
- Larger quantities of the sample can be handled for application, thus reducing the need for concentration step, which may be quite damaging in case of labile substances.
- The position of the plate during the densitometry scan becomes less critical as the composition of the compound is uniform in the entire area of the band.

13.5.1.5 SELECTION OF AN IDEAL MOBILE PHASE

The selection of the appropriate mobile phase is of prime importance in the development of a chromatogram and is primarily dependent on the components to be separated. Certain other factors such as proper elution, resolution, spot definition, symmetrical peak shapes, and R_f reproducibility of the analyte also play a significant role in the selection of the mobile phase. The interaction between the solute–mobile phase and solute–stationary phase will be determined by the number and nature of the functional groups in the solute. The old thumb rule "like dissolves like" is applicable in the selection of a suitable mobile phase. In case there is no suitable method found in literature, the mobile phases mentioned or reported for several classes of compounds can be tried out. There are guidelines which provide the scheme for the mobile phase optimization. Developing solvent usually is a mixture of nonpolar organic solvent (toluene) with a polar modifier such as methanol, ethyl acetate, acetone, methylene dichloride, and so forth, control the solvent strength and selectivity. The general strategy for optimizing the mobile phase is through trial and error in TLC. The solvent strength is adjusted by replacing a pure solvent by another, or by varying the proportions of the weak solvent and the strong solvent in a mixture so that the $\underline{R}_f$ values are in the range of 0.2–0.7. The solvent strength once optimized is kept constant and the composition of the solvent system is played with to get the desired separation. However, a binary solvent system may not work with a mixture of components. In such cases, ternary or quaternary solvent systems would be an ideal system. However, the solvent strength has to be kept constant (Fried and Sherma, 1994; Fried and Sherma, 1996).

13.5.1.6 SATURATION OF CHAMBER FOR DEVELOPMENT OF CHROMATOGRAM

Chamber saturation step plays an important role in the development of the chromatogram as it is reported that in case of unsaturated chambers solvent evaporation takes place at the solvent front. This effect is also referred as "edge effect" because the developing solvent evaporates more rapidly at the edge than at the center of the plate resulting into the curved solvent front (Fried and Sherma, 1996; Sethi, 2001). The loss of solvent also results in the requirement of larger volumes of solvents thereby increasing the R_f values.

In planar chromatography, the separation process occurs in a three-phase system – stationary, mobile, and vapor phase, all of which interact with one another and with the operating parameters. Selection of the chamber type and vapor space is offered only by planar chromatography, as the third dimension of the chromatographic parameters. Chambers used for separation are saturated with the solvent system used for separation so that the entire chamber gets saturated by the vapors of the mobile phase. Owing to chamber saturation, there is a uniform distribution of solvent vapors which minimizes the volume of solvent required for separation (Reich and Schibli, 2006).

13.5.1.7 DEVELOPING, DERIVATIZATION, AND DRYING

There are several modes of development of chromatograms such as ascending, descending, radial; two-dimensional and multidimensional modes are planned as per the nature and ease of technique for separation of components. Suitable chambers are selected for the selected mode of chromatogram development. For the analysis of botanicals, after development, the plates may or may not be derivatized. The plates are dried and then evaluated using densitometry scanning.

13.5.1.8 VISUALIZATION, DETECTION, AND QUANTIFICATION USING SCANNING DENSITOMETRY

TLC is a versatile technique, hence offers several modes for visualization and detection of separated components. An analyte can also be quantified by eluting the relevant band or spot from the sorbent followed by spectrophotometry. This is tedious to perform, time-consuming, prone to errors, and with poor accuracy and precision. Scanning densitometers overcome the tediousness of spectrophotometry and offer an accurate type of evaluation in HPTLC, particularly for the quantitation of marker compounds. It also allows spectral sensitivity. Densitometry is the measurement used to see the activity of the component to be separated. Absorbance or fluorescence of separated compounds is measured and evaluated against that of reference standards of a known quantity. For sensitive measurement, monochromatic light in the range of 190–800 nm can be tuned to the absorption/fluorescence maximum of the target compounds. Typical detection limits are in the low nanogram range (absorbance) or medium pictogram level (fluorescence). Densitometry can be performed prior to or after derivatization.

13.5.1.9 PARAMETERS INFLUENCED BY CHANGES IN CHROMATOGRAPHIC CONDITIONS

Retention factor: R_f is defined as the amount of separation due to solvent migration through the sorbent layer as shown in the formula. The factors affecting the R_f values are the time required for the development and the velocity of the solvent.

$$R_f = \frac{\textit{Migration distance of the solute}}{\textit{Distance traveled by the solvent from the point of the origin}}$$

Peak purity: The null hypothesis states that these spectra are identical and in this case the peaks obtained. During the purity test, the spectrum taken at the first peak slope is correlated with the spectrum of peak maximum and this is in turn correlated with the peak end or reference spectra. The error probability is rejected if P, 0.01 is greater than 2.576.

13.5.2 HPTLC METHOD DESIGN AND DEVELOPMENT

The first step of design and development begins with the purpose of the study with well-defined objectives. The objectives may be only qualitative analysis or both qualitative and quantitative estimates or may be to optimize time required for analysis. Designing a method for HPTLC begins with lots of permutations and combinations based on previously available literature or by trial and error (Reich and Blatter, 2004). The first and the most difficult task is to select a suitable stationary and mobile phase as the entire principle of chromatographic separation is based on these two factors. Mobile phase selection can be worked out with "PRISMA model" or the "four solvent approach" model for botanicals as very less is known about the analytes. The mobile phase selection is a three-tier process which begins basically with the selection of neat solvents at the first level for separation and selecting the solvents having average separation. In the second level, water or hexane is used to obtain the desired solvent strength. The third step involves trying mixtures of solvents from the first and second step and then optimizing the separation by introducing a modifier which may be an acid or an alkali. Silica gel is used as the stationary phase as it is suitable for separation of many analytes (Sethi and Charegaonkar, 2008). The final step of the method development is visualization and detection of the analyte. Fluorescence property or absorption is explored for visualization. Clear defined peaks which are symmetrical and well separated by slight modifications in the mobile phase is the end product of a successfully developed method design.

13.5.3 HPTLC METHOD VALIDATION

Validation is a formal proof that any designed method is actually viable and suited for its intended use. It is a formalized part of pharmaceutical industries regulated under good manufacturing practice thereby assuring the quality of the raw material or the product. Validation of a method leads to assurance and reliability to the analyst that the set analytical goals were achieved. Analytical method validation includes all the procedures required for proving the reliable facts for the method developed. Bioavailability, bioequivalence, and pharmacokinetic studies require reliable and validated methods so as to determine the drug concentration in the complex matrix such as biological fluids. Validation emphasizes the entire process from sampling, sample preparation, analysis, calculation, and evaluation of the result.

There are two kinds of HPTLC methods routinely used by the analyst for analysis of the analytes and these methods are validated separately.

- *Qualitative method* which is focused on the procurement and data collection of parameters such as R_f values, color zones, and sequences. The analysis is carried out irrespective of any prior knowledge of the analyte. Visual screening or densitometry is carried out based on the images obtained on the HPTLC plate. Validation can be done using a reference standard that can be run simultaneously with test sample/s or can be run on a separate plate.
- *The quantitative method* determines the amount well-separated known analytes. Peak areas/heights of the separated analytes are calculated using calibration plots using a standard reference compound in a purified form separated on the same plates.

Quantitative methods for plant-based drugs are validated like synthetic drugs following official guidelines are given in the International Conference on Harmonization (ICH), ISO. Two important documents by the ICH provide the framework for validation. The details of the key term used and the adopted methodology is described in the "Note for Guidance on Validation of Analytical methods Q2 (R1)" (Reich and Schibli, 2006).

KEYWORDS

- **secondary metabolites**
- **analytical tools**
- **high-performance liquid chromatography**
- **high-performance thin-layer chromatography**
- **validation**

REFERENCES

Barbosa Filho, V. M.; Waczuk, E. P.; Kamdem, J. P.; Abolaji, A. O.; Lacerda, S. R.; Costa, J. G. M. Phytochemical Constituents, Antioxidant Activity, Cytotoxicity Andosmotic Fragility Effects of Caju (Anacardium *microcarpum*) *Ind. Crops Prod.* [Online] **2014,** *55,* 280–288.

Boligon, A. A.; Janovik, V.; Frohlich, J. K.; Spader, T. B.; Froeder, A. L.; Alves, S. H. Antimicrobial and Cytotoxic Activities of Leaves, Twigs and Stem Bark of Scutia *Buxifolia* Reissek. *Nat Prod. Res.* **2012**, *26,* 939–944.

Boligon, A. A.; Kubica, T. F.; Mario, D. N.; de Brum, T. F.; Piana, M.; Weiblen, R. Antimicrobial and Antiviral Activity-Guided Fractionation from Scutia *Buxifolia* Reissek Extracts. *Acta Physiol. Plant* **2013**, *35,* 2229–2239.

British Pharmacopoeia (Ph. Eur. method 2.2.27). Thin Layer Chromatography. **2007**. Chan, E. C.; Wee, P. Y.; Ho, P. C. The Value of Analytical Assay that are Stability–Indicating. *Clin. cChim. Acta*, **1999**, 288, 47–-53.

Chan, C. C., Leo, Y. C., Lam, H. *Analytical Method Validation and Instrument Performance Validation;* Wiley Interscience: USA, 2004; Vol. 1.

Chitturi, S. R.; Bharathi, C. H.; Reddy, A. V. R.; Reddy, K. C.; Sharma, H. K.; Handa, V.; Dandala, R.; Bindu, V. M. Impurity Profle Study of Lopinavir and Validation of HPLC Method for the Determination of Related Substances in Lopinavir Drug Substance. *J. Pharma. Biomed. Anal.* **2008**, *48,* 1430–1440.

Colpo, E.; Dalton, D. A.; Vilanova, C.; Reetz, L. G.; Duarte, M. M.; Farias, I. L. Brazilian Nut Consumption by Healthy Volunteers Improves Inflammatory Parameters. *Nutrition* **2014**, *30,* 459–465.

Deng, S.; Brett, J. W.; Jensen, C. J.; Basar, S.; Westendorf, J. Development and Validation of an RPHPLC Method for the Analysis of Anthraquinones in Noni Fruits and Leaves. *Food Chem.* **2009**, *116,* 505–508.

Dolan, J. W. Peak Tailing and Resolution. *LCGC North Am.* **2002**, *20,* 430–436.

Elbarbry, F.; Wilby, K.; Alcorn, J. Validation of a HPLC Method for the Determination of p-Nitrophenol Hydroxylase Activity in Rat Hepatic Microsomes. *J. Chromatography-B* **2006**, *834,* 199–203.

Fan, X. H.; Cheng, Y. Y.; Ye, Z. L.; Lin, R. C.; Qian, Z. Z. Multiple Chromatographic Fingerprinting and Its Application to the Quality Control of Herbal Medicines. *Anal. Chim. Acta.* **2006**, *555,* 217–224.

FDA. *Guidance for Industry-Analytical Procedures and Method Validation;* Chemistry, Manufacturing, and Controls Documentation, Center for Drug Evaluation and Research (CDER) and Center for Biologics Evaluation and Research (CBER), 2000.

Fried, B.; Sherma, J. *Thin Layer Chromatography*, 4th ed; Marcel Dekker Inc.: New York, 1994; Vol. 81.

Fried, B.; Sherma, J. *Handbook of Thin Layer Chromatography, Chromatographic Science Series;* Marcel Dekker: NY, 1996; Vol. 81.

Goparaju, G.; Kaushal G. Significance of Stability-Indicating LC Methods in Pharmaceuticals. *Austin Chromatogr.* **2014**, *1,* 2.

Hernández, Y. S.; Sánchez, L. B.; Bedia, M. M. G.; Luis, T. G. Determination of Parthenin in Parthenium *Hysterophorus* by Means of HPLC-UV: Method Development and Validation. *Phytochem. Lett.* **2011**, *4,* 134–137.

Hill, A. R. C.; Reynolds, S. L. Guidelines for In-House Validation of Analytical Methods for Pesticide Residues in Food and Animal Feeds. *Analyst* **1999**, *124,* 953–958.

ICH Q2 (R1). In *Validation of Analytical Procedures: Text and Methodology*, International Conference on Harmonization, IFPMA: Geneva, 2005.

Janovik, V.; Boligon, A. A.; Athayde, M. L. Antioxidant Activities and HPLC/DAD Analysis of Phenolics and Carotenoids from the Barks of Cariniana Domestica (Mart.) Miers. *Res. J. Phytochem.* **2012**, *6,* 105–112.

Julia, T.; Mena, A. J.; Aucoin, M. G.; Kamen, A. A. Development and Validation of a HPLC Method for the Quantifcation of Baculovirus Particles. *J. Chromatography-B* **2011**, *879*, 61–68.

Khan, M. C.; Reddy, N. K.; Ravindra, G.; Reddy, K. V. S. R. K.; Dubey. P. K. Development and Validation of a Stability Indicating HPLC Method for Simultaneous Determination of Four Novel Fluoroquinolone Dimers as Potential Antibacterial Agents. *J. Pharm. Biomed. Anal.* **2012**, *59*, 162–166.

Kokate, C. K. Practical Pharmacognosy. Vallabh Prakashan: New Delhi, 1994; pp 107–113.

Krier, F.; Brion, M.; Debrus, B.; Lebrun, P.; Driesen, A.; Ziemons, E.; Evrard, B.; Hubert, P. Optimisation and Validation of a Fast HPLC Method for the Quantification of Sulindac and Its Related Impurities. *J. Pharm. Biomed. Anal.* **2011**, *54*, 694–700.

Martin, M.; Guiochon. G. Effects of High Pressure in Liquid Chromatography. J. *Chromatogr. A.* **2005**, *1090*, 16–38.

Miller, J. N.; Miller, J. C. *Statistics and Chemometrics for Analytical Chemistry Harlow;* Pearson Prentice Hall: Edinburgh Gate, England, 2005; p 263.

Mowafy, H. A.; Alanazi, F. K.; Maghraby, G. M. E. Development and Validation of an HPLC–UV Method for the Quantifcation of Carbamazepine in Rabbit Plasma. *Saudi Pharm. J.* **2012**, *20*, 29–34.

Nguyen, A. T.; Aerts, T.; Dam, D. W.; Deyn, P. P. D. Biogenic Amines and Their Metabolites in Mouse Brain Tissue: Development, Optimization and Validation of an Analytical HPLC Method. *J. Chromatography-B* **2010**, *878*, 3003–3014.

Prathap, B.; Dey, A.; Srinivasarao, G. II.; Johnson, P.; Arthanariswaran, P. A Review—Importance of RP-HPLC in Analytical Method Development. *Int. J. Novel Trends Pharma. Sci.* **2013**, *3*, 15–23.

Reich, E.; Blatter, A. *Handbook of Thin-Layer Chromatography*, 3rd ed.; Marcel Dekker: New York, 2003; pp 535–564.

Reich E.; Blatter A. Modern TLC: A Key Technique for Identification and Quality Control for Botanicals and Dietary Supplements. *Inside Laboratory Management, AOAC International*, May/June 2004, 14–18.

Reich, E.; Schibli, A. Standard Operating Procedure for HPTLC of Herbal Raw Materials and Preparations. In *High Performance Thin Layer Chromatography for the Analysis of Medicinal Plants;* Thieme: New York, 2006, pp 227–230.

Reis, E. M.; Schreiner, Neto F. W.; Cattani, V. B.; Peroza, L. R.; Busanello, A.; Leal, C. Q. Antidepressant-Like Effect of Ilex *Paraguariensis* in Rats. *Biomed. Res. Int.* **2014**, Article id: 958209, 1-9. http://dx.doi.org/10.1155/2014/958209.

Sasidharan, S.; Chen, Y.; Saravanan, D.; Sundram, K. M.; Yoga, Latha L. Extraction, Isolation and Characterization of Bioactive Compounds from Plants' Extracts. *Afr. J. Tradit. Complementary Altern. Med.* **2011**, *8*, 1–10.

Sethi, P. D.; Charegaonkar, D. Introduction. In *Identification of Drugs in Pharmaceutical Formulations by Thin Layer Chromatography,* 2nd ed.; CBS publishers and Distributors: New Delhi, 2008; pp 1–52.

Sethi, P. D. *HPTLC-Quantitative Analysis of Pharmaceutical Formulations*, 1st ed.; CBS Publishers: New Delhi, 2001.

Sivarajan, V. V. Introduction to the Principles of Plant Taxonomy. Cambridge University Press, 1991.

Shabir, G. A.; Lough, W. J.; Arain, S. A.; Bradshaw, T. K. Evaluation and Application of Best Practice in Analytical Method Validation. *J. Liq. Chromatogr. Relat. Technol.* **2007**, *30*, 311–333.

Staes, E.; Rozet, E.; Učakar, B.; Hubert, P.; Préat, V. Validation of a Method for the Quantitation of Ghrelin and Unacylated Ghrelin by HPLC. *J. Pharm. Biomed. Anal.* **2010,** *51,* 633–639.

Trani, M. T. T.; Katherine, M. P.; Marlyn, C. Matrix-Specific Method Validation for Quantitative Analysis of Vitamin C in Diverse Foods. *J. Food Compos. Anal.* **2012,** *26,* 12–25.

Ye, M.; Han, J.; Chen, H.; Zheng, J.; Guo, D. Analysis of Phenolic Compounds in Rhubarbs Using Liquid Chromatography Coupled with Electrospray Ionization Mass Spectrometry. *J. Am. Soc. Mass Spectrom.* **2007,** *18,* 82–91.

CHAPTER 14

ANALYTICAL TECHNIQUES IN ELEMENTAL PROFILING

ANDREW G. MTEWA[1,2,*] and ANNU AMANJOT[2]

[1]*Department of Chemistry, Institute of Technology, Malawi University of Science and Technology, Malawi, Tel.: +265 999643272/+256 794547811*

[2]*Department of Pharmacology and Therapeutics, Mbarara University of Science and Technology, Mbarara, Uganda*

*Corresponding author. E-mail: amtewa@must.ac.mw; andrewmtewa@yahoo.com
ORCID: https://orcid.org/0000-0003-2618-7451

ABSTRACT

Elemental analysis is a technique that either identifies and/or quantifies specific elements in matter. It involves the understanding of the nature of the elements, appropriate sample preparation techniques, analytical methods, and tools. Elements are the simplest form of matter that cannot be broken further. The most common of these are metals which are categorized according to their properties. The body's proper functioning requires metal elements called minerals at different levels for different functions and plants are their good natural sources. However, among the elements found in the plants and their phytomedicinal products are sometimes heavy metals that are toxic. It is therefore critical to establish the nature of elements and the amount present. These studies require proper techniques to minimize errors and avoid misinterpretation which could potentially be hazardous. This chapter puts together essential techniques in the elemental profiling of plants and plant products with a focus on inorganic metal elements and a brief introduction to techniques for organic elements.

14.1   INTRODUCTION

Plants remain one of the most natural sources of elements in the world, including minerals, as required for body functioning. However, they also contain toxic elements such as heavy metals (Helaluddin et al., 2016), which are principally accumulated through biochemical uptake from water, fertilizers, and soil (Pruszkowski and Bosnak, 2015; Husejnovic et al., 2016). There are various known limited guidelines on the intake of minerals which could cause harm. The determination of the amounts of elements, both toxic and essential minerals in plants and plant products is critically essential for the health of consumers.

There are classical methods and contemporary methods, with the latter having a better edge in terms of ease of operations, duration of analysis, concurrent multiple analyses, precision and control over errors and calibrations, among others. Although classical methods are still in use, they are largely being replaced by contemporary methods in both industry and academia.

In the determination of elemental contents, there are several stages that require attention. These include sample material handling, test sample matrix preparation (Pruszkowski and Bosnak, 2015), which involves digestion, analysis, and lastly reporting. These steps need to be systematic by the use of particular techniques to minimize errors and avoid reporting false results from costly analyses. This chapter outlines basic techniques in the elemental analysis of plants and plant products using contemporary methods as opposed to classical ones and ultimately serves to make experimental operations and analytical costs worthwhile. This chapter does not discuss the technical makeup and functions of the equipment used but the techniques for ensuring the best results possible.

14.2   MATRIX PREPARATION TECHNIQUES

The preparation of matrices is a crucial step to elemental analysis. They are prepared in different ways to suit a particular analytical technique being undertaken in order to get the purported data thereof. There are basic techniques for which matrices are prepared.

14.2.1   CLEANING

The plant sample materials are usually contaminated. The contamination can potentially affect the results of your analysis by giving you false information.

For example, if someone is looking at a microbial growth over a specific duration as done by Mtewa (2017), the person might end up registering microbial population on day 1 which is not necessarily from the formulation itself but rather pre-formulation contamination. The same applies to metal content determination, where one could register metal content from miniature soil particles or pollen from some random bees (Paslawski and Migaszewski, 2006) adsorbed on the surfaces of the plant material rather than the metals that are inherent in the plant. This is the reason why cleaning is vital for the starting plant material before derivation of your extracts.

Cleaning could be in a physical form, for example, dusting off and high-pressure air blowing. It could also be chemical by use of liquids to wash, mainly water. However, it should be appreciated that some researchers discourage washing particularly for plant materials that have now protective resins in fear of washing off important airborne particulates, waxes, and other elements from the surfaces (Paslawski and Migaszewski, 2006). Again, this decision will largely depend on what your target of analysis is, for the metals, most of which are significantly embedded in the structural framework of the plants, washing would not have a significant adverse effect if any. There are three basic ways used in cleaning plant sample materials as outlined below:

i.   **Machine washing:** The samples are put in tightly tied and knotted plastic bags containing deionized or distilled water. The bags are then put in tailor-designed washers with agitators inside for at least a complete cycle for washing or rinsing. There is no use of detergent or water at elevated temperatures to avoid affecting the chemical makeup of the plant material (Peacock, 1992).

ii. **Hand washing:** This involved directly washing the plant materials under running water or use of a series of washing sessions in containers called "beaker soaking" (Peacock, 1992). The containers may not necessarily be beakers and this method requires that washing water be changed regularly from one washing to the next. You may wish to use several beakers in a series with different clean water in them to minimize chances of contamination.

iii. **Colander washing:** Colanders are plastic or metallic bowl-shaped containers with perforations in them and are usually used to drain food in kitchens and to wash vegetables. Usually, there has to be a continuous supply of running water for manual washing. The advantage is that dirt does not sediment in the containers, they are washed away directly.

Challenges in cleaning can arise when the cleaning material itself is contaminated or has inherent composition as the composition of interest you are targeting in your material/matrix which can result in bloated concentrations. Generally, natural or tap water contains minerals in its own right and deionized water is reported to contain some traces of organic matter (Gorsuch, 1970); the researcher may wish to use distilled water depending on what fits the objectives of the research being undertaken. Alternatively, Saiki and Maeda (1982) reported a successful use of HCl (0.2 M) and distilled water rinsing technique which was successful (Peacock, 1992).

14.2.2 DRYING

The plant material for analysis may require appropriate drying techniques. Most researchers use heating method, either by the application of elevated temperature or by the use of natural sun-drying methods. It is very critical to carefully consider the potential composition of your research and the target compounds and study in advance the maximum temperatures at which the compounds of interest are stable in case they are labile at some elevated levels of temperature. Air-drying is another method that can be used (Paslawski and Migaszewski, 2006) to avoid thermal degradation of important features of your test materials, mostly so for materials with no coating resins (Peacock, 1992). These features include nature of certain compounds, taste, color, texture (from molecular bonding), and odor which you might want to maintain. Unless there is a need for much lower temperatures in drying, you may wish to dry your material to not more than 40°C (Peacock, 1992). Sometimes, to avoid damaging some vital components of the matrix, samples may be lymphorized (Zygmunt and Namiesnik, 2003) to below 21°C for about 18 h. The advantage with lymphorization is that you can work on ready-to-serve aqueous herbal formulations without complications of concentration determinations. Lymphorized samples may be taken directly to analysis if they are already extracted, if not, extraction in appropriate solvents is required.

14.2.3 MILLING

Milling of the samples is not mandatory and it depends on the type of analysis and target compound of the research. Other research objectives may require directly putting the materials in water but for the efficient evolution of compounds from the plant matrix, milling is the best way in order to take advantage of the high surface area thereof. Milling works best with leaves and shoots but for twigs, bark, and roots, consider chopping to as small pieces as possible, between 5 and 13 mm (Peacock, 1992), depending on the type of milling blades and sieves used. After milling, make the samples as homogenous as possible for representativeness of the whole. This can be done using a rotor or manually by putting in a sealed/tied plastic bag and shake vigorously for some time in almost all directions.

14.2.4 STORAGE

Samples prepared as above need good storage techniques to avoid losing important components of interest like volatile elements, for example, mercury. Make sure they are kept in tightly closed containers that cannot sweat after some time because moisture may take you back to a stage that requires drying. Polyvinyl chloride containers work very well. For short periods of storage in economy-strained situations, papers made from vegetation are the best. You may choose to store your samples at freezing temperatures or below room temperature according to the nature of the components of interest in your samples that needs to be well understood, prior to sample preparation.

14.3 EXTRACTION TECHNIQUES

Naturally, metal elements are usually found in chelate forms in plant tissue or in ionic forms in organic plants. To identify the content of the elements, there is need to free them from the rest of the plant matrix in techniques known as digestion. Digestion prevents the interaction between metal ions and organic substances from the plant matrix (Husejnovic et al., 2016), a case which avails the maximum possible number of metal elements to exposure to be identified. The most used digestion procedures are discussed below.

14.3.1 DRY ASHING

Muffle furnace maintaining temperatures between 200 and 600°C is used to vaporize volatile materials including water and burn organic substances. Crucibles are used and furnace temperatures should be maintained at 450°C for 8–10 h without the use of any catalytic ashing aids (Peacock, 1992). Besides being accurate, rapid, and precise, this method requires minimal attention of the analyst. Samples are protected from contamination with reagents which would otherwise potentially affect errors at some stage of analysis. This method is very inefficient in the determination of volatiles under the ashing temperature (Husejnovic et al., 2016). One can also employ combustion techniques in closed vessels like special combustion bombs where the inorganic analyte is recollected with minute amounts of acids (Begerow and Dunemann, 2001). The advantage of this technique over the furnace method is that volatile trace elements like mercury are contained within the test matrix. In the general control of interferences, ashing auxiliaries such as acids and salts can be added to the matrices during ashing to facilitate a rapid digestion while containing the original elements as they naturally are (Begerow and Dunemann, 2001).

14.3.2   WET DIGESTION

This method breaks down the organic matrix to free metal elements into aqueous solutions (Husejnovic et al., 2016). Weighed milled plant samples are transferred into a flask with oxidizing agents and strong acids, usually nitric, perchloric, and/or sulfuric acids, which are then heated until all organic material gets digested leaving only a solution with oxides of the metal elements (Gray et al., 2015). It is faster than dry-ashing and preserves volatiles much better in the solution. However, the process is long and tedious and requires the attention of the analyst at all times (Husejnovic et al., 2016). Other versatile wet digestion techniques like thermally convective pressure and photolysis (ultraviolet [UV]) can also be used where elevated pressure/ temperatures conditions and UV-facilitated radicals, respectively, get the organic matrices sufficiently oxidized (Begerow and Dunemann, 2001).

14.3.3   MICROWAVE DIGESTION

This is a closed system in which a solvent which is in contact with the sample is heated using microwave energy to form a solution at pressures ≥ 300 psi (~ 20 bar) and temperatures of up to 200°C (Gray et al., 2015). Being a nonionizing energy, microwaves do not change the overall structure of the molecules in the sample but may only rearrange bond patterns and orientations. This method uses minimal reagents and is very quick. Soylaki et al. (2004) reported that the microwave digestion method is the best in terms of operational requirements but in terms of comparative results, Husejnovic et al. (2016) reported no differences.

14.4 CONTEMPORARY ANALYTICAL TECHNIQUES

The analytical techniques being looked at in this chapter includes inorganic and basic organic elemental analysis.

14.4.1 INORGANIC ELEMENTAL ANALYSIS

Techniques that are mostly used are atomic absorption spectroscopy (AAS), inductively coupled plasma mass spectroscopy (ICP-MS), inductively coupled plasma optical emission spectroscopy (ICP-OES), atomic emission spectroscopy (AES), X-ray fluorescence (XRF), and neutron activation analysis (Tessadri, 2003; Helaluddin et al., 2016).

14.4.1.1 ATOMIC SPECTROSCOPY TECHNIQUES

The principle behind the AAS is based on the ability of an atom to have at least one of its electrons in the ground state gets excited to a less stable orbital when energy is supplied to it. Taking advantage of the instability of the excited atom, it spontaneously returns to the more stable state, thereby releasing photons (Helaluddin et al., 2016). This technique is similar for AAS, AES, and AFS (Helaluddin et al., 2016) with minor variations on the timing of photon release. Microwave plasma atomic emission spectroscopy is one of the best instruments in the atomic spectroscopy techniques (Perkel, 2012). It is an improvement from flame AAS which works by creating plasma from nitrogen, one of the most abundant gases in the world, rather than argon, thereby saving costs (Perkel, 2012). Graphite furnace AAS is generally the only AAS variant that is capable of analyzing samples in a micro-semisolid form (petro–online, 2014). They use graphite tubes as atomizers and they have very low chemical interferences (Helaluddin et al., 2016). Cold vapor AAS is a nonflame-use AAS technique that detects mercury by the use of radiation absorption at 253.7 nm. Stannous chloride or sodium borohydride as reducing agents are first used to reduce the mercury to its elemental state, then argon carrier gases position the mercury vapor along the light path of the spectrophotometer for detection (Mester and Sturgeon, 2003; Helaluddin et al., 2016).

14.4.1.2 INDUCTIVELY COUPLED PLASMA MASS SPECTROMETRY

ICP-MS is very sensitive in the determination of trace elements and it has an advantage of providing a very wide range of options to do away with potential interferences (Perkel, 2012). Elements are identified by their individual isotopic masses and fingerprints (LUCIDEON, 2017) through spiking with specific isotopes whose concentrations are known (internal and calibration standard) and the concentration of the unknown is determined by the change that follows in isotopic mass-to-charge ratios (Gray et al., 2015; LUCIDEON, 2017). Sample size is limited to the amounts required by the digestion process. The disadvantage of this technique is that it is too destructive for the sample (Perkel, 2012).

14.4.1.3 INDUCTIVELY COUPLED PLASMA OPTICAL EMISSION SPECTROSCOPY

This is an optical emission spectroscopy which is generally designed to minimize argon use in plasma generation (Perkel, 2012). It is capable of both qualitatively (identification) and quantitatively analyzing elements, and is very good with trace elements (LUCIDEON, 2017). This technique involves the introduction of samples into plasma at specific wavelengths which gets them dissolvated, ionized, and excited. The determination of output uses characteristic emission lines for qualitative analyses and intensity of the lines for quantity determination (Boss and Fredeen, 1997; LUCIDEON, 2017). Sample size is limited to the amounts required by the digestion process.

14.4.1.4 X-RAY FLUORESCENCE

A nondestructive method of analysis which uses X-rays to bombard the samples and the outcome X-rays characteristic signatures are observed for each element (Perkel, 2012). An atom is stuck with X-ray radiation (high intensity) which removes at least one of the strongly held electrons right from inner orbitals, making the atom very unstable. The inner orbital unoccupied gaps are then filled by an electron from a higher orbital, thereby releasing energy in the form of X-rays (Helaluddin et al., 2016). Within the XRF, there is the wavelength-dispersive X-ray fluorescence, which is a technically more complicated and precise piece of equipment and uses a series of optics with usually bright X-ray sources (Perkel, 2012; LUCIDEON, 2017). Another technique within the XRF is the energy-dispersed X-ray fluorescence where the whole energy spectrum is measured using a solid-state detector. The latter is much simpler and less precise (Perkel, 2012). Generally, XRF's sample preparations are very simple (Helaluddin et al., 2016). Inorganic solids- and powders-based materials of samples sizes 5 g for quantitative and 0.05 g for semiquantitative analyses can be analyzed (LUCIDEON, 2017).

14.4.1.5   NEUTRON ACTIVATION ANALYSIS

In this technique, a neutron flow is used to which a sample matrix is exposed to generate radioactive isotopes of the elements of interest. Element characteristic gamma-ray energies are released as the radioactive isotopes decay to lower states. The intensities of the gamma rays give quantitative measurements of the elemental concentrations (Helaluddin et al., 2016).

14.4.2   INTRODUCTION TO ORGANIC ELEMENTAL ANALYSIS TECHNIQUES

Apart from inorganic elements, among which metal elements are, plants also contain various structures, some of which are synthesized and used as industrial material processes. The structures include condensed heterocyclic, aromatic, polycyclic, carbonaceous structures (carbon and graphite blocks), organometallic, organophosphorous compounds among others (Fadeeva et al., 2008; Culmo, 2013). Organic elemental determination assists in the identification of the presence of the structures and their purity (Fadeeva et al., 2008). For organic substances, main elements are carbon, nitrogen, hydrogen, and sulfur usually denoted as CHNS (Fadeeva et al., 2008). Generally, techniques in organic elemental analyses employ the combustion of gases method giving water, carbon dioxide, and nitrogen gases from which the individual elements are determined (Jordi, 2017). These analyses use commercially available analyzers of different types depending on the nature of the test material and the intended target element. The analyzers chosen must demonstrate high performance by the use of efficient scrubbing reagents, which is an embedded system in some equipment (Culmo, 2013).

In heterocyclic compounds that have nitrogen in their ring or in the substituents such as nitrone, nitro, amine, and azide groups in specific concentrations (>30%), there is reported to be an incomplete conversion of elemental nitrogen from different forms of nitrogen which is one challenge with the technique (Fadeeva et al., 2008). Polyfluorinated compounds pose a more significant challenge which is due to the aggressive nature of HF and F formed during decomposition and this leads to damage of analytical instruments through corrosion. This challenge can be overcome through the use of more stringent decomposition conditions taking advantage of the thermal stability of F in the zone of combustion (Fadeeva et al., 2008). It is also important to note that ICP-OES is capable to determine CHNO elements but not at trace levels, just as it is for halogens (Boss and Fredeen, 1997).

14.5 REPORTING ELEMENTAL PROFILES

When reporting elemental profiles, the data should not present the data in a generic form. It should be noted that each and every plant being worked on is unique and has its own characteristics based on the conditions it has been exposed to. The samples, even from the same species, may have different elemental compositions due to differences in climatic environments, the geochemical profile of the land, and handling methods (preparation, storage containers, and duration before analysis) (Paslawski and Migaszewski, 2006). This entails that it is important to detail all the specifics about the plant being studied, including the type of extract it finally got to be. The profile should include the following information.

14.5.1 PLANT TAXONOMY

Enough details on the name (species, genus, and family) and technical identification of the plant under study should be provided. This should include the family, genus, and species of the plant and any physiological characteristics.

14.5.2 LOCATION

Consideration should be put on the variations among different soil profiles and environmental conditions from where the plants were sourced, it is imperative to mention the actual location of sample collection and where necessary, the conditions at which the analyses were conducted. Global positioning system information could be helpful in reporting elemental profiles. This becomes crucial when the information reported is to be carried on and used for the purposes of monograph development, where there lie risks of misrepresenting the data for a particular species. For monographs and similar reports, samples of the same species need to be studied from across a wide and well-traceable location for representativeness of the whole species under study and repeatability of sample collection and analysis, respectively.

14.5.3 METHODOLOGY AND EQUIPMENT USED

Results may differ from one another due to differences in methodologies and equipment used for the analysis. The researcher should be well conversant with the techniques involved in a particular analysis including equipment calibration protocols for quality assurance of the data. Sometimes, information about the testing unit used is critical to the reliability of the results. This is critically important when it comes to data profiles to be used for certifications, imports, and exports of products.

14.5.4 UNITS OF MEASURE

This should include the specific unit of measure from which the test sample results were calculated. It should be clear if the units are representing wet or dry basis results of the profile. Where necessary, conversion factors should be available for the readers to trace how the calculations went about. This guarantees the reliability of the data profiles being presented.

KEYWORDS

- **analytical techniques**
- **elemental profiling**
- **sample preparation**
- **extraction techniques**
- **atomic absorption spectroscopy**

REFERENCES

Begerow, J.; Dunemann, L. Sample Preparation for Trace Analysis. In *Handbook of Analytical Techniques;* Gunzler, H., Williams, A., Eds.; Wiley-VCH: Weinheim, 2001; Vol. 78, p 103.

Boss, C. B.; Fredeen, K. J. *Concepts, Instrumentation and Techniques in Inductively Coupled Plasma Optical Emission Spectrometry*, 2nd ed.; Perkin-Elmer Corp.: Waltham, USA, 1997.

Culmo, R. F. *The Elemental Analysis of Various Classes of Chemical Compounds Using CHN;* PerkinElmer, Inc.: Waltham, MA, 2013; pp 1–6.

Fadeeva, V. P.; Tikhova, V. D.; Nikulicheva, O. N. Elemental Analysis of Organic Compounds with the Use of Automated CHNS Analyzers. *J. Anal. Chem.* **2008,** *63*(11), 1197–1210.

Gorsuch, T. T. *The Destruction of Organic Matter. In International Series of Monographs in Analytical Chemistry;* Pergamon Press ltd: Oxford, 1970; Vol. 39, p 152.

Gray, P. J.; Mindak, W. R.; Cheng, J. Elemental Analysis Manual for Food and Related Products. Services. *US Food Drug Adm.* **2015,** *1*(1), 1–24.

Helaluddin, A. B. M.; Khalid, R. S.; Alaama, M.; Abbas, S. A. Main Analytical Techniques Used for Elemental Analysis in Various Matrices. *Trop. J. Pharm. Res.* **2016,** *15*(2), 427–434.

Husejnovic, M. J.; Cilovic, E.; Dautovic, E.; Ibisevic, M.; Dzambic, A.; Karabasic, E.; Beganovic, M. Preparation of Samples for the Determination of Heavy Metals in Medicinal Plants. Conference Proceedings of the Pharmacy Symposium, Tuzla Canton. **2016,** *3*, 45–52.

Jordi Labs. Combustion of Gases, "CHNO by Combustion". Mansfield, MA. [Online] 2017. https//jordilabs.com/lab-testing/technique/elemental-analysis/chno/ (accessed Dec 15, 2017).

LUCIDEON. Testing and Characterization-Chemical Analysis. https://www.lucideon.com/testing-characterization/analytical-techniques-chemical-analysis (accessed Dec 12, 2017)

Mester, Z.; Sturgeon, R. E. *Sample Preparation for Trace Element Analysis*, 1st ed.; Elsevier: Boston, 2003.

Mtewa, A. G. K. Antibacterial Potency Stability, pH and Phytochemistry of Some Malawian Ready-to-Serve Aqueous Herbal Formulations Used Against Enteric Diseases. *Int. J. Herb. Med.* **2017,** *5*(3), 1–5.

Paslawski, P.; Migaszewski, Z. M. The Quality of Element Determinations in Plant Materials by Instrumental Methods. *Polish J. Environ. Stud.* **2006,** *15*(2a), 154–164.

Peacock, T. R. *The Preparation of Plant Material and Determination of Weight Percent Ash;* U.S.D.I.G.S, Open File Report 92-345: Denver, CO., 1992; pp 1–9. https://pubs.usgs.gov/of/1992/0345/report.pdf

Perkel, J. M. New Analytical Techniques for the Analytical Chemistry Laboratory. In American Laboratory. [Online] March 6, 2012. http// www.americanlaboratory.com/914-Application-Notes/38746-New-Elemental-Analysis-Techniques-for-the-Analytical-Chemistry-Laboratory/ (accessed Dec 14, 2017)

Petro-Online. Overview of most Commonly Used Analytical Techniques for Elemental Analysis. Feb 25, 2014. https://www.petro-online.com/article/analytical-instrumentation/11/university-of-girona/overview-of-most-commonlynbspused-analytical-techniques-for-elemental-analysis/1571 (accessed Dec 13, 2017).

Pruszkowski, E.; Bosnak, C. *Analysis of Plant Materials for Toxic and Nutritional Elements with the NexION 350 ICP-MS;* PerkinElmer, Inc.: Shelton, CT, 2015; Vol. 012267_01.

Saiki, H.; Maeda, O. Cleaning Procedures for Removal of External Deposits from Plant Samples. *Environ. Sci. Technol.* **1982,** *16*(8), 536–539. DOI: 10.1021/es00102a020.

Soylaki, M.; Tuzen, M.; Narin, I; Sari, H. Comparison of Microwave, Dry and Wet Digestion Procedures for the Determination of Trace Metal Contents in Spice Samples Produced in Turkey. *J. Food Drug Anal.* **2004,** *12*(3), 254–258.

Tessadri, R. Analytical Techniques for Elemental Analysis of Minerals. In *Encyclopedia of Life Support Systems EOLSS*, UNESCO: www.eolss.net, **2003,** Vol. 3.

Zygmunt, B.; Namiesnik, J. Preparation of Samples of Plant Material for Chromatographic Analysis. *J. Chrom. Sci.* **2003,** *41,* 109–116. https//academic.oup.com/chromsci/article-abstract/41/3/109/286982. DOI: 10.1093/chromsci/41.3.109 (accessed Dec 14, 2017).

CHAPTER 15

PHYTOCHEMICAL TEST METHODS: QUALITATIVE, QUANTITATIVE AND PROXIMATE ANALYSIS

CHUKWUEBUKA EGBUNA[1,*], JONATHAN C. IFEMEJE[1], MARYANN CHINENYE MADUAKO[1], HABIBU TIJJANI[2], STANLEY CHIDI UDEDI[3], ANDREW C. NWAKA[1], and MARYJANE OLUOMA IFEMEJE[1]

[1]*Department of Biochemistry, Chukwuemeka Odumegwu Ojukwu University, Anambra State, Nigeria, Tel.: +2347039618485*

[2]*Natural Product Research Laboratory, Department of Biochemistry, Bauchi State University, Gadau, Nigeria*

[3]*Department of Applied Biochemistry, Nnamdi Azikiwe University (UNIZIK), Awka, Nigeria*

Corresponding author. E-mail: egbuna.cg@coou.edu.ng; egbunachukwuebuka@gmail.com; https://egbunac.com ORCID: https://orcid.org/0000-0001-8382-0693

ABSTRACT

Phytochemical analysis involves both qualitative and quantitative analysis. While qualitative analysis is concerned with the presence or absence of a phytochemical, quantitative analysis accounts for the quantity or the concentration of the phytochemical present in the plant sample. The first step in phytochemical analysis is preliminary phytochemical screening before quantitative analysis. Quantitative analysis is a more comprehensive and useful method compared to qualitative analysis because the results obtained from the studies can be useful for drug discovery, standardization of herbal drugs, explanation of the medicinal potentials of plants and determination of the toxicity levels in plants. This chapter details the various simplified methods for the qualitative and quantitative analysis of phytochemicals including proximate composition analysis. It also presents useful hints for reagent preparation, how to determine the concentration of plant extract and make dilute solutions for standard curve making. It also details how to calculate the half maximal inhibitory concentration (IC_{50}) of plant extracts on a given biological system among other calculations commonly encountered during phytochemical studies.

15.1 INTRODUCTION

Phytochemical test is an analytical procedure utilized for the detection and quantification of phytoconstituents in plants. The test could either be qualitative or quantitative. Qualitative analysis or simply phytochemical screening is a practice geared towards the detection of phytochemicals in plants. As the name implies, it only reports the presence or absence of a phytochemical. Over the years, different methods of analysis have been developed while research is constantly ongoing to identify new techniques or methods of analysis in order to increase the chances of success. The successes recorded so far in the detection of phytochemicals is largely based on the function of the functional groups of the phytochemicals present which reacts with a reagent to give a characteristic color. For instance, the presence of flavonoids is detected when a characteristic yellow color is produced when plant extracts are treated with NaOH and HCl. Another example is the ability of the plant extracts to react with $FeCl_3$ to give bluish-black color, which is an indication of the presence of phenols.

Once a phytochemical is found, the next in line will be to determine the quantity present – quantitative analysis. Many modern techniques have been employed in this regard but some are very expensive and are not readily available to researchers. Quantitative analysis is very important in the discovery of new drugs, standardization of herbal drugs, offering explanation about the medicinal potentials of plants and determining the toxicity level of plant natural products. Through this method, many novel compounds have been discovered. The need for new methods will for a long time persist because of the chemical diversity found in the plant kingdom.

15.2 REAGENT PREPARATION

Reagents are chemical substances that cause reactions to occur in a system. It can be a compound or a mixture which is usually an inorganic or organic molecule. The term "reagent" is quite different from the term "chemical". A reagent is usually a readily made compound or known mixture of compounds while a chemical is any specific chemical element or chemical compound.

The extraction and isolation of phytochemicals in plants are directly affected by the type and nature of reagent. Moreover, the ability to freshly prepare a reagent for use at the right time is a crucial step to a successful screening and quantification of phytochemicals. In order to prepare solutions of lower concentrations for qualitative and quantitative analysis, a calculated volume of the concentrated solution is taken from the stock solution and then added to a specific volume of distilled water or a specified solvent. However, such information to be taken depends on the information provided by the manufacturer on the label on the stock bottle.

15.2.1 COMMONLY ENCOUNTERED TERMS DURING REAGENT PREPARATION

1. **Solvent:** A solvent is a liquid in which a solute is dissolved to form a solution.
2. **Solute:** A solute is the minor component in a solution, dissolved in the solvent.
3. **Solution:** A solution is a homogeneous mixture of two or more substances.
4. **Standard solution:** A standard solution is a solution containing a precisely known concentration of a substance.
5. **Molar mass:** This implies the mass of one mole of an element or a compound.
6. **Concentration:** This refers to the relative amount of solute and solvent in a solution.
7. **Molarity:** Molarity is a concentration unit (M) defined as the number of moles of solute divided by liters of solution.
8. **Normality:** Normality is a concentration unit (N) defined as the number of equivalents of solute per liter of solution. For example, $1 \text{ M } H_2SO_4 = 2 \text{ N } H_2SO_4$.
9. **Distilled water:** Distilled water is water that has had many of its impurities removed through distillation. It is free of inorganic materials, and most organic contaminants. It has an electrical conductivity of not more than 11 µS/cm and total dissolved solids of less than 10 mg/L.
10. **Deionized water or demineralized water:** This is water that has had almost all of its mineral ions removed, such as cations and anions. Deionization produces highly pure water that is generally similar to distilled water with an advantage that most non-particulate water impurities are dissolved salts, as such the process is quicker and does not build upscale.

15.2.2   COMMONLY USED ABBREVIATIONS

The correct use of units is an important process to a successful reagent preparation. Some of the units were presented in Table 15.1.

TABLE 15.1   Some commonly encountered units.

Quantity	Units
Mass	g (gram)
Kilogram	Kg
Milligram	Mg
Percent	%
Normality	N
Liter	L
Volume	mL
Molar mass	g/mol
Molar Concentration	mol/L or mol/dm^3
Molarity	M

15.2.3   GUIDE TO REAGENT PREPARATION/CALCULATIONS

1.   Preparation of reagent in % w/v: The % w/v implies that a particular weight of a solute should be dissolved in a known quantity of solvent and made up to 100 mL.

   Note: 1 mL = 1 cm^3

   For example

   • To prepare 0.9% w/v NaCl, this means that 0.9 g of NaCl should be dissolved first in a little quantity of water and make up to 100 mL.
   • To prepare 0.3% ammonium thiocyanate, dissolve 0.3 g of ammonium thiocyanate in water and make up to 100 mL mark.

Note: Distilled water is recommended for preparation involving water and preparation should be done using volumetric flasks that have been calibrated. Other apparatus such as measuring cylinder, beakers, pipettes, and so forth, should be assembled before analysis begins. The calibration of equipment's and glassware's.

Precautionary measures are meant to be observed at all times by wearing lab coats, face masks, hand gloves, and most important chemicals in the fume cupboard. This is because most chemicals used in the phytochemical analysis are toxic and can be dangerous to health.

2.   Preparation of reagent in % v/v: This means that a particular volume of a solute (liquid) should be dissolved and made up to 100 mL of the solution.

For example, to prepare

- 80% v/v ethanol means to dissolve 80 mL of ethanol in water and make it up to 100 mL with water.
- 10% acetic acid in ethanol means to dissolve 10 mL of acetic acid in first small quantity of ethanol and make it up to 100 mL with ethanol. *Warning:* The principle of adding acid to water and not water into acid should be observed.
- 20% H_2SO_4 means 20 mL of stock or concentrated H_2SO_4 in some quantity of water and make it up to 100 mL with distilled water.

3.   Preparation of solutions involving molar concentration (v/v): Generally, the original molar concentration, C_M of a chemical substance of molar mass, M grams per mole in a commercial product of P % by mass and of density (or specific gravity) d gram per cm^3 is given as:

$$C_M = \frac{10 \times P \times d}{M}$$

where C_M=molar concentration of stock reagent; P=percentage purity (% purity); d=density or specific gravity; M=molar mass.

Note

1. C_M is sometimes represented on the label of the reagent bottle.
2.   The information needed for these calculations can be readily accessed from the label on the stock bottle. This is recommended because they usually differ from company to company. As a guide, information about some chemicals is presented in Table 15.2.

For example, to prepare 50 mL of 2 M solution of HCl from a stock solution of HCl with the following information on the label, specific gravity=1.18%, purity=36%, molar mass=36.5 g/mol.

Step 1: Determine the concentration of the chemical in the stock solution, that is, if not provided.

TABLE 15.2 Some Vital Information of Analytical Reagents/Chemicals.

Chemicals	Molarity (M)	% Purity	RMM (g/mol)	SG
Tetraoxosulfate (VI) acid (H_2SO_4)	18.00	97 or 98	98.00	1.82
Hydrochloric acid (HCl)	11.6	36	36.46	1.18
Nitric acid (HNO_3)	16.4	69	63.00	1.42
Acetic acid (CH_3COOH)	17.4	99	60.05	1.05
Perchloric acid ($HClO_4$)	11.7; 9.5	70; 61	100.46	1.71; 1.66
Hydrofluoric acid (HF)	27	48	20.01	1.29
Phosphoric acid (H_3PO_4)	15 M, 45 N	88	97.99	1.69
Ammonium hydroxide (NH_4OH)	14.50	28–30% NH_3	35.05	0.90
Potassium hydroxide (KOH)	11.7	45	56.12	1.46
Sodium hydroxide (NaOH)	19.4	50	40.00	1.54

RMM = relative molecular mass; SG = specific gravity[1].

$$C_M = \frac{10 \times P \times d}{M}$$

$$= \frac{10*36*1.18}{36.5}$$

$$= 11.64 \ M$$

Then, the amount of HCl required to prepare 2 M HCl in 50 mL can be expressed as follows:

$$C_1V_1 = C_2V_2$$

where

C_1 = Original concentration of the stock HCl undiluted = 11.64 M.
V_1 = Volume of the required stock solution needed to prepare the desired/diluted concentration =?
C_2 = Concentration desired = 2 M.
V_2 = Volume of the new/desired concentration required = 50 mL

---

[1]The specific gravity of 1.82 means that the stock solution is 1.82 times heavier than an equal volume of water. This implies that 1 mL of the stock solution weighs 1.82 g or that 1000 mL of stock solution weighs 1.82×1000=1800

Calculations

$$V_1 = \frac{C_2 V_2}{C_1}$$

$$V_1 = \frac{2 \times 50}{11.64}$$

$$= 8.59 \text{ mL}$$

Therefore, 8.59 mL of concentrated HCl will be required to prepare 2M of HCl in 50 mL of water.

Note: Standardization of the reagent for each preparation is important so as to be sure of the exact concentration.

4. Preparation of solutions involving molar concentration (w/v): If the starting material is in the solid form. For instance, NaOH, KOH pellets, and so forth. The following calculations apply:

$$Molar\ concentration\ (mol\,/\,dm^3) = \frac{Mass\ Concentration\,(g\,/\,dm^3)}{Molar\ mass(g\,/\,mol)}$$

As an example, prepare 0.1 M or 0.1 mol/dm^3 of NaOH.

You will need to calculate the mass of NaOH required to be dissolved in 1000 mL of water which will give 0.1 mol/dm^3. To get this, follow the following steps:

Desired molar concentration = 0.1 mol/dm^3

Molar mass of NaOH = 40 g/mol

Mass concentration (g/dm^3)
  = *Molar Concentration (mol/dm^3) × Molar mass (g/mol)*
  = 0.1 ~~mol~~/dm^3 × 40 g/~~mol~~
  = 4 g/dm^3

This implies that 4 g of NaOH should be dissolved in 1000 mL of water to make the concentration of 0.1 mol/dm^3.

However, if 1000 mL of it will be too much and you wanted 50 mL of 0.1 mol/dm^3 NaOH, you can simply cross multiply:

4 g → 1000 mL

x g → 50 mL

x g = 0.2 g

This implies that you should dissolve 0.2 g of NaOH and make up to 50 mL with water or appropriate solvent to obtain the same concentration of 0.1 mol/dm³ NaOH.

5.   Preparation of solution in normality: To make a solution involving Normality, you must first determine the equivalent mass of the chemical and then determine the gram needed of that chemical.

As an example, the steps involved in preparation of 250 mL of 1 N H_2SO_4 solution are:

Step 1: Calculate the equivalent mass which is the gram formula weight divided by the number of acid hydrogen in the compound.

In H_2SO_4, the gram formula weight = 98 g.

The acid hydrogen = 2

Dividing 98/2 = 49 g

Step 2: Calculate the number of grams of H_2SO_4 needed.

Gram of compound needed

= (N desired) × (equivalent mass) × (volume in liters desired)

Gram of H_2SO_4 needed = (1 N) × (49) × (0.250 L)

= 12.25 g

Step 3: The result in step 2 implies that a 1 N solution of H_2SO_4 will require 12.25 g of sulfuric acid powder, that is, if one existed, diluted in 250 mL of water. But since H_2SO_4 is a liquid, there will be a need to calculate the concentrated volume required for the preparation that will contain 12.25 g of it. The following formula applies:

$$Volume\ of\ concentrated\ acid\ needed = \frac{Gram\ of\ acid\ needed}{\%\ concentration\ x\ specific\ gravity}$$

$$= \frac{12.25\ g}{0.97\ x\ 1.82}$$

$$= 6.94\ mL$$

This means that 6.94 mL of concentrated sulfuric acid should be diluted to 250 mL of water to obtain 1 N H_2SO_4.

A simplified approach to the preparation of solution in normality:

Since, 1M Acid = (1 × Number of replaceable hydrogen) N Acid

Then, 1M H_2SO_4 = (1 × 2) N H_2SO_4 = 2N H_2SO_4

Now, to prepare 250 mL 1N H_2SO_4 as illustrated previously

Since, 1M H_2SO_4 = 2N H_2SO_4

xM = 1N H_2SO_4

This resolves to 0.5M H_2SO_4 as the equivalent of 1N H_2SO_4

This means that 1N H_2SO_4 can be prepared by simply preparing 0.5M H_2SO_4

Taking C_1 = 18M, V_1 = ?, C_2 = 0.5M, V_2 = 250mL

$$C_1V_1 = C_2V_2$$

$$V_1 = \frac{C_2 x\, V_2}{C_1}$$

$$= \frac{0.5\ x\ 250}{18}$$

$$= 6.94\ mL$$

This implies that 6.94 mL of concentrated H_2SO_4 should be diluted to 250 mL with water to obtain 1N H_2SO_4.

6. Determination of molarity from percent solutions: This can be possible if the density is known.

As an example, determine the molarity of 37.2% HCl with density of 1.19 g/mL

Step 1: Mass of solution = 1000 mL × 1.19 g/mL = 1.190 g

Step 2: Mass % = 37.2% = 0.372, that is, the decimal equivalent

Step 3: Molar mass of HCl = 36.46 g/mol

Step 4: Determine the number of moles by multiplying the mass (step 1) by the mass % (step 2) and divided by molar mass (step 3)

$$= \frac{1190\ g\ x 0.372}{36.46\ g\ /\ mol}$$

$$= 12.1\ mol$$

Step 5: Molarity=mol/liters=12.1 mol/1 L=12.1 M.

7. Determination of percent from molarity solutions: To convert from percent solution to molarity, multiply percent solution value by 10 to get g/L, then divided by the molar mass.

As an example, convert 2% HCl solution to molarity

Step 1: Multiply 2% by 10
Step 2: Divide by molar mass of HCl = 36.46 g/mol

$$= \frac{2\% \, x10}{36.46} = 0.55 \, M$$

8.   Preparation of Indicators: The preparation of indicators differ remarkably from indicators to indicators. Each indicator has a standard method of preparation. A few were presented below.

- **Methyl orange:** 0.01% in water
- **Methyl red indicator:** Dissolve 1.0 g of solid in 600 mL of ethanol, and dilute to 1 dm3 with water. or Dissolve 0.04 g of methyl red in 40 mL of ethanol and makeup to 100 mL with water
- **Phenolphthalein indicator:** Dissolve 1 g of powder in 500 mL of 50% alcohol
- **Phenol red:** Dissolve 0.1 g of phenol red in 400 mL of water and dilute to 500 mL

9.   Preparation of dilute concentration of plant extract: The preparation of dilute concentration from plant crude extract is an essential step in phytopharmacology. The diluted extract could be useful in many ways such as in making of a standard curve or where a desired concentration is intended to be made. The following details will be helpful in determining exact concentrations:

Dissolving 1 mg (0.001 g) of plant extract in 1 mL of solvent gives 1 mg/mL. But since it will be practically difficult to weigh 1 mg, one can weigh 10 mg (0.01 g) and dissolve in 10 mL which still gives 1 mg/mL or 1000 µg/mL.

To prepare 500, 250, 125, 62.5, 31.25 µg/mL, the procedure described below can be adopted. Alternatively, the dilution formula $C_1 V_1 = C_2 V_2$ can be used once a stock is prepared.

Step 1: Dissolve 10 mg of crude plant extract in 10 mL to give 1000 µg/mL stock = 1 mg/mL

Step 2: Take a fixed amount of the stock (say 5 mL) and add equal volume of same solvent (5 mL). This gives 500 µg/mL (A) = 0.5 mg/mL

Step 3: Take a fixed amount of (A) (say 5 mL) and add equal volume of same solvent (5 mL). This gives 250 µg/mL (B) = 0.25 mg/mL

Step 4: Take a fixed amount of (B) (say 5 mL) and add equal volume of same solvent (5 mL). This gives 125 µg/mL (C) = 0.125 mg/mL

Step 5: Take a fixed amount of (C) (say 5 mL) and add equal volume of same solvent (5 mL). This gives 62.5 µg/mL (D) = 0.0625 mg/Ml

Step 6: Take a fixed amount of (D) (say 5 mL) and add equal volume of same solvent (5 mL). This gives 31.25 µg/mL (E) = 0.03125 mg/mL

10.   Extrapolation of readings from a standard curve: The determination of the extract concentration from a standard curve should be calculated thus:

$$Phytochemical\ (mg\,/\,100g)=\frac{Concentration\ from\ curve\ x\ extract\ volume\ x\,100}{Aliquote\ volume\ x\ weight\ of\ sample}$$

11.   Determination of LD$_{50}$: The determination of LD$_{50}$ are usually carried out in two phases in which different concentration of extracts are administered to a model and observed for 24 hours for behavior as well as mortality. Phase 1 may involve the administration of 10, 100, 1000 mg extract/kg body weight to 3 groups of 3 animals each while phase 2 may involve the administration of 2000, 3000, 4000, 5000 mg extract/kg body weight to 4 groups of 1 animal each. The number of deaths and the behavior of the animals should be noted at each phase. The behavior of the animals could be reported as either normal or palpitating. The LD$_{50}$ can be calculated according to Lorke's method thus:

$$LD_{50}=\sqrt{Highest\ dose\ that\ gave\ no\ mortality\ x\ Lowest\ dose\ that\ produced\ mortality}$$

12.   Determination of the volume of extract to administer in an in vivo model: The following formula is applicable in determining the exact volume containing the right concentration to be administered:

$$Dose\ volume\ (mL)=\frac{Desired\ dose\ (mg\,/\,kg)\,x\,Weight\ of\ animal\ (kg)}{Stock\ (mg\,/\,mL)}$$

13.   Determination of IC$_{50}$ by the non-linear regression method: The half maximal inhibitory concentration (IC$_{50}$) is a measure of the potency of a substance in inhibiting a specific biological or biochemical function. It forms a fulcrum for comparison between the activities of two or more extracts on a biological system. The lower the IC$_{50}$ the better the inhibition of the extract.

IC$_{50}$ can be calculated by the logit and probit method (Box 15.1). By this method, the concentration of the extract is converted to Log 10, whereas % Inhibition of the extract on a biochemical process e.g. an interaction of the extract and DPPH is converted from percentage to probit using the probit chat (Table 15.3). A plot of probited values on Y-axis against log 10 concentration on the X-axis (Fig. 15.1) should be made. The equation of the graph should then be obtained and the IC_{50} calculated.

BOX 15.1 IC_{50} Calculations using probit chat

Concentration of extract (mg/ml)	Log 10 of extract concentration*	% Inhibition by extract	Probit of % Inhibition**
10	1	30	4.48
20	1.30103	60	5.25
30	1.477121	75	5.07
40	1.60206	90	6.28

Intercept	= 1.9376
Slope	= 2.4775

$$Y^{\dagger} = mx + C \quad x = 1.23$$
$$\text{Antilog } (10^{\wedge}) \quad IC_{50} = 16.98 \text{ mg/ml}$$

** Probit serves as y-axis while *log 10 values serves as x-axis. The Linest excel function can be used to determine the slope and the intercept. †Since IC_{50} is to be determined, the value 50 should by probited which gives 5 i.e. the Y (see Table. 15.3). This method of IC_{50} determination is called non-linear regression method.

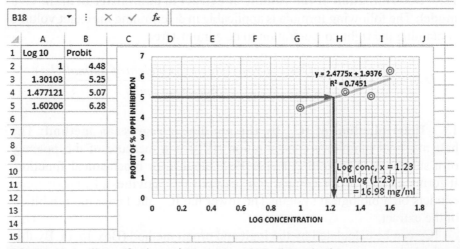

FIGURE 15.1   (See color insert.) Illustration of IC_{50} determination.

TABLE 15.3 Transformation of percentages to probit.

%	0	1	2	3	4	5	6	7	8	9
0	-	2.67	2.95	3.12	3.25	3.36	3.45	3.52	3.59	3.66
10	3.72	3.77	3.82	3.87	3.93	3.96	4.01	4.05	4.08	4.12
20	4.16	4.19	4.23	4.26	4.29	4.33	4.36	4.39	4.42	4.45
30	4.48	4.50	4.53	4.56	4.59	4.61	4.64	4.67	4.69	4.72
40	4.75	4.77	4.80	4.82	4.85	4.87	4.90	4.92	4.95	4.97
50	5.00	5.03	5.05	5.08	5.10	5.13	5.15	5.18	5.20	5.23
60	5.25	5.28	5.31	5.33	5.36	5.39	5.41	5.44	5.47	5.50
70	5.52	5.55	5.58	5.61	5.64	5.67	5.71	5.74	5.77	5.81
80	5.84	5.88	5.92	5.95	5.99	6.04	6.08	6.13	6.18	6.23
90	6.28	6.34	6.41	6.48	6.55	6.64	6.75	6.88	7.05	7.33
-	0.0	0.1	0.2	0.3	0.4	0.5	0.6	0.7	0.8	0.9
99	7.33	7.37	7.41	7.46	7.51	7.58	7.65	7.75	7.88	8.09

15.3 QUALITATIVE PHYTOCHEMICAL ANALYSIS

Phytochemical screening are usually carried out to identify the presence or absence of phytochemicals in plants crude extract. Usually, findings are reported as either present (positive [+]) or absent (negative [−]).

15.3.1 TESTS FOR ALKALOIDS

The following tests can be adopted for the detection of the presence of alkaloids. Usually, it is good to employ two or three of the methods as a counter check. The crude extracts can be prepared by dissolving the dried powdered sample in dilute hydrochloric acid and filtered with cotton wool or filter paper.

Mayer's test: The filtrates obtained should be treated with Mayer's reagent (potassium mercuric iodide). The formation of a yellow colored precipitate indicates the presence of alkaloids (Prashant et al., 2011).

Wagner's test: Aliquot of 2 mL of extract should be treated with Wagner's reagent (iodine and potassium iodide). The formation of reddish brown precipitate indicates the presence of alkaloids (Kumar et al., 2014).

Hager's test: The filtrates were treated with Hager's reagent (saturated picric acid solution). The presence of alkaloids is confirmed by the formation of yellow colored precipitate (Prashant et al., 2011).

Dragendroff's test: To the filtrate, treat with few drops of Dragendroff's reagent (solution of potassium bismuth iodide). The formation of red precipitate indicates the presence of alkaloids (Prashant et al., 2011).

Dragendroff's test by thin-layer chromatography: Apply extract on pre-coated thin-layer chromatography (TLC) plates developed in chloroform: methanol (9:1) as the mobile phase. After movement of solute in the mobile face, dry and spray it with Dragendroff's reagent. The appearance of orange-red spot at room temperature indicates the presence of alkaloid (Chakraborthy, 2011).

With Tannic Acid: To 1 mL of extract, add 2–3 drops of the tannic acid solution reagent, the appearance of amorphous or crystalline precipitate indicates the presence of alkaloid (Harsha et al., 2013).

15.3.2   TESTS FOR FLAVONOIDS

Lead acetate test: To 3 mL of aqueous extract, add 1 mL of 10% lead acetate solution. The formation of a yellow or white precipitate indicates a positive result for flavonoids (Kumar et al., 2014; Pradeep et al., 2014).

Shinado's test: To the extract in alcohol, add a few magnesium turnings and few drops of concentrated hydrochloric acid and boil for 5 min. A red coloration indicates the presence of flavonoids (Kagbo and Ejebe, 2009; Salna et al., 2011).

NaOH test: To 2 mL of extract, add 2 mL of aqueous NaOH and dilute HCl. The formation of a yellow-orange color which changes to colorless on the addition of dilute HCl indicates the presence of flavonoids (Trease and Evans, 2002).

H_2SO_4 test: Treat a fraction of the extract with concentrated H_2SO_4 and observe for the formation of orange color which indicates the presence of flavonoids (Kumar et al., 2014).

Aluminum chloride test: To the extract, add a few drops of 1% aluminum solution. The formation of a yellow coloration indicates the presence of flavonoids (Edeoga et al., 2005).

Ammonium solution test: To the extract, add a few drops of 1% NH3 solution. The formation of a yellow coloration indicates the presence of flavonoids (Krishnaiah et al., 2009).

15.3.3   TESTS FOR SAPONINS

Froth test: Boil 2 g of the powdered sample with 20 mL of distilled water in a water bath and filter. Mix 10 mL of the filtrate with 5 mL of distilled water and shake vigorously for a stable persistent froth. Add three drops of olive oil to the froth and shake vigorously. The formation of emulsion indicates the presence of saponins (Kagbo and Ejebe, 2009).

Saponin test by thin-layer chromatography: Apply sample on TLC plates developed in chloroform–methanol–water (60:35:5) as mobile phase and dry. Spray plates with 1% vanillin and 5% sulfuric acid reagent and dry at 110°C for few minutes. Glycosides appear as dark bluish to black spot (Chakraborthy, 2011).

Heamolysis test: Treat 1 g of the extract with distilled water and add 2 mL of aqueous NaCl solution and 2 mL of the filtrate. Then add three drops of an animal blood to the test tube by means of syringe and mix gently by inverting the tube (no shaking) and allow to stand for 15 min. The settling down of the red blood cells denotes the presence of saponins (Yusuf et al., 2014).

15.3.4   TESTS FOR PHENOLS

Ferric chloride test (Brayer's test): Treat extract with three to four drops of ferric chloride solution. The formation of bluish-black color indicates the presence of phenols (Prashant et al., 2011).

Liebermann test: Add 1 mL of extract and heat briefly with $NaNO_3$, H_2SO_4 and dilute with water. Add excess of dilute NaOH and observe the formation of deep red or green or blue color which indicates the presences of phenols (Kumar et al., 2014).

Folin–Ciocalteu test: Add 1 mL of extract to a clean test tube, followed by the addition of 1 mL of Folin–Ciocalteu plus 1 mL of 20% Na_2CO_3, the presence of dark blue color shows the presence of phenol.

15.3.5   TESTS FOR TANNINS

Ferric chloride test: To the extract, add few drops of 0.1% ferric chloride and observe for brownish green or a blue-black coloration for a positive result (Trease and Evans, 2002).

Gelatin test: To the extract, add few drops of 1% gelatin solution containing sodium chloride. The formation of white precipitate indicates the presence of tannins (Prashant et al., 2011).

Lead acetate test: To 2 mL of extract, add few drops of 1% lead acetate. A yellowish precipitate shows the presence of tannins (Harsha et al., 2013).

Bromine water test: Add three drops of bromine water to the filtrate. A buff colored precipitate indicates the presence of condensed tannins while hydrolyzable tannins may give none (Yusuf et al., 2014).

15.3.6   TEST FOR PHLOBATANNINS

HCl test: Aqueous extract of the plant sample should be boiled with aqueous hydrochloric acid. The presence of red precipitate indicates the presence of phlobatannins (Abdullahi et al., 2014).

15.3.7   TESTS FOR STEROIDS

Salkowski test: To 2 mL of aqueous extract, add 2 mL of chloroform and 2 mL of H_2SO_4. Shake the solution well. This will result in the formation of red chloroform layer and greenish-yellow fluorescence in the acid layer (Harsha et al., 2013).

H_2SO_4 test: To 1 g of the test substance, add a few drop of acetic acid, acetic anhydride, warm, and cool under the tap water. Then add drops of concentrated sulfuric acid gently along the sides of the test tube. The presence of green color indicates the presence of steroids (Salna et al., 2011).

TLC test: Apply extract to TLC plates developed in benzene–methanol (95:5) as the mobile phase. Spray 5% alcoholic sulfuric acids reagent on the plate. A bluish-green spot indicates the presence of steroids (Chakraborthy, 2011).

15.3.8   TESTS FOR TERPENOIDS

Test for terpenoids: Take 3 mL of the extract and dissolve in 2 mL of chloroform and evaporate to dryness. Add 2 mL of concentrated sulfuric acid and heat for 2 min. The formation of greyish color indicates the presence of terpenoids (Pradeep et al., 2014).

Liebermann–Burchard test: Treat 1 mL of the extract with ethanol, acetic anhydride, and few drops of H_2SO_4. The formation of pink to violet color indicates the presence of terpenoids (Sofowora, 1993).

15.3.9   TESTS FOR TRITERPENOIDS

Noller's test: Warm the extract with tin and thionyl chloride. A purple coloration indicates the presence of triterpenoids (Salna et al., 2011).

Triterpenoids Test by TLC: Apply sample extract on TLC plate impregnated with silver nitrate and then developed in butanol-2M ammonium hydroxide (1:1) as the mobile phase. Spray the plate with antimony trichloride. A purplish spot indicates the presence of triterpenoids (Chakraborthy, 2011).

15.3.10   TEST FOR TERPENES

H_2SO_4 test: To 0.5 g of extract, add 3 mL of chloroform, shake, and filter. Add 10 drop of acetic anhydride followed by 2 drops of concentrated sulfuric acid. A reddish brown coloration at the interface shows a positive result for the presence of terpenes (Kagbo and Ejebe, 2009).

15.3.11   TEST FOR DITERPENES

Copper acetate test: Dissolve extract in water and treat with three to four drops of copper acetate solution. The formation of emerald green color indicates the presence of diterpenes (Prashant et al., 2011).

15.3.12   TESTS FOR ANTHRAQUINONE

Borntrager's test (for free anthracene derivatives): Measure 0.5 g of powdered sample and add 5 mL of chloroform. Shake for 5 min and filter. To the filtrate, add equal volume of 10% ammonia solution. A pink, red, or violet color in the aqueous layer after shaking indicates the presence of free anthraquinone (Sofowora, 1993).

Modified Borntrager's test (for combined anthracene derivatives): To 1 g of the powdered sample, add 5 mL of 10% hydrochloric acid and boil for 3 min. Filter the hot solution, cool, and extract gently with 5 mL of benzene. Pipet off the upper benzene layer and shake gently in a test tube with half its volume of 10% ammonium hydroxide solution. A rose pink to cherry red color in the ammonia layer indicates the presence of anthraquinone (Trease and Evans, 2002).

15.3.13   TEST FOR CYANOGENIC GLYCOSIDES

Sodium picrate test: Suspend 1 g of the powdered sample in a beaker containing water. Then suspend the sodium picrate paper by means of a thread in the beaker. Heat for 1 h and observe for color change. The change in color from yellow to brick red indicates a positive result (Hegnauer, 1986).

15.3.14   TESTS FOR CARDIAC GLYCOSIDES

Keller-Killani test: Treat 5 mL of extract with 2 mL of glacial acetic acid containing one drop of ferric chloride solution. Underlay the mixture with 1 mL of concentrated sulfuric acid. A brown ring at the interface indicates a deoxysugar characteristic of cardenolides. A violet ring may appear below the brown ring, while in the acetic acid layer, a greenish ring may form just gradually throughout thin layer (Edeoga et al., 2005).

Legal's test: Treat extract with sodium nitroprusside in pyridine and sodium hydroxide. The formation of pink to blood red color indicates the presence of cardiac glycosides (Prashant et al., 2011).

15.3.15   TESTS FOR GLYCOSIDES

Borntrager's test: To 3 mL of aqueous extract, add dilute sulfuric acids, boil, and filter the solution. Treat the filtrate with an equal volume of benzene and shake well. Decant the organic layer formed into a test tube. Add equal volume of dilute ammonia solution. The ammonia layer will turn pink showing the presence of glycosides (Harsha et al., 2013).

Bromine water test: Dissolve extract in bromine water and observe for the formation of yellow precipitate to show a positive result for the presence of glycosides (Satheesh et al., 2012).

15.3.16   TESTS FOR QUINONE

NaOH test: To the test substance, add sodium hydroxide. A blue-green or red color indicates the presence of quinone (Salna et al., 2011).

HCl test: Treat a small amount of the extract with concentrated HCl and then observe for the formation of yellow colored precipitate which indicates the presence of quinones (Kumar et al., 2014).

Alcoholic potassium hydroxide test: Treat 1 mL of each of the extract with alcoholic potassium hydroxide solution. Quinines gives coloration ranging from red to blue (Kumar et al., 2013).

15.3.17 TEST FOR COUMARIN

NaOH test: To the test sample, add 10% of sodium hydroxide and chloroform. The formation of a yellow color indicates the presence of coumarin (Salna et al., 2011).

15.3.18 TEST FOR GUM

Test for gum: To the test substance, add few mL of water and shake well. The formation of swells or adhesives indicates the presence of gum (Salna et al., 2011).

15.3.19 TESTS FOR ANTHOCYANIN

Test for anthocyanins: To 2 mL of aqueous extract, add 2 mL of 2N HCl and ammonia. The appearance of pink-red which turns to blue-violet indicates the presence of anthocyanin (Harsha et al., 2013).

Test for anthocyanin and betacyanin: To 2 mL of the extract, add 1 mL of 2N NaOH and heat for 5 min at 100°C. The formation of bluish green color indicates the presence of anthocyanin while the formation of yellow color indicates the presence of betacyanin (Kalpana et al., 2014).

Test for leucoanthocyanins: To 5 mL of aqueous extract, add 5 mL of isoamyl alcohol. The formation of color in the upper layer indicates the presence of leucoanthocyanins (Harsha et al., 2013).

15.3.20 TEST FOR FATTY ACIDS

TLC method: Apply the samples on a pre-coated TLC plates, dry, and develope in hexane-ethyl acetate (95:5) as mobile phase. Spray with 5% alcoholic potassium permanganate solution. The appearance of dark brown spots indicates the presence of fatty acids (Chakraborthy, 2011).

15.3.21 TEST FOR ESSENTIAL OILS

TLC method: Pre-coat the TLC plate and obtain chromatogragh with the solvent system, methelyne-di-chloride-chloroform-ethyl acetate-n-propanol

(47:45:2:2.5) as the mobile phase. Spray the TLC plates with vanillin sulfuric acids reagent dried at 105°C for 2 min. The appearance of pink-brown color spots shows the presence of essential oils (Chakraborthy, 2011).

15.3.22   TEST FOR CARBOXYLIC ACIDS

Test for carboxylic acids: To 1 mL of the extract, add few mL of sodium bicarbonate solution. A reaction involving effervescence (due to the liberation of carbon dioxide) indicates the presence of carboxylic acids (Kumar et al., 2013).

15.3.23   TEST FOR RESINS

Test for resins: To 1 mL of extract, add few drops of acetic anhydride solution followed by 1 mL of concentrated H_2SO_4. The formation of orange to yellow coloration indicates a positive result (Kumar et al., 2013).

15.3.24   TEST FOR OXALATE

Test for oxalate: To 3 mL portion of extract, add a few drops of ethanoic/ glacial acetic acid. A greenish black coloration indicates the presence of oxalates (Solomon et al., 2013).

15.3.25   TESTS FOR PROTEINS AND AMINO ACIDS

Several testing options are available for the detection of amino acids and proteins. They include:

Biuret test: To the test solution, add Biuret reagent. The blue reagent turns violet in the presence of proteins (Salna et al., 2011).

Xanthoproteic test: To 1 mL of extract add 1 mL of concentrated H_2SO_4. This would result in the formation of white precipitate which on boiling turns yellow. To the yellow precipitate, add NH4OH, the change from yellow to orange indicates a positive result (Harsha et al., 2013).

Million's test: Treat the crude extract with 2 mL of Million's reagent and mix. The formation of a white precipitate which turns red upon gentle heating indicates the presence of protein (Yadav and Munin, 2011).

Ninhydrin test: Boil the crude extract with 2 mL of 0.2% solution of Ninhydrin. The formation of a violet color indicates the presence of amino acid and proteins (Yadav and Munin, 2011).

TLC test: Spot the extract on the TLC plate using n-butanol–acetic acid–water (12:3:5) as the mobile phase. After subjecting it to solvent system and the generation of TLC fingerprint on plates, spray the plate with 0.2% Ninhydrin in acetone, dry briefly at 105°C for 1–2 min. The presence of violet color to pink color indicates (Chakraborthy, 2011).

15.3.26   TESTS FOR CARBOHYDRATE

Dissolve extract in 5 mL of distilled water and filter. Use the filtrate for carbohydrate test.

Benedict's test: Treat filtrates with Benedict's reagent and heat gently. An orange-red precipitate indicates the presence of reducing sugar (Prashant et al., 2011).

Molisch's test: Add few drops of Molisch's reagent to the extract and dissolve in distilled water. Then add 1 mL of concentrated H_2SO_4 by the side of the test tube. Allow mixture to stand for 2 min and then dilute with 5 mL of distilled water. The formation of red or dull violet color at the interphase of the two layers shows positive test for the presence of carbohydrates (Sofowora, 1993).

Barfoed's test: Pipette 1 mL of filtrate and mix with 1 mL of Barfoed's reagent. Heat the sample on water bath for about 2 min. A reddish precipitate of cuprous oxide indicates the presence of monosaccharides (Sofowora, 1993).

Iodine test: Treat crude extract with a mixture of 2 mL of iodine solution. A dark blue or purple coloration indicated the presence of starch.

15.3.27   TEST FOR REDUCING SUGAR

Fehling's test: Mix the test sample with equal volumes of Fehling's A and B solutions and heat in a water bath. The formation of red color indicates the presence of reducing sugars (Salna et al., 2011).

15.3.28   TEST FOR VITAMIN C

2,4-dinitrophenylhydrazine test: Treat test substance with dinitrophenylhydrazine dissolved in concentrated sulfuric acid. The formation of yellow precipitate indicates the presence of vitamin C (Satheesh et al., 2012).

15.3.29   TEST FOR EMODINS

Test for emodins: Add 2 mL of NH_4OH and 3 mL of benzene to sample extract. The appearance of red color indicates the presence of emodins.

15.3.30   TEST FOR PHYTATE

Phytate is the principal storage form of phosphorus in many plant tissues. Structurally, it is cyclic in nature and referred to as inositol hexakisphosphate (IP6) or inositol polyphosphate. There has not been a defined qualitative determination method for phytate, largely because it is usually found in a bound state which may require hydrolysis before the free phosphorus could be released for a phosphorous test to be conducted. However, since phytate is known as a chelating agent by binding metals, this property can be utilized for the test for phytate in which a metallic precipitate of its mixture can be taken as a positive result. The method described by Garcia-Villanova et al. (1982) could be useful. By this method, measure an equivalent of sample containing 6.6–52.8 mg of phytate in water. Take 20 mL and add 0.4 M HCl, 20 mL 0.02 M iron (III) solution, and 20 mL of 20% sulfosalicylic acid solution in a 100-mL test tube. Shake gently and seal the tube with a rubber cork through which passes a narrow 30 cm long glass tube, to prevent evaporation. Place the tube in a boiling water bath for 15 min then allow it to cool or cool it with tap water. If a white precipitate forms, this could be taken as a positive test for the qualitative analysis of phytate.

15.3.30.1   TEST FOR PHYTATE: METHOD 2

The following procedure outlined by Zhejiang Orient Phytic acid Co., Ltd., may be helpful.

   To the aqueous solution (1→10) of the additive, which is neutralized by sodium hydroxide solution, add three drops of phenolphthalein solution followed by the addition of silver nitrate solution (1→100). A white colloidal precipitate indicates a positive result. Note that it will be proper to first hydrolyze the sample in acid before the test.

15.3.31   TEST FOR IRIDIODS

Add trim hill reagent (1 mL) to 2 ml of methanolic plant extract. If solution turns blue then iridiods, a cyclopentanopyran monoterpenoid is present.

15.3.32 TEST FOR LIGNANS

Add 2% furfuraldheyde to 2 ml of methanolic plant extract concentrated. Acidify with hydrochloric acid. The development of red colour indicates a positive result for lignans.

15.4 QUANTITATIVE ANALYSIS BY SPECTROPHOTOMETRIC METHODS

1. **Determination of phenolics:** Weigh 0.5 g of sample into 50 mL beaker and add 20 mL of acetone with proper mixing for about 1 h. Filter the mixture with a Whatman filter paper into another container. Pipette 1 mL of the extract into a 50 mL volumetric flask, add 20 mL distilled water, 3 mL of phosphomolybdic acid, 5 mL of 23% (w/v) $NaCO_3$, and make up to the mark with distilled water. Allow the mixture to stand for about 10 min to develop a bluish-green color, which should be read spectrophotometrically at 510 nm. Prepare a standard phenolic solution with the concentration range of 0–10 mg/ml, from the stock and treat similarly as sample (Harborne, 1973). Percentage phenolic content can be calculated using the formula:

$$\% \, Phenolic = \frac{Absorbance \times Gradient \; factor \times Dilution \; factor}{Weight \; of \; sample \times 10000}$$

2. **Determination of triterpenes:** Weigh 5 g of sample and extract successively with petroleum ether and chloroform. Both extracts contain triterpenoids and triterpenes, respectively. Concentrate the sample and dry the sample at about 100°C. Dissolve in concentrated sulfuric acid and warm at about 70°C for 60 min. Read the absorbance at 310 nm (Simonyan et al., 1972). Prepare a calibration curve of ursolic acid at concentration of 0.10–0.40 mg/mL. Triterpenes concentration is determined from the ursolic acid standard curve.

3. **Determination of anthraquinones:** Weigh 2 g of sample and reflux in 30 mL of distilled water for about 15 min. Separate the aqueous layer by centrifuging at 4000 rpm for 10 min. Pipette 10 mL of the supernatant and add 20 mL of 10.5% $FeCl_3$, reflux for 20 min, and add 1 mL of concentrated HCl and reflux again for another 20 min. Extract with 25 mL of ether and separate the ether layer. Wash with 15 mL of distilled water and extract again with 100 mL ether.

Evaporate the solvent and add 10 mL of 0.5% magnesium acetate in methanol, read absorbance at 515 nm (Rizwan et al., 2011). Prepare standard anthraquinone solution (0–5 mg/ml) from the stock anthraquinone for reference calculation of anthraquinones.

4. **Determination of alkaloids:** Weigh 0.1 g of sample and extract with 10 mL of 80% ethanol. Filter the extract and centrifuge at 5000 rpm for 10 min. Pipette 1 mL of the supernatant, mix with 1 mL of 0.025 M $FeCl_3$ in 0.5 M HCl and 1 mL of 0.05 M 1,10-phenanthroline in ethanol. Incubate the reaction mixture in hot water bath for about 30 min. Allow to cool with a red color complex and read the absorbance at 510 nm against the reagent blank (Singh et al., 2004). Prepare a calibration curve of colchicine for estimation of alkaloid.

5. **Determination of saponins:** Weigh 1 g of sample into 250 mL beaker and add 100 mL of isobutyl alcohol. Shake the mixture for about 5 h to allow for uniform mixing and filter using a Whatman filter paper into a 100 mL beaker. Add 20 mL of 40% (w/v) saturated solution of magnesium carbonate. The mixture obtained with saturated $MgCO_3$ should again be filtered through a Whatman filter paper to obtain a clear and colorless solution. Pipette 1 mL of the colorless solution into 50 mL volumetric flask and add 2 mL of 5% (w/v) $FeCl_3$ solution, making it up to the mark with distilled water. Allow to stand for about 30 min for a blood red color to develop. Similarly, prepare standard saponin solutions (0–10 mg/mL) from saponin stock solution and treat as above with 2 mL of 5% $FeCl_3$ solution. Read their absorbance after color development at 380 nm (Brunner, 1984). Calculate the percentage saponin using the expression:

$$\% \, Saponin = \frac{Absorbance \times Gradient \; factor \times Dilution \; factor}{Weight \; of \; sample \times 10000}$$

6. **Determination of flavonoid by the aluminum chloride colorimetric assay:** Measure an aliquot (1 mL) of extracts or standard solution of quercetin (20, 40, 60, 80 and 100 mg/L) into 10 mL volumetric flask containing 4 mL of deionized water. Add 0.3 mL 5% $NaNO_2$. After 5 min, add 0.3 ml 10% aluminum chloride. Further, to it at 6th min, add 2 mL 1M sodium hydroxide and bring the total volume to 10 ml with deionized water. Mix the solution and measure the absorbance against prepared reagent blank at 510 nm. Total flavonoids content should be expressed as mg quercetin equivalents QE/100 g crude drug.

7. **Determination of tannin:** Measure 1 g of the dry test sample into 50 mL of distilled water and shake for 3 min in a shaker. Filter the mixture and keep the filtrate. Take 5 mL of the extract into 50 mL volumetric flask and dilute with 35 mL of distilled water. Similarly, take 5 mL of the standard tannic acid solution and 5 mL of distilled water separately. Add 1 mL of Follins—Dennis reagent into the flask followed by 2.5 mL of saturated sodium carbonate solution (35%). Make up the content with distilled water and incubate for 90 min at room temperature. Measure absorbance at 760 nm with the reagent blank at zero. Calculate tannin content (Pearson, 1976).

$$\%\text{Tannin} = \frac{100}{W} \times \frac{AU}{AS} \times \frac{C}{1000} \times \frac{Vf}{Va} \times D$$

where,
W = weight of sample analyzed; AU = Absorbance of the test sample; AS = Absorbance of standard tannic solution; C = Concentration of standard in mg/mL; Vf = Volume of filtrate analyzed; Va = Volume of extract used; D = Dilution factor where applicable.

8. **Determination of cyanogenic glycoside:** Weigh 5 g of each sample and add 50 mL of distilled water in a conical flask and allow to stand overnight. To 1 mL of the sample filtrate in a corked test tube, add 4 mL of alkaline picrate and incubate in a water bath for 5 min. Measure the absorbance of the samples at 490 nm and that of a blank containing 1 mL distilled water and 4 mL alkaline picrate solution. Prepare cyanide standard curve and extrapolate the concentration. Note that the change in color from yellow to reddish brown after incubation for 5 min in a water bath indicates the presence of cyanide (Onwuka, 2005). This can also be used as a qualitative test for cyanides.

9. **Determination of trypsin inhibitor:** Weigh 1 g of the sample into a screw cap centrifuge tube and 10 mL of 0.1 M phosphate buffer. Shake the content for about 1 h at room temperature and centrifuge at 5000 rpm for 5 min. Filter to separate the residue from the super- natant using Whatman filter paper (No. 42). Adjust the volumes to 2 mL with phosphate buffer. Place the test tubes in a water bath at 37°C. To it, add 6 mL of 5% TCA solution except for the blank sample. Add 2 mL of casein solution to all samples and incubate them for the next 20 min until the formation of a blood red color. Prepare a standard trypsin with concentrations of 0–10 mg/L from stock and treat similarly with 2 mL of 5% $FeCl_3$ solution. After 20 min add

6 mL of TCA to the tubes and mix properly. Maintain the reaction at room temperature for the next 1 h. Filter the resulting solution with a Whatman filter paper (No. 42). Read absorbance of the filtrate and trypsin standard solution at 280 nm (Kakade et al., 1969). Trypsin inhibitor is calculated using the formula:

$$Trypsin\ inhibitor\ (mg\ /\ g) = \frac{A\ standard - A\ sample \times Dilution\ factor}{0.1g \times sample\ weight\ in\ grams}$$

where, A = Absorbance

10. **Determination of steroids:** Weigh 0.5 g of the sample into a 100 mL beaker and extract with 20 mL chloroform–methanol (2:1) for about 30 min. Filter the extract using a Whatman filter paper (No. 1) into a dry 100 mL flask. Repeat this procedure until the sample is free of steroid. Pipette 1 mL from the extract and add 5 mL of alcoholic KOH and shake the mixture properly to ensure homogeneous mixture. Place the mixture in a water bath at 40°C for about 90 min, cool at room temperature and add 10 mL of petroleum ether, followed by 5 mL of distilled water. Evaporate the resulting mixture to dryness on a water bath. Add 6 mL of Liebermann–Burchard reagent to the residue and read absorbance at 620 nm (Wall et al., 1952). Prepare standard steroids concentration of 0–4 mg/mL and treat similarly as the sample. Calculate the percentage steroid using the formula:

$$\%\ Steriod = \frac{Absorbance \times Gradient\ Factor \times Dilution\ factor}{Sample\ weight\ in\ grams \times 10000}$$

11. **Determination of proanthocyanidins:** Weigh 10 mg of sample and dissolve in 10 mL of methanol to prepare a 1 mg/mL concentration of the sample. Pipette 0.5 mL and vortex with 3 mL of 4% v/v vanillin-methanol and 1.5 mL of hydrochloric acid. Allow to stand for 15 min at room temperature and read absorbance at 500 nm (Sun et al., 1998). Prepare a varying gallic acid (mg/ml) concentration to use as equivalents of total proanthocyanidin content from the standard curve.

15.5   QUANTITATIVE ANALYSIS BY GRAVIMETRIC METHODS

1. **Determination of alkaloid:** Weigh 5 g of the sample into a 250 mL of 10% acetic acid in ethanol, cover and allow to stand for 4 h. Filter and concentrate on a water bath to one-quarter of its original

volume. Add concentrated ammonium hydroxide dropwise to the extract until the precipitation is complete. Allow the whole solution to settle and collect the precipitate. Wash the precipitate with dilute ammonium hydroxide and then filter (Harborne, 1973). The residue is the alkaloid, which is obtained by drying and weighing.

$$\% \, Alkaloids = \frac{W_2 - W_1}{Weight \, of \, sample} \, x100$$

where W_1 = Weight of empty filter paper; W_2 = Weight of filter paper + Alkaloid

2. **Determination of flavonoid by the methods of Boham and Kocipai (1994):** Add 50 mL of 80% aqueous methanol to 2.50 g of sample in a 250 mL beaker, covered, and allowed to stand for 24 hours at room temperature. Discard the supernatant, and re-extract the residue three times with the same volume of ethanol. Filter the solution with Whatman filter paper number 42 (125 mm). Transfer the sample filtrate into a crucible and evaporate to dryness over a water bath. Cool the content in the crucible in a desiccator and weigh until a constant weight is obtained. The percentage of flavonoid was calculated as

$$\% \, Flavonoid = \frac{W_2 - W_1}{Weight \, of \, sample} \, x100$$

Where, W_1 = Weight of empty crucible; W_2 = Weight of crucible + Flavonoid

3. **Determination of saponin:** Weigh 5 g of sample for double extraction and mix with 50 mL of 20% aqueous ethanol solution. Heat the mixture in a water bath at 55°C for 90 min with periodic agitations and then filter through Whatman filter paper (No. 42). Extract the residue with 50 mL of 20% ethanol and combine the double extractions. Reduce the volume of the extract to about 40 mL by heating at 90°C, transfer to a separating funnel, and add 40 mL diethyl ether with vigorous shaking. The two layers of ethyl ether and water are separated and the process of extraction repeated severally until the aqueous layer is clear. Saponins are then extracted with 60 mL of normal butanol, washed with 5% sodium chloride solution and evaporated to dryness in a crucible with known weight. Dry the extract at 60°C in an oven and re-weigh the crucible after allowing it to cool in

a desiccator (Obadoni and Ochuko, 2001). Repeat the procedure and calculate the average for accurate results. The quantity of saponin are then determined using the expression;

$$\% \ Saponin = \frac{W_2 - W_1}{Weight \ of \ sample} \ x100$$

where, W_1 = Weight of empty crucible; W_2 = Weight of crucible + saponin

4. **Determination of steroid:** Weigh 5 g of sample and hydrolyze it by boiling for 30 min in a 50 mL hydrochloric acid solution. Filter the solution using Whatman filter paper and transfer into a separating funnel. Add equal volume of ethyl acetate to it, mix well and allow to separate into layers. Recover the ethyl acetate layer fraction and discard the aqueous fraction or keep for other analysis if required. Dry the ethyl acetate layer fraction for 5 min at 100°C in a steam bath and extract the steroids by heating with concentrated amyl alcohol. The resulting mixture becomes turbid. Weigh it using Whatman filter paper, cool in a desiccator and reweigh again (Harborne, 1973). Repeat the process and obtain the average weights in each experiment. Percentage steroid in the sample is then determined using the expression;

$$\% \ Steroid = \frac{W_2 - W_1}{Weight \ of \ sample} \ x100$$

where, W_1 = Weight of empty crucible; W_2 = Weight of crucible + steroid

5. **Determination of percentage lipid composition:** Weight 5 g of sample and sample holder for extraction in Soxhlet extractor chamber. Add 100 mL of petroleum ether into the reflux chamber and extract exhaustively for about 3 h by heat at 50°C. Distillate off the petroleum ether and reweigh the sample holder and its content (AOAC, 1984). Calculate the percentage lipid composition using the expression;

$$\% \ Lipid = \frac{W_2 - W_1}{Weight \ of \ sample} \ x100$$

where, W_1 = Weight of empty sample holder; W_2 = Weight of sample holder + steroid.

15.6   QUANTITATIVE ANALYSIS BY OTHER METHODS

1. **Determination of total phenolic by Folin–Ciocalteu method:** Add 2.5 mL of 10% Folin–Ciocalteu reagent and 2 mL of 2% solution of Na_2CO_3 to 1 mL of plant extract. Incubate the resulting mixture at room temperature for 15 min. Measure the absorbance at 765 nm. Use gallic acid as standard (1 mg/ml). Determined the result from the standard curve and express as gallic acid equivalent (mg/g of extracted compound) (Spanos and Wrolstad, 1990).

$$\% \text{ phenol} = \frac{100}{W} \times \frac{AU}{AS} \times \frac{C}{1000} \times \frac{VF}{Va} \times D$$

where, W = weight of sample analysed; AU = absorbance of the test sample; AS = absorbance of standard tannic solution; C = concentration of standard in mg/ml; Vf = volume of filtrate analysed; Va = volume of extract used; D = dilution factor where applicable.

2. **Determination of tannin by Prussian blue spectrophotometer method:** Weigh 0.2 g of the dry test sample and dissolve in 6.9 mL distilled water, 1 mL of 0.008 M potassium ferric cyanide, 1 mL of 0.2 M ferric chloride in 0.1 M HCl. Measure the absorbance of the blue color formed at 760 nm with the reagent blank at zero (Graham, 1992). Calculate tannin content from a standard calibration curve.

3. **Determination of cyanogenic glycoside by titration method:** Weigh 1 g of sample into 200 mL distilled water and allowed to stand for about 2 h. Distill the whole sample in 250 mL conical flask with 20 mL of 2.5% Sodium hydroxide (NaOH) after adding tannic acid as an antifoaming agent. Measure 100 mL of the cyanogenic glycoside, 8 mL of 6 M ammonium hydroxide (NH_4OH), 2 mL of 5% potassium iodide (KI), and add to the distillate, with mixing, followed by titration with 0.02 M silver nitrate ($AgNO_3$) noting turbidity of the solution as the endpoint for the titration (Amadi et al., 2004; Ejikeme et al., 2014). The cyanogenic glycoside content is determined using the expression:

$$Cyanogenic\ glycoside\ (mg\,/\,100g) = \frac{Titre\ value\ (mL) \times 1.08 \times exact\ volume}{Aliquot\ volume\ (mL) \times sample\ weight\ (g)} \times 100$$

4. **Determination of oxalate by titration method:** Weigh 2 g of sample and boil in 40 mL distilled water for 30 min. Add 10 mL of 20% Na_2CO_3 and boil for another 30 min. Extract the liquid and wash

the residue with hot water until no trace of alkaline reactions in the washed water. This should then be concentrated to a small volume by heating and allowed to cool. Add HCl to the concentrate with constant stirring, until the final mixture becomes acidic. Add 10 mL of 6 M HCl solution and digest at 100°C for 1 h. Cool the sample and make up to 250 mL mark of the flask with distilled water and re-acidified with acetic acid. Add 10 mL of calcium chloride solution and stir until induced calcium oxalate precipitate is visible. Allow the precipitate to settle overnight. Filter the sample through a Whatman filter paper (No. 42) without disturbing the precipitates. Dissolve the precipitate in HCl (1:1). Adjust the pH with ammonium hydroxide (NH$_4$OH) solution (dropwise) to re-precipitate oxalic acid. Boil the content and allow settling overnight. Take aliquots of 125 mL of the filtrate, heat until near boiling and then titrate against 0.05 N standardized KMnO$_4$ solutions to a pink color which persisted for 30 seconds. Calculate the oxalate contents of each sample (Fasset, 1966).

5. **Determination of phytic acid by titration method:** Weigh 2 g of the sample into 250 mL conical flask and add 100 mL of 2% hydrochloric acid (HCl) and soak for 3 h. Filter using a double layer filter paper. From the filtrate, transfer 50 mL into a 250 mL beaker and add 107 mL of distilled water to it. Use 10 mL of 0.3% ammonium thiocyanate solution as indicator and titrate the solution with standard iron chloride at 0.00195 g iron per mL. Note the endpoint, which is slightly brownish-yellow which persist for about 5 min during the titration process (Lucas and Markakas, 1975). Calculate the percentage phytic acid using the formula:

$$\% \, Phytic \, acid = \frac{Titre \, value \, x \, 0.00195g \, x \, 1.19}{Weight \, of \, sample} x \, 100$$

15.7 PROXIMATE COMPOSITION ANALYSIS

Proximate composition analysis describes useful methods used in estimating the various micronutrients available in food and foodstuff. They are generally categorized into six; moisture content, total ash, crude protein, crude lipid, crude fiber, and nitrogen-free extract, thus, proximate analysis is only a fraction of nutrient analysis (Fig. 15.2). The methods (ASEAN, 2011) for the listed nutrients are summarized.

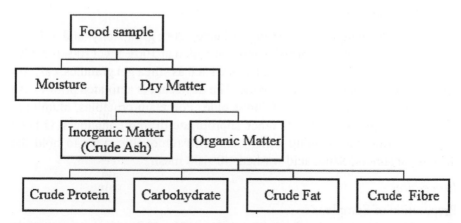

FIGURE 15.2 An illustration of the parameters involved in the proximate composition determination.

1. Determination of moisture content by air oven

Definition

The moisture content of food samples can be defined as the amount of free water and volatile substances that are lost by drying food samples under controlled temperature in an air oven. This method is not suitable for products that decompose during drying.

Aim

The method is used for determining quantitatively the amount of moisture in all foods except food samples high in sugar and fat (> 10%). It is required to express the nutrient content per dry weight basis. In some foods, moisture is used to indicate their quality. Standard values of moisture are indicated in food notification or regulation. Food samples with high moisture content spoil/deteriorate faster than those with little moisture content.

Principle

Moisture content determination by air oven employs the principle of drying food sample under controlled temperature until constant weight is obtained. Food samples are subjected to a temperature of 100–105°C for some hours until a constant weighed is obtained. The number of hours subjected often differ from the nature of the food sample (i.e., whether solid or liquid).

Material/Apparatus

Food sample, analytical weighing balance, 200 g capacity and 0.1 mg sensitivity, air oven (capable of being controlled at $100 \pm 5°C$ (100–105°C)), desiccator with desiccant stationed inside such as silica gel granules, calcium chloride or dry phosphorus pentoxide. The desiccant is activated prior to use by heating in an oven at 100°C until blue. Porcelain crucibles, aluminum dishes or weighing bottles or other appropriate drying containers. Others: Tongs, Stirring rod. Boiling water bath with removable rings to hold the drying containers, Sand, acid washed, 40–100 mesh

Procedures

Preparation of Sample

1. Place container in the drying oven at $100 \pm 5°C$ until constant weight (1–2 h). Cool in a desiccator for about 30 min and weigh (W_1). For liquid or semisolid sample, prepare drying container with 15–20 g acid washed sand and a stirring rod.

2. Grind sample until homogenous (40–100 mesh screen) to increase the surface area. Samples are recommended to be analyzed immediately after preparation. If for one reason or the other samples cannot be analyzed on the same day, samples should be kept in a screw cap bottle in a freezer. For samples intended for analysis of vitamins or other labile nutrients, samples are flushed with nitrogen before storing.

Analysis

1. For dry sample: Thaw sample at room temperature. Mix sample thoroughly by turning the tightly closed bottle up and down three times. Weigh accurately 2 g (or usually 2–5 g) sample using standard analytical balance in triplicate, into a pre-weighed drying container and weigh (W_2).

2. For liquid/wet/slurry sample: Samples are mixed thoroughly and weighed (5–15 g for slurry sample and 20 g for liquid sample) into a pre-weighed drying container with acid washed sand and stirring rod (W_2). For liquid samples, dry to a consistency of a thick paste over a boiling water bath before drying in an oven.

3. Place container with the sample in the air oven pre-heated to $100 \pm 5°C$ for 2–3 h.

4. Transfer the container with the dried sample into a desiccator, cool for 30 min and weigh (W_3).

5. Repeat the heating procedure until constant weight. The difference in weight between two consecutive weighing should not be more than 5 mg.
6. Calculations

$$Moisture\,(g/100g) = \frac{(W_2 - W_3)}{(W_2 - W_1)} \, x100$$

while,

$$Total\ Solid\ (\%) = 100 - \%\ Moisture\ w/w$$

where

W_1 = Weight of container or empty dish (g),
W_2 = weight of container + sample before drying (g),
$W_2 - W_1$ = weight of sample (g),
W_3 = weight of container + sample after drying (g),
$W_2 - W_3$ = loss of weight (g)

It is expressed in g per 100 g sample or in percentage.
Precaution: Do not carry hot material with bare hands rather use tongs.

2. Determination of crude protein by the simplified Kjeldahl method

Definition
The crude protein content of food sample is the total nitrogen content multiplied by protein factor. The nitrogen content of food sample is primarily available from protein and to a lesser extent from all organic containing non-protein. For practical purposes, non-protein nitrogen is assumed to be negligible or of little significance. The Kjeldahl method is a means of determining the nitrogen and protein content of organic and inorganic substances

Aim
Quantitative determination of crude protein. The crude protein shows the total uncategorized protein which is usually difficult to obtain directly in the laboratory.

Principle
This technique employs three steps for the determination of total nitrogen before multiplying with the protein factor. These steps include digestion, distillation, and titration.

Digestion: This involves the use of sulfuric acid (H_2SO_4) in the presence of catalyst to release nitrogen from protein to form ammonium tetraoxosulfate (VI) ($(NH_4)_2SO_4$). Ammonia gas (NH_3) is further liberated upon addition of excess alkali such as concentrated Sodium Hydroxide (NaOH).

Distillation: Ammonia gas liberated is collected through a condenser attached to the apparatus and distilled off into a standard boric acid solution to form ammonium–borate complex.

Titration: The distillate is titrated against a standardized hydrochloric acid and the end point determined through a color change.

The percentage of nitrogen in the sample is determined from the milligram equivalent of the acid used and converted to crude protein by multiplying with a protein conversion factor.

Material/Apparatus

Kjeldahl flask, 250 mL or 500 mL capacity, electrothermal heater, analytical weighing balance, 200 g capacity with 0.1 mg sensitivity, Liebig condenser with ice cold water, round bottom flask, Erlenmeyer flask or conical flask, 250 mL or 500 mL, steelhead adaptor and receiving adaptor, burette, pipette, retort stand, and clamp, measuring cylinder.

Reagents

1. Concentrated sulfuric acid-free from nitrogen.
2. A suitable catalyst: mix and grind together 0.5 g $CuSO_4$ + 10 g Na_2SO_4 or 500 g K_2SO_4 +
3. 15 g $CuSO_4 0.5H_2O$ + TiO_2.

   Note: Catalyst involving Mercury should be avoided because of environmental and health concerns.

4. Sodium hydroxide, 40%. Weigh 40 g NaOH, dissolve in distilled water and makeup to 100 mL.

   Note: since the reaction of NaOH is exothermic, place it in the basin of ice cold water.

5. Boric acid, 2%. Weigh 2 g of boric acid, dissolve it in hot distilled water, cool and makeup to 100 mL.
6. Double indicator (methyl red-methylene blue combination). Preparation: methylene blue, 0.2% in 95% ethanol and methyl red, 0.2% in ethanol (1:2). Or simply 1% double indicator.
7. Standardized hydrochloric acid, 0.01M. Dilute 9.0 mL analytical grade HCl with distilled water and make 1 L. It is then standardized

by titrating against 0.1 N anhydrous Na_2CO_3 solution using methyl red as indicator.

Note: Methyl red indicator is prepared thus: Dissolve 1 g of methyl red in 600 mL of ethanol and dilute with 400 mL water.

8. Boiling chips/bumping chips/glass beads.
9. Blank: Prepare 50 mL of 2% boric acid and add 4 drops of the double indicator into the boric acid solution and keep for titration.

Procedures

Digestion:

1. Grind and thaw sample until homogeneous. Weigh in duplicate 1 g of the sample depending on the protein content (could be 1–10 g) into a nitrogen-free filter paper and drop into the Kjeldahl digestion flask.
2. Add a few boiling chips to prevent the solution from frothing and add 3.0 g of digestion catalyst and 25.0 mL of concentrated H_2SO_4.
3. Heat the flask by placing it on the electrothermal heater or digestor at an initial lower temperature in a slanting position with a clamp on a retort stand until frothing has ceased and the content has liquefied completely. Tilt the flask intermittently to pick up undissolved particle and increase the temperature until a clear light-green color appears. When clear, heat for another hour after the liquid has become clear to complete breakdown of all organic matter. Stop heating and allow to cool at room temperature and dilute to 100 mL with distilled water.

Note: when heating, if the digest is still yellowish, cool the digest and add an additional 5–10 mL sulfuric acid and continue heating until a clear light-green color appears.

Distillation:

1. Place a 250 mL Erlenmeyer/conical flask containing 50 mL of 2% boric acid and add 4 drops of the double indicator into the boric acid solution as the receiver on the distillation unit.
2. Add 20 mL of the diluted digest into a 250 mL round-bottomed distillation flask.
3. Grease and connect the steelhead carrying the Liebig condenser on the flask and hold the distillation flask in position with a retort stand.
4. Position the boric acid at the collection adaptor terminal of the Liebig condenser.

5. Inject 40 mL of 40% NaOH into the flask already containing 20 mL of the diluted digest through a syringe attached to the corked end of the steelhead above the distillation flask.

    Note: Ensure enough NaOH was added to neutralize sulfuric acid so as to ensure complete release of NH_3.

6. Apply heat to the distillation flask to evolve NH_3 and collect it through the condenser into the boric acid solution. The entry of NH_3 into the boric acid solution containing indicator triggers a change in color from pink to green. From the point when boric acid turns green, 10 min should be allowed for complete distillation of the NH_3 present.

    Note: Ensure the ice cold water runs through the Liebig condenser for effective condensation of the ammonia gas.

7. After distillation, rinse the delivery tube with water and allow the washings to drain into the flask.

Titration:

1. Titrate the distillate with the standardized 0.10 M HCl back to a pink color. Moreover, titrate the blank differently with 0.10 M HCl.
2. Note and record the volume of the acid used (titre value) to the nearest 0.05 mL.
3. Calculate for the % nitrogen and crude protein as shown below:

% Nitrogen

$$= \frac{(Titre\ of\ 0.1\ N\ HCl\ in\ Sample - Titre\ of\ 0.1\ N\ HCl\ in\ Blank)\ mL\ x\,0.0014\ x\ N\ HCl}{Weight\ of\ Sample\,(g)}\ x100$$

% Crude protein=% Nitrogen × appropriate protein conversion factor (Table 15.4).

3. Determination of crude fat by acid hydrolysis method using Soxhlet

Definition

The crude fat content of food sample gives the overall estimate of fats present. Fat is also known as triglyceride. It is an ester of three fatty acid chain and a glycerol backbone. It can be saturated or unsaturated (oil).

Aim

To estimate quantitatively the crude fat content of food sample including milk and milk products, raw and cooked foods, natural, or processed food products.

TABLE 15.4   Nitrogen Conversion Factors to Protein.

Food	Factor*
Meat and fish	6.25
Gelatin	5.55
Milk and milk products	6.38
Casein	6.40
Human Milk	6.37
Butter and margarine	6.38
Eggs: whole	6.25
Vitellin	6.32
Albumin	6.12
Wheat: whole meal or floor	5.83
Bran	6.31
Marcaroni, spaghetti, wheat paste	5.70
Embryo	5.80
Rice and rice floor	5.95
Barley, oats, rye, and flour	5.83
Soybean	5.71
Castor bean	5.30
Nuts and seeds	
Peanuts, Brazil nuts, groundnuts	5.46
Almonds	5.18
Coconuts, cashew nuts, and other nuts	5.30
Sesame seeds, sunflower seeds and all other seeds	5.30
All other foods	6.25

*Source: Modified from WHO, 1973; Onyeike and Osuji, 2003; ASEAN, 2011.

Principle
The principle is based on extracting fat with non-polar solvent and usually petroleum ether, diethyl ether, or other suitable solvents. Extracted fat substance is then calculated.

Material/Apparatus
Soxhlet apparatus, heating mantle, oven, analytical weighing balance, desiccator, Erlenmeyer flask or conical flask, 250 mL or 500 mL, measuring cylinder, beakers, cotton wool free of fat

Reagents
Petroleum ether, or diethyl ether or n-hexane.

Procedures

1. Grind and homogenize the food sample into fine particle/flour.
2. Rinse all glassware with petroleum ether, drain and dry in an oven at 102°C.
3. In 100 mL beaker, place a piece of cotton wool in the bottom. Moreover, put a plug of cotton wool in the bottom of the thimble and stand the thimble in the beaker.
4. Weigh 2–5 g of the sample and wrap in a porous filter paper (Whatman No. 1 filter paper).
5. Place the wrapped sample into the thimble and dry in an oven for about 7 h at 100°C in an oven to first remove any traces of moisture that could affect the final result.
6. After oven drying, remove the thimble in the beaker containing the sample together with the cotton wool from the beaker and place them over pre-weighed Soxhlet flask (W_1). Add 250 mL of the extractant. Note: the cotton wool is previously added to drain out any traces of oil dripping out during oven drying. Acid washed sand can also be added together with the sample in the thimble to facilitate the extraction. An exception of acid-washed sand usage is for meat sample.
7. Before reflux, rinse the beaker twice with the extractant (petroleum ether or diethyl ether as the case may be) and add the rinsing to the Soxhlet.
8. Set up the extraction unit over either an electric heating mantle or a water bath.
9. Heat the solvent in the flask until it boils. Adjust the heat source so that solvent drips from the condenser into the sample chamber at the rate of about 6 drops per seconds.
10. Continue the extraction for 6 h.
    Note: when the extraction solvent reduces depending on the set-up, the solvent can intermittently refilled.
11. Switch off the heat source and detach the extractor from the condenser. Replace the flask with the heat source and evaporate off all the solvents.
    Note: The solvent may be distilled and recovered.
12. Dry the flask in an oven at 102°C and dry the contents until a constant weight is reached for 1–2 h.
13. Allow the flask to cool the flask in a desiccator and weigh the flask and contents (W_2).

Calculations,

$$\% \ Crude \ fat = \frac{W_2 - W_1}{Weight \ of \ sample} \ x100$$

Where,

W_1 = Weight of empty flask (g)

W_2 = Weight of flask + extracted fat (g)

4. Determination of crude fiber content of food sample

Definition

Crude fiber is somewhat different from dietary fiber. Crude fiber refers to the fibrous food residue that is left over after it has been dissolved in the laboratory with certain harsh chemical solvents such as sulfuric acid and sodium hydroxide while, dietary fiber refers to complex mixture of different components; it may or may not include the fibrous structure.

Aim

To estimate quantitatively the crude fiber content of food sample. This method gives the crude fiber content of the sample after it has been digested in sulfuric acid and sodium hydroxide solutions and the residue calcined.

Principle

The principle is based on obtaining insoluble residue by acid hydrolysis followed by an alkaline one.

Material/Apparatus

Muffle Furnace, 600 mL flat-bottomed, Condensation unit for flask, Buchner funnel, Filtration crucible, Whatman filter paper, Dryer, Oven, Crucible furnace

Reagents

1. 10% H_2SO_4
2. Petroleum ether (boiling point 40–60°C) or diethyl ether or n-hexane
3. 10% NaOH 0.313N, free of sodium carbonate
4. Antifoam (e.g., octyl alcohol or silicone)
5. Alcohol or Ethyl alcohol at 95% (v/v)
6. Chlorhydric acid solution at 1% (v/v)
7. Cotton wool free of fat

Procedures

1. Weigh out 2–3 g of sample.

    Note: For samples rich in fat, defat by placing the sample into a conical flask and stir with petroleum ether. The process can be repeated two to three times and allowed to dry at room temperature. Soxhlet method can also be used to defat the sample.

2. Add the weighed sample to 200 mL boiling solution of 1.25% sulfuric acid.

    Note: On adding the acid, 50 mL should be added first, followed by another 150 mL through a dispenser.

3. Add 5–6 drops of antifoam and bring to boiling within 1–2 min. Boil gently for exactly 30 min, maintaining the volume of distilled water constant and swirling the flask periodically to remove particles adhering to the sides.

    Note: A cold-finger condenser can be used so as to ensure the solvent is returned/recycled and not allowed to dry off.

4. Set-up the Buchner funnel with the filter paper and pre-heat with boiling water. At the same time, at the end of the boiling period, remove the flask, let rest 1 min and filter the contents carefully, using suction. Filtration should be carried out in less than 10 min. Wash the filter paper with boiling water.

5. For the second time, transfer the residue in a flask and boil for 30 min using 200 mL of boiling NaOH solution.

6. After boiling allow to stand for 1 min, then filter the hydrolyzed mixture into a crucible that was preheated with boiling water and dried.

7. The residue obtained is washed with boiling water and the water discarded. Wash with HCl solution and again with boiling water and discard. Yet again, wash thrice with petroleum ether. Place the crucible in an oven (105°C) for 12 h then cool in a dryer.

8. The weight of the crucible with the residue inside is obtained (W_2) before placing the crucible with content in the furnace at 550°C for 3 h for ashing. After ashing, leave to cool in a dryer and weigh again (W_1).

Calculation

$$\% \ Crude \ Fibre = \frac{W_2 - W_1}{Weight \ of \ sample} \ x100$$

Where,
W_1 = Weight of ash (g)
W_2 = Weight of insoluble matter (g)

5. Determination of ash content of food sample by gravimetric method

Definition
The ash content of a sample represents the overall estimate of the mineral composition of the food sample. Sometimes it is the first step for elemental analysis.

Aim
To quantitatively determine the mineral composition of the sample.

Principle
This method involves the incineration of sample/organic matter in a furnace at <555°C. The residue left after incineration is the ash content of the sample.

Material/Apparatus
Muffle furnace capable of been controlled from 100°C to 560°C, desiccator containing silica gel as desiccant, electric hot plate, analytical weighing balance, crucible or porcelain dish

Procedures
1. Grind and homogenize the sample into fine particle/flour.
2. Heat the crucible at low temperature of about 180°C and transfer the crucibles into a desiccator, cool for 30 min and weigh (W_1).
3. Weigh 2–4 g of dry samples and 10 g for wet samples into the weighed crucible and reweigh to determine W_2.
4. It is important to char dry samples initially at low temperature to avoid spattering. Increase the temperature gradually until smoking ceases.
   Note: charring is a chemical process of incomplete combustion of applying high heat to drive off hydrogen and oxygen.
5. For wet or liquid samples, pre-dry over a boiling water bath until samples are dry. Char the sample as in step 4.
6. Place the charred samples in a furnace at 550°C until the residue is uniformly white or nearly white. This could take 3 h or more depending on the sample. If ash is not completely white, it can be moist with a few drops of water or diluted acid and continued heating.

Note: Do not open the furnace while hot. Allow to cool before opening.

7. Reduce the temperature of the furnace to 180°C and transfer the crucibles into a desiccator, cool for 30 min and weigh (W_3).

Calculations

$$\% Ash = \frac{W_3 - W_1}{W_2 - W_1} \times 100$$

Where,

W_1 = Weight of empty crucible
W_2 = Weight of crucible + sample
W_3 = Weight of crucible + ash

6. Determination of total carbohydrate content

The total carbohydrate content of each sample may be estimated by 'difference'. In this, the sum of the percentages of other proximate components should be subtracted from 100.

Total carbohydrate (%) = 100−(% moisture + % crude protein + crude fiber + % crude fat + % ash)

15.8 CONCLUSION

Phytochemical analysis is key tools in the discovery of active compounds from plants and related materials. We have presented different methods that are important in the qualitative and quantitative estimation of phytochemicals. The basic principles required for reagent preparations and calculations are highlighted for fresher. The various definitions, aims, principles, required apparatus, and procedures for the estimation of plant proximate analysis were also presented. This will be very handy for fresher in the biological, chemical and other science fields.

KEYWORDS

- phytochemical analysis
- qualitative analysis
- quantitative analysis
- reagent preparation
- proximate composition

REFERENCES

Abdullahi, D. K.; Michael, O. O.; Indabawa I. I. Antibacterial Activities and Phytochemical Screening of Aloe Vera (*A. Babardenis*), Galic (*A. Sativum*) and Ginger (*Z Officinale*). *J. Emerging Trends Eng. Appl. Sci. (JETEAS)* **2014**, *5*(3), 172–178.

Amadi, B. A.; Agomuo, E. N.; Ibegbulem, C.O. *Research Methods in Biochemistry;* Supreme Publishers: Owerri, Nigeria, 2004.

ASEAN (The Association of Southeast Asian Network). Manual of Food Analysis, 1st ed.; Regional Centre of ASEAN Network of Food Data System, Institute of Nutrition: Mahidol University, Thailand, 2011.

Association of Official Analytical Chemists (AOAC). *Official Methods of Analysis, Association of Official Analytical Chemists,* 14th ed.; Washington, DC, USA, 1984.

Boham, B. A. and Kocipai, A. R. Flavonoids and condensed Tannins from Leaves of Hawaiian Vaccinium vaticulatum and V. calycinium. *Pacific Science,* **1994**, *48*, 458–463.

Brunner, J. H. Direct Spectrophotometric Determination of Saponins. *Anal. Chem.* **1984**, *34*, 1314–1326.

Chakraborthy, G. S. Phytochemical Screening of Mirabilus Jalap Linn Leaf Extract by TLC. *Res. J. Pharm. Biol. Chem. Sci.* **2011**, *2*(1), 521–524.

Edeoga, H. O.; Okwu, D. E.; Mbaebie, B. O. Phytochemical Constituents of Some Nigerian Medicinal Plants. *Afr. J. Biotechnol.* **2005**, *4*(7), 685–688.

Ejikeme, C. M.; Ezeonu, C. S.; Eboatu, A. N. Determination of Physical and Phytochemical Constituents of Some Tropical Timbers Indigenous to Niger Delta Area of Nigeria. *Eur. Sci. J.* **2014**, *10*(18), 247–270.

Fasset, D. W.; Oxalate, J. *Toxicants Occurring Naturally in Foods;* National Academy of Science/Natural Resources Council: Washington D.C., 1966.

Garcia-Villanova, R.; Garcia-Villanova, R.J.; Ruiz de Lope, C. Determination of phytic acid by complexometric titration of excess of iron. *Analyst.* **1982**, *107*: 1503–1506.

Graham, H. D. Stabilization of the Prussian Blue Color in the Determination of Polyphenols. *J. Agric. Food Chem.* **1992**, *40*(5), 801–805.

Harborne, J. B. *Phytochemical Methods, A Guide to Modern Techniques of Plant Analysis;* Chapman and Hall, Ltd: London, 1973; pp 49–188.

Harsha, N.; Sridevi, V.; Lakshmi, C.; Rani, K.; Vani, N. D. S. Phytochemical Analysis of Some Selected Spices. *Intl. J. Inno. Res. Sci. Eng. Tech.* **2013**, *2*(11), 6618–6621.

Hegnauer, R. *Chemotaxonomie der Pflanzen;* Birkhauser: Basel, 1986; Vol. 7, p. 345.

Kagbo, H.; Ejebe, D. Phytochemistry and Preliminary Toxicity Studies of the Methanol Extract of the Stem Bark of *Garcinia kola* (Heckel). *Int. J. Toxicol.* **2009**, *7*(2).

Kakade, M. I.; Rachis, J. J.; Meghee, J. E.; Puski, G. Determination of Trypsin Inhibitor Activity of Soy Products: A Collaboration Analysis of Improved Procedure. *Cer. Chem.* **1969**, *51*(3), 151–376.

Kalpana, D. R.; Subramani, V. I.; Nakulan, V. R.; Annamalai, P. Qualitative and Quantitative Phytochemical Analysis in Four Pteridophytes. *Int. J. Pharm. Sci. Rev. Res.* **2014**, *27*(2), 408–412.

Krishnaiah, D.; Devi, T.; Bono, A.; Sarbatly, R. Studies on Phytochemical Constituents of Six Malaysian Medicinal Plants. *J. Med. Plants Res.* **2009**, *3*(2), 67–72.

Kumar, R. S.; Balasubramanian, P.; Govindaraj, P.; Krishnaveni, T. Preliminary Studies on Phytochemicals and Antimicrobial Activity of Solvent Extracts of *Coriandrum sativum* L. Roots (Coriander). *J. Pharmacogn. Phytochem.* **2014**, *2*(6), 74–78.

Kumar, R. S.; Venkateshwar, C.; Samuel, G.; Gangadhar, S. R. Phytochemical Screening of Some Compounds from Plant Leaf Extracts of *Holoptelea integrifolia* (Planch.) and *Celestrus emarginata* (Grah.) used by Gondu Tribes at Adilabad District, and Hrapradesh, India. *Int. J. Eng. Sci. Invent.* **2013**, *2*(8), 65–70.

Lucas, G. M.; Markakas, P. Phytic Acid and Other Phosphorus Compounds of Beans (*Phaseolus vulgaris*). *J. Agric. Ed. Chem.* **1975**, *23*, 13–15.

Obadoni, B. O.; Ochuko, P. O. Phytochemical Studies and Comparative Efficacy of the Crude Extracts of Some Homostatic Plants in Edo and Delta States of Nigeria. *Global J. Pure Appl. Sci.* **2001**, *8b*, 203–208.

Onwuka, G. *Food Analysis and Instrumentation: Theory and Practice,* 3rd Ed.; Naphohla Prints. A Division of HG Support Nigeria Ltd.: 2005; pp 133–161.

Onyeike, E. U.; Osuji, J. O.; Ed. *Research Techniques in Biological and Chemical Sciences;* Springfield Publishers Ltd: Nigeria, 2003; pp 228–229.

Pearson, D. *Chemical Analysis of Food,* 7th ed.; Churchill Livingstone: Edinburg, UK, 1976. p 575.

Pradeep, A.; Dinesh, M.; Govindaraj, A.; Vinothkumar, D.; Ramesh, B. N. G. Phytochemical Analysis of Some Important Medicinal Plants. *Int. J. Biol. Pharm. Res.* **2014**, *5*(1), 48–50.

Prashant, T.; Bimlesh, K.; Mandeep, K.; Gurprect, K.; Harleen, K. Phytochemical Screening and Extration: A Review. *Int. Pharm. Sci. Int. Peer Rev. J.* **2011**, *1*(1), 98–106.

Rizwan, A.; Kushagra, N.; Tekeshwar, K.; Mukesh, S.; Dhansay, D. Phytochemical Estimation of Anthraquinones from Cassia Species. *Int. J. Res. Ayurveda Pharm.* **2011**, *2*(4), 1320–1323.

Salna, K. P.; Sreejith, K.; Uthiralingam, M.; Mithu, A. P.; John, M. M. C.; Albin, T. F. A Comparative Study of Phytochemicals Investigation of Andrographis Paniculata and Murraya Koenigii. *Int. J. Pharm. Pharm. Sci.* **2011**, *3*(2), 291–292.

Satheesh, K. B.; Suchetha, K. N.; Vadisha, S. B.; Sharmila, K. P.; Mahesh, P. B. Preliminary Phytochemical Screening of Various/Extracts of Punica Granatum Peel, Whole Fruit and Seeds. *Nitte Univ. J. Health Sci.* **2012**, *2*(4), 34–38.

Simonyan A. V.; Shinkarenko A. L.; Oganesyan E. T. Quantitative Determination of Terterpenoids in Plants of the Genus Thymus. *Pyatigotak Pharm. Inst.* **1972**, *3*, 292–295.

Singh, D. K.; Srivastva, B.; Sahu, A. Spectrophotometric Determination of *Rauwolfia alkaloids*, Estimation of Reserpine in Pharmaceuticals. *Anal. Sci.* **2004**, *20*, 571–573.

Sofowora, A. *Medicinal Plants and Traditional Medicinal in Africa,* 2nd ed.; Spectrum Books Ltd.: Sunshine House, Ibadan, Nigeria Screening Plants for Bioactive Agents; 1993; pp 134–156.

Solomon, C. U.; Arukwe, U.; Onuoha, I. Preliminary Phytochemical Screening of Different Solvent Extracts of Stem Bark and Roots of *Dennetia tripetala* G. Baker. *Asian J. Plant Sci. Res.* **2013**, *3*(3), 10–13.

Spanos, G. A.; Wrolstad, R. E. Influence of Processing and Storage on the Phenolic Composition of Thompson Seedless Grape Juice. *J. Agric. Food Chem.* **1990**, *38*, 1565–1571.

Sun, J. S.; Tsuang, Y. W.; Chen, J. J.; Huang, W. C.; Hang, Y. S.; Lu, F. J. An Ultra- Weak Chemiluminescence Study on Oxidative Stress in Rabbits Following Acute Thermal Injury. *Burns* **1998**, *24*, 225–231.

Trease, G. E.; Evans, W. C. *Pharmacognosy,* 15th ed.; Saunders Publishers: London, 2002.

Wall, M. E.; Eddy, C. R.; McClenna, M. L.; Klump, M. E. Detection and Estimation of Steroid and Sapogenins in Plant Tissue. *Anal. Chem.* **1952**, *24*, 1337–1342.

World Health Organization (WHO). Report of a Joint FAO/WHO Ad Hoc Expert Committee on Energy and Protein Requirements, WHO Technical Report Series No. 522, WHO, Geneva, 1973.

Yadav, R. N. S.; Munin, A. Phytochemical Analysis of Some Medicinal Plants. *J. Phytol.* **2011**, *3*(12), 10–14.

Yusuf, A. Z.; Zakir, A.; Shemau, Z.; Abdullahi, M.; Halima. S. A. Phytochemical Analysis of the Methanol Leaves Extract of *Paullinia pinnata* Linn. *J. Pharm. Phytother.* **2014**, *6*(2), 10–16.

Zhejiang Orient Phytic Acid Co., Ltd. Testing Method for Phytic Acid 50%. http://www.phytics.com/for_details.html. Accessed: Jan 20, 2018.

Suggested Reading

Greenfield, H.; Southgate, D. A. T. Food Composition Data: Production, Management and use. Elsevier Applied Science: UK, 1992.

Horwitz, W.; Ed. Official Method of Analysis of Association of Official Analytical Chemists (AOAC) International. 17th Edition. AOAC. International, Maryland, USA, 2000.

Kirk, R. S.; Sawyer, R. Pearson's Composition and Chemical Analysis of Foods, 9th ed.; Longman Scientific & Technical, Essex: England, 1991.

Meat Technology- Information Sheet. Crude Fat Determination- Soxhlet Method. http://www.meatupdate.csiro.au/infosheets/Crude%20Fat%20Determination%20-%20Soxhlet%20Method%20-%201998.pdf (accessed Oct 12, 2016).

CHAPTER 16

ANIMAL MODELS IN PHYTOPHARMACOLOGY

AHMED A. ADEDEJI[1], MULKAH O. AJAGUN-OGUNLEYE[2], and MARTA VICENTE-CRESPO[3,*]

[1]*Department of Pharmacology and Toxicology, Faculty of Medicine and Surgery, University of Gitwe, Rwanda*

[1]*Foresight Institute of Research and Translation, Eleyele, Ibadan, Nigeria*

[2]*Department of Biochemistry, School of Biomedical Sciences, Kampala International University Western Campus, Uganda*

[3]*Department of Biochemistry, School of Medicine, St. Augustine International University, Kampala, Uganda*

[3]*DrosAfrica Trust, UK, Tel.: +256 (0) 775609697*

*Corresponding author. E-mail: mvicentecrespo@drosafrica.org

ABSTRACT

The variety of species that the animal kingdom provides has remarkably helped in the advancement of scientific investigations, leading to land-breaking discoveries that have made life better for the world inhabitants. In the process of drug discovery, the use of animal models is an inevitability; they provide the needed platform that will help reveal, to a large extent, the physiological functions of phytochemical compounds. In this chapter, we review the various animal methods commonly used in evaluating candidate drugs from phytochemicals, the method of obtaining the models and the different disease conditions successfully modeled. Special attention is given to *Drosophila melanogaster*. We give an introduction to the biology of this model organism and an overview to its use to model human diseases and plagues. We describe the general process of using *Drosophila* in phyto-pharmacology studies and provide a compilation of resources that will help anyone wishing to utilize this organism.

16.1   INTRODUCTION

Phytochemicals are the natural chemicals considered to be of great value to healthcare and wellness of the people in the world today. With increasing challenge to efficacy of old and new synthetic drugs for treatment of diseases, phytochemicals are greatly explored as an alternative. Over the decades, huge scientific exploration focusing on phytochemical are emerging, describing extracts and possible activities through in vitro screening, organ and tissue effect analysis, constituent analysis, identification, and characterization but many have limited information on mechanistic evaluation and preclinical relevance.

This inability to completely evaluate the phytochemical in most cases is due to lack of comprehensive information or protocol on diseases or physiological models that can help in high-throughput analysis. We provide in this chapter the basic model that can be explored in understanding the biological importance of phytochemicals. In addition, we advance suggestions to improve quality of phytochemical research arguing that the component of value to wellness of people should be an important consideration in reporting primary or secondary metabolite phytochemicals.

Phytochemicals are biologically active compounds obtained from plants and are used for medicine and food. The biological activities of these substances are essential to understand their roles in healthy living and drug development. The components of phytochemicals associated with health are phenolics, carotenoids, organic acids, and other bioactive compounds such as saponins and steroids. Due to poor understanding of the roles of phytochemicals in health, there arose the need to validate anecdotal claims, usefulness, and medicinal values in human diseases treatment. The safety of phytochemical concoctions, mechanism of action, health interventions, and valuable potential role in disease amelioration and physiological modification are important to document.

Unlike synthetic drugs which take a number of years to get to market due to regulatory and scientific processes involved for safety reasons, phytochemicals are appearing on market as nutraceutics and other forms of pharmaceutics now, hence the need to scrutinize them for careful benefit versus harm they could subject human.

In order to carry out this exploration of the potential treatment or disease management values of any phytochemicals, primary experimentation in animals or cells are important. This chapter will be concerned with the use of animals as a model for exploration of phytochemicals.

16.2   USE OF ANIMAL MODEL

The use of animals in scientific investigation has been an important practice in biology and medicine but not without concerns, generating frequent debate in present-day society. There are remarkable anatomical and physiological similarities between human and the animals, especially mammals, and had been instrumental to investigations on disease pathology and mechanisms of drug action. Importantly, when new molecules are intended to be used in human, the phase of preclinical investigation uses animals or animal models to create safety profile before such discoveries are used in human.

Although there has been immense contribution of animal experiments to our understanding of mechanism of diseases, effectiveness of treatment in human, judging from animal research data have remained controversial (Hackam and Redelmeier, 2006; Hackam, 2007; Perel et al., 2007; Barré-Sinoussi and Montagutelli, 2015). Arguments have been raised against the use of animals by animal rights advocacy groups with the claims that animals are harmed in the process. Despite this challenge, it is arguable that animals remain useful for research purposes where the balance for its use outweighs the risks to life or impossibility of carrying out such studies in human, and where the benefit to human is significant. Animal studies have contributed to unique developments in medical and scientific researches that benefit both animals and humans. The unavoidable use of animals, however, has compelled researchers to ensure that, though these creatures are animals, there is respect, care, and compassion in treatment of the animals for research, as they pursue ethical, judicious, and responsible research activities.

The animal kingdom provides a variety of species that have remarkably helped in the advancement of scientific investigations leading to land-breaking discoveries. Such discoveries have made life better for the world inhabitants. These important learning subjects range from small worms, insects, and fishes to higher mammals. The species that have been extensively used, especially as models, included *Caenorhabditis elegans*, *Drosophila melanogaster*, *Danio rerio* (Zebra fish), *Mus musculus* (house mouse) *Rattus norvegicus* (brown rats), and others.

16.3 ANIMAL MODELS FOR HUMAN DISEASES

In most diseases conditions, the distinct physiological and anatomical changes that occur are complex involving highly integrated and regulated functional alterations. There are many circulating factors, network of biomolecules such as neurochemical transmitters, hormones, cell to cell talking across compartments, and other complex activities involved. The functional alterations in health and disease conditions would require biological interrogation to understand multilevel molecular, cellular, tissue and organ involvements, and mechanism of disease establishment. Although there are in vitro methods available to explore health and diseases states including use of cell cultures and three-dimensional (3D) analytical techniques that have potentially been presented to replace use of animals, there still remains the need to understand physiological functions and systemic interactions between organs in real-time exploration (Barré-Sinoussi and Montagutelli, 2015). This necessitated the use of whole organism, hence the relevance of animal model of these diseases.

Since phytochemicals are purposefully going to alter physiology or ameliorate pathological conditions, it is important that we understand the physiological functions of these promising molecules. Animal models provide curious engagement that will help reveal, to a large extent, the values of phytochemicals in question.

16.4 HIGHLIGHTS ABOUT MOUSE AND RAT MODELS

16.4.1 THE MICE MODEL

The mice model of human diseases was among first disease model available to scientists for investigation and understanding of mechanism (s) underlying establishment of diseases. The phylogenic relatedness and physiological similarity to human, ease of maintaining and breeding mouse in the laboratory, and availability of many inbred strains made *M. musculus* available as models for human biology and diseases (Morse, 2007). Just as available to most important models, the susceptibility to manipulation of their genome, creating transgenics, knockout and knockin mice provided tools for mouse research (Waterston et al., 2002; Brown and Hancock, 2006; Fox et al., 2007) and proved valuable in preclinical trials. It is, therefore, possible to use the model for phytochemical screening.

The models available are not without limitation that must be considered in attempts to use them for phytochemical screening. Responses to experimental interventions of mice have shown remarkable difference, often time, compared to response in human (Perlman, 2016). Candidate drugs in pipeline have come out with poor response in human despite successful cure of diseases, like cancer, in mouse models (Adams, 2012). With reference to cancer, as an example, substances that normally are carcinogenic to mice are not in human, and vice versa. The factors that have been identified responsible for the difference include lineage divergence from common ancestral species being several years, adaptation to different environment resulting in evolution of differing developmental processes, and modification in both mice and human system physiology (Elsea and Lucas, 2002; Springer and Murphy, 2007). Thus, activities of phytochemicals, though may be screened using mouse, must be interpreted and extrapolated to human with caution.

Earlier efforts on mouse models showed that since disease processes are not all determined by heritable gene dysfunction and due to influence of injury, infection, aging, cancer, neural degeneration, and neural regeneration on genes, mouse models may provide very interesting leads on a range of diseases. This understanding has been explored to improve utility and relevance of mouse model. The diseases of interest for which genetically modified mouse model (mutants) exist are diabetes, obesity, sensory (hearing and vision), neurological disorder (neuronal growth, differentiation, and plasticity), neurobehavioral conditions, cardiovascular disease, cancer, ageing disorders, and musculoskeletal (myopathy) conditions (Gibson et al., 1995; Ohl and Keck, 2003; Carrol et al., 2004; Takahashi and Smithies, 2004; Usera et al., 2004; Shelton and Engvall, 2005).

More recent argument, however, is raising more concern on many non-successful explorations of the animal model research especially due to failure of application of mice model breakthroughs in human diseases. An example was demonstrated from the analysis of reputed contribution of mouse experiment to human type 2 diabetes research by Chandrasekera and Pippin (2013). The failures recorded were not only in diabetes research but also in discordance in pattern of gene expression in human and mice experiencing severe inflammatory human disorder of trauma, sepsis, and burns, with about 150 successful treatment in mice failing in human (Seok et al., 2013); spinal cord injury (Tator, 2012), and in cancer (Hutchinson, 2011; Prinz, 2011; Begley, 2012).

16.4.2   THE RAT MODEL

With similar advantages of using mouse, rats were the first mammalian species to be domesticated about 150 years ago as animal model of human disease (Iannaccone and Jacob, 2009). The introduction of the first transgenic mouse in 1987 caused the shift of attention of many scientists away from rat (Capecchi, 2001). However, relevant considerations of the advantage that support the use of rats include their physiological history that is richer than those of mice and that these animals are bigger than mice making them more suitable for performing surgeries, drug studies that require serial drawing of blood, and transplantation studies (Ellenbroek and Youn, 2016). As new rat models are becoming available, the already available transgenic ones can be used in screening phytochemicals. The rats have been shown to demonstrate more advance utilization for cognition and memory studies, capable of learning a wider variety of tasks that provide landmark results in series of investigations over the years (Quillfeldt, 2016). Other areas of investigation that has employed rat models are autism-related disorder, Phelan-McDermid syndrome (Harony-Nicolas et al., 2017), autoimmune disease such as multiple sclerosis (Storch et al., 1998) and diabetes mellitus (King 2012, Takeda et al., 2017). For those conditions in which the results have shown valuable extrapolation to human, phytochemical research will benefit from the use of such models.

16.5   OBTAINING PRECLINICAL DATA

Animal models have been used in many circumstances to first experiment an hypothesis. Data collected had found profound usefulness in shaping the designs of studies in human and eventual development of life-saving approaches. Although the appropriateness of extrapolation of findings from use of animal models remained argued, variety of scientific questions has been answered through use of animals as earlier mentioned; from basic science to development and assessment of therapy and vaccines (Barré-Sinoussi and Montagutelli, 2015). Observations and testing on animal models have recorded breakthroughs as it was when Banton and McLeod first established the treatment of type 1 diabetes with insulin in 1921 and in the case of cellular therapies for tissue regeneration (Klug et al., 1996). All these point to the fact that preclinical trials would remain valuable using the animal model.

It is expected that phytochemicals that would find their ways into compendium of drugs for treatment of diseases should undergo preclinical evaluations. Animal model would provide useful resource. This notwith-standing, it is argued that certain considerations are important when using the animal. The limit of variation in the biology of the two subjects, animal and human, must be taken into account when designing the trial studies; genetic and physiological differences. Other consideration would be in respect of adequate internal validity (differences observed between groups of animals allocated to different interventions), proper randomization to prevent selection bias, genuine blinding which makes the investigator unable to influence the outcome, and appropriate sample size without neglecting the ethical need to keep the number of animals small. Phytochemicals need to be evaluated for a range of biochemical and physiological variables ranging from effects on blood, systems function – renal, liver, cardiac, gastrointestinal, reproductive, respiratory, and brain. Toxicity studies are crucial with clear determination of toxicity index for the particular phytochemicals. This preliminary evaluation will give clues to what therapeutic advantage the phytochemical presents.

On completion of extraction of phytochemicals from source plant, it is important to conduct bioassays in small animal model. This extraction process must be quality assured as it may affect results of the bioassay. The toxicological assay would primarily focus on the sensitive indicators of hepatocellular damage, serum alanine transaminase and aspartate aminotransferase. Depending on which biological target a phytochemical is intended or reported, active several tests can be conducted and may include activities assessment as anti-inflammatory, antimicrobial, antitumor, antidiabetic, and so forth.

16.6 DEFINING DYNAMICS AND KINETICS OF PHYTOCHEMICALS

An important aspect of evaluation of phytochemicals is getting to know what the phytochemicals do to the body and how the body handles it. Before large trials in human subjects, animal models provide opportunity to evaluate these phenomena. The concept that the phytochemicals do react with appropriate receptors to illicit actions desired or undesired, constitute an aspect of phytochemical studies that may be referred to as "sphytochemi-codynamic." This will entail studies using animal models that examine the relationship between phytochemicals and responses they produce following introduction to the body of the animals. Structural activity, receptor reaction, and responses are defined by what the phytochemical contains.

The other phenomenon is the concept that evaluates how the body of the animal or human eventually handles the phytochemical, a phenomenon that may be referred to as "phytochemicokinetics." This phenomenon is a time-course analysis of movement of the phytochemical through the phases of absorption, distribution, metabolism, and excretion or elimination.

Often time, studies found reporting phytochemical activities are selective of what they report and a comprehensive evaluation is rarely reported. The time is fast changing that effective evaluation would be accepted for publication in reputable journals which demonstrate a clear picture of the importance of the phytochemical in question. Thus, it is imperative that those who will investigate phytochemicals should apply broader investigation techniques.

The availability of high-tech instruments like high-performance liquid chromatography, mass spectrophotometer, and photon-driven analyzing equipment are providing a lead to understand chemical activities in the body. Basic kinetic information are easily obtainable; area under the concentration-time curve, phytochemical concentration at different times, elimination half-life, as may be affected by route of administration, formulation, animal species, age, body condition, gender, and physiological status. Such has been described in respect of antimicrobial agents (Zhao et al., 2016).

In case of phytochemicals for treatment of infection, common models are available as outlined by Zhao et al. (2016). These common models include models for thigh infection, acute bacterial pneumonia, chronic bacterial pneumonia, skin and soft tissue infection, septicemia, meningitis, urinary tract infection, infectious endocarditis, and intraperitoneal infection. It is expected that many more will be available in the course of disease modeling exploration. Also, the dynamics of protein binding and influence on the kinetic parameter can be assessed in respect of administered phytochemical. Most chemicals bind to proteins such as α, β, and γ globulins, acid glycol proteins, lipoproteins, and erythrocytes when introduced to the animal body. It is well known that the unbound phytochemicals are those presenting the activities that are observed. Although this segment is not intended to be a detail exploration of the dynamics and kinetics of phytochemicals, it emphasizes the possibility provided by animal models to support detail investigation into how phytochemicals work and what the body of animals or human may handle it.

16.7   ANIMAL MODELS IN DIFFERENT HUMAN DISEASE CONDITIONS

Several disease conditions of human require evaluating therapeutic efficacy and safety of old drugs or new ones in pipeline to which phytochemicals are a group. These diseases may include, but not limited to, hypertension, anxiety disorders, clinical pathology conditions such as asthma and chronic bronchitis, cardiac ischemia. inflammation and arthritis, peripheral and visceral pain, depression, schizophrenia, attention deficit hyperactivity disorder, eating disorders, dementia, epilepsy, Parkinson's disease, diabetes, gastrointestinal disorders like ulcer, renal insufficiency, urogenital dysfunction, inflammatory bowel disease, systemic lupus erythematosus, pulmonary fibrosis, and cancer. To all these, there are several animal models that have been developed over the years. Phytochemical studies will benefit not only in determining the toxicity profile of their constituent molecules but also in understanding the clinical potential of the molecules. As earlier mentioned, there are limitations to direct extrapolation of findings in animal models but knowledge derived from the genetic, biochemical, and histological studies in human of the disease conditions may be compared to those obtained from animal data in order to determine how appropriate the animal model might be for that particular mechanistic approach. It is in this manner that the false negative results that may come from experimentation with animals may be reduced. The animal model of choice will have to respond to phytochemicals that are to be evaluated for pharmacological activities in a manner similar to the effects of standard or established therapeutic agents (control) for a particular disease.

The chemicals that are clinically inactive of new compounds in drug development pipelines, such as phytochemicals, may have shown activities in animal models causing a false positive condition. This further emphasizes the need to take cautionary steps in deploying animal models for activity studies. Therefore, it is important to appreciate the limitations of a model to ensure effective use within the context of understanding peculiarity of diseases for which cure is sought.

In order to appreciate the models, typical example of the disorders, diabetes – a metabolic disorder, cancer, and neurodegenerative disorders are summarily presented in this chapter with accessories of models for evaluation of effects of phytomedicine.

16.7.1 DIABETES MELLITUS

Diabetes mellitus is a chronic disease characterized by a relative or absolute lack of insulin, leading to hyperglycemia condition. It has remained one of the global health concern affecting children and adults. When chronic, hyperglycemia can lead to a variety of complications such as neuropathy, nephropathy, and retinopathy and increased risk of cardiovascular disease (King, 2012). It is established that the two types of diabetes, type 1 (an autoimmune disease leading to the destruction of the insulin-producing pancreatic β cells in the islets of Langerhan) and type 2 (associated with insulin resistance, and a lack of appropriate compensation by the β cells leads to a relative insulin deficiency) are importantly pathologic disorder that would continuously require investigation in respect of appropriate therapy and improved management. Although a type 2 diabetes can be managed with improving weight reduction and exercise (Solomon et al., 2008), when such intervention fails, drugs that are available are used to treat the diabetes (Krentz et al., 2008). These drug categories include drugs that stimulate insulin production from the β cells (e.g., sulphonylureas), drugs that reduce hepatic glucose production (e.g., biguanides), drugs that delay carbohydrate uptake in the gut (e.g., α-glucosidase inhibitors), drugs that improve insulin action (e.g., thiazolidinediones), and drugs that target the GLP-1 axis (e.g., GLP-1 receptor agonists or DPP-4 inhibitors). These classes of drug may require improvement and further understanding of their mechanisms of action. Animal models provide a unique opportunity to search for more relevant molecules from phytochemical; screening them for activities.

The lack of insulin production in type 1 diabetes is due to autoimmune destruction of the pancreatic β cells. It is important to simulate this condition in animal for pytochemical screening and evaluation. The deficiency in insulin production can be achieved using different approaches; using chemical ablation of the β cells and genetic modification that allows rodents develop autoimmune diabetes.

16.7.1.1 CHEMICAL INDUCTION MODEL

In this model, chemicals are used to generate high percentage of the endogenous β cells destruction to allow only little insulin to be endogenously produced. There are two main compounds that can be used to induce diabetes. These are streptozotocin (STZ) and alloxan. The two are similar in structure to glucose (Bansal et al., 1980), hence compete with glucose. The relative instability of alloxan and STZ make it important that the solution should ideally be prepared when just about to inject the chemical into the animals.

Following the administration of STZ through intraperitoneal or intravenous route, it enters the pancreatic β cell through the Glut-2 transporter and causes alkylation of the DNA, a reduction in cellular adenosine triphosphate, and inhibition of insulin production. It also generates free radicals that can also contribute to DNA damage and subsequent cell death. This can be achieved on administration of a single high dose, for example, 100–200 mg/ kg in mice or 35–65 mg/kg in rats, or as multiple low doses, range from 20–40 mg/kg/day over 5 days to induce insulitis in mice or rats depending on strain (Lukic et al., 1998; Wang and Gleichmann, 1998; Srinivasan and Ramarao, 2007; Dekel et al., 2009).

These animals following administration would present with weight loss and hyperglycemia. In the analysis of a phytochemical, this will be a simple model to create in the laboratory and possibly cheap. The animal may be left for a minimum of 5 days to be sure of stable hyperglycemia. Objectively, this procedure will find high value in experiment in which the suspected mechanism of action is lowering of blood glucose through non-β-cell-dependent pathway and in transplantation therapies with the goal to lower blood glucose level (Sheshala et al., 2009; Deeds et al., 2011). An important caution is to ensure that evaluation of the graft-bearing kidney and endogenous β cells for reactivation of activities are done. Although the chemical induction may be useful, it carries high risk of being injurious or toxic to other organs of the body and may result in changes in the activities of Cyt P450 isozymes in the liver, kidney, lungs, intestines, and brain (Lee et al., 2010).

Alloxan, on the other hand, is rapidly taken up by the β cells, reduced to dialuric acid, and then reoxidized back to alloxan. This process creates a redox cycle for the generation of superoxide radicals that undergo dismutation to form hydrogen peroxide and thereafter highly reactive hydroxyl radicals that can destroy the DNA (Nerup et al., 1994; Szkudelski, 2001). The protective capacity of the liver shields it from the reactive oxygen species when it takes up alloxan, preventing liver damage (Mathews and Leiter, 1999). There are other mechanisms of induction of β cell damage by alloxan. The report showed that oxidation of the –SH groups of enzymes like glucokinase and disturbance of intracellular calcium homeostasis are possible (Kim et al., 1994; im Walde et al., 2002). A dose range of 50–200 mg/kg in mice and 40–200 mg/kg in rats, depending on the strain, would just be enough diabetogenic doses beyond which general toxicity of the kidney may occur (Szkudelski, 2001).

16.7.1.2   AUTOIMMUNE MODEL

The common autoimmune models of type 1 diabetes models are produced from mouse as nonobese diabetic (NOD) mouse and rats as biobreeding (BB) rats. The NOD mice develop insulitis in about 3–4 weeks (Hanafusa et al., 1994). NOD mice develop insulitis at around 3–4 weeks of age with the pancreatic islets infiltrated by predominately CD4[+] and CD8[+] lymphocytes, while B cells and NK cells are present (Yoon and Jun, 2001). About 90% of pancreatic insulin is lost at around 10–14 weeks to continuous destruction from insulinitis that was initiated and may be sustained for 30 weeks of age. A pathogen-free cage may be required to maintain the NOD mouse due to negative association of these animals to exposure to infectious microbes. Chemicals can also be used to induce NOD in mice with use of cyclophosphamide (Caquard et al., 2010). Other means are also available (Christianson et al., 1993; Rydgren et al., 2007).

The BB rats were derived from outbred Wistar rats and the lines were sustained through successful crossings and used for experiment (Mordes et al., 2004). There are other models such as genetically induced insulin dependent diabetes Akita mice and virus-induced models and models by pancreatectomy or STZ.

Type 2 diabetes models are characterized by insulin resistance and β-cell failure – inability of the β cell to sufficiently compensate. The animals are obese and thus reflect the human condition where obesity is closely linked to type 2 diabetes development. This obesity may be naturally occurring or genetically manipulated or high-fat feeding of the animal. The most widely used monogenic models of obesity have defective leptin signaling, lack of functional leptin, loss of satiety response, causing hyperphagia and subsequent obesity. Examples of these models include the Lep[ob/ob]mouse (deficient in leptin), the Lepr[db/db] mouse, and Zucker diabetic fatty rat (deficient in the leptin receptor).

The polygenic models of obesity are much more related to human condition with variety of conditions modeling obesity, glucose intolerance and diabetes. These allow for a variety of genotypes and susceptibilities to be investigated. Models available for such investigations are the KK mice (Clee and Attie, 2007), the Otsuka Long-Evans Tokushima Fat rat, the New Zealand obese mouse, the Tallyho mouse (naturally occurring model of obesity and type 2 diabetes) recently shown to help as model for diabetic wound healing (Buck et al., 2011), the high-fat feeding C57BL/6 mice that can present with obesity, hyperinsulinemia, and altered glucose homeostasis due to insufficient compensation by the islets (Winzell and Ahren, 2004), the desert gerbil (*Psammomys obesus*), the Nile grass rat (*Arvicanthis niloticus*) recently suggested as a model for metabolic syndrome (Noda et al., 2010), the Goto–Kakizaki rats (Goto et al., 1976) which are wistar rats with the poorest glucose tolerance and are lean model of type 2 diabetes.

All these models will be useful in studying phytochemicals that can influence disorders of the related metabolic syndrome.

16.7.2   CANCER

Cancer has remained one of the diseases that has sprouted more concern of scientists to search natural products including phytochemicals for more treatment molecules, given the challenges associated with existing therapeutics. Inducing carcinogenesis in animal models has provided templates for screening new molecules. With some 30 substances that were first shown to cause cancer in animals which may be genotoxic and nongenotoxic and linked to human cancer through epidemiologic studies, models of animal cancer are easy to create in the laboratory.

These substances include estrogen, formaldehyde, diethylstilbestrol, dichlorodiphenyltrichloroethane, vinyl chloride, 2,3,7,8-TCDD, radon gas, beryllium, asbestos, 4-aminobiphenyl, bis (chloromethyl) ether, and 1,3 butadiene (Huff, 1993; Rall, 2000). Comparing cancer susceptibility in human and rodent, low cancer rates occur in human's liver, kidney, forestomach, and thyroid gland than in rodents but high in both species in the lung, mammary gland, the hematopoietic system, bladder, oral cavity, and skin. In humans, cancer rate is high for prostate gland, pancreas, colon/rectum, and cervix/uterus compared to rodents. A careful bioassay of carcinogen and interaction of phytochemicals to prevent development and reduce carcinogen actions would depend on evidence that such cancer can be induced using same chemicals in human, mechanisms of action, threshold levels, and dose–response patterns of test compounds. It is also possible to generate models of cancer in animals using genetic engineering (see Kemp, 2015). The use of genetically engineered models would be additional logical approach to unravelling interactions between phytochemicals and induced cancers in animal models, for example, p53 gene knockout mice that can be used for spontaneous lymphomas and sarcomas tumors (Donehower et al., 1992). Several protocols are available to induce different tumors in animal model. An example is induction of lung tumor in mice using urethane or N-ethyl-N-nitrosourea (Gurley et al., 2014a,b).

16.7.3   NEURODEGENERATIVE DISORDERS

There are yet unsuccessful searches for new and effective therapies for neurodegenerative disorders. This makes the advances for new therapies from phytochemicals relevant. Evaluating potential advantages will be done through use of models that are readily available. With increasing understanding of the pathogenic mechanisms underlying major neurodegenerative conditions, mechanisms governing the pathological aggregation of the key proteins, the nature and processes of neuronal damage associated with protein aggregate formations, and the role of neuroinflammation in fuelling the neurodegenerative processes are abundantly elucidated. Most designs to correct the biochemical or molecular defect are tested in animal models. A summary of the diseases and models available are shown in Table 16.1.

16.8 GENERAL PHYTOPHARMACOLOGICAL EVALUATION HINT

The animals, when deciding to use them for phytochemical assays, must be properly identified and their health status should be characterized. Choice of which animal model to use, as earlier mentioned, will depend on the research question and the ability of the model to provide near answers. The species must be well identified and properly handled. There will be a need to determine if young or adult animals will be used, male or female, pregnant or nonpregnant depending on the analysis to be conducted. The weight of the animals must be recorded as it is important in administering the phytochemical doses and dose determination. If animals were just brought from elsewhere into the laboratory, it is important to acclimatize them for specific days not less than a week. The experimental procedure can thereafter commence. The research ethic principles on the handling of animals must be respected at all times.

In case of plants, that investigator suspects have compounds of interest, a large quantity of fresh parts of the plants at the beginning are usually collected, identified by experts, and given a voucher specimen number. The processing of the plan through washing, drying under specified condition, and for a specified duration is undertaken using established protocol. The pulverized plant samples may be macerated in methanol or any other solvent depending on the procedure and other processes untill a crude extract is obtained and gel-like solid is produced. The extracts can be administered with the aid of a gavage acting as an orogastric tube with utmost care taken not to inflict oral or esophageal injuries on the animal. Another method of administering phytochemical may be employed, including intraperitoneal route.

Toxicity activities of the phytochemicals are usually the first step and are embarked upon by determining 50% lethal dose (LD50) and acute toxicity using standard protocols. Subchronic and acute toxicity assessment may also be done. At this point, all observations including clinical sign and mortality are essential to document. Changes in biochemical activities may be monitored by obtaining blood samples for analysis and behavioral response are also monitored.

TABLE 16.1 A Summary of the Neurodegenerative Diseases and Models Available.

Disease/Disorder	Model Basis	Repository of Animal Model
Alzheimer's disease and tauopathies (leading to dementia)	Virtually all AD models are based on the use of transgenic methodologies targeting APP, presenilin, tau or AOPE genes, mostly in mice.	The Jackson Laboratory (JAX®mice), Taconic, QPS Austria Neuropharmacology
Amyotrophic lateral sclerosis	Targeted genes include those encoding superoxide dismutase 1, (TAR)-DNA-binding protein 43, and DNA/RNA-binding protein Fused in Sarcoma. A toxic model based on the systemic administration of neurotoxic amino acid β-methylamino-L-alanine has also been described. Invertebrate models that replicate some aspects of the ALS pathology are also available	The Jackson Laboratory (JAX®mice), Taconic, QPS Austria Neuropharmacology
Huntington' disease	Toxic models based on the use of neurotoxins, such as mitochondrial toxin 3-nitropropionic acid or excitotoxins (kainate, ibotenate, quinolinate), that can induce selective degeneration of striatal GABAergic projection neurons, without affecting striatal interneurons giving a neuropathological lesion of HD. From genetics, numerous transgenic models targeting the *huntingtin* (Htt) gene have been developed	The Jackson Laboratory (JAX®mice), QPS Austria Neuropharmacology.
Parkinson's disease	Both *toxic* and *transgenic* models are available Toxic models are generated from use of compounds acting as mitochondrial toxins and/or pro-oxidant agents, with selective toxicity for dopaminergic neurons (i.e., MPTP, paraquat, rotenone, 6-hydroxydopamine, etc.). These compounds can be administered to the animals, directly into the nigrostriatal pathway (i.e., 6-hydroxydopamine). Depending on the compound and the route of administration, different sets of PD-like pathological and phenotypic features can be reproduced. Transgenic models are also available.	The Jackson Laboratory (JAX®mice), Taconic, QPS Austria Neuropharmacology

16.8.1   THE 3RS CONCEPT

The 3Rs concept (replacement, reduction, refinement) is developed to mini-mize animal use and address suffering or harms to animal. It is a framework that supports high-quality science and translation. As earlier mentioned in respect of difficulty in extrapolating findings from animal models, model validity and appropriateness may be a contributory factor, especially in complex disease modeling where harms are caused to animals. In order to minimize such problems, the 3Rs concept was streamlined into scientific efforts. Currently, the investments and activities in the 3Rs are delivering new research models, tools, and approaches with reduced reliance on animal use (Box 16.1). It has also improved animal welfare and scientific and predictive value of research (Graham and Prescott, 2015).

BOX 16.1 Comparison between *in vitro*, vertebrate and invertebrate models. +++: very good; ++: good; +: possible but not easy; -: hard or disadvantageous			
	In vitro models	**Invertebrate** models	**Vertebrate** models
Cost	-	+++	-
Handling	++	+++	+
Genetics	++	+++	+ (mice) /- (rat)
Analysis of mechanism	++	+++	+
High-throughput drug scree	+++	++	-
Conservation	++	++	+++

It is important to understand the research question for which answers are being sought using a model. The investigators of the phytochemicals would benefit from 3Rs principle through clear understanding of what is the objec-tive of their investigation and may wisely decide to reduce on or avoid animal use. With new research models, tools, and approaches being developed, this concept has found relevance in conducting high-quality bioscience that addresses the concerns of poor reproducibility of animal studies and high rates of attrition in drug development. Thus, assessment of phytochemical activities may be open to extended tools and not restricted to animal model studies alone. There are other whole organism models that satisfy greatly the framework of the 3Rs principle. These include *D. melanogaster* which has a wide range of cutting-edge technologies built around it and being used to develop robust approaches for the study of human biology, diseases, and treatments. Other technologies in pipeline with 3Rs potentials include stem cell technologies, 3D tissue constructs, and bioprinting mathematical and *in silico* modeling (Graham and Prescott, 2015).

16.9 *DROSOPHILA MELANOGASTER* IN PHYTOPHARMACOLOGY STUDIES

"You get 10 times more biology for a dollar invested in flies that you get in mice"

—Hugo Bellen

16.9.1 THE FLY AS A MODEL

"most of what we know that is relevant for understanding basic human biology and how it can go wrong in disease was discovered with simpler organisms. These basic mechanisms have been very well conserved in evolution and thus this has been a very efficient, cost-effective and ethical way to gain this knowledge"

—Gerald Rubin

D. melanogaster has been a key player in genetics and developmental biology since the beginnings of both sciences. A member of the family Drosophilidae, in the taxonomic order Diptera, *D. melanogaster* appeared in Sub-Saharan Africa some 2–3 million years ago, differentiating from its close relative *simulans* somewhere in Eastern West Africa (reviewed in David and Capy (1988)). Both species are widely spread in wild and urban ecosystems of the African continent. Biogeography studies in the 1970s and 1980s suggest that, as the species separated, *D. melanogaster* colonized Central and West Africa while *Drosophila simulans* remained confined to the East of the Cameroon mountains (Lachaise et al., 1988). The first trip out of Africa seems to have occurred between 10,000 and 15,000 years ago when it emigrated to Asia and Europe.

D. melanogaster belongs to the order Diptera, in the Drosophilidae family, and was first described in 1830 (Meigen, 1830; EOL, 2017). It is also known as *the fruit fly,* alias that has led to dangerous misconceptions when it is mistaken for one of the other fruit flies, *Ceratitis* spp. and others, which causes great economic losses as a plague of fruits in places as far away as Spain, Uganda, and Australia. To avoid this confusion one can refer to it as the vinegar fly, nickname that emanates from the habit of this little fly to feed on fermented fruit. After spending many years confined to Equatorial Africa, the fly found in humans the perfect vehicle to spread all over the globe and is now common and commensal all over the planet (Keller, 2007).

Flies have a short life cycle (8 days from egg to sexually active adult). This short generation span, together with the capacity of each female to produce hundreds of eggs and their inexpensive way of life, make it suitable to conquer, not only the kitchens of all corners of the world but also the shelves of scientists pursuing the secrets of life. Most people have heard the story of the pioneer of genetics, Thomas Hunt Morgan, taking on the study of flies in the early 1900s but few know that it was an entomologist, Charles Woodworth, who first reared them (Markow, 2015). Another entomologist, Frank Lutz, was the one who introduced *D. melanogaster* to Morgan who would embrace the organism as an experimental model and with it performed work worth a nobel prize (Morgan, 1910). In 2017, researchers Jeffrey C. Hall, Michael Rosbash, and Michael W. Young received the nobel prize "for their discoveries of molecular mechanisms controlling the circadian rhythm," a work done in flies. And that makes five nobel prizes made in flies (The Nobel Assembly, 2017) and many other fundamental discoveries (Letsou and Bohmann, 2005; Stephenson and Metcalfe, 2013; Markow, 2015).

It is more than numbers that make *D. melanogaster* a workhorse for the biological sciences. Flies are small and feed on fruit, which makes them easy and cheap to rear. Their short generation time and high fecundity allow obtaining big numbers in a short time. Their genome is structured in only four pairs of chromosomes and is highly compact (175 Megabases) facilitating genetics and -omics studies. In a more technical note, male flies do not show meiotic recombination, making it easier to preserve chromosomes intact during genetic studies. All these would make for any organism to be easy to study but the skeptics would still say that there is no worth on studying an insect like a harmless fly. Thanks to the fly, though, we know more about ourselves than it would be possible to know depending on expensive mammalian experimental animals. Study after study have shown that key processes and genes found in flies are playing similarly important roles in our own biology. The principles of genetics like heredity (Morgan's 1933 Nobel) and mutagenesis (Muller's 1946 Nobel), key processes in developmental biology like axis determination and the segmentation genes (1995 Nobel for Nusslein-Volhard and Wieschaus), the core pathway in innate immunity (Nobel for Hoffman in 2011) were first discovered in flies and then found to be conserved in humans.

D. *melanogaster* makes for a very multifaceted model in biology and also in medicine, especially since the publication of the human genome humbled the genetic superiority aspirations of our species (reviewed in Bellen et al., 2010; Jennings, 2011; Wangler et al., 2015 and many others). Fields like cancer research or neurobiology rely heavily on findings made in flies (Notch, Hedgehog, TGFb, circadian rhythms). The biomedical relevance of fly research is highlighted by a few numbers: the human genome contains predicted homologues of over 60% of the fly proteome and only 7% of vertebrate-specific protein families (Lander et al., 2001) and the fly genome contains homologues of 75% of the human disease-related genes (Reiter et al., 2001).

And if the biology of the fly and its degree of conservation was not enough, fly research also has a cultural component that makes this organism a great one to work with. A century of work has produced an enormous amount of tools and the fly community shares them readily. Stock collections, databases, protocols (Table 16.2), are pooled together, organized, and made easy to find and request (Bilder and Irvine, 2017).

To keep to the scope of this chapter, we will not analyze all the existing fly models. Fly researchers have been particularly successful in modeling noncommunicable diseases (Jennings, 2011; Millburn et al., 2016; Wangler et al., 2017). Research on neurodegenerative disorders like Parkinson, Alzheimer's disease, or Huntington (Lenz et al., 2013), myotonic dystrophy (Fernandez-Costa et al., 2013), cholesterol homeostasis (Niwa and Niwa, 2011), cancer (Sonoshita and Cagan, 2017), diabetes (Graham et al., 2017), autism (Wise et al., 2015), microcephaly (Yamamoto et al., 2014), kidney disorders (Fu et al., 2017), and many others has benefited from work done in flies. Also, infectious disorders have been studied using flies (Dionne and Schneider, 2008), including bacteria host–pathogen interactions (Igboin et al., 2012), fungi (Hamilos et al., 2012), and viruses (Hughes et al., 2012). And if it has been a great model to study human physiology and disease, it is in an even better position to be a good model to study the biology of disease and plague-causing insects (Dimopoulos, 2003; Salvemini et al., 2011).

16.9.2 USING D. MELANOGASTER IN DRUG DISCOVERY

High-throughput drug screen has traditionally been done using in vitro and cell culture models which provide easiness of automation but often fall short in biological relevance. D. *melanogaster* among a few invertebrate models offer a good balance between ease of experimental use and biological

TABLE 16.2 Some of the Resources Available for the Fly Researcher. All Websites Included were Accessed on December 10, 2017.

	Description and Link
Stock collections	Bloomington Stock Center flystocks.bio.indiana.edu/ and their list of stocks related to human diseases and orthologous to genes of relevance flystocks.bio.indiana.edu/Browse/HD/HDintro.htm
	Kyoto Stock Center dgrc.kit.ac.jp/
	VDRC Stock Center stockcenter.vdrc.at/control/main
Web resources	The flybase–A database of Drosophila genes and genomes http://flybase.org with their Human Disease Report List flybase.org/static_pages/FBhh/browse.html
	The Berkeley Drosophila Genome Project fruitfly.org/
	The FlyMove–videos of fly development flymove.uni-muenster.de/
	The Drosophila as a Model for Human Diseases Section of The Interactive Fly: sdbonline.org/sites/FLY/modelsystem/aamodelsystem.htm
	The Drosophila page in the Model Organism Encyclopedia of DNA Elements http://modencode.sciencemag.org/drosophila/introduction
	An introduction to flies by the Berg lab depts.washington.edu/cberglab/wordpress/outreach/an-introduction-to-fruit-flies/
	Drosophila RNAi Screening Center fgr.hms.harvard.edu/including a tool to identify CRISPRs
	Drosophila models of human disease blog by Stephanie Mohr, PhD http://flydiseasemodels.blogspot.ug/
References	Fly development:
	The Development of Drosophila melanogaster. Bates, M and Martinez-Arias, A. Ed. Cold Spring Harbor Laboratory Press, Cold Spring Harbor, NY, 2000
	Lawrence, P. A. The making of a fly. Blackwell Scientific Publications, Oxford, 1992
	Fly Protocols:
	Sullivan W, Ashburner M, and Hawley RS. Drosophila Protocols. Cold Spring Harbor Laboratory Press, Cold Spring Harbor, NY, 2000

TABLE 16.2 *(Continued)*

	Description and Link
	Greenspan RJ. Fly pushing: The theory and practice of Drosophila genetics. Cold Spring Harbor Laboratory Press, Cold Spring Harbor, NY, 2004
	Fly Genetics:
	Roote and Prokop, 2013
	The Genome of *Drosophila melanogaster*, Lindsley DL and Zimm GG Ed. Academic Press, San Diego, 1992
Other resources	The Fly Community: flybase.org/static_pages/community_html
	The Manchester Fly Facility: flyfacility.manchester.ac.uk
	DrosAfrica: drosafrica.org and researchgate.net/project/DrosAfrica
	Trend in Africa: trendinafrica.org
	Fly Indonesia: flyindonesia.wordpress.com/
	Nigerian Drosophila Research Community: researchgate.net/project/Nigerian-Drosophila-Research-Community
	GSA Genes to Genome Drosophila posts: genestogenomes.org/tag/drosophila/

relevance for high-throughput screen (Ségalat, 2007; Strange, 2016). Several reviews have covered the use of *Drosophila* as a model in drug discovery (Giacomotto and Ségalat, 2010; Kasai and Cagan, 2010; Pandey and Nichols, 2011; Ségalat, 2007; Ziehm et al., 2017). For that reason, in the interest of clarity, we will limit this section to describing the key points to take into consideration in the major steps to follow when using flies for drug discovery (Fig. 16.1).

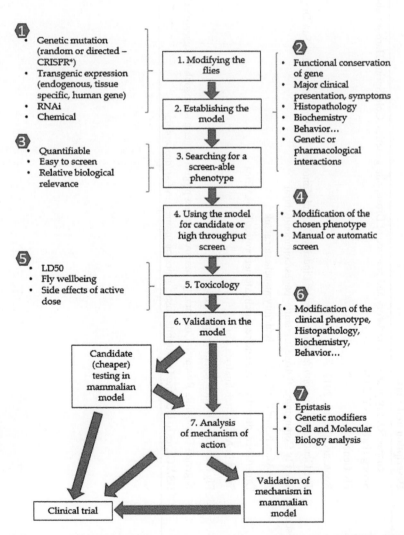

FIGURE 16.1 Workflow using *Drosophila melanogaster* in drug screen. CRISPR: Clustered Regularly Interspaced Short Palindromic Repeats; RNAi: RNA interference; LD50: lethal dose at which 50% of flies die within a short period of time.

One of the major advantages of working with *Drosophila* is the availability of techniques and tools to genetically modify the flies. Depending on the disease, it may be of interest to knockout the function of a particular gene to mimic the loss of function that originates a disease. This is the case, for example, of the models of Parkinson *DJ1-alpha* or *parkin* (Julienne et al., 2017; Lavara-Culebras and Paricio, 2007). Loss of function alleles have traditionally been generated through random chemical mutagenesis (e.g., using EMS) or P-element mobilization (Rubin and Spradling, 1982). With the advent of molecular biology techniques, the use of RNAi and site-directed mutagenesis have become a routine exercise (Basset and Liu, 2014; Sharma and Rao, 2009). When the loss of function of a gene is lethal, flies still offer the possibility to study the situation in vivo by inducing mutant clones in an otherwise heterozygous fly. These clones of mutant cells are generated via mitotic recombination often using the FRT/Flipase system (Xu and Rubin, 1993). In some cases, though, it is necessary to express proteins or RNA sequences that are not found in the fly. Several models of Alzheimer's have been obtained after expression of mutated forms of β-amyloid peptide (Prübing et al., 2013) and amyotrophic lateral sclerosis has been reproduced in flies by expressing the mutated form of human TDP-43 associated with the disease (Krug et al., 2017). This non-endogenous expression, like the expression of the RNAi constructs, has been made possible by the workhorse of *Drosophila* transgenics: the Gal4/UAS system (Brand and Perrimon, 1993). This system, based in the specific recognition of the UAS sequences by the yeast transcription factor Gal4, allows for the expression of any sequence of interest in any particular group of cells at any particular point in time (Roote and Prokop, 2013). Diseases can also be modeled by inducing a similar phenotype through exposure to drugs or toxicants (Betarbet et al., 2002; Coulom and Birman, 2004). This technique allows for a less rigorous analysis of the genetic mechanism but provides a quick way to test a hypothesis before wasting too much time generating tools without having a clue of whether the model will reproduce the disease or not. It also helps in analyzing the mechanism by which exposure to some chemicals induces diseases that mimic other genetic disorders.

Once the flies have been modified, there is need to establish the conservation of the gene function and the known clinical and cellular events found in human patients. The functional conservation is often tackled with "rescue experiments" in which the human gene is introduced in the fly lacking the function of the fly gene. If the function is conserved, the human gene will be able to ameliorate, "rescue," the problems observed in the loss of function mutant (Monferrer and Artero, 2006). The fly proteins can also be expressed in mammalian cell culture to show that they are capable of interacting with known partners of the human homolog (Vicente-Crespo et al., 2008). Fly models need to mimic disease-like events that can be informative of what happens in humans, for example, neurodegeneration and tau tangles in models of tauopathies or polyglutamin and RNA aggregates in triplet repeat expansion disorders. General phenotype, histopathology – including cellular and molecular events – developmental processes, and behavior should be analyzed to establish the level of parallelism with the modeled condition. When the involvement of other genes has been described, genetic interactions with the loss and gain of function of those genes should also be tested. The goal at this stage is to demonstrate that the fly reproduces certain events that characterize the human disorder. It is important to keep in mind that not all the defects found in humans are found in flies and it is not necessary that everything is reproduced for the model to be useful or of interest. A model of myotonic dystrophy, for example, can reproduce muscular defects but will not develop cataracts, since there is no lens in flies.

The defects found in flies can be used to understand the underlying molecular mechanism and also as markers of drug effect when testing some candidate drugs (Sanz et al., 2017). Most of the disease-related phenotypes, though, are too cumbersome for high-throughput screens. When it comes to screening tens or hundreds, even thousands of compounds, it is better to use a phenotype that is easy to observe and quantify. Lethality, for example, or sterility are easily observable since one only has to look if there is any fly coming out of the vial. The capture and analysis of some behaviors like negative geotaxis – the natural tendency of flies to climb up when left alone – larval locomotion, or even social behavior can be automated to facilitate the detection of a treatment that induces changes (Aleman-Meza et al., 2015; Dankert et al., 2009). Image analysis techniques can also help to detect drugs that reduce the size of tumors generated in a fly (Willoughby et al., 2013). The selection of the phenotype determines the method of screen, which is why it is so important to select a quantifiable trait. Those compounds that ameliorate the phenotype are selected for further analysis. Since we are talking about using an insect as a screening tool, we can also be interested in compounds that kill the flies if we are looking for compounds that help fight against plagues or disease-transmitting insects.

The candidate compounds should undergo a thorough toxicology test determining the lethal dose (LD50) in short and long exposure. When there is no previous information on the appropriate dose needed, these toxicology studies can provide a safe range to start with, but in the case of drug libraries, it is not really feasible to perform a thorough toxicological study of all compounds included in the collection. The trade-off between safety and activity will determine if the compound has the potential to become a medicine. Beyond the LD50, flies allow for analysis of the possible mutagenic effects of the drugs (Graf et al., 1984), as well as a wide range of side effects, from general health and well-being (measured with impact in life span and climbing activity) to effects on neurocognitive function (learning and memory), locomotion or social behavior. With a safe and active dose, the researcher goes back to the model, testing the capacity of the drug to ameliorate the disease-related phenotypes. Thanks to its short generation span and high fertility, *Drosophila* allows for many tests to be run with organisms of similar genetic background. Drugs can be tested individually or in a combinatorial manner, looking for drug synergy or to study possible harmful drug interactions.

Despite the conservation, it is important to understand the limitations of the model. Differences in pharmacokinetics and pharmacodynamics of molecules can lead to significantly different drug levels and tissue distribution (Pandey and Nichols, 2011). *Drosophila* is a powerful tool to identify potential candidates and screen for activity and safety within a much smaller budget, but results obtained in flies need to be validated in mammalian systems. Numerous studies have shown that findings in flies have great potential to be relevant for mammalian physiology and can help not only reducing the costs but also speeding up the rate of findings. Flies have been used to screen chemical libraries of different nature, from already FDA-approved compounds (Ziehm et al., 2017) to combinations of peptides specifically designed for a particular drug target (Garcia-Lopez et al., 2008). The strong background of knowledge about *Drosophila* development and genetics also make it a model of choice for those in the field of personalized medicine (Kasai and Cagan, 2010) and it is already giving positive results in the search for combinatorial therapeutics (Agrawal et al., 2005).

The role of flies in drug discovery does not end with the switch to rodent models for validation. Once the effect of the drug is validated in mammals, *Drosophila* still offers a great opportunity to study the mechanism of action of the compound. The availability of genetic tools allows for the dissection of genetic modifiers and epistatic interactions in a way hardly possible in any other system. In short, once a drug is found to ameliorate the phenotype of a particular disease model, the genetic model can be modified to determine which genes are necessary for that amelioration to happen. The field of drug discovery using flies may be just emerging but has already shown that it can fly to great heights (Gonzalez, 2013; Pandey and Nichols, 2011).

16.9.3   UNVEILING PHYTOPHARMACOLOGICALLY ACTIVE PRINCIPLES USING D. MELANOGASTER

Having been at the core of so many breakthroughs in Biology and Pharmacology, there is no reason why flies should not play an important part in modern Phytopharmacological studies. During its life cycle, *Drosophila* goes through four stages. The embryo develops for 24 h at 25°C (all times double if flies are kept at 18°C) and then hatches as a larva. Three 1-day-long larval stages eat their way through to a 4-day pupation in which most larval tissues are destroyed and adult structures arise from the imaginal discs, groups of cells that form early in the embryonic development and remain quiescent until metamorphosis (Bate and Martinez-Arias, 1993; Ashburner et al., 2005). Each of these phases is a model in itself and the Phytopharmacology researcher will need to get familiar with their biology to make the most out of the fly.

Using *Drosophila* for Phytopharmacological studies is not very different to other models with more tradition in the field like mice of rats, but it brings the advantage of a large number of animals that can be used and still work in an affordable budget. The steps described in the previous section also apply here without many changes. There are a few issues that the researcher needs to take into consideration, though, when beginning to work with flies for Phytopharmacology studies (Fig. 16.2).

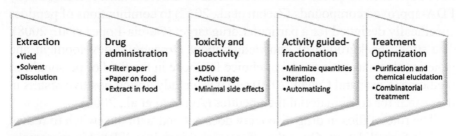

FIGURE 16.2   'Milestones in the use of *D. melanogaster* in Phytopharmacology'

The extraction procedures and parameters to take into account when juicing out the active principles of a plant are covered in detail elsewhere in this book. In brief, when the goal is to give those extracts to our small flying friends, the researcher needs to take into account that, even though one fly will not need much extract, the large numbers involved in an experiment with a significant number of replicas may require a good yield. It is also key to work with an extract clean of toxic solvents, as it is always, and work with a control that is exposed to the same concentration of solvents that may remain in the final extract. Finally, many of the administrative procedures require that the extract is dissolved in an aqueous solution. Researchers working with extracts rich in essential oils or with a high lipid profile may need to troubleshoot the drug administration step.

The most common route of drug administration is feeding but, depending on the developmental stage used, permeability, injection or inhalation may also be used (Abolaji et al., 2013). When it comes to feeding, the extract can be applied on a filter paper that is introduced in an empty vial where the flies will be placed. It is a common practice to starve the flies for six to ten hours before exposure to the extract to increase intake and it is also recommended to add glucose, in a concentration of 1–5% to awaken the flies appetite. Some extract may be specially bitter or repellant for the flies and may require even up to 10% of glucose. A simple essay with bromophenol blue can be used to visualize that the flies are taking the extract (Wong et al., 2009). The filter paper can also be placed on top of a vial with food to avoid desiccation and use the smell of the food as an attractant. Filter paper procedures are the best option for single exposure protocols but when a longer exposure to the extract is needed, the option of choice is to dissolve it in the food. The extract can be dissolved in a small portion of the water that will be used to prepare the food and added in a later stage to avoid overheating. The volume of extract needs to be significant with respect to the food to facilitate a homogeneous distribution of the extract in the food.

As we discussed in the previous section, it is key to select a quantifiable and easy-to-screen phenotype. When working with extracts, one also has to keep in mind the yield available for bioactivity essays. The essay chosen has to be easy to observe, quantifiable, and require minimum levels of extract to be used. Given the big differences between insect and mammalian metabolism, it is not so important to work on a range relative to the human dose as it is to work in the safe dose determined for the fly. LD50 determination and effect of serial dilutions in life span are often a good indicator of the range of concentration that can be given to the fly without inducing toxicity. Still, approximations of grams per kilo can be made determining the average weight of the developmental stage to which the extract is being administered.

The active extracts shall then be further fractionated to identify the fraction containing the bioactive compound(s). In some instances in which toxicity is detected, it is still worth analyzing the bioactivity and toxicity of the fractions since the two could be originating in different compounds and, therefore, it could be possible to separate them (at least in theory). In any case, the activity-guided fractionation needs to be performed keeping in mind that many times it is the combination of phytochemicals present in a plant, and not just one of them, that gives a particular biological activity. Following the same steps described above, the phytopharmacology researcher can use the different models available to test the activity of their extract against a variety of disease models and use the body of knowledge about *Drosophila* development and genetics to dissect the mechanism of action of the bioactive components. Thanks to the inexpensive nature of fly experiments, combinatorial treatments with some but not all of the fractions obtained from an active extract are feasible. This gives the researcher the opportunity to work out which phytochemicals should be included and which should be discarded in an optimal herbal remedy.

Phytopharmacology researchers have started using flies and the model is paying back. Flies have been used to test the efficacy of traditional remedies against neurodegenerative diseases (reviewed in Lee et al., 2014), as anti-fungal agents (Pinho et al., 2016), or antioxidants (Manasa and Ashadevi, 2015). With the long tradition of Chinese phytopharmacology recent turn to flies, the opening of a fly facility in India, and the growing interest of the African scientific community in the use of *D. melanogaster*, it is expected that the number and quality of works will only grow in the next few years. Flies have revolutionized scientific fields (cancer, personalized medicine, neuroscience) and have shaped the scientific landscape of countries (Arias, 2008; Martinez-Arias, 2009). We think that *D. melanogaster* can also bring phytopharmacology to a different level.

KEYWORDS

- animal model
- fly as a model
- *Drosophila melanogaster*
- mice model
- rat model

REFERENCES

1. References to the General Section on Animal Models

Adams, D. J. The Valley of Death in Anticancer Drug Development: a Reassessment. *Trends Pharmacol. Sci.* **2012**, *33*, 173–180.

Bansal, R.; Ahmad, N.; Kidwai, J. R. Alloxan-Glucose Interaction: Effect on Incorporation of 14C-Leucine Into Pancreatic Islets of Rat. *Acta Diabetol. Lat.* **1980**, *17*, 135–143.

Barré-Sinoussi, F.; Montagutelli, X. Animal models are essential to biological research: issues and perspectives. *Future Science OA* **2015**, *1*(4), FSO63. http://doi.org/10.4155/fso.15.63.

Begley, C. G.; Ellis, L. M. Raise Standards for Preclinical Cancer Research. *Nature* **2012**, *483*, 531–533.

Brown, S. D. M.; Hancock, J. M. The Mouse Genome. In *Vertebrate Genomes.* Volff J.N. Ed.; Karger: Basel, **2006**, pp 33–45.

Buck, D. W.; Jin, D. P.; Geringer, M.; Jong, H. S.; Galiano, R. D.; Mustoe, T. A. The Tallyho Polygenic Mouse Model of Diabetes: Implications in Wound Healing. *Plast. Reconstr. Surg.* **2011**, *128*, 427e–437e.

Capecchi, M. R. Generating Mice with Targeted Mutations. *Nat. Med.* **2001**, *7*, 1086–1090.

Caquard, M.; Ferret-Bernard, S.; Haurogne, K.; Ouary, M.; Allard, M.; Jegou, D.; Bach, J.; Lieubeau, B. Diabetes Acceleration by Cyclophosphamide in the Non-Obese Diabetic Mouse is Associated with Differentiation of Immunosuppressive Monocytes Into Immunostimulatory Cells. *Immunol. Lett.* **2010**, *129*, 85–93.

Carroll, L.; Voisey, J.; van Daa, I. A. Mouse Models of Obesity. *Clin. Dermatol* **2004**, *22*, 345–349.

Chandrasekera, P. C.; Pippin, J. J. Of Rodents and Men: Species-Specific Glucose Regulation and Type 2 Diabetes Research. *ALTEX* **2013**, *31*, 157–176.

Christianson, S. W.; Shultz, L. D.; Leiter, E. H. Adoptive Transfer of Diabetes Into Immunodeficient Nod-Scid/Scid Mice. Relative Contributions of Cd4+ and Cd8+ T-Cells from Diabetic Versus Prediabetic Nod.Non-Thy-1A Donors. *Diabetes* **1993**, *42*, 44–55.

Clee, S. M.; Attie, A. D. The Genetic Landscape of Type 2 Diabetes in Mice. *Endocr. Rev.* **2007**, *28*, 48–83.

Deeds, M. C.; Anderson, J. M.; Armstrong, A. S.; Gastineau, D. A.; Hiddinga, H. J.; Jahangir, A.; Eberhardt, N. L.; Kudva, Y. Single Dose Streptozotocin-Induced Diabetes: Considerations for Study Design in IsletTransplantation Models. *Lab. Anim.* **2011**, *45*, 131–140.

Dekel, Y.; Glucksam, Y.; Elron-Gross, I.; Margalit, R. Insights Into Modeling Streptozotocin-Induced Diabetes in Icr Mice. *Lab. Anim.* **2009**, *38*, 55–60.

Donehower, L. A.; Harvey, M.; Slagle, B. L.; McArthur, M. J.; Montgomery, C. A.; Butel, J. S.; Bradley, A. Mice Deficient for p53 are Developmentally Normal But Susceptible to Spontaneous Tumours. *Nat.* **1992**, *356*, 215–221.

Ellenbroek, B.; Youn, J. Rodent Models in Neuroscience Research: Is it a Rat Race? *Dis. Model Mech.* **2016**, *9*(10):1079–1087. doi:10.1242/dmm.026120.

Elsea, S. H.; Lucas, R. E. The Mousetrap: What We Can Learn When the Mouse Model Does Not Mimic the Human Disease. *ILAR J.* **2002**, *43*, 66–79.

Fox, J. G., Barthold, S. W., Davisson, M. T., Newcomer, C. E., Quimby, F. W., Smith, A. L., Eds.; *The Mouse in Biomedical Research.* Elsevier: Amsterdam, **2007**.

Goto, Y.; Kakizaki, M.; Masaki, N. Production of Spontaneous Diabetic Rats by Repetition of Selective Breeding. *Tohoku J. Exp. Med.* **1976**, *119*, 85–90.

Graham, M. L.; Prescott, M. J. The Multifactorial Role of the 3Rs in Shifting the Harm-Benefit Analysis in Animal Models of Disease. *Euro. J. Pharmacol.* **2015**, *759*, 19–29.

Gibson, F., Walsh, J., Mburu, P., Varela, A., Brown, K.A., Antonio, M., Beisel, K.W., Steel, K.P., Brown, S.D. A Type VII Myosin Encoded by the Mouse Deafness Gene Shaker-1. *Nature* **1995**, *374*, 62–4.

Gurley, K. E.; Moser, R. D.; Kemp, C. J. Induction of Liver Tumors in Mice with N-ethyl-N-nitrosourea or N-nitrosodiethylamine. *Cold Spring Harb. Protoc.* **2014b**, DOI: 10.1101/pdb.prot077438.

Gurley, K. E.; Moser, R. D.; Kemp, C. J. Induction of Lung Tumors in Mice with Urethane. *Cold Spring Harb. Protoc.* **2014a**, DOI: 10.1101/pdb.prot077446.

Hackam, D. G. Translating Animal Research Into Clinical Benefit. *BMJ* **2007**, *334*, 163–164.

Hackam, D. G.; Redelmeier, D. A. Translation of Research Evidence from Animals to Humans. *JAMA* **2006**, *296*, 1731–1732.

Hanafusa, T.; Miyagawa, J.; Nakajima, H.; Tomita, K.; Kuwajima, M.; Matsuzawa, Y.; Tarui, S. The NOD Mouse. *Diabetes Res Clin Pract.* **1994**, 24(Suppl.), S307–S311.

Harony-Nicolas, H.; Kay, M.; du Hoffmann, J.; Klein, M. E.; Bozdagi-Gunal, O.; Riad, M. et al. Oxytocin Improves Behavioral and Electrophysiological Deficits in a Novel Shank3-Deficient Rat. Mason, P., Ed. *eLife.* **2017**, *6*, e18904. DOI: 10.7554/eLife.18904.

Huff, J. Chemicals and Cancer in Humans: First Evidence in Experimental Animals. *Environ. Health Perspect.* **1993**, *100*, 201–210.

Hutchinson, L.; Kirk, R. High Drug Attrition Rates-Where are We Going Wrong? *Nat. Rev. Clin. Oncol.* **2011**, *8*, 189–190.

im Walde, S. S.; Dohle, C.; Schott-Ohly, P.; Gleichmann, H. Molecular Target Structures in Alloxan-Induced Diabetes in Mice. *Life Sci.* **2002**, *71*, 1681–1694.

Iannaccone, P. M.; Jacob, H. J. Rats! *Dis. Model Mech.* **2009**, *2*(5-6), 206–210. http://doi.org/10.1242/dmm.002733.

Kemp, C. J. Animal Models of Chemical Carcinogenesis: Driving Breakthroughs in Cancer Research for 100 Years. 2015, Cold Spring Harbor Laboratory Press.

Kim, H. R.; Rho, H. W.; Park, B. H.; Park, J. W.; Kim, J. S.; Kim, U. H.; Chung, M. Y. Role of Ca2+ in Alloxan-Induced Pancreatic Beta-Cell Damage. *Biochim. Biophys. Acta* **1994**, *1227*, 87–91.

King, A. J. F. The Use of Animal Models in Diabetes Research. *Br. J. Pharmacol.* **2012**, *166*(3), 877–894.

Klug, M.G.; Soonpaa, M.H.; Koh, G.Y.; Field, L.J. Genetically Selected Cardiomyocytes from Differentiating Embryonic Stem Cells from Stable Intracardiac Grafts. *J Clin Invest.* **1996**, *98*, 216–224.

Krentz, A. J.; Patel, M. B.; Bailey, C. J. New Drugs for Type 2 Diabetes Mellitus: What is Their Place in Therapy? *Drugs* **2008**, *68*, 2131–2162.

Lee, J. H.; Yang, S. H.; Ho, J. M.; Lee, M. G. Pharmacokinetics of Drugs in Rats with Diabetes Mellitus Induced by Alloxan Or Streptozocin: Comparison with Those in Patients with Type I Diabetes Mellitus. *J. Pharm. Pharmacol.* **2010**, *62*, 1–23.

Lukic, M. L.; Stosic-Grujicic, S.; Shahin, A. Effector Mechanisms in Low-Dose Streptozotocin-Induced Diabetes. *Dev. Immunol.* **1998**, *6*, 119–128.

Mathews, C. E.; Leiter, E. H. Constitutive Differences in Antioxidant Defense Status Distinguish Alloxan-Resistant and Alloxan-Susceptible Mice. *Free Radical Biol. Med.* **1999**, *27*, 449–455.

Mordes, J. P.; Bortell, R.; Blankenhorn, E. P.; Rossini, A. A.; Greiner, D. L. Rat Models of Type 1 Diabetes: Genetics, Environment, and Autoimmunity. *ILAR J.* **2004**, *45*, 278–291.

Morse, H. C. I. Building a Better Mouse: One Hundred Years of Genetics and Biology. In *The Mouse in Biomedical Research;* Fox, J. G., Ed.; Elsevier: Amsterdam, 2007, pp 1–11.

Nerup, J.; Mandrup-Poulsen, T.; Helqvist, S.; Andersen, H. U.; Pociot, F.; Reimers, J. I. On the Pathogenesis of IDDM. *Diabetologia* **1994**, *37*(Suppl. 2), S82–S89.

Noda, K.; Melhorn, M. I.; Zandi, S.; Frimmel, S.; Tayyari, F.; Hisatomi, T.; AlMulki, L.; Pronczuk, A.; Hayes, K. C.; Hafezi-Moghadam, A. An Animal Model of Spontaneous Metabolic Syndrome: Nile Grass Rat. *FASEB J.* **2010**, *24*, 2443–2453.

Ohl, F.; Keck, M.E. Behavioural Screening in Mutagenised Mice: In Search for Novel Animal Models of Psychiatric Disorders. *Eur J Pharmacol.* **2003**, *480*, 219–28.

Perel, P.; Roberts, I.; Sena, E.; Wheble, P.; Briscoe, C.; Sandercock, P.; Macleod, M.; Mignini, L. E.; Jayaram, P.; Khan, K. S. Comparison of Treatment Effects Between Animal Experiments and Clinical Trials: Systematic Review. *BMJ* **2007**, *334*, 197.

Perlman, R. L. Mouse Models of Human Disease: An Evolutionary Perspective. *Evol. Med. Public Health* **2016**, *1*, 170–176.

Prinz, F.; Schlange, T.; Asadullah, K. Believe it or Not: How Much Can We Rely on Published Data on Potential Drug Targets? *Nat. Rev. Drug Discov.* **2011**, *10*, 712. DOI: 10.1038/nrd3439-c1.

Quillfeldt, J.A. Behavioral Methods to Study Learning and Memory in Rats. In *Rodent Model as Tools in Ethical Biomedical Research*; Andersen, M. L., Tufik, S, Ed; SpringerInternational Publishing: Switzerland, 2016; pp 271–311.

Rall, D.P. Laboratory Animal Tests and Human Cancer. *Drug Metab. Rev.* **2000**, *32*, 119–128.

Rydgren, T.; Vaarala, O.; Sandler, S. Simvastatin Protects Against Multiple Low-Dose Streptozotocin-Induced Type 1 Diabetes in Cd-1 Mice and Recurrence of Disease in Nonobese Diabetic Mice. *J. Pharmacol. Exp. Ther.* **2007**, *323*, 180–185.

Ségalat, L. Invertebrate animal models of diseases as screening tools in drug discovery. *ACS Chem. Biol.* **2007**, *2*(4), 231-6.

Seok, J.; Warren, H. S.; Cuenca, A. G.; Mindrinos, M. N.; Baker, H. V.; Xu, W. et al Genomic Responses in Mouse Models Poorly Mimic Human Inflammatory Diseases. *Proc. Natl. Acad Sci.* **2013**, *110*, 3507–3512.

Shelton, G. D.; Engvall, E. Canine and Feline Models of Human Inherited Muscle Diseases. *Neuromuscular Disord.* **2005**, *15*, 127–138.

Sheshala, R.; Peh, K. K.; Darwis, Y. P. Characterization, and in Vivo Evaluation of Insulin-Loaded Pla-Peg Microspheres for Controlled Parenteral Drug Delivery. *Drug Dev. Ind. Pharm.* **2009**, *35*, 1364–1374.

Solomon, T. P.; Sistrun, S. N.; Krishnan, R. K.; Del Aguila, L. F.; Marchetti, C. M.; O'Carroll, S. M.; O'Leary, V. B.; Kirwan, J. P. Exercise and Diet Enhance Fat Oxidation and Reduce Insulin Resistance in Older Obese Adults. *J. Appl. Physiol.* **2008**, *104*, 1313–1319.

Springer, M. S.; Murphy, W. J. Mammalian Evolution and Bio-Medicine: New Views from Phylogeny. *Biol. Rev. Cambridge Philos. Soc.* **2007**, *82*, 375–392.

Srinivasan, K.; Ramarao, P. Animal Models in Type 2 Diabetes Research: an Overview. *Indian J. Med. Res.* **2007**, *125*, 451–472.

Storch, M. K.; Stefferl, A.; Brehm, U.; Weissert, R.; Wallström, E.; Kerschensteiner, M.; Olsson, T.; Linington, C.; Lassmann, H. Autoimmunity to Myelin Oligodendrocyte Glycoprotein in Rats Mimics the Spectrum of Multiple Sclerosis Pathology. Brain Pathol. 1998, 8, 681–694.

Szkudelski, T. The Mechanism of Alloxan and Streptozotocin Action in B Cells of the Rat Pancreas. *Physiol. Res.* **2001**, *50*, 537–546.

Takahashi, N.; Smithies, O. Human Genetics, Animal Models and Computer Simulations for Studying Hypertension. *Trends Genet.* **2004,** *20,* 136–145.

Tator, C. H.; Hashimoto, R.; Raich, A.; Norvell, D.; Fehlings, M. G.; Harop, J. S.; Guest, J.; Aarabi, B.; Grossman, R. G. Translational Potential of Preclinical Trial of Neuroprotection Through Pharmacotherapy for Spinal Cord Injury. *J. Neurosurg. Spine* **2012,** *17*(1 Suppl), 157–229.

Usera, P. C.; Vincent, S.; Robertson, D. Human Phenotypes and Animal Knockout Models of Genetic Autonomic Disorders. *J. Biomed. Sci.* **2004,** *11,* 4–10.

Wang, Z.; Gleichmann, H. Glut2 in Pancreatic Islets: Crucial Target Molecule in Diabetes Induced with Multiple Low Doses of Streptozotocin in Mice. *Diabetes* **1998,** *47,* 50–56.

Waterston, R. H.; Lindblad-Toh, K.; Birney, E.; Rogers, J.; Abril, J. F.; Agarwal, P. et al Initial Sequencing and Comparative Analysis of the Mouse Genome. *Nature* **2002,** *420,* 520–562.

Winzell, M. S.; Ahren, B. The High-fat Diet-fed Mouse: A Model for Studying Mechanisms and Treatment of Impaired Glucose Tolerance and Type 2 Diabetes. *Diabetes* **2004,** *53*(3), S215–S219.

Yoon, J. W.; Jun, H. S. Cellular and Molecular Pathogenic Mechanisms of Insulin-Dependent Diabetes Mellitus. *Ann. N. Y. Acad. Sci.* **2001,** *928,* 200–211.

Zhao, Y.; Chen, J.; Freudenberg, J.M.; Meng, Q.; Rajpal, D.K.; Yang, X. Network-Based Identification and Prioritization of Key Regulators of Coronary Artery Disease Loci. *Arterioscler. Thromb. Vasc. Biol.* **2016,** *36,* 928–941.

2. References to the Section on Drosophila as a Model

Abolaji, A. O.; Kamdem, J. P.; Farombi, E. O.; Rocha, J. B. T. *Drosophila melanogaster* in Toxicological Studies. *Arch. Bas. App. Med.* **2013,** *1,* 33–38.

Agrawal, N.; Pallos, J.; Slepko, N.; Apostol, B. L.; Bodai, L.; Chang, L. W.; Chiang, A. S.; Thompson, L. M.; Marsh, J. L. Identification of Combinatorial Drug Regimens for Treatment of Huntington's Disease Using *Drosophila*. *PNAS* **2005,** *102*(10), 3777–3781.

Aleman-Meza, B.; Jung, S. K.; Zhong, W. An Automated System for Quantitative Analysis of *Drosophila* Larval Locomotion. *BMC Dev. Biol.* **2015,** *24*(15):11. DOI: 10.1186/s12861-015-0062-0.

Arias, A. M. *Drosophila melanogaster* and the Development of Biology in the 20Th Century. *Methods Mol. Biol.* **2008,** *420,* 1–25. DOI: 10.1007/978-1-59745-583-1_1.

Ashburner, M.; Golic, K. G.; Hawley, R. S. *Drosophila: A Laboratory Handbook,* 2nd ed.; Cold Spring Harbor Laboratory Press: New York, 2005, p 1409.

Bassett, A. R.; Liu, J. L.; CRISPR/Cas9 and Genome Editing. *J. Genet. Genomics* **2014,** *41*(1), 7–19. DOI: 10.1016/j.jgg.2013.12.004.

Bate, M.; Martinez-Arias, A. The Development of *Drosophila melanogaster*, Cold Spring Harbor Laboratory Press, Science, **1993,** p 1558

Bellen, H. J.; Tong, C.; Tsuda, H. 100 Years of *Drosophila* Research and Its Impact on Vertebrate Neuroscience: A History Lesson for the Future. *Nat. Rev. Neurosci.* **2010,** *11,* 514–522.

Betarbet, R.; Sherer, T. B.; Greenamyre, J. T. Animal Models of Parkinson'S Disease. *Bioessays* **2002,** *24,* 308–318.

Bilder, D.; Irvine, K. D. Taking Stock of the *Drosophila* Research Ecosystem. *Genetics* **2017,** *206*(3), 1227–1236. DOI: 10.1534/genetics.117.202390.

Brand, A. H.; Perrimon, N. Targeted Gene Expression as a Means of Altering Cell Fates and Generating Dominant Phenotypes. *Development* **1993,** *118*(2), 401–415.

Coulom, H.; Birman, S. Chronic Exposure to Rotenone Models Sporadic Parkinson'S Disease in *Drosophila melanogaster*. *J. Neurosci.* **2004,** *24,* 10993–10998.

Dankert, H.; Wang, L.; Hoopfer, E. D.; Anderson, D. J.; Perona, P. Automated Monitoring and Analysis of Social Behavior in *Drosophila*. *Nat. Methods.* **2009,** *6*(4), 297–303. DOI: 10.1038/nmeth.1310.

David, J. R.; Capy, P. Genetic Variation of *Drosophila melanogaster* Natural Populations. *Trends Genet.* **1988,** *4*(4), 106–111, DOI: 10.1016/0168-9525(88)90098-4.

Dimopoulos, G. Insect Immunity and Its Implication in Mosquito-Malaria Interactions. *Cell Microbiol.* **2003,** *5*(1), 3–14.

Dionne, M. S.; Schneider, D. S. Models of Infectious Diseases in the Fruit Fly *Drosophila melanogaster*. *Dis. Models Mech.* **2008,** *1*(1), 43–49. DOI: 10.1242/dmm.000307.

EOL. Encyclopedia of Life. http://eol.org/pages/733739/overview (accessed Dec 10, 2017).

Fernandez-Costa, J. M.; Garcia-Lopez, A.; Zuniga, S.; Fernandez-Pedrosa, V.; Felipo-Benavent, A.; Mata, M. et al. Expanded CTG Repeats Trigger Mirna Alterations in *Drosophila* That are Conserved in Myotonic Dystrophy Type 1 Patients. *Hum. Mol. Genet.* **2013,** *22*(4), 704–716.

Fu, Y.; Zhu, J.; Richman, A.; Zhao, Z.; Zhang, F.; Ray, P. E.; Han, Z. A. *Drosophila* Model System to Assess the Function of Human Monogenic Podocyte Mutations That Cause Nephrotic Syndrome. *Hum. Mol. Gen.* **2017,** *26*(4), 768 DOI: 10.1093/hmg/ddw428.

Garcia-Lopez, A.; Monferrer, L.; Garcia-Alcover, I.; Vicente-Crespo, M.; Alvarez-Abril, M. C.; Artero, R. D. Genetic and Chemical Modifiers of a CUG Toxicity Model in *Drosophila*. *PLoS One* **2008,** *3*(2), e1595. DOI: 10.1371/journal.pone.0001595.

Giacomotto, J.; Ségalat, L. High-Throughput Screening and Small Animal Models, Where are We? *Br. J. Pharmacol.* **2010,** *160*(2), 204–216. DOI: 10.1111/j.1476-5381.2010.00725.x.

Gonzalez, C. *Drosophila melanogaster*: A Model and a Tool to Investigate Malignancy and Identify New Therapeutics. *Nat. Rev. Cancer* **2013,** *13*(3), 172–183. DOI: 10.1038/nrc3461.

Graf, U.; Würgler, F. E.; Katz, A. J.; Frei, H.; Juon, H.; Hall, C. B.; Kale, P.G. Somatic Mutation and Recombination Test in *Drosophila melanogaster*. *Environ. Mutagen.* **1984,** *6*(2), 153–188.

Graham, P.; Pick, L. *Drosophila* as a Model for Diabetes and Diseases of Insulin Resistance. *Curr. Top. Dev. Biol.* **2017,** *121,* 397–419. DOI: 10.1016/bs.ctdb.2016.07.011.

Hamilos, G.; Samonis, G.; Kontoyiannis, D. P. Recent Advances in the Use of *Drosophila melanogaster* as a Model to Study Immunopathogenesis of Medically Important Filamentous Fungi. *Int. J. Microbiol.* **2012,** DOI: 10.1155/2012/583792.

Hughes, T. T.; Allen, A. L.; Bardin, J. E.; Christian, M. N.; Daimon, K.; Dozier, K. D.; Hansen, C. L.; Holcomb, L. M.; Ahlander, J. *Drosophila* as a Genetic Model for Studying Pathogenic Human Viruses. *Virology* **2012,** *423*(1), 1–5. DOI: 10.1016/j.virol.2011.11.016.

Igboin, C. O.; Griffen, A. L.; Leys, E. J. The *Drosophila melanogaster* Host Model. *J. Oral. Microbiol.* **2012,** *4.* DOI: 10.3402/jom.v4i0.10368.

Jennings, B. *Drosophila*: A Versatile Model in Biology and Medicine. *Materials Today* **2011,** *14*(5), 190–195.

Julienne, H.; Buhl, E.; Leslie, D. S.; Hodge, J. J. L. Drosophilapink1 and Parkin Loss-Of-Function Mutants Display a Range of Non-Motor Parkinson's Disease Phenotypes. *Neurobiol. Dis.* **2017,** *104,* 15–23. DOI: 10.1016/j.nbd.2017.04.014.

Kasai, Y.; Cagan, R. Drosophila as a Tool for Personalized Medicine: a Primer. *Per Med.* **2010,** *7*(6), 621–632.

Keller, A. *Drosophila melanogaster's* History as a Human Commensal. *Curr. Biol.* **2007,** *17*(3), R77–R81.

Krug, L.; Chatterjee, N.; Borges-Monroy, R.; Hearn, S.; Liao, W. W.; Morrill, K.; Prazak, L.; Rozhkov, N.; Theodorou, D.; Hammell, M.; Dubnau, J. Retrotransposon Activation Contributes to Neurodegeneration in a *Drosophila* TDP-43 Model of ALS. *PLoS Genet.* **2017,** *13*(3), e1006635. DOI: 10.1371/journal.pgen.1006635.

Lachaise, D.; Cariou, M. L.; David, J. R.; Lemeunier, F.; Tsacas, L.; Ashburner,. M. Historical Biogeography of the *Drosophila melanogaster* Species Subgroup. *Evol. Biol.* **1988,** 159–225.

Lander, E. S.; Linton, L. M.; Birren, B.; Nusbaum, C.; Zody, M. C.; Baldwin, J. et al. International Human Genome Sequencing Consortium. Initial Sequencing and Analysis of the Human Genome. *Nature* **2001,** *409*(6822), 860–921.

Lavara-Culebras, E.; Paricio, N. *Drosophila* DJ-1 Mutants are Sensitive to Oxidative Stress and Show Reduced Lifespan and Motor Deficits. *Gene* **2007,** *400*(1–2), 158–165.

Lee, S.; Bang, S. M.; Lee, J. W.; Cho, K.S. Evaluation of Traditional Medicines for Neurodegenerative Diseases Using *Drosophila* Models. *Evidence. Based Complementary Alternat. Med.* **2014.** DOI: 10.1155/2014/967462.

Lenz, S.; Karsten, P.; Schulz, J. B.; Voigt, A. Drosophila as a Screening Tool to Study Human Neurodegenerative Diseases. *J. Neurochem.* **2013,** *127*(4), 453–460. DOI: 10.1111/jnc.12446.

Letsou, A.; Bohmann, D. Small Flies – Big Discoveries: Nearly a Century of *Drosophila* Genetics and Development. *Dev. Dyn.* **2005,** *232,* 526–528.

Manasa, N.; Ashadevi, J. S. Impact of Phyllanthus amarus Extract on Antioxidant Enzymes in *Drosophila melanogaster*. *J. Appl. Biol. Biotechnol.* **2015,** *3*(6), 43–047.

Markow. ELife. **2015,** *4,* e06793.

Martinez-Arias, A. A Perspective on the Development of Genetics in Spain During the XX Century. *Int. J. Dev. Biol.* **2009,** *3,* 1179–1191, DOI: 10.1387/ijdb.082811am.

Meigen, J. W. Systematische Beschreibung der Bekannten Europäischen Zweiflügeligen Insekten. Schulzische Buchhandlung, Hamm, 1830, *6,* iii-xi + 1–401 + 24 unnumbered pages.

Millburn, G. H.; Crosby, M. A.; Gramates, L. S.; Tweedie, S.; the Flybase Consortium. Flybase Portals to Human Disease Research Using *Drosophila* Models. *Dis. Model. Mech.* **2016,** *9,* 245–252. DOI: 10.1242/dmm.023317.

Monferrer, L.; Artero, R. An Interspecific Functional Complementation Test in *Drosophila* for Introductory Genetics Laboratory Courses. *J. Hered.* **2006,** *97*(1), 67–73.

Morgan, T. H. Sex-Limited Inheritance in *Drosophila*. *Science* **1910,** *32,* 120–122.

Niwa, R.; Niwa, Y. S. The Fruit Fly *Drosophila melanogaster* as a Model System to Study Cholesterol Metabolism and Homeostasis. *Cholesterol.* **2011,** 176802. DOI: 10.1155/2011/176802.

Pandey, U. B.; Nichols, C. D. Human Disease Models in *Drosophila melanogaster* and the Role of the Fly in Therapeutic Drug Discovery. *Pharmacol. Rev.* **2011,** *63*(2), 411–436. DOI: 10.1124/pr.110.003293. (Barker EL Ed.)

Pinho, F.V.; da Cruz, L. C.; Rodrigues, N. R.; Waczuk, E. P.; Souza, C. E.; Coutinho, H. D.; da Costa, J. G.; Athayde, M. L.; Boligon, A. A.; Franco, J. L.; Posser, T.; de Menezes, I. R.; Composition, P. Antifungal and Antioxidant Activity of Duguetia Furfuracea A. St.-Hill. Oxid. Med. Cell. Longev. **2016,** 7821051. DOI: 10.1155/2016/7821051.

Prübing, K.; Voigt, A.; Schulz, J. B. *Drosophila melanogaster* as a Model Organism Foralzheimer's Disease. *Mol. Neurodegener.* **2013,** *8,* 35. DOI: 10.1186/1750-1326-8-35.

Reiter, L. T.; Potocki, L.; Chien, S.; Gribskov, M.; Bier, E. A Systematic Analysis of Human Disease-Associated Gene Sequences in *Drosophila melanogaster*. *Genome Res.* **2001,** *11,* 1114–1125.

Roote, J.; Prokop, A. How to Design a Genetic Mating Scheme: A Basic Training Package for Drosophila Genetics. *G3 (Bethesda)* **2013**, *3*(2), 353–358. DOI: 10.1534/g3.112.004820.

Rubin, G. M.; Spradling, A. C. Genetic Transformation of *Drosophila* with Transposable Element Vectors. *Science* **1982**, *218*(4570), 348–353.

Salvemini, M.; Mauro, U.; Lombardo, F.; Milano, A.; Zazzaro, V.; ArcÃ, B.; Polito, L. C.; Saccone, G. Genomic Organization and Splicing Evolution of the Doublesex Gene, a DrosophilaRegulator of Sexual Differentiation, in the Dengue and Yellow Fever Mosquito Aedes Aegypti. *BMC Evol. Biol.* **2011**, *10*(11), 41. DOI: 10.1186/1471-2148-11-41.

Sègalat, L. Invertebrate animal models of diseases as screening tools in drug discovery. *ACS Chem Biol.* **2007**, *2*(4), 231-236.

Sanz, F. J.; Solana-Manrique, C.; Munoz-Soriano, V.; Calap-Quintana, P.; Molto, M. D.; Paricio, N. Identification of Potential Therapeutic Compounds for Parkinson's Disease Using *Drosophila* and Human Cell Models. *Free Radic. Biol. Med.* **2017**, *108,* 683–691. DOI: 10.1016/j.freeradbiomed.2017.04.364.

Sharma, S.; Rao, A. Rnai Screening: Tips and Techniques. *Nat. Immunol.* **2009**, *10*(8), 799–804. DOI: 10.1038/ni0809-799.

Sonoshita, M.; Cagan, R. L. Modeling Human Cancers in *Drosophila. Curr. Top. Dev. Biol.* **2017**, *121,* 287–309. DOI: 10.1016/bs.ctdb.2016.07.008.

Stephenson, R.; Metcalfe, N. H. *Drosophila melanogaster*: A Fly Through Its History and Current Use. *J. R. Coll. Physicians Edinburgh* **2013**, *43,* 70–75. DOI: 10.4997/JRCPE.2013.116.

Strange, K. Drug Discovery in Fish, Flies, and Worms. *ILAR J.* **2016**, *57*(2), 133–143. DOI: 10.1093/ilar/ilw034.

The Nobel Assembly at Karolinska Institutet. All Nobel Laureates in Physiology or Medicine. www.nobelprize.org/nobel_prizes/medicine/laureates/index.html (accessed on Dec 10, 2017).

Vicente-Crespo, M.; Pascual, M.; Fernandez-Costa, J.M.; Garcia-Lopez, A.; Monferrer, L.; Miranda, M. E.; Zhou L; Artero, R. D. *Drosophila* Muscleblind is Involved in Troponin T Alternative Splicing and Apoptosis. *PLoS One* **2008**, *3*(2), e1613. DOI: 10.1371/journal. pone.0001613.

Wangler, M. F.; Hu, Y.; Shulman, J. M. *Drosophila* and Genome-Wide Association Studies: a Review and Resource for the Functional Dissection of Human Complex Traits. *Dis. Model Mech.* **2017**, *10*(2), 77–88. DOI: 10.1242/dmm.027680.

Wangler, M. F.; Yamamoto, S.; Bellen, H. J. Fruit Flies in Biomedical Research. *Genetics* **2015**, *199,* 1–15.

Willoughby, L. F.; Schlosser, T.; Manning, S. A.; Parisot, J. P.; Street, I. P.; Richardson, H. E.; Humbert, P. O.; Brumby, A. M. An *in Vivo* Large-Scale Chemical Screening Platform Using *Drosophila* for Anti-Cancer Drug Discovery. *Dis. Model. Mech.* **2013**, *6*(2), 521–529. DOI: 10.1242/dmm.009985.

Wise, A.; Tenezaca, L.; Fernandez, R. W.; Schatoff, E.; Flores, J.; Ueda, A.; Zhong, X.; Wu, C. F.; Simon, A. F.; Venkatesh, T. *Drosophila* Mutants of the Autism Candidate Gene Neurobeachin (rugose) Exhibit Neuro-Developmental Disorders, Aberrant Synaptic Properties, Altered Locomotion, and Impaired Adult Social Behavior and Activity Patterns. *J. Neurogenet.* **2015**, *29,* 2–3, 135 143. DOI: 10.3109/01677063.2015.1064916.

Wong, R.; Piper, M. D. W.; Wertheim, B.; Partridge, L. Quantification of Food Intake in *Drosophila. PLoS One* **2009**, *4*(6), e6063. DOI: 10.1371/journal.pone.0006063.

Xu, T.; Rubin, G. M. Analysis of Genetic Mosaics in Developing and Adult *Drosophila* Tissues. *Development* **1993**, *117*(4), 1223–1237.

Yamamoto, S.; Jaiswal, M.; Charng, W. L.; Gambin, T.; Karaca, E.; Mirzaa, G. et al. A *Drosophila* Genetic Resource of Mutants to Study Mechanisms Underlying Human Genetic Diseases. *Cell* **2014,** *159*(1), 200–214. DOI: 10.1016/j.cell.2014.09.002.

Ziehm, M.; Kaur, S.; Ivanov, D. K.; Ballester, P. J.; Marcus, D.; Partridge, L.; Thornton, J. M. Drug Repurposing for Aging Research Using Model Organisms. *Aging Cell* **2017,** *16*(5), 1006–1015. DOI: 10.1111/acel.12626.

CHAPTER 17

TOXICOLOGICAL TESTING OF PLANT PRODUCTS

MONICA NEAGU[1,*] and CAROLINA CONSTANTIN[2]

[1]Victor Babes National Institute of Pathology, Bucharest, Romania, Tel.: +40213194528

[2]Pathology Department, Colentina University Hospital, Bucharest, Romania

*Corresponding author. E-mail: neagu.monica@gmail.com
ORCID: https://orcid.org/0000-0001-9339-2805

ABSTRACT

The biodiversity of natural chemical compounds derives from the continuous natural adaptation of organisms and the pharmaceutical industry has recently (re) focused on natural-derived compounds. Although historically used, toxicities related to natural/plant products are reported as appending to intrinsic (direct) and extrinsic (indirect) factors. Direct toxicity refers to the presence of active molecule (s) that initiates a biological intended effect, and the evaluation of this direct toxicity is the subject of the present chapter. Hence, this chapter details the main toxicological tests at molecular/cellular levels in an in vitro systems and the in vivo approaches. These tests are intended for predicting the potential toxicity of plant-derived drug candidates. Toxicological studies drive the decision if a new drug through human clinical use. The data provided by the in vitro and in vivo toxicity evaluations on medicinal plants are at the core of future use of pharmaceuticals.

17.1 INTRODUCTION

17.1.1 PLANT-ORIENTED DRUGS

Human evolution records its medical history based on natural-derived products. Before the "synthetic era," at the beginning of 20th century, 80% of all medicines were obtained from roots, barks, and leaves. Moreover, when synthetic chemistry gained field in the past couple of decades, research into natural products declined (McChesney et al., 2007). A re-invigoration of the research in this domain came when pharmaceutical discovery acknowledged that agents of natural origin derive from the phenomenon of biodiversity. This biodiversity of natural chemical compounds derived from the continuous natural adaptation of organisms one to another and to a dynamic environment. Therefore, the complex natural molecules are a direct result of the natural evolution of enhancing organism's survival and competitiveness potential (Waterman, 1992). Nature's combinational chemistry leads to a myriad of natural chemical structures with complex stereochemistry that designs special auto-regulating functional groups that interact with biological target molecules (McChesney et al., 2007).

It was revised that over 200,000 natural products of plant origin are already known, but large numbers are still to be discovered (Ifeoma and Oluwakanyinsola, 2013; Kinghorn et al., 2011; WHO, 2011). For example, for cardiac glycosides of plant origin, there are still no alternative drugs, thus the need to study and develop plant/natural-based drugs is essential (WHO, 2011). The research in this domain focuses on two main branches, one that identifies new plant-based active components for human and animal diseases and one that seeks to develop synthetic molecules that are inspired from the plant/natural components (Harvey, 2008).

Natural components have inspired around 80% of the active ingredients in the most common drugs, either directly using the compound or mimicking a natural one, thus emphasizing on the importance of natural products in human drugs discovery (Harvey, 2001; Harvey, 2007). Amidst the drugs that were introduced in a 20 year time frame (1981–2002), 28% of the 868 new chemical molecules were natural products or derived from natural products. In the same time range, over 850 drug types (24%) were designed having their pharmacophore[1] derived from a natural product (Newman et al., 2003). In 2004, there were reported 70 natural product-related compounds that had

---

[1]Pharmacophore is the molecular structure (s) that is responsible for a particular biological or pharmacological interaction.

open clinical trials (Butler, 2005). Afterward, a plethora of compounds of plant origin entered in the medical therapeutical approaches. Hence, to give just few examples, chemotherapy uses taxol, that was actually obtained from the Pacific yew (*Taxus brevifolia*), vinca alkaloids vincristine/vinblastine vindesine, vinorelbine, present in the Madagascar periwinkle (*Vinca rosea*) (Bishayee and Sethi, 2016), taxanes (paclitaxel, docetaxel) were isolated from genus *Taxus* (yews), podophyllotoxin and its derivatives (etoposide, teniposide) were isolated from the roots and the rhizomes of *Podophyllum* species, camptothecin, and its derivatives (topothecan, irinothecan) were isolated from the bark and stem of *Camptotheca acuminata*, anthracyclines (doxorubicin, daunorubicin, epirubicin, idarubicin) were isolated from *Streptomyces* spp. (Bhanot et al., 2011). Thus, anticancer drugs have a plethora of natural agents, including phytochemicals. These molecules have already passed all the clinical trials and are actively introduced in human therapy. Other molecules are still in clinical trials and in combination therapy with standard chemotherapeutic agents (Bishayee and Sethi, 2016).

As a consequence of new technologies emerging in the last years (e.g., genetic techniques for the production of secondary plant metabolites, synthesis based on combinatorial techniques and high-throughput screening) we will witness a large number of bioactive natural compounds in both prevention and therapy of human diseases. Moreover, exploring natural products bioactivity and the intracellular pathways that are triggered by these compounds will give researchers new information regarding novel chemical scaffolds for new drug patents (Chin et al., 2006).

As compounds of natural/plant origin and their bioactive molecules are subject of intense and continuous research, there is also apprehension that within the compounds there can be also a potentially harmful effect of these products. This concern is not new, and the first acknowledged potential harmful effect was reported 2000 years ago by Galen, a Greek pharmacist, and physician, that has shown that there is also the toxicity of herbs not only medicinally beneficial constituents (Cheng and Zhen, 2004). In the USA, in 2003, over 1500 herbal products were sold as nutraceuticals,[2] these category being exempted from tests evaluating preclinical efficacy and toxicity as stipulated by US Food and Drug Administration (Bent and Ko, 2004). In the European Union, food legislation obeys European Food Safety Authority, these rules focusing on "food supplements" and other substances with a beneficial nutritional effect and regulated by Directive 2002/46/EC on food

---

[2]Nutraceutical is a pharmaceutical-grade and standardized nutrient, that in USA, is not a regulatory category, being assimilated as dietary supplements and food additives.

supplements. In Canada and Australia, nutraceuticals are regulated more as a medicine than a food additive (Bagchi, 2008).

Therefore, in order to speak a common worldwide legislative language, the first step is to globally harmonize standards of toxicity testing methods in plant/natural-derived compounds with intended drug action. Toxicological studies drive the decision if a new drug can enter human clinical use. The data provided by in vitro and in vivo toxicity evaluation on medicinal plants are at the core of future use of pharmaceuticals.

This chapter will tackle the main toxicological tests at molecular and cellular levels for in vitro testing and the in vivo models that are intended to predict the potential toxicity of plant-derived drug candidates and the challenges arising from testing these complex natural compounds.

17.1.2 TOXICITY OF NATURAL PRODUCTS

Using natural products in traditional medicines since the dawn of humanity have shown that there is not only one molecular compound with biological activity. There are estimated more than 10^{60} compounds with low molecular weights (under 500 Da) that are comprised in the natural products and that can trigger complex biological activities and probably much more is to be discovered (Boufridi and Quinn, 2017).

One main target to harness the biological activity of natural products is to test their levels of toxicity in the biological systems that will represent their future medical target.

Toxicities related to natural/plant products are reported as appending to intrinsic (direct) and extrinsic (indirect) factors (Drew and Myers, 1997). Hence, direct toxicity refers to the presence of active molecule(s) that pursue(s) the biological intended effect; for example, ephedrine-type alkaloids to be found in plants of the *Ephedra* type (www.ashp.org) can have an intrinsic toxicity effect. Extrinsic factors that sustain indirect toxicity are related to contamination, adulteration, and misidentification of plant products, thus foreign toxic substances sustain the extrinsic toxicity (Shing et al., 2012), but this is not the subject of the presented chapter.

Bioassays technologies that speeded up in the last years have led to the development of new isolation, purification, and testing methods (Littleton et al., 2005; Rollinger et al., 2006). The main outline is that once a biological activity has been confirmed in a primary screen, the further step is to isolate, purify, and to determine the chemical structure of the active constituent using several separations methods and structure elucidation technology

(McChesney et al., 2007). The main separation technology is based on high-performance chromatography methods and countercurrent partition chromatography (Pauli, 2006). After separation, structure elucidation is based on high-field nuclear magnetic resonance (NMR) spectrometry and other various versions of mass spectrometry (Deng and Sanyal, 2006). For complex natural products, the structural identification applies to two-dimensional NMR techniques, a technique that has a rapid identification rate. Recently, mass spectrometry analyses coupled with liquid chromatography provides a good methodological approach for separation and structure identification for bioactive plant compounds (de Rijke et al., 2006).

Toxicology research has to establish, besides the overall toxicity of the compound, the biological and physiological routes that are influenced by a certain compound or by a group of biologically active compounds. The worldwide pharmaceutical industry is interested in the discovery and development of new pharmaceuticals based on natural products (Vuorela, 2004).

17.2 INCREASING REQUIREMENT OF TOXICOLOGICAL TESTS

Toxicology is the branch of pharmacology that evaluates bioactive substance, testing them on biological systems for identification of their unwanted effects prior to becoming a drug (Bruin et al., 2009). There are complex networks for standard testing of compounds, tests types being controlled by licensed regulatory bodies. All these evaluations are based on accurate and effective methods that identify and predict the toxicity of thousands of compounds. In the last years, high-throughput screening (HTS) was developed to test large numbers of chemical compounds for their toxicological pattern in conjunction with their biological effect.

HTS tests can identify multiple toxicity mechanisms for different compound concentrations or combination of compounds (as seen in plant products). HTS can cover the evaluation at different times of exposure and evaluate complex experimental models. The development of HTS techniques is intended to evaluate complex cellular physiology affected by the tested compound, starting from the membrane integrity, mitochondria and endoplasmic reticulum, intracellular pathways deregulation, nuclear damage, just to mention the main intracellular known targets. Extensive databases should be put to use in order to establish new molecular connections triggered by the possible drug and thus drive once again the complexity of the tests. Computational and bioinformatics methods are used to evaluate compound databases for toxicity, developing tailored quantitative structure-activity relationship models. Developing these predictive models can lead to better technological approaches in testing complex plant-derived drugs (Wills, 2017).

Investigating toxicological area with bioinformatics-based methods was very important in establishing the possible interaction of molecules with their specific receptor(s) and identifying the specific one, rather than a family of receptors. In the plant-derived drugs discovery, computing is the basis of a high throughput, selective and specific tests. Pharmaceutical development is focusing on natural-derived molecules because nature is the main source of inimitable chemical structures and drug industry can develop new assaying methodologies for identifying their potential pharmaceutical utility (Vuorela, 2004).

An outline of the technological flow that a natural compound is subjected to is presented in Figure 17.1

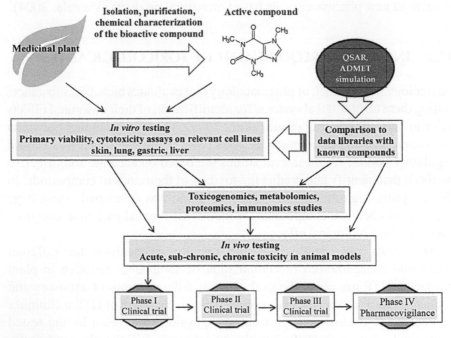

FIGURE 17.1   Flow of toxicological tests for natural compounds.

17.2.1   IN VITRO TESTS

In vitro tests have the main goal to establish the concentration–effect relationship for a certain compound or combination of compounds.

Conducting screening on the cytotoxicity profile of complex herbal mixtures is a prerequisite for drug discovery. This attempt could be assessed by in vitro approaches relying on certain cellular functional characteristics such as viability, metabolic activity, cellular growth, or morphological features (size, shape, cell membrane disruption events, and so forth).

The effect of plant extracts upon cell physiology could be considered through the type of cell death potentially induced and this effect could be classified based on some specific intracellular events (e.g., deoxyribonucleic acid [DNA] damage, reactive oxygen species association and so forth) (Agarwal et al., 2014; Cobb, 2013; Matei et al., 2014). When inquiring cytotoxic, antitumor or protective effects of a natural mixture, in vitro methods are the first steps to be applied in studying toxicological portrait, and the first parameter to be determined is the cytotoxic concentration of the respective compound.

For example, in a recent study where nanoparticles (NPs) of poly (methyl methacrylate) were evaluated for the incorporation capacity of plant extracts with antitumor activity, the toxicological profile was assessed. *Piper cabralanum* (PCA-HEX) extract was tested in polymeric NPs and its cytotoxicity was tested using MTT assay upon K562 cell lines. To cross-validate the cytotoxicity profile, trypan blue assay[3] was used. Moreover, it should be kept in mind that natural compounds can interfere with the testing methods, thus cross-validation through several methods would offer a more accurate toxicological profile of the compound(s) (Nogueira et al., 2017). This approach should be followed by a cross-validation of all the in vitro toxicological tests and always ensuring that the toxicological profile is sustained by several complementary methods. Our own experience in the in vitro toxicological testing led us to the conclusion that several classical methods for toxicological assays should always be complemented with a newer one. For example, the cellular impedance measurement can complement MTT, lactate dehydrogenase (LDH), and trypan blue tests (Tampa et al., 2016).

There are a great number of in vitro approaches that addressed to cytotoxic profile depiction of herbal/natural mixtures. It is mandatory to measure the efficacy of natural compounds in drug discovery area either as isolated compounds or as complex plant extracts (Bunel et al., 2014).

In Table 17.1 are presented several types of cellular in vitro methods classified according to a specific measured functional parameter.

---

[3]Trypan blue assay – test that uses Trypan blue dye to distinguish live and dead cells because this dye does not enter viable cells, while staining cells with injured cell membrane; the test can be found also denominated as dye exclusion method.

TABLE 17.1 Main Methods Used for in Vitro Toxicological Testing of Natural-Derived Compounds.

Functional parameter	Types of in vitro evaluation	Specific comments
Cellular viability		
Metabolic activity	Tetrazolium salts–based assays Resazurin (Alamar blue) assay Neutral red assay Adenosine triphosphate content assay	The most popular techniques for assessing cell viability are tetrazolium salts-based ones, where a tetrazolium salt (e.g., MTT, XTT, MTS, or WSTs) is reduced by cellular metabolites (e.g., NAD (P) H) to formazan derivatives. The spectrophotometry assessment of formazan's concentration would provide the percentage of living cells subjected to a certain natural compound action.
Plasma membrane integrity	LDH release assay Trypan blue exclusion Fluorescence staining	LDH, a cytoplasmic enzyme that converts lactate to pyruvate, is extracellular released when the cell membrane is damaged. The amount of LDH released in cell culture media is further detected by spectrophotometric measurement and is directly related to the proportion of damaged cells cultivated with a specific compound (Kim et al., 2009).
Cellular growth/cellular proliferation	Cell counting Cell cycle analysis DNA synthesis measurement Clonogenic assay	Deoxyribonucleic acid (DNA) synthesis could be measured by BrdU or ^{3}H-thymidine uptake which are the most common approaches to assess DNA synthesis through the S phase of the cell cycle and thus represent a direct indicator of cellular proliferation. However, it may be necessary to synchronize the cells in a certain phase as proliferative capacity to be measured in the same point of cell cycle; for instance, either by accumulates cells in G_1 phase by serum removal from cell culture or by arresting cells in S phase with different (ribo) nucleosides, structural analogs of (ribo) nucleosides or DNA disruptors such as hydroxyurea (Adan et al., 2016).
Cellular morphology	Cell size and shape evaluation Videomicroscopy Cell detachment evaluation	Cellular morphology including cell detaching could be assessed by microscopy evaluation. Moreover, a real-time evaluation by video microscopy although requiring a specific equipment could measure individual cells gathering data related to important cellular functions such as invasiveness potential (Evensen et al., 2013).

TABLE 17.1 *(Continued)*

Functional parameter	Types of in vitro evaluation	Specific comments
Cellular death		
Apoptosis/necrosis	Annexin V/propidium iodide (PI) binding	PI could be both a marker for early apoptosis (externalization of PI on cell membrane) or necrosis/late apoptosis (membrane disruption).
	Caspase 3 activity	Caspase 3 activity reveals the apoptotic rate
	DNA damage assessment (terminal deoxynucleotidyl transferase dUTP nick end labeling, Comet assay etc.)	
Autophagy	Fluorescence staining	Staining with acridine orange of autophagic vacuoles and measuring thus the level of vacuole accumulation.
Anoikis (apoptosis form by which a cell is being detached from the extracellular matrix/ support)	DNA fragmentation assay enzyme-linked immunosorbent assay kits to assess apoptosis key factors	Anoikis evaluation is particularly useful in testing the anti-cancer potential of an herbal compound/mixture, as tumor cells acquire the ability for support-independent growth.

17.2.2   IN VIVO TESTS

After establishing the in vitro outline of the natural compound toxicity, it is mandatory to conduct an in vivo test. In the in vivo settings, the toxicological characterization seeks to establish the acute high-dose exposure effects, chronic low-dose toxicity tests and specific cellular, organ and system-based toxicity assessments. These primary in vivo tests are followed by local toxicity studies if the compound is intended for local administrations; allergenic potential and hypersensitivity tests are to be followed. If the administration is intended for a longer period of time, genotoxicity and carcinogenicity tests should be added to the in vivo testing panel.

For acute systemic toxicity testing, the Organization for Economic Co-operation and Development (OECD) has issued several documents that are the pillar documents for in vivo toxicity testing in the European Area (ICCVAM, 420; ICCVAM, 423; ICCVAM, 425; ICCVAM, 508). As OECD guidelines regulate, in order to identify the safety and efficiency of a new compound, in vivo toxicological studies are undertaken in animal models using standard strains of mice, rat, pig, dog, rabbit, monkey, and so forth, under various conditions of drug application. By applying these tests, the therapeutic index, calculated using the formula: Maximum tolerated dose/Minimum curative dose, establishes if a certain compound and/or combinations of compounds are safe for use; smaller ratio of the formula shows a better safety of the compound.

For acute toxicity testing, the general indication is that the compound should be tested in two different species (rodent and non-rodent) in a unique dose by gavage (through a stomach tube or using a suitable intubation cannula). If the single dose cannot be delivered, the dose can be administered in smaller fractions over a period but not exceeding 24 h (ICCVAM, 423).

Acute Oral Toxicity-Up-and-Down Procedure (ICCVAM, 425) is a version of the acute toxicity testing where lethal dose 50 (LD_{50}) is estimated within a couple of days. In this version of testing, single animal dosage should be given at 48 h intervals. The in vitro tests have oriented the LD_{50} used in in vivo tests; thus, the first animal is dosed immediately below the best preliminary estimates of the LD_{50}. If the first tested animal dies, the second one receives a lower dose or if the first animal survives, the second one receives a higher dose. Animals are observed during the first 4 and 24 h afterward, in general for 2 weeks. Several types of information can be obtained in these tests, hence weight, biochemical parameters, morphological and pathological changes should be registered. All the animals that were tested should be subjected to necropsy and within this testing, a target organ for toxicity can be established.

Repeated dose studies or subacute or chronic toxicity would establish the maximum tolerated dose and the nature of the chronic induced toxicity if any. This test uses also two species (rodent and non-rodent) and preferably both sexes. In these tests, the compound is administered for a long duration namely 30–180 days using at least three doses. In these studies, the dose should be done as intended for future therapeutical human use, for example, daily. Moreover, the administration route should be done as it will be tested in human clinical trials, for example, orally. During these tests, several parameters will be followed: behavioral pattern of the animals, physiological and pathological alterations, biochemical parameters and, after tests completion, necropsies will give information regarding alterations at tissues and organs levels. The mean of 90-day sub-chronic test should estimate the level of non-toxicity (ICCVAM, 407).

If a chronic evaluation is intended, over 90-days administration is performed providing data for the long-time effect of the tested compound(s).

Refining in vivo studies for local administrations of plant extracts according to the intended use, several routes of testing can be conducted. Thus, if the dermal administration is sought, the direct skin toxicity can be evaluated on rats and rabbits following some clear dermatological signs as erythema, edema, and finally cutaneous histological examination, for example, inflammatory signs. If dermato-phototoxicity is tested for particular compounds, for example, a photosensitizing natural agent (Constantin and Neagu, 2017), the preferred animal model is the guinea pig. In this case, besides erythema, edema evaluation, the histology of the skin can evaluate the penetration of the photosensitizers. A recent method that is evaluating in vivo models for skin toxicity is the in vivo confocal microscopy that can evaluate long-term skin toxicity, regeneration, and skin histology in only one imagistic, noninvasive test (Ghiţă et al., 2017).

Other local toxicity tests can involve testing vaginal toxicity that can be assessed on rabbits or dogs. Within the test, macroscopic swelling is followed and, on the histopathology level, the vaginal mucosa is investigated. For testing rectal tolerance also rabbits or dogs are the best animal models. Within the test, pain, blood, or mucus appearance is followed and on the histopathology level, the rectal mucosa is investigated. Another local toxicity investigation in animal models can be ocular administration tested manly in Albino rabbit. In these tests changes in the cornea, iris, and aqueous humor are investigated. Upon test ends, the histopathology of the eye is investigated. These prior presented topical administration of natural compounds are quite frequent. Nevertheless, less frequent are natural compounds delivered as aerosols, where inhalation toxicity studies should be performed. For example, a plant extract (*Cistus incanus*) with rich polymeric polyphenols, exhibited antiviral activity for avian influenza A virus (H7N7). Thus, in H7N7 mouse infection models, an aerosol formulation of this herb was tested (Droebner et al., 2007). Upon administration, several parameters were followed: body temperature, motor activity, respiratory rate. In the end, histological examination of the respiratory passages and lung tissue was examined for any alterations of the bronchiolus epithelial cells. Except for the isolated compounds from plants, but far less frequent than the inhalation of plant extract, the parenteral administration of plant extracts has also some in vivo toxicological outlines. Parenteral administration can be done intravenously, intramuscularly, subcutaneous, or intradermally by inoculation. For example, an alcoholic extract of chamomile was inoculated in neonatal calves to study if this extract influences the capacity to absorb immunoglobulin G from colostrum (Mokhber Dezfouli et al., 2011). In this test, the sites of inoculation were observed for any local reaction and in the end, the histopathology of the inoculation site is studied besides other target tissues and organs.

Hypersensitivity/allergenic potential of natural compounds is frequently tested. The testing is usually performed in guinea pigs where the focus is to determine the maximum nonirritant dose or minimum irritant dose. After evaluation of local erythema and edema, a local lymph node assay can be performed. This last test can be done on mice ears and after 5 days the auricular lymph nodes can be extracted and the radioactive ^{3}H-thymidine incorporation[4] test can be used to evaluate the proliferation within the local lymph node.

Genotoxicity studies are intended to evaluate if the long-term effect of the compound(s) can induce alteration of the nuclear material within the cells of the animal subjected to the test. The standard test is the micronucleus assay that evaluates the chromosomes changes in rodent hematopoietic cells (Luzhna et al., 2013).

Carcinogenicity studies are intended to evaluate if a certain compound, or even better combinations of compounds, can induce on very long time of exposure, matching sometimes the lifespan of the animal, any carcinogenic effects. These studies are performed for drugs intended to be

---

[4]Thymidine incorporation assay – assay used to determine the extent of cell division that has occurred in response to a test agent; radioactive nucleoside, ^{3}H-thymidine, is incorporated into new strands of chromosomal DNA during mitotic cell division. A scintillation beta-counter is used to measure the radioactivity in DNA recovered from the cells.

used over 6 months or for chronic diseases. For rats, these studies have a 24-months span, while for mice 18-months span so that matches the animal's life period. The overall physiological alterations are followed along with tumor appearance registered in time. In carcinogenicity type of studies, the valuable indication can come from the actual structure of the compound that can indicate per se a carcinogenic potential. For example, *Aristolochia* genus, used as medicinal Chinese remedies, contains aristolochic acid, a naturally carcinogenic compound, inducing a high rate of mutations (Hoang et al., 2013).

An example of an in vivo study developed on Swiss albino mice with natural extract was recently published where the repeated dosage of two concentration of plant extracts (400 and 600 mg/kg) was orally administered daily for 2 weeks. Physical parameters, biochemical parameters, and liver toxicity were studied and, at the end, histopathological studies were assessed for organ-specific toxicity (Rajalakshmi et al., 2014).

In vivo studies in toxicology can provide a series of important added data that can bring valuable information for future in vitro testing. Thus, a mere example of evaluating in in vivo studies the cytokine pro/anti-inflammatory pattern developed by a certain drug can lead to the development of new in vitro tests for establishing the inflammatory pattern of the active molecule (Surcel et al., 2017).

17.3 CONCLUSION

Plants and their derivatives are at the basis of human medicines from the dawn of humanity. Their activity was tested for thousands of years, and now with the advent of using less synthetic drugs, research is switching its interests to natural products discoveries. The need to thoroughly evaluate the effect of plant-derived molecules used in the treatment of various diseases is increasing as the medical world is focusing its attention on this domain. The fact that these drugs have been in use for as long as the human history and classified as non-toxic is not always sustained by modern technologies testing. Thus, safety issues are raised especially for new molecules isolated and purified from plants/herbs. In this respect, there is a logical testing flow of the newly identified molecules. Therefore, primary screenings focus on in vitro systems using validated methodologies. This primary screening will assess the potential toxicities. Results obtained in in vitro settings should be thoroughly interpreted, because in an in vivo settings, there is a significant influence of pharmacokinetics, the rate of absorption, distribution, and metabolism of the biological system in which the future intended drug will be introduced. From this point of view, the conclusions obtained from the in vitro tests can drive the in vivo tests at one point or can explain the failure of the in vivo systems tests. There is still a lack of serious information regarding metabolism and ADME for a large panel of plant-derived drugs. The issues can have an explanation also in the highly complex mixtures of active plant-derived molecules, these complex mixtures can have different inference in the standard in vitro assays. One modality to overcome these issues is to develop new in vitro, more complex assays, and the other is to develop predictive mathematical models of complex interactions that can drive new technological discoveries better suited to plant-derived drugs testing.

Besides the domain that uses directly plant active molecules, another branch of plant-derived drugs is the one that synthesizes a plant-derived molecule, as natural compounds can be synthetically shaped/tailored to better address to a specific human pathology. For example, baccatin III isolated from *Taxus baccata* (yew tree), was modified in the wide known anticancer drug taxol (Erdogan, 2014).

Natural compounds are an inexhaustible collection of grounds for future drug discovery and the current involvement of drugs of natural origin is above question. Consequently, the research in this domain and the proper interpretation of the results obtained should be based on a comprehensive understanding of the principles and limitations of applied tests for natural products.

ACKNOWLEDGMENT

This chapter was partially supported by grant COP A 1.2.3., ID: P_40_197/2016, grant of the Romanian National Authority for Scientific Research and Innovation.

KEYWORDS

- **nutraceuticals**
- **metabolites**
- **intracellular pathways**
- **natural-derived compounds**
- **nuclear magnetic resonance**

REFERENCES

Adan, A.; Kiraz, Y.; Baran, Y. Cell Proliferation and Cytotoxicity Assays. *Curr. Pharm. Biotechnol.* **2016,** *17*(14), 1213–1221.

Agarwal, A.; D'Souza, P.; Johnson, T. S.; Dethe, S. M.; Chandrasekaran, C. Use of in vitro Bioassays for Assessing Botanicals. *Curr. Opin. Biotechnol.* **2014,** *25,* 39–44.

Bagchi, D. *Nutraceutical and Functional Food Regulations in the United States and Around the World.* Academic Press, 2008; pp 115–364.

Bent, S.; Ko, R. Commonly Used Herbal Medicines in the United States: A Review. *Am. J. Med.* **2004,** *116*(7), 478–485.

Bhanot, A.; Rohini, S. R.; Noolvi, M. N. Natural Sources as Potential Anti-cancer Agents. *Int. J. Phytomed.* **2011,** *3,* 09–26.

Bishayee, A.; Sethi, G. Bioactive Natural Products in Cancer Prevention and Therapy: Progress and Promise. *Semin. Cancer Biol.* **2016,** *40–41,* 1–3.

Boufridi, A.; Quinn, R. J. Harnessing the Properties of Natural Products. *Annu. Rev. Pharmacol. Toxicol.* **2017.** DOI: 10.1146/annurev-pharmtox-010716-105029. [Epub ahead of print].

Bruin, Y. et. al. Testing methods and toxicity assessment (Including alternatives); Academic Press: *Elsevier, 2009; pp 497–514.*

Bunel, V.; Ouedraogo, M.; Nguyen, A. T.; Stévigny, C.; Duez, P. Methods Applied to the in vitro primary Toxicology Testing of Natural Products: State of the Art, Strengths, and Limits. Planta Med. **2014,** *80(14), 1210–1226.*

Butler, M. S. Natural Products to Drugs: Natural Product Derived Compounds in Clinical Trials. *Nat. Prod. Rep.* **2005,** *22,* 162–195.

Cheng, Z. F.; Zhen, C. *The Cheng Zhi-Fan Collectanea of Medical History;* Peking University Medical Press: Beijing; China, 2004.

Chin, Y.-W.; Balaunas, M. J.; Chai, H. B.; Kinghorn, A. D. Drug Discovery from Natural Sources. *AAPS J.* **2006,** *8,* E239–E253.

Cobb, L. Cell Based Assays: the Cell Cycle, Cell Proliferation and Cell Death. *Mater Methods.* **2013,** *3,* 172.

Constantin, C; Neagu, M. Chapter 1 Photosensitizers Imprinting Intracellular Signaling Pathways in Dermato-oncology Therapy. In *Photomedicine–Advances in Clinical Practice;* Tanaka, Y., Ed.; Intech, 2017; pp 1–27; ISBN 978-953-51-3156-4.

de Rijke, E.; Out, P.; Niessen, W. M.; Ariese, F.; Gooijer, C.; Brinkman, U. A. Analytical Separation and Detection Methods for Flavonoids. *J. Chromatogr.* **2006,** *A 1112*(1–2), 31–63.

Deng, G.; Sanyal, G. Applications of Mass Spectrometry in Early Stages of Target Based Drug Discovery. *J. Pharm. Biomed. Anal.* **2006,** *40*(3), 528–538.

Drew, A. K.; Myers, S. P. Safety issues in herbal medicine: Implications for the health professions. *Med. J. Aust.* **1997,** *166,* 538–541.

Droebner, K.; Ehrhardt, C.; Poetter, A.; Ludwig, S.; Planz, O. CYSTUS052, a Polyphenol-rich Plant Extract, Exerts Anti-influenza Virus Activity in Mice. *Antiviral Res.* **2007,** *76*(1), 1–10.

Erdogan, O. I. E. Pharmacognosy: Science of Natural Products in Drug Discovery. *Bioimpacts* **2014,** *4*(3), 109–110.

Evensen, N. A.; Li, J.; Yang, J.; Yu, X.; Sampson, N. S.; Zucker, S.; Cao, J. Development of a High-throughput Three-dimensional Invasion Assay for Anti-Cancer Drug Discovery. *PLoS One* **2013,** *8*(12), e82811.

Ghiţă, M. A; Căruntu, C.; Rosca, A. E.; Căruntu, A.; Moraru, L.; Constantin, C.; Neagu, M.; Boda, B. Real-Time Investigation of Skin Blood Flow Changes Induced by Topical Capsaicin. *Acta. Dermatovenerol. Croat.* **2017,** *25*(3), 223–227.

Harvey, A. L. *Natural Product Pharmaceuticals: A Diverse Approach to Drug Discovery*; PJB Publications: Richmond, Surrey, UK, 2001.

Harvey, A. L. Natural Products as a Screening Resource. *Curr. Opin. Chem. Biol.* **2007,** *11,* 480–484.

Harvey, A. L. Natural Products in Drug Discovery. *Drug Discovery Today.* **2008,** *13*(19/20), 894–901.

Hoang, M. L.; Chen, C. H.; Sidorenko, V. S.; He, J.; Dickman, K. G.; Yun, B. H.; Moriya, M.; Niknafs, N.; Douville, C.; Karchin, R.; Turesky, R. J.; Pu, Y. S. Vogelstein, B.; Papadopoulos, N.; Grollman, A. P.; Kinzler, K. W.; Rosenquist, T. A. Mutational Signature of Aristolochic Acid Exposure as Revealed by Whole-exome Sequencing. *Sci. Transl. Med.* **2013,** *5,* 197ra102.

ICCVAM, OECD 420, https://ntp.niehs.nih.gov/iccvam/suppdocs/feddocs/oecd/oecd_gl420.pdf.

ICCVAM, OECD 423, https://ntp.niehs.nih.gov/iccvam/suppdocs/feddocs/oecd/oecd_gl423.pdf.

ICCVAM, OECD 508, https://ntp.niehs.nih.gov/iccvam/suppdocs/feddocs/oecd/oecd_gl425-508.pdf.

ICCVAM, OECD doc. 407, https://ntp.niehs.nih.gov/iccvam/suppdocs/feddocs/oecd/oecdtg 407-2008.pdf.

Ifeoma, O.; Oluwakanyinsola, S. Chapter 4 Screening of Herbal Medicines for Potential Toxicities, In *New Insights into Toxicity and Drug Testing INTECH Book*; Croatia: Rijeka, 2013; pp 64–88.

Kim, H.; Yoon, S. C.; Lee, T. Y.; Jeong, D. Discriminative Cytotoxicity Assessment Based on Various Cellular Damages. *Toxicol. Lett.* **2009,** *184*(1), 13–17.

Kinghorn, A. D.; Pan, L.; Fletcher, J. N.; Chai H. The Relevance of Higher Plants in Lead Compound Discovery Programs. *J. Nat. Prod.* **2011,** *74*(6), 1539–1555.

Littleton, J.; Rogers, T.; Falcone, D. Novel Approaches to Plant Drug Discovery Based on High Throughput Pharmacological Screening and Genetic Manipulation. *Life Sci.* **2005,** *78,* 467–475.

Luzhna, L.; Kathiria, P.; Kovalchuk, O. Micronuclei in Genotoxicity Assessment: from Genetics to Epigenetics and Beyond. *Epigenomics Epigenet.* **2013,** *4,* 131.

Matei, C.; Tampa, M.; Caruntu, C.; Ion, R.-M.; Georgescu, S.-R.; Dumitrascu, G. R.; Constantin, C.; Neagu, M. Protein Microarray for Complex Apoptosis Monitoring of Dysplastic Oral Keratinocytes in Experimental Photodynamic Therapy. *Biol. Res.* **2014,** *47,* (1), 33–41.

McChesney, J. D.; Venkataraman, S. K.; John T.; Henri, J. T. Plant Natural Products: Back to the Future or into Extinction? *Phytochemistry* **2007,** *68,* 2015–2022.

Mokhber Dezfouli, M. R.; Mohammadi, H. R.; Nadalian, M. G.; Nazem Bokaee, Z.; Hadjiakhoondi, A.; Nikbakht Borujeni, G. R.;Tajik, P.; Jamshidi, R. Influence of Parenteral Administration of Chamomile (Matricaria recutita L.) Extract on Colostral IgG Absorption in Neonatal Calves. *Int. J. Vet. Res.* **2011,** *5*(3), 169–171.

Newman, D. J.; Cragg, G. M.; Snader, K. M. Natural Products as Sources of New Drugs Over the Period 1981–2002. *J. Nat. Prod.* **2003,** *66,* 1022–1037.

Nogueira, M. A.; Alves, F. L.; Pimentel, S. M. R.; Moreno, B. G.; Holandino, C; de Lima M. D.; Pinto, J. C.; Nele, M. Encapsulation of *Piper cabralanum* (Piperaceae) Nonpolar Extract in Poly(methyl methacrylate) by Miniemulsion and Evaluation of Increase in the Effectiveness of Antileukemic Activity in K562 Cells. *Int. J. Nanomed.* **2017,** *12,* 8363–8373.

Pauli, G. Countercurrent Chromatography of Natural Products. CCC 2006. In *The 4th International Conference on Countercurrent Chromatography*, August 8–11, 2006, Bethesda, MD.

Rajalakshmi, A.; Jayachitra, A.; Gopal, P.; Krithiga, N. Toxicity Analysis of Different Medicinal Plant Extracts in Swiss Albino Mice. *Pharmacol. Toxicol. Res.* **2014**, *1*(1), 1–6.

Rollinger, J. M.; Langer, T.; Stuppner, H. Strategies for Efficient Lead Structure Discovery from Natural Products. *Curr. Med. Chem.* **2006**, *13*(13), 1491–1507.

Shing, C.; Woo, J.; See Han Lau, J.; El-Nezami, H. Herbal Medicine: Toxicity and Recent Trends in Assessing Their Potential Toxic Effects. In *Advances in Botanical Research*; Lie-Fen, Shyur, Allan, S. Y. Lau, Eds.; Academic Press: Burlington, 2012; Vol. 62, pp 365–384.

Surcel, M.; Constantin, C.; Caruntu, C.; Zurac, S.; Neagu, M. Inflammatory Cytokine Pattern is Sex-dependent in Mouse Cutaneous Melanoma Experimental Model. *J. Immunol. Res.* **2017**, Article ID 9212134, 10 pages.

Tampa, M.; Matei, C.; Caruntu, C.; Poteca, T.; Mihaila, D.; Paunescu, C.; Pitigoi, G.; Georgescu, S.-R.; Constantin, C.; Neagu, M. Cellular Impedance Measurement – Novel Method for in Vitro Investigation of Drug Efficacy. *Farmacia* **2016**, *64*(3), 430–434.

Vuorela, P. Natural Products in the Process of Finding New Drug Candidates. *Curr. Med. Chem.* **2004**, *11*(11), 1375–1389.

Waterman, P. G. Secondary Metabolites: Their Function and Evolution. In *Ciba Foundation Symposium*, Wiley: Chichester England, 1992; Vol. 171, pp 255–275.

WHO. The world Medicines Situation 2011. Traditional medicines: Global situation, issues and challenges. WHO/EMP/MIE/2011.2.3.http://apps.who.int/medicinedocs/documents/s18063en/s18063en.pdf. (Accessed Nov 5, 2017).

Wills, L. P. The Use of High-throughput Screening Techniques to Evaluate Mitochondrial Toxicity. *Toxicology* **2017**. pii: S0300-483X(17)30226-3.

www.ashp.org The American Society of Health-System Pharmacists. Archived from the original on 2017-09-08. Retrieved Nov 2017.

CHAPTER 18

ROLE OF BIOSTATISTICS IN PHYTOCHEMICAL RESEARCH: EMPHASIS ON ESSENTIAL OIL STUDIES

S. ZAFAR HAIDER*, GAURAV NAIK, HEMA LOHANI, and NIRPENDRA K. CHAUHAN

Centre for Aromatic Plants (CAP), Industrial Estate Selaqui-248011, Dehradun, Uttarakhand, India, Tel.: +91-9450743795

*Corresponding author. E-mail: zafarhrdi@gmail.com; zafarhaider.1@rediffmail.com
ORCID: https://orcid.org/0000-0002-3061-9264

ABSTRACT

The trend of statistics is increasing immensely and being used in almost all the fields such as scientific research, market research, business, industry, medicine and so forth. Biostatistics is instrumental in collecting, organizing, analyzing, interpreting, and presenting scientific data in order to draw significant conclusions from scientific results in research problems. It is applied in all the scientific sectors such as phytochemical, biological, biochemical, and biomedical fields for appropriate interpretation of results. In recent years, biostatistics has become a widely adopted technique in the studies involving phytochemicals. For instance, scientific data are being summarized using bivariate statistics (analysis of variance, correlation, t-test, and so forth), descriptive statistics, linear regression, cluster analysis and factor analysis, and so forth. A number of statistical software such as Statistical Package for the Social Sciences, SAS, R, XLSTAT, STATA, and Statistica and so forth are used by researchers for data interpretation. This chapter is a brief discussion of the various statistical tools using essential oil as a case study.

18.1   INTRODUCTION

Biostatistics is the branch of statistics which is applied for the proper interpretation of scientific data generated in the biology, biomedicine, phytochemical, and biochemical sciences. Biostatistics plays a vital role in data collecting, organizing, analyzing, interpreting, and presenting in order to make significant elucidation of scientific results. There are two major branches of biostatistics, that is, descriptive and inferential. Descriptive statistics is applied to describe and summarize raw data to get significant information and inferential statistics is functional for estimation of population parameters, testing of statistical hypotheses and meaningful conclusions.

Biostatistical measures are extensively used in all kind of research because its rational leads to significant descriptions and precise conclusions. Sometimes, it is not easy to interpret large results without using biostatistics. Following the proper statistical procedure, a complex and complicated data can be summarized significantly with accurate predictions and results can be interpreted in good ways. Thus, the trend of application of biostatistics in modern phytochemical and biological research is rising and widely adopted technique in various fields. The scientific context is essential, and the key to accurate statistical analysis is to bring analytic methods into close correspondence with scientific questions (Kass et al., 2016). Good experimental design can be considered as the strategy, prior to analysis. Statistical methods rely on the implicit assumption that the design is correct (Lovell, 2013). There is a vast application of biostatistics in the studies related to essential oils. Many researchers have applied statistical parameters such as analysis of variance (ANOVA), correlation, regression, cluster, and principal component in the studies on chemical diversity, essential oil variability, chemical polymorphism, and similarity for a meaningful and realistic conclusion.

The present chapter focuses on the role of biostatistics in phytochemical research with emphasis on essential oil studies.

18.2   USEFUL STATISTICAL SOFTWARE FOR PHYTOCHEMICAL STUDIES

A number of statistical software packages are used by the researchers of various fields. Software programs which are mostly used in the field of phytochemical, biochemical, biological, and biomedical sciences are Statistical Package for the Social Sciences (SPSS), SAS, R, XLSTAT, STATA, and Statistica. Several other useful software programs are Minitab, JMP,

MATLAB, S-PLUS, SigmaStat, Systat, GraphPad Prism, InStat, MLwiN, Statmate WinBUGS, and so forth. Statistical software packages help the researchers to execute required statistical techniques such as one and two-way ANOVA, t-tests, descriptive statistics, regression, nonparametric comparisons, analysis of contingency and so forth. A number of software packages support necessary statistical applications for data analysis, while some have been designed to apply modern methods for analyzing data and plotting of graphs. The details of necessary and useful software applied in phytochemical researches are given in Table 18.1.

18.3 BIOSTATISTICS APPLIED IN THE STUDIES ON ESSENTIAL OILS

Researchers have explored the composition of essential oils, gas chromatography fingerprinting, chemical diversity, chemotype variation, and polymorphism in various plant species from different parts of the world and biostatistics methods were applied in their data for justified conclusion, as described in Table 18.2. ANOVA technique was applied to study the effect of seasonal and tree girth size variation in the essential oils of *Cupressus torulosa* and quantitative occurrence of the major compounds was determined. Some major compounds were significantly influenced by different seasons and tree girth, but the variations were found non-significant in small, medium, and big trees (Lohani et al., 2014). ANOVA was also applied to conclude the findings of antimicrobial potential of various essential oils (Rahman et al., 2011; Sitarek et al., 2012; Hasika et al., 2014; Shirazi et al., 2014; Maria et al., 2015; Louail et al., 2016; Taghreed et al., 2017). Intraspecific and interspecific chemical diversity and chemotypes have been observed in various essential oils isolated from aromatic plant species. These chemical variations were statistically defined using cluster analysis, principal component analysis, and so forth. Sometimes these analyses also defined the similarity and uniqueness in various essential oils (Joshi et al., 2009; Rezende et al., 2013; Gwari et al., 2016). Gwari et al. (2016) studied the chemical diversity in the oils of *Perilla frutescens* populations and data were subjected to cluster analysis and principal component analysis (PCA) using the SPSS software. Statistical analysis separated the populations into two major groups on the basis of the essential oil components of various populations. The oils from one group were rich in perilla ketone and isoegomaketone, while other group separated from former due to the presence of trans-caryophyllene. Some other statistical procedures such as correlation

TABLE 18.1 Software Useful for Applications of Biostatistics in Phytochemical Studies.

S/No.	Common software	Description and websites*
1.	Statistical Package for the Social Sciences (SPSS) (IBM SPSS Statistics)	SPSS software is commonly used in the studies of social sciences and also useful in phytochemical, biological, biomedical researches, and market survey data analysis, and so forth. The software supports bivariate statistics (analysis of variance [ANOVA], correlation, t-test etc.), descriptive statistics, linear regression, cluster analysis, factor analysis, and so forth. Website: https://www.ibm.com/products/spss-statistics
2.	Statistical Analysis Software (SAS)	SAS is used for statistical application in the fields of phytochemistry, biology, biochemistry, medicine, pharmacy and having modern methods for analyzing data such as ANOVA analysis, correlation, regression analysis, cluster analysis, factor analysis, and so forth. SAS also having advanced data management tools and understand any type of data. Website: https://www.sas.com/en_us/software/stat.html
3.	Minitab	Minitab is a command and menu-driven software package for statistical analysis and very useful in biostatistics. The software is having basic data analysis functions such as ANOVA, t-test, chi-square, variance tests, correlation, linear regression and also functional for creating a graph, histogram, box plot, scatter plot and bar chart, and so forth. Website: http://www.minitab.com/en-us/
4.	XLSTAT	XLSTAT is built-in excel function where all necessary statistical applications viz. ANOVA, correlation, fisher, f test, t-test, quartile, standard deviation, standard error and so forth. are available. Website: https://www.xlstat.com/en/
5.	JMP	JMP is the data analysis tool for analysis of routine and difficult statistical problems. It is instrumental in the univariate statistical analysis, bivariate scatter plot, one-way ANOVA, simple logistic regression, correlations, multivariate analysis, principal components, clustering, and so forth. The software is very useful for application of statistics in phytochemical and biological researches. Website: https://www.jmp.com/en_us/home.html
6.	MATLAB	MATLAB, a programming software, is used for data analysis and scientific graphics. It is more useful for mathematical and computation researches. Website: https://www.mathworks.com/

TABLE 18.1 *(Continued)*

S/No.	Common software	Description and websites*
7.	R	R is both statistics and programme software and can be applied in data manipulation, calculation, and graphical display. It allows users to add additional modern statistical functions. R is an open source software freely available under the GNU General Public License. Website: https://www.r-project.org
8.	S-PLUS	S-PLUS is a modern implementation of the S programming language as well as statistics. To perform advanced statistical analysis on large datasets S-PLUS is used by researchers from biological, biomedical fields as well as industries. Website: http://www.solutionmetrics.com.au/products/splus/default.html
9.	STATA	STATA software is made especially for the researchers those are working in the fields of biomedicine, and also economics and sociology. It is general-purpose statistical software that enables researchers to analyze data and also produce graphical visualizations of data. Website: https://www.stata.com/
10.	Statistica	Statistica, with advanced analytics software provides data analysis, data mining and data visualization procedures. Website: http://statistica.io/
11.	SigmaStat	SigmaStat is a statistical software package having many statistical applications namely principal components analysis (PCA), one-way analysis of covariance, one-sample t-test, and Cox regression and also profile plots for multi-factor ANOVA. These statistical procedures are widely used by the researchers in the field of phytochemical, biochemical, and biological science. Website: https://systatsoftware.com/
12.	Systat	SYSTAT is designed as statistical graphics software for making two-dimensional and three-dimensional charts and graphs. It analyses principal components analysis, cluster, multidimensional scaling, factor, linear variance, and regression models. Website: https://systatsoftware.com/

TABLE 18.1 *(Continued)*

S/No.	Common software	Description and websites*
13.	Excel	Excel is a spreadsheet program developed by Microsoft. It comes with Microsoft office package. It is a descriptive, parametric, and extremely useful software for making calculations and graphs. Its wide usage could be attributed to its compatibility with many statistical packages. Website: https://products.office.com/en-us/excel
14.	PSPP	GNU PSPP is an open source software for statistical analysis of sampled data. It is freely available under GNU license. PSPP bears close resemblance to the proprietary program SPSS but with few exceptions. Website: http://www.gnu.org/software/pspp/
15.	RegressIt	Regress is a freely available Excel add-in which can perform multivariate descriptive data analysis and linear regression analysis. It is a good add-in for creating high-quality table and chart output in native Excel format. Website: http://regressit.com/

*All website link provided were accessed on the 20th January, 2018.

TABLE 18.2 Biostatistics Applied in the Studies on Essential Oils of Various Plant Species.

S/No.	Biostatistics Applied	Description	References
1.	ANOVA using SPSS software	The content of major compounds in *Cupressus torulosa* essential oil namely α-pinene, sabinene, limonene, γ-terpinene, terpinen-4-ol and umbellulone were significantly influenced by different seasons and tree girth ($P=0.05$; CD values 0.41–1.79).	Lohani et al. (2014)
2.	ANOVA using SPSS	The antioxidant, antimicrobial and cytotoxicity (IC_{50}) activities of *Tagetes minuta* and *Ocimum basilicum* oils examined and the data were expressed as the means ± standard deviations (SD) of three independent experiments. The significant differences at $P<0.01$ between treatments were analyzed by one-way ANOVA.	Shirazi et al. (2014)
3.	ANOVA using the SAS	ANOVA was performed to determine the antimicrobial potential of the essential oils of cinnamon, oregano, thyme, clove and so forth and showed strong antimicrobial activities. A significant difference in mean values of oils (MICs and MBCs) was observed at $P \le 0.05$.	Hasika et al. (2014)
4.	ANOVA using Minitab statistical software	Antimicrobial and antioxidant properties of *Bursera graveolens* essential oils were examined. In the result, moderate to high antimicrobial and good antioxidant activity was found. All the data were analyzed by ANOVA. The significance of differences between means was determined by Tukey at $P<0.05$.	Mendez et al. (2017)
5.	ANOVA using Statistica software	In *citrus* essential oils, significant variations in concentration of limonene and other major compounds were observed with respect to different drying conditions of the plant material ($P<0.05$). All the data were recorded as mean±SD.	Kamal et al. (2011)
6.	One-way ANOVA	The essential oil of *Ammodaucus leucotrichus* showed the broad spectrum antimicrobial activity against fungi and bacteria and the minimum inhibitory concentration ranged from 0.37–0.92 mg/ml. The data were presented as mean ± SD of three replicates. Statistical significance was declared at $P<0.05$.	Louail et al. (2016)
7.	ANOVA and post hoc Tukey test using SPSS	The antimicrobial potential of essential oils of *Ocimum tenuiflorum* against *Streptococcus aureus* different strains was checked. ANOVA followed by post hoc Tukey test was applied in data for determination of statistical significance.	Yamani et al. (2016)

TABLE 18.2 *(Continued)*

S/No.	Biostatistics Applied	Description	References
8.	ANOVA by Tukey's HSD test (P<0.05) and Spearman's coefficient of correlation using SAS	The antimicrobial activities of the essential oils of *Cymbopogon flexuosus*, *Ocimum basilicum*, *Origanum vulgare*, *Cinnamomum zeylanicum and Laurus nobilis* were tested against food-borne bacteria and statistically evaluated the MIC and MBC value using Tukey's HSD test (P<0.05) and correlation coefficient.	Silveira et al. (2012)
9.	Tukey test at the 5% of probability level	The minimum inhibitory concentrations of *Thymus vulgaris*, *Cymbopogon citratus*, and *Laurus nobilis* essential oils were determined against various bacterial strains and the results were concluded using Tukey's test at the 5% of probability level. The experimental design was completely randomized in a factorial outline with three repetitions.	Millezi et al. (2012)
10.	Descriptive statistics/ CROSSTABS using SPSS	SPSS, based on CROSSTAB analysis, afforded the seasonal variation factors to use the relative amount (%) with different tree girth stages of *Cupressus torulosa*. Missing compounds and the compounds with maximum percentage were also reported.	Lohani et al. (2014)
11.	Cluster analysis using the SPSS software (ver. 13.0).	Cluster analysis was applied in the essential oil composition of *Perilla frutescens* populations. The nearest-neighbor method was used for cluster definition and euclidean distance was selected as a measure of similarity. Dendrogram differentiated oils into two major groups; group-1 possessed perilla ketone + isoegomaketone rich oils, while group-2 having perilla ketone + trans-caryophyllene.	Gwari et al. (2016)
12.	Cluster analysis by BD-Pro software.	Simple-average method was used as the basis of the cluster and Bray-Curtius was selected as the similarity measure. Cluster analysis grouped essential oils of plant species of Lauraceae family into two categories namely, furan-containing genera and mono- and sesquiterpenoid-rich genera.	Joshi et al. (2009)
13.	Hierarchical cluster analysis according to Ward's variance minimizing method by using SAS and Statistica software	Cluster analysis employing Ward's method was applied to study similarity relationship among essential oils of *Syzygium jambos* and the oils showed high variations within the essential oils.	Rezende et al. (2013)

TABLE 18.2 *(Continued)*

S/No.	Biostatistics Applied	Description	References
14.	PCA	Grouping of the *Perilla frutescens* population on the basis of chemical compositions showed that different populations fall in the two major classes based on PCA.	Gwari et al. (2016)
15.	95% Confidence interval	Statistical range of citral and other compounds along with 95% confidence interval of the difference were observed in lemongrass (*Cymbopogon flexuosus*) oil. The range is considered between first and third quartile of oil samples. The lower limit and upper limit of citral were considered as 72.8 and 74.2%, respectively on the basis of the confidence interval of the difference (95%).	Chauhan et al. (2017)
16.	Multiple Regression	The relationship between the components found in leaf essential oils (dependent variables) from *Syzygium jambos* and the environmental factors (independent variables) were investigated	Rezende et al. (2013)
17.	Probit regression using Bio-Stat Pro software	The toxicity study on *Nigella Sativa* essential oils was conducted for determination of LD50 based on probits regression mortalities according to the logarithms essential oils. The result on the basis of regression showed that the essential oil has significant larvicidal properties.	Adil et al. (2016)
18.	Student's t-test, one-way ANOVA	The cytotoxicity and genotoxicity of different essential oils on human embryo lung cells were assessed and found that none of the oils induced significant de-oxyribonucleic acid damage in vitro after 24 h. All data, represented statically in means ± SD were assessed by Student's t-test and one way ANOVA.	Puskarova et al. (2017)
19.	Student's t-test, correlation and regression analysis using MS-Excel program	The antimicrobial activity of essential oil and extract of *Pelargonium graveolens* against bacteria and fungi strains showed broad-spectrum antimicrobial activity. The significant difference in activity of essential oil and extract was calculated by Student's t-test, correlation and regression analysis using MS-Excel program.	Hsouna et al. (2012)
20.	Paired t-test using SPSS	Paired t-test was applied to compare the differences of mean values of MIC and MBC of essential oils of *Melissa officinalis* and *Dracocephalum moldavica* and it showed that *M. officinalis* oil has more antimicrobial potential.	Ehsani et al. (2017)

TABLE 18.2 *(Continued)*

S/No.	Biostatistics Applied	Description	References
21.	Least Significant Difference (LSD)	LSD (at 0.05%) applied in the data and it was observed that essential oil content of in *Cymbopogon citrates* leaves varied significantly with different drying methods namely fresh, sun, shade, and oven drying.	Hanaa et al. (2012)
22.	Duncan's Multiple Range Test (DMRT) using one-way ANOVA	Among the eight essential oils (clove, betel, cinnamon, lemongrass, vetiver, calamus, lime, pine), clove and betel oils were the strongest antioxidant agents in comparison to the control with non-significant differences observed by Duncan's Multiple Range Test at the significance level of 0.05.	Utakod et al. (2017)
23.	Pearson's correlation coefficient	Antioxidant activity of eight essential oils (clove, betel, cinnamon, lemongrass, vetiver, calamus, lime, pine) was carried out. Among different assays, DPPH, ABTS, and FRAP showed high positive correlation with each other with coefficients ranging from 0.808 to 0.989.	Utakod et al. (2017)

coefficient, confidence interval, multiple regression, probit regression, least significant difference, Duncan's Multiple Range Test (DMRT) in essential oils and antimicrobial studies were also applied by various workers (Hanaa et al., 2012; Hsouna et al., 2012; Rezende et al., 2013; Adil et al., 2016; Chauhan et al., 2017; Utakod et al., 2017). Many workers conducted antimicrobial studies on essential oils and the findings were described by using ANOVA, Tukey's test, student's t-test, paired t-test, regression analysis and multivariate analysis and so forth. (Chaudhary et al., 2012; Gomes et al., 2012; Hsouna et al., 2012; Millezi et al., 2012; Costa et al., 2017; Ehsani et al., 2017; Tsasi et al., 2017).

18.4 CONCLUSION

Biostatistics plays a significant role in many phytochemical researches where large data cannot easily be processed manually or without using any statistical technique. Biostatistics is instrumental in designing of phytochemical experiments and analyzing data from research problems. A well-implemented good experimental design produces a statistically significant conclusion and strong results. Application of biostatistics using statistical software makes data processing more appropriate. Biostatistics also plays a vital role in the preparation of standard research publications and patents.

KEYWORDS

- **biostatistics**
- **phytochemical**
- **essential oil**
- **statistical software**
- **analysis of variance**

REFERENCES

Adil, B.; Tarik, A.; Abderahim, K.; Khadija, O. The Study of the Insecticide Effect of the Essential Oil of *Syzygium aromaticum* L. Against Larvae of *Tuta absoluta. Int. J. Innovations Sci. Res.* **2016,** *20*(1), 188–194.

Chaudhary, L. K. D.; Jawale, B. A.; Sharma, S.; Sharma, H.; Kumar, C. D. M.; Kulkarni, P. A. Antimicrobial Activity of Commercially Available Essential Oils Against *Staphylococcus* Mutant. *J. Contemp. Den. Pract.* **2012**, *13*(1), 71–77.

Chauhan, N.; Sah, S.; Yadav, R.; Bartwal, S.; Sagar, S. L. Acclimatization of Lemongrass Cultivation in Agro-Climatic Conditions of Uttarakhand. *J. Essent. Oil Bear. Plants* **2017**, *20*(3), 855–859.

Costa, C. B.; Sendra, E.; Fernandez-Lopez, J.; Perez, A. J.; Viuda, M. M. Assessment of Antioxidant and Antibacterial Properties on Meat Homogenates of Essential Oils Obtained from Four *Thymus* Species Achieved from Organic Growth. *Foods* **2017**, *6*(59), 1–11.

Ehsani, A.; Alizadeh, O.; Hashemi, M.; Afshari, A.; Aminzare, M. P., Antioxidant and Antibacterial Properties of *Melissa officinalis* and *Dracocephalum moldavica* Essential Oils. *Vet. Res. Forum.* **2017**, *8*(3), 223–229.

Gomes, G. A.; Caio, M. O. M.; Senra, T. O. S.; Zeringota, V.; Calmon, F.; Matos, R. S.; Daemon, E.; Gois, R. W. S.; Santiago, G. M. P.; Carvalho, M. G. Chemical Composition and Acaricidal Activity of Essential Oil from Lippia Sidoides on Larvae of Dermacentor Nitens (Acari: Ixodidae) and Larvae and Engorged Females of *Rhipicephalus microplus* (Acari: Ixodidae). *Parasitol. Res.* **2012**, *111*(6), 2423–2430.

Gwari, G.; Lohani, H.; Bhandari, U.; Haider, S. Z.; Singh, S.; Andola, H.; Chauhan, N. Chemical Diversity in the Volatiles of *Perilla frutescens* (L.) Britt. Populations from Uttarakhand Himalaya (India). *J. Essent. Oil Res.* **2016**, *28*(1), 49–54.

Hanaa, A. R. M.; Sallam, Y. I.; El-Leithy, A. S.; Aly, S. E. Lemongrass (*Cymbopogon citratus*) Essential Oil as Affected by Drying Methods. *Ann. Agric. Sci.* **2012**, *57*(2), 113–116.

Hasika, M.; Dure, R.; Delcenserie, V.; Zhiri, A.; Daube, G.; Clinquart, A. Antimicrobial Activities of Commercial Essential Oils and Their Components Against Food-Borne Pathogens and Food Spoilage Bacteria. *Food Sci. Nut.* **2014**, *2*(4), 403–416.

Hsouna, A. B.; Hamdi, N. Phytochemical Composition and Antimicrobial Activities of the Essential Oils and Organic Extracts from *Pelargonium graveolens* Growing in Tunisia. *Lipids Health and Dis.* **2012**, *11*(167), 1–7.

Joshi, S. C.; Padalia, R. C.; Bisht, D. S.; Mathela, C. S. Terpenoid Diversity in the Leaf Essential Oils of Himalayan Lauraceae Species. *Chem. Biodiversity* **2009**, *6*, 1364–1373.

Kamal, G. M.; Anwar, F.; Hussain, A. I.; Sarri, N.; Ashraf, M. Y. Yield and Chemical Composition of Citrus Essential Oils as Affected by Drying Pretreatment of Peels. *Int. Food Res. J.* **2011**, *18*(4), 1275–1282.

Kass, R.; Caffo, B.; Davidian, M.; Meng, X.; Yu, B.; Reid, N. Ten Simple Rules for Effective Statistical Practice. *PLoS Comput. Biol.* **2016**, *12*, e1004961. https://doi.org/10.1371/journal.pcbi.1004961.

Lohani, H.; Kumar, A.; Bhandari, U.; Haider, S. Z.; Singh, S.; Chauhan, N. Effect of Seasonal and Tree Girth Size Variation on *Cupressus torulosa* D. Don Leaves Essential Oil Composition Growing in Uttarakhand. *J. Essent. Oil Bear. Plants* **2014**, *17*(6), 1257–1267.

Louail, Z.; Kameli, A.; Benabdelkader, T.; Bouti, K.; Hamza, K.; Krimat, S. Antimicrobial and Antioxidant Activity of Essential Oil of *Ammodaucus leucotrichus* Coss. & Dur. Seeds. *J. Mater. Environ. Sci.* **2016**, *7*(7), 2328–2334.

Lovell, D. P. Biological Importance and Statistical Significance. *J. Agric. Food Chem.* **2013**, *61*, 8340–8348.

Maria, F.; Athanasios, K.; Ioanna, M.; Stavros, P.; Irene, T.; Virginia, P.; Ioannis, K.; Maria, P.; Elisavet, S.; Eugenia, E. B.; Athanasios, A. Antimicrobial Activity of Essential Oils of Cultivated Oregano (*Origanum vulgare*), Sage (*Salvia officinalis*) and Thyme (*Thymus vulgaris*) Against Clinical Isolates of Escherichia Coli, *Klebsiella Oxytoca* and *Klebsiella Pneumonia. Microb. Ecol. Health Dis.* **2015,** 26.

Mendez, A. H. S.; Cornejo, C. G. F.; Coral, M. F. C.; Arnedo, M. C. A. Chemical Composition, Antimicrobial and Antioxidant Activities of the Essential Oil of *Bursera graveolens* (Burseraceae) from Peru. *Ind. J. Pharm. Edu Res.* **2017,** *51*(3), 429–436.

Millezi, A. F.; Caixeta, D. S.; Rossoni, D. F.; Cardoso, M. G.; Piccoli, R. H. Invitro Antimicrobial Properties of Plant Essential Oils *Thymus vulgaris, Cymbopogon citratus* and *Laurus nobilis* Against Five Important Food Borne Pathogens. *Campinas* **2012,** *32*(1), 167–172.

Puskarova, A.; Buckova, M.; Krakova, L.; Pangallo, D.; Kozics, K. The Antibacterial and Antifungal Activity of Six Essential Oils and Their Cyto/genotoxicity to Human HEL 12469 Cells. *Sci Rep.* **2017,** *7*(1), 8211.

Rahman, L. A.; Shanta, Z. S.; Rashid, M. A.; Parvin, T.; Afrin, S.; Khatun, M. K.; Sattar, M. A. In vitro Antibacterial Properties of Essential Oil and Organic Extracts of *Premna integrifolia. Arabian J. Chem.* **2011,** *9,* S475–S479.

Rezende, W. P.; Borges, L. L.; Alves, N. M.; Ferri, P. H.; Paula, J. R. Chemical Variability in the Essential Oils from Leaves of *Syzygium jambos. Rev. Bras. Farmacogn.* **2013,** *23*(3), 433–440.

Shirazi, M. T.; Gholami, H.; Kavoosi, G.; Rowshan, V.; Tafsiry, A. Chemical Composition, Antioxidant, Antimicrobial and Cytotoxic Activities of *Tagetes minuta* and *Ocimum basilicum* essential Oils. *Food Sci. Nutr.* **2014,** *2*(2), 146–155.

Silveira, S. M.; Cunha, A.; Scheuermann, G. N.; Secchi, F. L.; Vieira, C. R. W. Chemical Composition and Antimicrobial Activity of Essential Oils from Selected Herbs Cultivated in the South of Brazil Against Food Spoilage and Food Borne Pathogens. *Cien. Rur.* **2012,** *42*(7), 1300–1306.

Sitarek, P. B.; Rijo, P.; Garcia, C.; Skaba, E.; Kalemba, D.; Biabas, A. J.; Szemraj, J.; Pytel, D.; Toma, M.; Wysokinska, H.; Uliwi, N. T. Antibacterial, Anti-inflammatory, Antioxidant, and Antiproliferative Properties of Essential Oils from Hairy and Normal Roots of *Leonurus sibiricus* L. and Their Chemical Composition. *Oxi. Med. and Cell. Long.* **2012,** *47*(5), 1–12.

Taghreed, A. I.; Atef, A. H.; Hala, M. H.; Areej, M. T.; Shagufta, P. Chemical Composition and Antimicrobial Activities of Essential Oils of Some Coniferous Plants Cultivated in Egypt. *Iran J. Pharm. Res.* **2017,** *16*(1), 328–337.

Tsasi, G.; Mailis, T.; Daskalaki, A.; Sakadani, E.; Razis, P.; Samaras, Y.; Skaltsa, H. The Effect of Harvesting on the Composition of Essential Oils from Five Varieties of *Ocimum basilicum* L. Cultivated in the Island of Kefalonia, Greece. *Plants (Basel)* **2017,** *6*(3), 41.

Utakod, N.; Laosripaiboon, W.; Chunhachart, O.; Issakul, K. The Efficiency and the Correlation Between Testing Methods on Antimicrobial and Antioxidant Activities of Selected Medicinal Essential Oils. *Int. Food Res. J.* **2017,** *24*(6), 2616–2624.

Yamani, H. A.; Pang, E. C.; Mantri, N.; Deighton, M. A. Antimicrobial Activity of Tulsi (*Ocimum tenuiflorum*) Essential Oil and Their Major Constituents Against Three Species of Bacteria. *Front. Microbiol. 7,* 681.

PART III
Computational Phytochemistry

CHAPTER 19

COMPUTATIONAL PHYTOCHEMISTRY IN DRUG DISCOVERY: DATABASES AND TOOLS

SUGUMARI VALLINAYAGAM[1], KARTHIKEYAN RAJENDRAN[1,*], and VIGNESHKUMAR SEKAR[1]

[1]*Mepco Schlenk Engineering College, Sivakasi, Tamil Nadu 626005, India*

Corresponding author. E-mail: rkarthi@mepcoeng.ac.in.

ABSTRACT

Plant-derived chemicals have found broad application in the treatment of several diseases. Due to the slow recovery and lack of evidence on their medicinal properties, the synthetic drugs appear to be more preferred. However, the synthetic drugs are now considered unsafe due to their side effects. Recently, World Health Organization (WHO) estimated that 80% of the people worldwide now rely on herbal medicine for some aspects of their primary healthcare needs. However, the use of these herbals will require scientific explanations which could also lead to the synthesis of new drugs or lead compounds. To reduce the time spent in the laboratory-scale experiment for studies involving the discovery of new therapeutic compounds, computational tools were invented which have been successfully applied. Moreover, results obtained will need to be validated in the laboratory before clinical trials. This chapter discusses various database tools involved in computational phytochemistry.

19.1 INTRODUCTION

Herbal-based targeted drug delivery is an emerging scenario in the medical world. The Ayurvedic medicine is a traditional medicine or folk medicine practices based on the exploit of plants and their extracts (Aggarwal et al., 2006). This kind of medicinal practice is also called the complementary and alternative medicine therapy, which helps for efficient treatment of patients of many distinct diseases. Many of them hesitate to use Ayurveda medicine due to lack of traditional knowledge in drug formulation. In the modern world, people are basically in need of immediate relief from the disease state. Synthetic drugs will do just that but not without issues in the internal pathways, mainly the body immune system. To overcome this issue, nowadays numerous healthcare practitioners practicing modern medicine widely recommend herbs and herbal products. There has been a revival in the use of herbs since the synthetic drugs cause side effects, numerous chronic diseases, and microbial resistance to the patients. The extraordinary investment in pharmaceutical research and development also motivate the herbal medicinal research (Duraipandi et al., 2015). Likewise, the global pharmaceutical companies equipped with contemporary science and technology will embark on to revive herbs as a future source of new drugs. They provided the transformed stage to herb and carried out different approaches in favor of natural product drug development and discovery (Pan et al., 2014). Raspberries and blackberries contain several essential phytochemicals, besides containing proteins, fats, carbohydrates, vitamins, and minerals.

The *Charaka Samhita* was the first proof critique that briefly explained the concepts and practices of Ayurveda 5000 years ago. The Sumerians also described the well-recognized medicinal uses for many herbs. Traditional Chinese and Indian medicinal practices are the major systems, which follow the phytochemical-based drug designing (Suzuki, 2004; Chung et al., 2014). At present, researchers are trying to understand the exact facts and basic mechanisms of traditional remedies to treat and prevent diseases. Computational phytochemistry studies are torching the way to the regeneration of herbal medicines (Bushkov et al., 2016).

19.2 COMPUTATIONAL PHYTOCHEMISTRY

Computational phytochemistry can aid the process of drug discovery to a greater extent. It can cram up a 10-year work of drug discovery to just 1 year. These in silico methods can simplify the steps in successive in vitro and in vivo processes that are involved in drug discovery (Bushkov et al., 2016). The activity of small molecules (phytochemicals) can be predicted by the developed in silico model. Also, it provides the structural insights into the individual features of various phytochemical categories. During drug development study, a researcher may use some computational tools (Fig. 19.1) in the different steps such as phytochemical characterization, structure analyses, separation of phytochemicals, toxicity prediction, analogy structure prediction, QSAR screening, molecular docking, molecular simulation, and drug-likeness property (Bhattacharjee et al., 2012). Algorithm-based software development is most helpful for various tools to advance drug discovery process. There are plenty of advanced tools used in computational phytochemistry. Molecular docking and simulation are most significant. Molecular docking method is the structure-based drug designing that works with the ligand and protein molecule. It is used to predict the binding conformation of ligands with active site of targets which is involved in the disease (Dammalli et al., 2015). The central processing unit (CPU) and graphics processing unit (GPU) are by far the most important components for bioinformatics-related programs. Because these programs are well threaded and parallel, the most important thing is to pick a CPU with a high core count. The more cores, the better performance, also lesser time to run simulations needed to run the computational tools. This means that on a single CPU system, there is no performance increase beyond a GTX 1070 and therefore, it recommends this card on the single one. For not much needed, one could try the usual Nvidia 750 as it is the best for the working of apps similar to this. It can stay away from upgrading the power supply for the program. RAM should be as high as multiple of 2 GB with the number of cores (<8). CPU system, NAMD, LAMMPS, and GROMACS can be fairly memory hungry, so defaulting the single and dual CPU systems to 32 and 64 GB of RAM are highly recommended, respectively. If the simulation work to be carried out is very large and/or complex, it is likely one will need a memory of 128–256 GB.

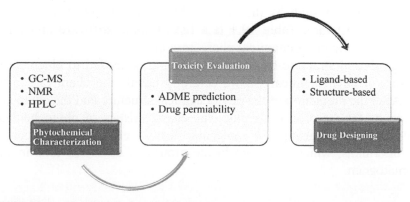

FIGURE 19.1 Workflow in drug development.

19.2.1   PHYTOCHEMICAL CHARACTERIZATION

The structure of a phytochemical can be identified by different equipment with the help of different software. Mass spectrometry (MS) has become the systematic method of preference in plant metabolites analysis. However, metabolite annotation remains a major challenge and involves the integration of structural searches in compound libraries with biological understanding attendant from metabolite-directive study (Harborne, 1998; Sermakkani and Thangapandian, 2012). In the gas chromatography–mass spectrometry (GC-MS) analysis, bioinformatics database-related search narrates integrative move towards the process and develop a prosperous structural information by understanding the patterns of high-resolution liquid chromatography–mass spectrometry (LC-MS) report (Cavalli et al., 2004; González-Gómez et al., 2010). A mass spectral database search could help to identify the phytochemicals (National Institute of Standards and Technology/Environmental Protection Agency/National Institutes of Health, NIST/EPA/NIH) followed by an assessment with the obtained MS data to find out the degree of matching. Nuclear magnetic resonance spectroscopy (NMR) is the most accepted method to compare and study the metabolites of the plant. This is one of the most generally used metabolomic approaches involved in the computational phytochemistry, which helps in the structure-based drug discovery approach. Every molecule has the unique character in their structural bonding by that way of characterization in which the high-performance liquid chromatography (HPLC) plays a major role. HPLC is used for analyzing herbal drugs and dietary supplements and to predict primary and secondary plant metabolites (González-Gómez et al., 2010). In the HPLC, the data from the samples are usually composed by a workstation such as the Agilent Mass Hunter Workstation Data acquisition software. Table 19.1 is a list of some software and online tools used in the phytochemical characterization.

Ligand- and structure-based drug designing is needed to elucidate the structure of phytochemicals so we carefully handle the chemicals in this step. After the prediction of the phytochemical structure and the characters, we can go for the drug designing. The characteristics of phytochemicals were achieved by using the molecular feature extraction and correlation algorithms, which is placed in the groups of covariant ions in each chromatogram.

TABLE 19.1 List of Software and Online Tools used in the Prediction of Phytochemical Characters.

Analysis	Software or online tool
Nuclear magnetic resonance spectroscopy	https://www.nmrdb.org/predictor/
	http://mestrelab.com/software/mnova/nmr-predict/
	http://www.acdlabs.com/products/adh/nmr/nmr_pred/
	http://www.cheminfo.org/Spectra/NMR/Predictions/1H_Prediction/index.html
	http://www.ch.ic.ac.uk/local/nmrs/
High-performance liquid chromatography	ChromNAV 2.0- https://jascoinc.com/products/chromatography/hplc/hplc-software/
	LC/MS/MS Screening Software- https://www.shimadzu.com/an/data-net/labsolutions/insight/library_screening/index.html
	Empower 3 Software- http://www.waters.com/waters/en_IN/Empower-3-Chromatography-Data-Software/
	ChromSwordAuto- http://www.indtechinstruments.com/chromsword-method- development. Html
	Chromeleon™ 7.2- https://www.thermcfisher.com/order/catalog/product/CHROMELEON7
	ChromLab Software – NGCTM
Gas chromatography–mass spectrometry	Agilent's MassHunter Workstation
	Analyst® Software- SCIEX
	TargetQuan 3 Software
	TraceFinder™ Software
	MetFrag- R package CAMERA

19.2.2 TOXICITY EVALUATION

Phytochemical usage in the drug development is an exploratory one because of its unknown activities in the human metabolic pathways. So many researchers eliminate the perilous compound at the earlier stage. Absorption, distribution, metabolism, excretion, and toxicity (ADME/T) properties of the drug decide the side effect and effects of the drug in the human body (Gombar et al., 2003). There are several methods used in drug selection process to check for ADME property, drug-likeness property, and intestinal absorption (Van De Waterbeemd and Gifford, 2003). Computational tools were programmed based on the scores which were obtained from the laboratory experiments. Programming codes compare our drug molecule with the already available background program and produce the drug-likeness data (Khanra et al., 2017).

Caco-2 model and MDCK cell are referred to as in vitro model for prediction of drug absorption, where the drug has been administered orally. Permeability value is between 4 and 70 denotes that the molecule has intermediate permeability. MDCK cell refers to Madin-Darby canine kidney cell. While MDCK cells lifespan is less than the lifespan of Caco-2 cells, the relationship between these cells should be high. The intestinal absorption is significant to find the potential candidate, and ADME/T helps to finds the absorption in percentage (Gombar et al., 2003). Well-absorbed compounds return 70–100%. Skin permeability factor is significant in case of cosmetics for transdermal delivery of drugs. Predicting whether drugs pass across the blood–brain barrier is critical in the pharmaceutical field because the central nervous system (CNS)-active compounds are the only substances which must cross the barrier. This can help avoid the CNS side effects in the brain. The drug has very low absorbance to CNS. Plasma protein binding of a drug gives information on not only the drug action but also its efficacy and disposition (Van De Waterbeemd and Gifford, 2003).

A list of software and online database for the toxicity prediction and drug-likeness property is presented in Table 19.2. The OSIRIS Property Explorer is useful for drawing chemical structures and for the calculation on-the-fly the various drug-relevant properties (cLogP, solubility, molecular weight, toxicity risk assessment, overall drug score, etc.) whenever a structure is valid. Prediction results are valued and color coded. Properties with high risks of undesirable effects like mutagenicity or a poor intestinal absorption will appear in red, whereas a green color indicates drug-conformation behavior (Ghosh et al., 2006; Pan et al., 2014).

TABLE 19.2 List of the Software and Online Database for the Toxicity Prediction and Drug-Likeness Property.

Software	DSSTox
	The Carcinogenic Potency Database (CPDB)
	MDL®Toxicity Database
	ADME/Toxicity Property Calculator
	MetaSite
	Tsar 3.2
	ChemTree
	MedChem Designer™
	QikProp
	FAFDrugs3
	PROTOX
Online tools	ToxPredict
	DrugLogit
	Pre ADME/T
	Molinfo
	MetaPrint2D
	Aggregator Advisor
	ALOGPS

The phytochemicals would be selected based on the screening of their toxicity and drug-likeness profile for the drug development. Lipinski's rule of five is a rule of thumb to estimate drug-likeness. Phytochemicals with a specific pharmacological activity are most favorable for drug designing. These properties would make it a likely orally active drug in humans. The rules explain molecular properties significant for drug pharmacokinetics in the human body as well as its ADME.

19.2.3 DRUG DESIGNING

Computational phytochemistry uses various tools to enhance the process of drug discovery. There are a plethora of tools used in computational phytochemistry. Molecular docking and simulation are most significant. Molecular docking is a prevalent method for structure-based drug designing. It is used to predict the binding conformation of ligands with suitable targets (Ashfaq et al., 2013). In silico tools are well integrated into the drug development process and are considered a complementary approach to experimental methods and has proved to identify ligand–target interactions successfully. Available for one compound are called bioactivity profiles can be generated (Binder et al., 2004).

19.2.3.1   STRUCTURE-BASED DRUG DESIGNING

The protein sequences of enzymes are downloaded from Protein Data Bank (PDB) (http://www.rcsb.org/pdb). PDB is a structural library for biological macromolecules which encompasses all the structural information of macromolecules as determined by X-ray crystallography, NMR studies, and so forth RasMol is a molecular graphics program intended for the visualization of proteins, nucleic acids, and small molecules (Vijesh et al., 2013). RasMol runs on extensive range of architectures and operating systems including Microsoft Windows, Apple Macintosh, UNIX, and VMS systems. The PubChem Compound Database contains validated chemical depiction information provided to describe substances (Gombar et al., 2003). Structures stored within PubChem are pre-clustered and cross-referenced by uniqueness and comparison of groups. Otherwise the two-dimensional (2D) chemical structures of the ligands can be drawn using ChemDraw Virtual screening software for computational drug discovery that is used to partition libraries of the compound against potential drug targets. To perform the docking model, the AutoDock 4.0 suite molecular-docking tool can be used, and the methodology is applied by many researchers (Trott and Olson, 2010). PyRx permits medicinal chemists to run virtual screening for many number of programming platform and helps the user in all steps of drug discovery process from data preparation to job submission and analysis of the results. The prepared ligands can be undergone in energy minimizations with Chem3D Ultra and saved in portable document format. PyMol is a molecular modeling program that is particularly effective for the construction and 3D visualization of macromolecules, including proteins and protein–ligand complexes. Kollman-united atom charges, salvation parameters, and polar hydrogens can be added to the receptor for the preparation of a protein in docking simulation. Since ligands are not peptides, the Gasteiger charge could be assigned, and then nonpolar hydrogens could be merged (Shannon et al., 2003). AutoDock requires precalculated grid maps for all the atoms present in the ligand being docked and it stores the potential energy arising. Other than this, many numbers of software and online tools are available for drug designing (Oda et al., 2007). Molecular mechanics force fields are used in the estimation of binding affinity between the target molecule and drug molecule that has been docked. The different mechanism is contributing to the binding free energy. It can be written as:

$$\Delta G_{bind} = \Delta G_{solvent} + \Delta G_{conf} + \Delta G_{int} + \Delta G_{rot} + \Delta G_{tor} + \Delta G_{vib}$$

Every compound consists of solvent effects, conformational changes in the target molecule and drug molecule, free energy due to target–drug interactions, internal rotations, association energy of target molecule and drug molecule to form a single complex and free energy due to changes in vibration modes. The best conformation was chosen based on the docking score and glide energy. The addition of all energy such as rotatable bond counts, lipophilic, metal interaction, hydrogen bonding, and salvation contribute to the docking score. The glide energy is binding free energy intended based on the optimized potentials for liquid simulations-all atom (OPLS-AA) force field. The paramount compound can be selected based on the least glide energy/docking score/both (Bushkov et al., 2016). Docked complexes were further analyzed using molecular dynamics (MD) simulation under episodic boundary setting in all guidelines to simulate the entire molecular system. Figure 19.2 explains the steps involved in the docking with AutoDock (PyRx).

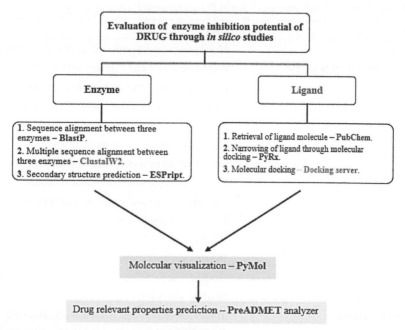

FIGURE 19.2   Steps in molecular docking.

19.2.3.2   LIGAND-BASED DRUG DESIGNING

The quantitative structure–activity relationship (QSAR) studies are incredibly helpful for the calculation of biological activities, especially in drug design. The study is based on the statement that variations in the properties of the compounds can be concurrent with changes in their molecular characteristics (Santana et al., 2006). QSAR model both enhances our understanding of the specificity of drug action and afford a theoretical establishment for lead optimization (SchuÈttelkopf and Van Aalten, 2004). However, the results have to be validated using in vitro studies before it could be established that drug has better specific inhibitory property for particular target molecules and could then be explored as lead drug molecule for the treatment. Predominant tools used in the MD simulation are LQTAgrid, UCSF Chimera, CoMFA, and CoMSIA, QPLD in Schrödinger suite, Molegro Virtual Docking software, Weka, SYBYL software, CDK tools, and QSARpro (Contrera et al., 2005). From the structural similarity score analog to the drug compound can be found by the researcher. After docking, the dynamic studies would need to be carried out on the docked compound (Contrera et al., 2008). Some software tools used in drug discovery are listed in Table 19.3.

TABLE 19.3   List of Software and Uses in Computational Phytochemistry.

Tools	Uses
KEGG	Metabolic pathways, phytochemical classification
SWISS-MODEL Repository	Protein structure and function information
GenBank	Protein structure and function information
Expasy	Protein structure and function information
CATH-Gene3D database	Protein structure and function information
Ligand Expo	Ligand structure and function information
BindingDB	Ligand structure and function information
RCSB PDB	Ligand structure and function information
BioLiP	Ligand structure and function information
Biostars	Binding site prediction
FunFOLD	Binding site prediction
3DLigandSite	Binding site prediction
Active Site prediction IITD	Binding site prediction
Cofactor or COACH	Binding site prediction
Protein Data Bank	3D shapes of proteins, nucleic acids, and complex assemblies

TABLE 19.3 *(Continued)*

Tools	Uses
PubChem	Chemical molecules
MDL Drug Data Report	Chemical molecules
World of Molecular Bioactivity Database	Chemical molecules
ChEMBL Medicinal Chemistry Database	Chemical molecules
LigandScout	Pharmacophore-based investigation
Discovery Studio	Pharmacophore-based investigation
PharmaDB	Pharmacophore study
PharmMapper	Pharmacophore study
OMEGA 2.3.2	PDB file converter
Dundee PRODRG2 server	Energy minimization
Discovery Studio 3.5	Molecular dynamics (MD) studies
Toxtree v2.6.6	Docking studies
FRED 2.1	OMEGA pre-generated structure
GOLD	Docking studies
SwissDock	Docking studies
Molsoft ICM	Docking studies
Molsoft ICM	Docking studies
Molegro virtual docker	Docking studies
Cluspro	Docking studies
Scigress-Dock	Docking studies
iGEMDOCK	Docking studies
HomDock	Docking studies
Rosetta 3.1	Docking studies
ArgusLab	Docking studies
Hex	Docking studies
Zdock	Docking studies
PASS	Bioactivity spectrum predictions
MOE2010	Docking process
AMBER12	MD simulations
Tremolo-X	MD simulations
LAMMPS	MD simulations
TINKER	MD simulations
XenoView	MD simulations
COSMOS	MD simulations
YASARA	MD simulations

TABLE 19.3   *(Continued)*

Tools	Uses
DL-POLY	MD simulations
Ascalaph Designer	MD simulations
SHARC molecular dynamics	MD simulations
Zinc Database	Ligand retrieval
PHASE	3D-QSAR analysis
TCM database	Protein information
Ligplot	ADME analysis
PyMol	Visualize the molecular
GroGUI 0.5.2 version of GROMACS MD	MD studies
MOLA.	Molecular docking
Docking Server	Online Docking
CAST P	Binding site prediction

19.3   MOLECULAR DYNAMICS SIMULATION

MD simulation studies are used for simulating biomolecules in explicit solvent/membrane, geometry optimization, and conformational search. Numerous numerical algorithms and tools were developed for integrating the equations of motion for MD programming. There are many simulation softwares available and among them is GROMACS, a freeware and most widely used in the drug development research (Abraham et al., 2015). It is a multipurpose package to carry out MD studies, which simulates the Newtonian equations of motion for systems with hundreds to millions of particles. GROMACS can write coordinates using compression, which provides a very compact way of storing trajectory data (Lee et al., 2015), and can be run using either the standard MPI communication protocol or other protocol. Molecular simulation of the protein consisted of energy minimization in the CHARM force field. The method of minimization depends on the size of the root mean square gradient. The lowest energy model is then selected for further analysis and validation. The binding site will then be predicted by the receptor cavity method (Eraser algorithm). The development of parameter sets is a very laborious work that needs some extensive optimization. Simulations can be carried out with tools, such as NAMD, GROMACS, Discovery Studio, and Schrödinger tools (Abraham and Gready, 2011).

19.4 CONCLUSION

Computational phytochemistry is a necessary lead for everyone concerned with the identification, extraction, and application of dynamic agents from natural products. Thus, this chapter briefly discussed the computational tools involved in drug discovery, which includes the information about the software and database; behind this, many advanced algorithms are available in computer languages. A researcher who is working on drug development has to understand the principles behind the tools and modify that for various applications in research.

KEYWORDS

- computational phytochemistry
- drug design
- ADME
- medicine
- herbs

REFERENCES

Abraham, M. J.; Gready, J. E. Optimization of Parameters for Molecular Dynamics Simulation Using Smooth Particle-Mesh Ewald in GROMACS 4.5. *J. Comput. Chem.* **2011**, *32,* 2031–2040.

Aggarwal, B. B.; Ichikawa, H.; Garodia, P.; Weerasinghe, P.; Sethi, G.; Bhatt, I. D.; Pandey, M. K.; Shishodia, S.; Nair, M.G. From Traditional Ayurvedic Medicine to Modern Medicine: Identification of Therapeutic Targets for Suppression of Inflammation and Cancer. *Expert Opin. Ther. Targets* **2006**, *10,* 87–118.

Ashfaq, U. A.; Mumtaz, A.; ul Qamar, T.; Fatima, T. Maps Database: Medicinal Plant Activities, Phytochemical and Structural Database. *Bioinformation* **2013**, *9,* 993.

Bhattacharjee, B.; Vijayasarathy, S.; Karunakar, P.; Chatterjee, J. Comparative Reverse Screening Approach to Identify Potential Anti-Neoplastic Targets of Saffron Functional Components and Binding Mode. *Asian Pac. J. Cancer Prev.* **2012**, *13,* 5605–5611.

Binder, K.; Horbach, J.; Kob, W.; Paul, W.; Varnik, F. Molecular Dynamics Simulations. *J. Phys. Condens. Matter* **2004**, *1,* S429.

Bushkov, N. A.; Veselov, M. S.; Chuprov-Netochin, R. N.; Marusich, E. I.; Majouga, A. G.; Volynchuk, P. B.; Shumilina, D. V.; Leonov, S. V.; Ivanenkov, Y. A. Computational Insight Into the Chemical Space of Plant Growth Regulators. *Phytochemistry* **2016**, *122,* 254–264.

Cavalli, J. F.; Tomi, F.; Bernardini, A. F.; Casanova, J. Combined Analysis of the Essential Oil of Chenopodium Ambrosioides by GC, GC-MS and 13C-Nmr Spectroscopy: Quantitative Determination of Ascaridole, a Heat-Sensitive Compound. *Phytochem. Anal.* **2004,** *15,* 275–279.

Chung, V. C.; Ma, P. H.; Lau, C. H.; Wong, S.; Yeoh, E. K.; Griffiths, S. M. Views on Traditional Chinese Medicine Amongst Chinese Population: A Systematic Review of Qualitative and Quantitative Studies. *Health Expect.* **2014,** *17,* 622–636.

Contrera, J. F.; Matthews, E. J.; Kruhlak, N. L.; Benz, R. D In Silico Screening of Chemicals for Bacterial Mutagenicity Using Electrotopological E-State Indices and MDL QSAR Software. *Regul. Toxicol. Pharmacol.* **2005,** *43,* 313–323.

Contrera, J. F.; Matthews, E. J.; Kruhlak, N. L.; Benz, R. D In Silico Screening of Chemicals for Genetic Toxicity Using MDL-QSAR, Nonparametric Discriminant Analysis, E-State, Connectivity, and Molecular Property Descriptors. *Toxicol. Mech. Methods* **2008,** *18,* 207–216.

Dammalli, M.; Naika, H. R.; Lingaraju, V. K.; Navya, P.; Chandramohan, V.; Suresh, D. Molecular Docking and Dynamic Studies of Bioactive Compounds from Naravelia Zeylanica (L.) DC Against Glycogen Synthase Kinase-3β Protein. *J. Taibah University Sci.* **2015,** *9,* 41–49.

Duraipandi, S.; Selvakumar, V.; Er, N. Y. Reverse Engineering of Ayurvedic Lipid Based Formulation, Ghrita by Combined Column Chromatography, Normal and Reverse Phase HPTLC Analysis. *BMC Complementary Altern. Med.* **2015,** *15,* 62.

Ghosh, S.; Nie, A.; An, J.; Huang, Z. Structure-Based Virtual Screening of Chemical Libraries for Drug Discovery. *Curr. Opin. Chem. Biol.* **2006,** *10,* 194–202.

Gombar, V. K.; Silver, I. S.; Zhao, Z. Role of ADME Characteristics in Drug Discovery and Their in Silico Evaluation: in Silico Screening of Chemicals for Their Metabolic Stability. *Curr. Top. Med. Chem.* **2003,** *3,* 1205–1225.

González-Gómez, D.; Lozano, M.; Fernández-León, M. F.; Bernalte, M. J.; Ayuso, M. C.; Rodríguez, A. B. Sweet Cherry Phytochemicals: Identification and Characterization by HPLC-DAD/ESI-MS in Six Sweet-Cherry Cultivars Grown in Valle del Jerte (Spain). *J. Food Compos. Anal.* **2010,** *23,* 533–539.

Harborne, A. Phytochemical Methods a Guide to Modern Techniques of Plant Analysis. Springer: Netherlands, 1998, Vol.14, 1–302.

Khanra, R.; Dewanjee, S.; Dua, T. K.; Bhattacharjee, N. Taraxerol, a Pentacyclic Triterpene from Abroma Augusta Leaf, Attenuates Acute Inflammation Via Inhibition of NF-κB Signaling. *Biomed. Pharmacother.* **2017,** *88,* 918–923.

Lee, J.; Cheng, X.; Swails, J. M.; Yeom, M. S.; Eastman, P. K.; Lemkul, J. A.; Wei, S.; Buckner, J.; Jeong, J. C.; Qi, Y. CHARMM-GUI Input Generator for NAMD, GROMACS, AMBER, OpenMM, and CHARMM/OpenMM Simulations Using the CHARMM36 Additive Force Field. *J. Chem. Theory Comput.* **2015,** *12,* 405–413.

Oda, A.; Okayasu, M.; Kamiyama, Y.; Yoshida, T.; Takahashi, O.; Matsuzaki, H. Evaluation of Docking Accuracy and Investigations of Roles of Parameters and Each Term in Scoring Functions for Protein–Ligand Docking Using ArgusLab Software. *Bull. Chem. Soc. Jpn.* **2007,** *80,* 1920–1925.

Pan, S. Y.; Litscher, G.; Gao, S. H.; Zhou, S. F.; Yu, Z. L.; Chen, H. Q.; Zhang, S. F.; Tang, M. K.; Sun, J. N.; Ko, K.-M. Historical Perspective of Traditional Indigenous Medical Practices: the Current Renaissance and Conservation of Herbal Resources. *Evidence-Based Complementary Altern. Med.* **2014,** *2014,* 525340.

Santana, L.; Uriarte, E.; González-Díaz, H.; Zagotto, G.; Soto-Otero, R. Méndez-Álvarez, E. A QSAR Model for in Silico Screening of MAO-A Inhibitors Prediction, Synthesis, and Biological Assay of Novel Coumarins. *J. Med. Chem.* **2006**, *49,* 1149–1156.

SchuÈttelkopf, A. W.; Van Aalten, D. M. PRODRG: A Tool for High-Throughput Crystallography of Protein–Ligand Complexes. *Acta Crystallogr. Sect. D: Biol. Crystallogr.* **2004**, *60,* 1355–1363.

Sermakkani, M.; Thangapandian, V. GC-MS Analysis of Cassia Italica Leaf Methanol Extract. *Asian J. Pharm. Clin. Res.* **2012**, *5,* 90–94.

Shannon, P.; Markiel, A.; Ozier, O.; Baliga, N. S.; Wang, J. T.; Ramage, D.; Amin, N.; Schwikowski, B. Ideker, T Cytoscape: A Software Environment for Integrated Models of Biomolecular Interaction Networks. *Genome Res.* **2003**, *13,* 2498–2504.

Suzuki, N. Complementary and Alternative Medicine: A Japanese Perspective. *Evidence-Based Complementary Altern.* **2004**, *1,* 113–118.

Trott, O.; Olson, A. J. AutoDock Vina: Improving the Speed and Accuracy of Docking with a New Scoring Function, Efficient Optimization, and Multithreading. *J. Comput. Chem.* **2010**, *31,* 455–461.

Van De Waterbeemd, H.; Gifford, E. ADMET in Silico Modelling: Towards Prediction Paradise? *Nat. Rev. Drug Discovery* **2003**, 2, 192–204.

Vijesh, A.; Isloor, A. M.; Telkar, S.; Arulmoli, T.; Fun, H. K. Molecular Docking Studies of Some New Imidazole Derivatives for Antimicrobial Properties. *Arabian J. Chem.* **2013**, *6,* 197–204.

CHAPTER 20

STEMNESS MODULATION BY PHYTOCHEMICALS TO TARGET CANCER STEM CELLS

PREM PRAKASH KUSHWAHA[1], PUSHPENDRA SINGH[2], and SHASHANK KUMAR[1,*]

[1]School of Basic and Applied Sciences, Department of Biochemistry and Microbial Sciences, Central University of Punjab, Bathinda 151001, Punjab, Tel.: +91-9335647413

[2]Tumor Biology Laboratory, National Institute of Pathology (ICMR), New Delhi, India

*Corresponding author. E-mail: shashankbiochembch@gmail.com ORCID: *https://orcid.org/0000-0002-9622-0512

ABSTRACT

Cancer stem cells (CSCs) are a small subpopulation of cells identified in a variety of tumors that are capable of self-renewal, differentiation, and have the unique property to evade radiotherapy and chemotherapy. CSCs are a very likely cause of resistance to current cancer treatments, and relapse in patients. ATP-binding cassette transporters and DNA repair capacity of CSCs determines the drug resistance in these cells. *Withania somnifera* (Solanaceae) also known as ashwagandha is a medicinal plant that has been utilized in traditional medicine. Different studies revealed various medicinal properties of this herb including anticancer. *W. somnifera* has the ability to modulate mitochondrial function, regulate apoptosis, reduce inflammation, and enhance endothelial function. There is no significant literature available regarding the role of *W. somnifera* phytoconstituents in cancer cell stemness and chemotherapy drug resistance. Keeping this in our mind we did in silico study to find out the potential of *W. somnifera* phytoconstituents against cancer cell stemness.

20.1   INTRODUCTION

Cancer is the main cause of death throughout the world; however, other death-causing diseases have knowingly reduced since last some millennia (Siegel et al., 2016). Genetic mutation, lifestyle, and microenvironment are the leading causes of the cancer development. Most of the cancer-causing factors stimulate the internal regulatory proteins which lose the control from the proper development of cell and promote cancer progression. Current therapies comprise the development of targeted strong inhibitors which affects cancer cell proliferation and tumor survival (Coates et al., 2015). Cancer cell holds the property for continuous mutation and abnormal function which causes them to adopt an aggressive nature and drug resistance against drug treatment (Moore et al., 2011; Colak et al., 2014). Cancer stem cells (CSCs) involve property of self-renewal and give rise to offspring which have the capability to differentiate freely (Wu and Izpisua Belmonte, 2016). CSCs require some specific factors and cytokines for proliferation and fail to maintain proper homeostasis. CSCs also have an excellent capacity to organize and educate the neighboring cells to deliver the healthy nutrition and form the favorable environment for the tumor progression and combat for the immune system. CSCs also provides heterogeneous cell populations with higher plasticity potential, stressful factors resistance, surrounding tumor microenvironment (hypoxic condition), or cell death induction by chemotherapeutic drug (Plaks et al., 2015). Phytochemicals are known to possess potential against CSCs markers. Different mechanism targeting CSCs are given in Table 20.1.

20.2   MECHANISM OF SELF-RENEWAL

The Wnt/β-catenin pathway regulates cell fate decisions as well as stem cell pluripotency during the development. These developmental cascades assimilate signals from several other pathways, including bone morphogenetic protein, retinoic acid, fibroblast growth factor, and transforming growth factor β within different cell types and tissues. Secreted glycoprotein (Wnt ligand) binds to Frizzled receptors and leads to the formation of a larger complex with lipoprotein receptor-related proteins 5/6 (LRP5/6). E3 ubiquitin ligase zinc and ring finger 3 (ZNRF3) and its homolog ring finger 43 (RNF43) provide ubiquitination of Frizzled receptor. ZNRF3 and RNF43 activity are inhibited by R-spondin binding to LRP5/6. In this fashion, R-spondins increase the sensitivity of cells to the Wnt ligand. Activation of

TABLE 20.1 Specific Molecular Mechanisms by Which Phytochemicals Able to Kill the Cancer Stem Cells.

Molecular Mechanism	A	B	C	D	E	F	G	H	I
Inhibits Wnt signaling									
Decreases ALDH1 activity									
Induces apoptosis									
Activating caspase 3									
Downregulates β-catenin									
Induces CSC differentiation									
Decreases number of mammospheres									
Decreases number of CD44⁺									
Decreases number of CD133⁺, CD166⁺ cells									
Induces G2/M phase arrest									

Different color represents a different type of cancer cell.

Red = Breast cancer; Green = Pancreatic cancer; Blue = Neuroblastoma; Violet = Colorectal cancer; Yellow = Prostate cancer; Cyan = Colon Cancer.

A = EGCG, B = Piperine, C = Sulforaphane, D= β-Carotene, E = Quercetin, F = Resveratrol, G =Genistein, H = Curcumin, I =*Sasa quelpaertensis* extract.

the Wnt receptor complex triggers dislocation of the multifunctional kinase glycogen synthase kinase-3 β (GSK-3β) from a regulatory APC/Axin/GSK-3β complex. In the absence of Wnt-signal, CK1 and the APC/Axin/GSK-3β complex provide coordinated phosphorylation of β-catenin and transcriptional coregulator resulting to its ubiquitination and proteasomal degradation through the β-TrCP/Skp pathway. In the presence of Wnt ligand, the coreceptor LRP5/6 is brought in complex with Wnt-bound Frizzled. This primes to the activation of dishevelled protein by sequential phosphorylation, poly-ubiquitination as well as polymerization, which relocates GSK-3β from APC/Axin via an uncertain mechanism that may include substrate trapping and/or endosome sequestration. Stabilized form of β-catenin moves toward the nucleus through Rac1 and several other factors where β-catenin binds to transcription factors lymphoid enhancer-binding factor/T-cell factor. Binding of β-catenin to transcription factors results in transposition of corepressors and enlisting supplementary coactivators to the Wnt-specific target genes. In addition, β-catenin cooperates with various other transcription factors to regulate specific targets. Prominently, investigators have found that β-catenin point mutations in human tumors that prevent GSK-3β phosphorylation and thus lead to its anomalous accumulation. R-spondin, Axin, APC, and E-cadherin mutations have also been documented in tumor samples, emphasizing the deregulation of Wnt pathway in cancers. Wnt signaling also promotes nuclear accumulation of other transcriptional regulator implicated in cancer, such as TAZ and Snail1. Pathways involved in self-renewal of cancer cells are depicted in Figure 20.1.

20.3   PHYTOCHEMICAL AND MIRNA REGULATION

MicroRNA is small non-coding RNA molecule which helps in gene silencing and post-transcriptional regulation of gene expression in eukaryotes and in some viruses. MicroRNAs are endogenous in origin and encoded by RNA polymerase II and RNA polymerase III. Processing of miRNA is completed into the nucleus as well as cytosol. In the nucleus, the precursor of miRNA is synthesized, known as pri-miRNA having a double-stranded helix. Drosha along with pasha or DGCR8 recognize pre-miRNA and form a complex called microprocessor complex. In this complex, drosha liberate hairpin from pre-miRNA and produce the overhanging 3-OH end. About 16% of a pre-miRNA is processed into the nucleus and further processing is completed into cytoplasm with the help of dicer and RISC complex. Exportin-5 helps in the transportation of pri-miRNA, using GTP as an energy source. Exportin-5 is a member of karyopherin superfamily. In the cytoplasm, pri-miRNA is cleaved by DICER and converted into mature miRNA: miRNA complex about 22 nucleotides in length. Although both strand of a duplex potentially acts in silencing, only one strand is incorporated into RISC complex where miRNA and its target mRNA interact. Micro RNA binds to 3-OH UTR region of a mRNA and leads to silencing of that gene.

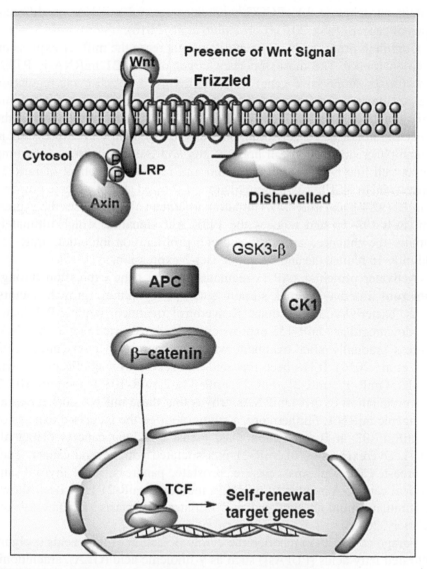

FIGURE 20.1   Pathway involved in self-renewal of the cancer cells.

Green tea extract possesses (-)-Epigallocatechin-3-O-gallate (EGCG), a polyphenolic compound that shows high anticancer activities (Shammas et al., 2006). A study reported that 67-kDa laminin receptor (67LR) recognized as a cell surface receptor for EGCG (Tachibana et al., 2004). Binding of EGCG to cell surface receptor explores its anticancer effects of EGCG (Kumazoe et al., 2013). EGCG also inhibits cancer progression by stimulating signaling pathways (intracellular), cAMP/protein kinase A (PKA)/ protein phosphatase 2A. EGCG modulates several miRNAs in different types of cancer (Table 20.2) (Carotenuto et al., 2016).

Curcumin produced by *Curcuma longa* increase the miR-21 expression in colon cancer. The most important target of miR-21 miRNA is PTEN gene (tumor-suppressive gene) which is involved in cell cycle regulation and proliferation inhibition. Oncogenic miR-21 miRNA has outstanding antiapoptotic activity in human cancer cell lines. One study showed the effect of difluorinated curcumin on miR-200 and miR-21 expression in human pancreatic cancer cell lines. Zhang and Bai (2014) treated the lung cancer cell line (A549) with curcumin and reported the effect of miR-21 expression. In NSCLC, curcumin treatment showed anti-oncogenic property of miR-192–5p and miR-215. Curcumin treatment also increases the expression miR-192–5p and reduces the PI3K/Akt signaling which ultimately initiates the enhanced apoptosis and cell proliferation inhibition. miR-15a and miR-16 reduce the anti-apoptotic Bcl-2 expression.

Activator protein 1 (AP-1) regulates several gene expression through numerous internal/external stimuli such as cytokines, growth factors, stress, bacterial/viral infections. Resveratrol treatment target AP-1 factor and downregulates miR-155 expression. A study reported that 22 miRNAs express gradually after treatment with resveratrol in colon cancer cells (Tili et al., 2010). It has been reported that resveratrol significantly downregulates miR-17, miR-21, miR-25, miR-92a-2, miR-103-1, and miR-103-2. Downregulation of these miRNAs proves that these miRNAs behave as an oncogenic miRNA. Furthermore, a study reported the increased expression of miR-17-92 in B-cell lymphomas, breast and lung cancers (Tiliet al., 2007). Overexpression of MiR-21 is associated with several cancers such as breast, CRCs, gliomas, gastric, prostate, pancreas, lung, thyroid, and cervical cancer. A number of miRNAs including miR-21 have been shown to stimulate multiple signaling and initiates metastasis (Krichevsky and Gabriely, 2009).

Faragó et al. (2011) reported the cytotoxic action of fatty acids (polyunsaturated fatty acids [PUFAs]) such as γ-linolenic acid (GLA), arachidonic acid (AA) and docosahexaenoicacid. Treatment of PUFA/temozolomide

TABLE 20.2 miRNA Regulated by Different Phytochemicals.

Epi-gallocatechin-3-gallate	Curcumin	Resveratrol	n3-polyunsaturated fatty acids	Common
miR-200c, miR-210, miR-222, miR-335–3p, let-7d, let-7g, let-7e, let-7bn, miR-322, miR-101a/b, miR-107, miR-290–3p, miR-302a/d, miR-128, miR-294, miR-29a/b, let-7a, miR-93, miR-24, miR-92, miR-106b, miR-18a/b, miR-194, miR-122, miR-185, let-7c, miR-34b, let-7f, miR-192, miR-221, miR-16, miR-25, miR-21, miR-181a, miR-146b, miR-34a	let-7a, miR-93, miR-24, miR-92, miR-16, miR-25, miR-21, miR-181a, miR-146b, miR-34a, miR-192, miR-221, miR-203, miR-27a, miR-9n, let-7i, miR-195, miR-215, miR-15a, miR-103, miR-19a, miR-20a, miR-17, miR-26a, miR-125b	miR-15a, miR-155, miR-103, miR-19a, miR-20a, miR-17, miR-26a, miR-93, miR-24, miR-92, miR-16, miR-25, miR-21, miR-181a, miR-146b, miR-34a, miR-106b, miR-194, miR-122, miR-185, 18a/b, miR-194, miR-122, miR-185, let-7c, miR-34b, miR-19b-1/b-2, miR-92a-1/a-2, miR-106a, miR-1915, miR-483–5p, miR-100–1/2, miR-363, miR-424, miR-497, miR-483, miR-146, miR-424, miR-497, miR-483, miR-146, miR-20b, miR-206, miR-29c, miR-34c	miR-34b, let-7f, miR-192, miR-221, miR-16, miR-25, miR-21, miR-181a, miR-146b, miR-34a, miR-20a, miR-17, miR-26a, miR-125b, miR-146, miR-20b, miR-206, miR-29c, miR-34c, miR-143, miR-145	miR-16, miR-25, miR-21, miR-181a, miR-146b, miR-34a

downregulates several miRNA (cox2, irs1, irs2, ccnd1, itgb3, bcl2, sirt1, tp53inp1, and k-ras) in cancer cells. In addition to this, another study reported by Mandal et al. (2012), omega-3 PUFA to regulate breast tumor CSF-1 (colony stimulating factor-1) expression through miR-21 modulation.

20.4   DNA REPAIR MECHANISM

The mammalian cell uses four types of DNA repair mechanism. The genes involved in these repair mechanism are shown in Table 20.3.

1. Base excision repair (BER).
2. Nucleotide excision repair (NER).
3. Mismatch repair (MMR).
4. Double-strand break repair which includes:
    a) Homologous recombination (HR).
    b) Non-homologous end joining (NHEJ).

TABLE 20.3   Enzymes Involved in DNA Repair.

Repair mechanism	Gene involved
Base excision repair	DNA glycosylase, APE1, XRCC1, PNKP, Tdp1, APTX, DNA polymerase β, FEN1, DNA polymerase δ or ε, PCNA-RFC, PARP
Mismatch repair	MutSα (MSH2-MSH6), MutSβ (MSH2-MSH3), MutLα (MLH1-PMS2), MutLβ (MLH1-PMS2), MutLγ (MLH1-MLH3), Exo1, PCNA-RFC
Nucleotide excision repair	XPC-Rad23B-CEN2, UV-DDB (DDB1-XPE), CSA, CSB, TFIIH, XPB, XPD, XPA, RPA, XPG, ERCC1- XPF, DNA polymerase δ or ε
Homologous recombination	Mre11-Rad50-Nbs1, CtIP, RPA, Rad51, Rad52, BRCA1, BRCA2, Exo1, BLM-TopIIIα, GEN1-Yen1, Slx1- Slx4, Mus81/Eme1
Non-homologous end-joining	Ku70-Ku80, DNA-PKc, XRCC4-DNA ligase IV, XLF

20.4.1   BASE EXCISION REPAIR

It involves the removal of the damaged base through excision of a short piece of DNA and resynthesized with a DNA polymerase. This repair is used to correct many minor damages like alkylation and deamination resulting from exposure to mutagenic chemicals or rays. DNA glycosylate initiate this repair process. It does not cleave phosphodiester bonds, instead, cleave the glycosidic bonds. DNA glycosylase liberates the altered base and generates AP sites (an apurinic and pyrimidine site). Another enzyme called AP endonuclease introduce chain break by the cleaving of the phosphodiester bond at AP sites. This bond cleavage initiate excision repair system with the help of three another enzymes – an exonuclease, DNA polymerase I, and DNA ligase.

20.4.2   NUCLEOTIDE EXCISION REPAIR

NER is almost similar to BER but do not proceed by the removal of the damaged base. This repair system includes the removal of the phosphodiester bond on either side of the lesion, on the same strand, resulting in the excision of an oligonucleotide. This excision creates a gap which is filled by some ligases.

This repair system is best studied in *Escherichia coli*. ABC exonuclease which is the key enzyme regulate all the repair system and is made up of three subunits, these subunits are transcribed by uvrA, uvrB, and uvrC genes. ABC exonuclease first binds to DNA at the site of the lesion. First, uvrA and uvrB binds to the damaged site of the gene. uvrA recognizes the damaged site. The departure of uvrA allows uvrC to bind, forming uvrBC dimer which cleaves the damaged strand at the phosphodiester bond. uvrD is a helicase helps to unwind the DNA to allow the release of the single strand between the cuts. The resulting gap is filled in by DNA polymerase I and sealed by ligase.

20.4.3   MISMATCH REPAIR

This repair system is present at the time of replication and completes into three steps. In the first step, MMR enzymes recognize MMR base pair. In the second step, enzymes determine which base is incorrect one in the mismatch. And in the third step enzymes excise incorrect base and completes the repair. MMR occurs only on daughter strand. Due to an methylate or hemimethylate of daughter strand excision repair enzymes recognize only daughter strand. There are three match repair system in *E. coli*, long patch, short patch, and very short patch. In long-patch system, there are Mut proteins involved in MMR encoded by *but* genes. The Mut proteins are MutH, MutL, MutS. Mainly MutH and MutS are involved in repair system.

20.4.4 REPAIR OF DOUBLE-STRANDED DNA BREAK

Mutagenic agents, radiations, and replication errors may cause a double-stranded break in DNA. Two different mechanisms are involved in this type of repair – homologous and NHEJ. Only one of both joining system is used by the cell and it depends on cell cycle phase. G0 and G1 phase choose NHEJ while S and G2 choose homologous end joining.

a) **HR:** In homologous end joining, some special recombination proteins recognize the area of DNA sequence matching between the two chromosomes and bring them together. An undamaged chromosome is used as a template for transferring genetic information to the broken chromosome, repairing with no change in the DNA sequence.

b) **NHEJ:** In NHEJ, the broken end is recognized by a heterodimer Ku70 and Ku80. This heterodimer allows DNA-dependent protein kinase (DNAPK) and Artemis to act. Artemis shows both endonuclease and exonuclease activity and trims the DNA ends. The final joining is carried out by DNA ligase IV in association with XRCC4.

Poly (ADP-ribose) polymerase (PARP) family (nuclear proteins) of proteins actively involved in DNA damage recognition. These proteins frequently bind with single-strand breaks. During the synthesis of poly(ADP-ribose) (pADPr) chains, PARP also binds with glutamate, aspartate, and lysine amino acids. PARP family has 17 isoforms. They are well classified by Krishnakumar and Kraus (2010), on the basis of their functional multi-domain architecture and cellular localization. PARP family helps in all DNA repair pathways such as BER, HR, NER, and NHEJ.

PARP protein inhibits pADPr chain synthesis and stops the employment of supplementary repair factors. PARP inhibition results in failure to release of PARP recognizing protein from the DNA damage sites which results in no access to further recruitment of additional repair factors. The first PARP inhibitor drug is olaparib (AZD-2281) which got approved by Food and Drug Administration. Another PARP inhibitor is talazoparib (BMN 673) which have the potential to inhibit both the isoforms such as PARP1 and PARP2 (Cardnell et al., 2013). Another PARP1 selective inhibitor known as NMS-P118 has outstanding absorption, distribution, metabolism, and excretion profile. A study showed that NMS-P118 has high effectiveness in triple-negative breast cancer with a BRCA1 mutation. In BRCA2 deficient pancreatic cancer xenograft models, a combination of NMS-P118 with temozolomide showed remarkable effects. Gossypol (natural phenol derived compound) acts as an inhibitor of PARP1-BRCA1 C terminus (BRCT) domain interaction, which explores new opportunities for the development of precise PARP1 inhibitors.

Soy isoflavones such as genistein and daidzein are a type of bioflavonoids commonly found in soy products. These compounds exert a cytotoxic effect in various cancer cell lines (Kingsley et al., 2011). Soy isoflavones treatment increases the DNA-repair enzyme activities in lung cancer cell lines. Both daidzein and genistein exhibit conflicting properties. Genistein showed enhanced metastasis while daidzein suppresses the metastasis in the lymph nodes by affecting APE1/Ref-1 and the levels of other TFs in prostate cancer cell lines (Singh-Gupta et al., 2010). Resveratrol treatment reduces the AP-1 and nuclear factor-kappa B (NF-kB) DNA-binding activity. AP-1 DNA-binding activity of APE1/Ref-1 is fully dependent on the dose of resveratrol. Another wonderful natural molecule known as curcumin stops the downstream signaling cascades of AP-1 and NF-kB by inhibiting APE1/Ref-1 redox function. An elevated level of APE1/Ref-1 showed drug resistance and treatment with curcumin decreases APE1/Ref-1 levels in cancer patients (Scapagniniet al., 2006). Rosmarinic acid and luteolin increases DNA repair capacity and protects DNA from oxidative damage in Caco-2 and HeLa cells (Ramos et al., 2010).

Checkpoint kinase 1 has been found as a new therapeutic target for neuroblastoma. A pharmacologic inhibitor of CHK1 known as CCT244747 showed remarkable potential activity in MYCN-driven neuroblastoma (Lainchbury et al., 2012).TNBC and MYCN-driven neuroblastoma sensitivity to CHK1 inhibitors shown association with CHK1 and p53 level (Ma et al., 2012). Both CHK1 and CHK2 inactivation induces sensitization to another inhibitor such as mitogen-activated protein kinase (MAPK) 1/2 inhibitor, SRC family kinases inhibitor, WEE1 inhibitor, and antimitotic potential (Fig. 20.2) (Chen et al., 2012).

Herbal medicine commonly known as botanical medicine comprises the use of parts of a plant or whole plant to treat a life-threatening disease. Ayurvedic, homeopathic, as well as naturopathic medicines, use the phytochemicals presents in the herb/plant. Different parts of the plant such as seeds, leaves, stems, bark, roots, and flowers have been used in natural medicine. *Withania somnifera* commonly known as ashwagandha, a prevailing herb used in India, Middle East, and some parts of North Africa since more than two millennia.

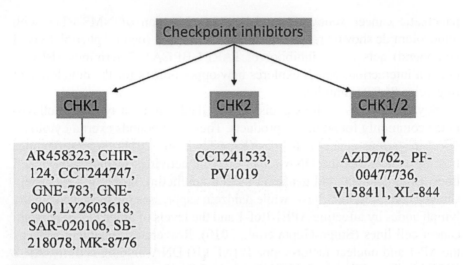

FIGURE 20.2   CHK2 or CHK1 inhibitors as radiosensitizing and/or chemosensitizing agents.

20.5   CLASSIFICATION OF *WITHANIA SOMNIFERA*

Kingdom: Plantae
Subkingdom: Tracheobionta
Superdivision: Spermatophyta
Division: Magnoliophyta
Class: Magnoliopsida
Subclass: Rosidae
Order: Solanales
Family: Solanaceae
Genus: *Withania*
Species: *somnifera*

20.6   PHYTOCONSTITUENTS PRESENT IN *W. SOMNIFERA*

Most of the withanolide class of compound, flavonoids, and many more active principles present in the root were presented in Figure 20.3. Steroidal lactones or withanolides provides earthy odor and flavor of *W. somnifera*. Some of the other alkaloids present in *W. somnifera* are somniferine, somnine, somniferinine, withananine, pseudo-withanine, tropino, pseudotropine, choline, cuscohygrine, isolettetierine, anaferine, anhydride, 3-alpha-gloyloxy tropane, and so forth.

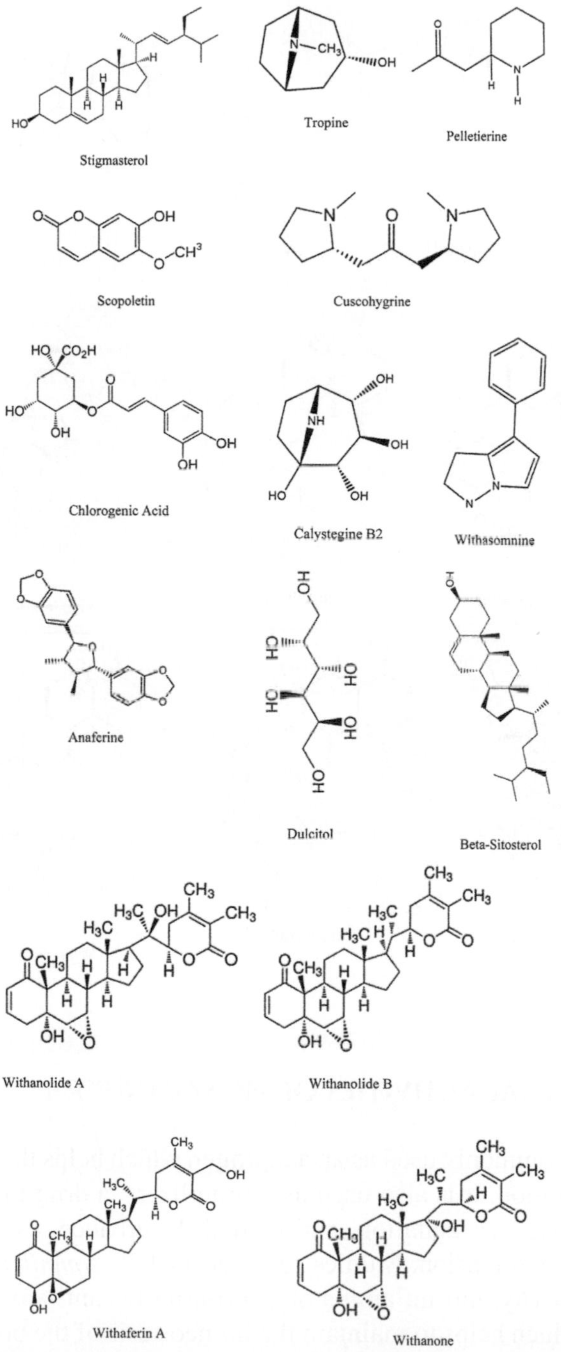

FIGURE 20.3 Structure of the phytoconstituents present in the *Withania somnifera*.

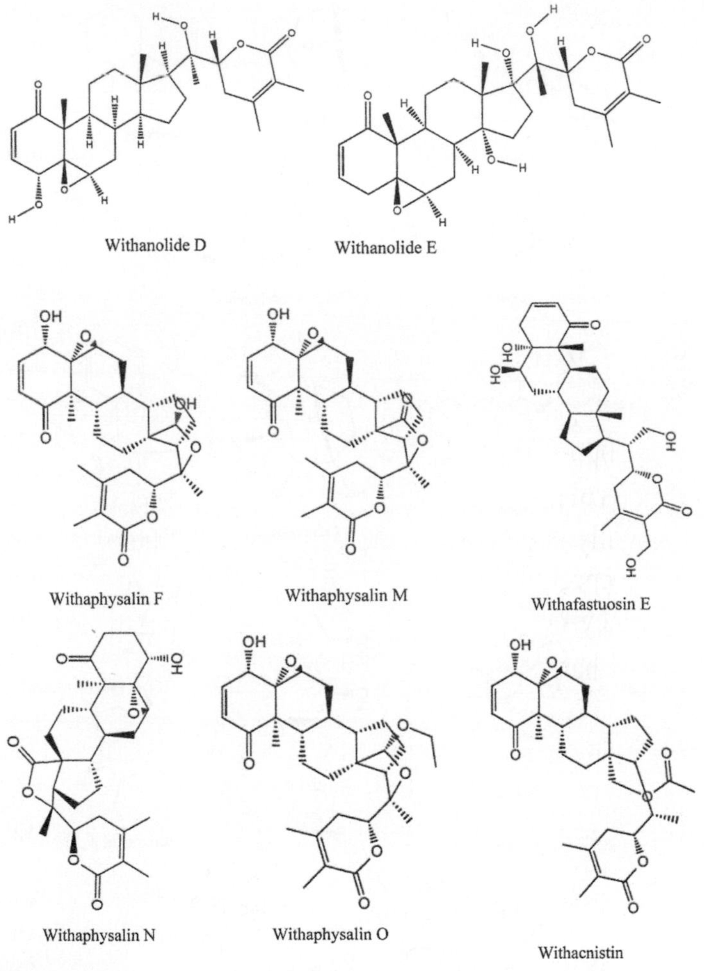

Withanolide D   Withanolide E

Withaphysalin F   Withaphysalin M   Withafastuosin E

Withaphysalin N   Withaphysalin O   Withacnistin

FIGURE 20.3   *(Continued)*

20.7   POTENTIAL ACTIVITIES OF *W. SOMNIFERA*

W. somnifera commonly used as an adaptogen which helps the body to adopt the stress condition. It is also used as tranquilizers, a drug to overcome the tension, anxiety, fear, agitation, and mental disturbance, exactly to reduce anxiety states and tension. Studies reported that *W. somnifera* have potent antioxidant activity, anti-inflammatory, anti-arthritic, anti-anxiety calmative, anti-tussive which helps to maintain the homeostasis of the body. It nurtures the nervous system, responds anxiety and stress to encourage a peaceful state of mind. It develops and consolidates female reproductive and hormonal system. *W. somnifera* helps in the improvement of blood circulation, clears mucus, enhances metabolism, and stimulates the digestive system for proper digestion.

Apart from the all above properties, it has excellent chemoprevention activity. Chemoprevention is a type of approach to prevent/postpone the progressiveness of cancer using natural/synthetic drugs. Chemoprevention term was initially used by Dr. Michael B. Sporn during his study. Sporn et al. (1976) reported the natural forms of vitamin A/synthetic analogs have the potency to delay the cancer development. Till now much more phytochemical has been reported with chemopreventive activity against cancer cell lines and animal cancer model. Various dietary compounds such asisothiocyanates from cruciferous vegetables, polyphenols from green and black tea, and flavonoids from soybeans also possess noteworthy chemopreventive effects. *W. somnifera* also showed remarkable chemopreventive properties. In addition to this, the chemopreventive activity of *W. somnifera* extract may be due to its detoxifying and antioxidant activity. Numerous phytochemicals and *W. somnifera* modulates molecular basis of chemopreventive potential. *W. somnifera* regulates cellular signaling cascades facilitated by nuclear factor E2-related factor 2 (Nrf2), NF-kB, activator protein-1 (AP-1), cyclooxygenases-2 (COX-2), MAPKs, and inflammatory mediator-related pathways. In perspective of DNA repairs mechanism, these signaling cascades play a crucial role. Both proper cellular signaling and DNA repair escape the chance to develop cancer.

Besides the cellular signaling cascade, genomic instability also helps in the development of cancer. Genomic instability may be due to the attainment of mutations in tumor suppressor genes, oncogenes, and DNA repair genes (Heinen et al., 2002). A defect in the DNA repair pathways and cell cycle checkpoint controls also leads to the progression of cancer. Normally defects in the genome and in their machinery activate the DNA repair genes which help to maintain the cell development. To capture this beneficial point in the cancer cell, many of the studies showed remarkable output to combat cancer progression. In addition to this, several inhibitors have been developed such as poly(ADP-ribose) polymerase (PARP) inhibitors which target faults in double-strand break repair in breast cancer. Some of the other developed inhibitors for the apurinic/apyrimidinic endonuclease-1 (APE1), ataxia-telangiectasia mutated (ATM), DNA repair protein RecA homolog (RAD51), and DNAPK are listed in Table 20.4.

TABLE 20.4 Dietary Factors Involved in Histone Acetylation and DNA Damage Signaling.

Compound	Act as	Ultimately Results	Comments
EGCG, curcumin, Se, ITC, allium, I3C, genistein, parthenolide, quercetin	HDAC inhibitors	Alteration of histone code	-
Genistein	HAT activators	Alteration of histone code	-
EGCG, curcumin, anacardic acid	HAT inhibitors	Alteration of histone code	-
Resveratrol	SIRT activators	Alteration of histone code	-
Genistein	SIRT inhibitor	Alteration of histone code	-
EGCG, curcumin, resveratrol, Se, ITC, allium, I3C, genistein, parthenolide, quercetin, anacardic acid	Activation of gamma H2AX, Histone acetylation, ATM/ ATR, GADD, Chk1/2, Cdc25c, p53, KAP1	Sustained damage signaling which makes DNA sensitive to UV, IR, and chemotherapeutics	EGCG, curcumin, resveratrol, Se, ITC, allium, I3C, genistein, parthenolide, quercetin and anacardic acid helps in DNA damage
Curcumin, resveratrol, quercetin	Inhibition of DNA-PK, Ku70, 80, MTA1/NuRD, BRCA1/2, FA, HR, and NHEJ pathways	Defective DNA repair become sensitive to UV, IR, and chemotherapeutics	Curcumin, resveratrol, and quercetin are the repair inhibitor

20.8 *W. SOMNIFERA* AS POTENTIAL TARGET FOR CANCER

Both in vitro and in vivo model studies showed that *W. somnifera* holds high antitumorigenic properties. For the first time in 1967, researcher explores experimentally that the root of *W. somnifera* has potential to prevent the cell proliferation in vitro (Shohat et al., 1967). Two main components of the *W. somnifera* extract namely withaferin A and withanolide derivatives showed highest activity comparison to others. Different studies also reported the valuable properties of the other components of the *W. somnifera*. Different parts of the *W. somnifera* such as root, leaf, shoot, and stem showed note-worthy cancer-fighting properties (Yadav et al., 2010). Whole *W. somnifera* plant and especially active ingredient withaferin A have been shown as a very excellent hepato-protective agent (Jadeja et al., 2015).Withaferin A downregulates antiapoptotic protein Bcl-2 and initiates apoptosis (Rah et al., 2015). One of the earlier studies showed that leaf extract of *W. somnifera* prevents the tumor formation in nude mice subcutaneously injected with fibrosarcoma HT1080 cells (Widodo et al., 2007).Withanolides showed antiangiogenic effect both in vitro and in vivo (Mohan et al., 2004). Another study reported that *W. somnifera* as a potent inhibitor of angiogenesis in vascular endothelial growth factor (VEGF)-induced neovascularization model in vivo (Mathur et al., 2006). Computation approach and molecular docking studies clear that withaferin A directly binds to VEGF and inhibit angiogenesis (Saha et al., 2013). A study in pancreatic cancer showed that withaferin A bind HSP90 to inhibit its chaperone activity through an ATP-dependent mechanism (Yu et al., 2010).Withaferin A also has a strong potential to induce the oxidative stress facilitated by the reactive oxygen species generation (Grogan et al., 2013).Withaferin A directly binds with cysteine 179 residue of IKK-β which proves the anti-inflammatory potential of withaferin A through in inhibition of the NF-kB signaling (Heyninck et al., 2014).Withaferin A also has a capability to inhibit the COX-2 enzymes in different experimental models (Min et al., 2011).

20.9 IN SILICO STUDY

In this chapter, we reported first time the in silico approach to target DNA repair pathway proteins by phytochemical present in *W. somnifera*. The three-dimensional structure of the target receptor mismatch and errors repair (MGMT) (PDB ID: 1EH8), cell cycle checkpoint proteins (Chk1) (PDB ID: 2WMW), cell cycle checkpoint proteins (Chk2) (PDB ID: 3I6U), BER (APE1) (PDB ID: 3U8U) and BER (PARP1) (PDB ID: 3L3L) was downloaded from RCSB-protein data bank in.pdb format. The *W. somnifera* phytoconstituents and standard inhibitor structure of the target were retrieved from NCBI PubChem compounds database in.sdf format. Offline docking tool such as AutoDock Tools 1.5.6 (ADT) was used for to study the drug-protein interaction. Results of the docking studies are shown in Table 20.5. Table 20.6 shows the different ADMET properties of the *W. somnifera* constituents. ADMET properties of *W. somnifera* phytochemicals were retrieved from the PreADMET online server.

The interaction pattern of the *W. somnifera* lead phytochemicals and targeted DNA repair pathway proteins are shown in Figure 20.4. The interaction is depicted in the form of surface structure. PyMOL molecular visualization system was used for visualization of the interaction pattern in the drug-protein complex. Schematic representation of the different type of interactions (hydrogen bonds and hydrophobic interactions) among lead compounds and targeted proteins was developed using LigPlot+v.1.4.5 and results are depicted in Figure 20.5.

TABLE 20.5 Binding Energy of *Winthania somnifera* Phytoconstituents and Standard Inhibitors with Different ProteinsInvolved in DNA Repair Pathways.

S. No.	Withania Phytoconstituents	PubChem ID	G-Score for different proteins				
			MGMT	CHK1	CHK2	PARP1	APE1
1	Withanolide D	161671	−8.5	−9.8	−9.6	−10.5	−9.7
2	Withaferin A	265237	−8	−8.4	−9.5	−8.4	−9.1
3	Withanolide E	301751	−8	−9.1	−9.7	−10.8	−9.7
4	Withafastuosin E	387980	−7.8	−8.6	−8.7	−8.6	−7.9
5	Withasomnine	442877	−6.9	−7.1	−7	−7.7	−6.5
6	Wiyhaphysalin M	10096775	−8.7	−8.7	−9.7	−11.6	−9.9
7	Withaphysalin O	10436447	−7.9	−7.9	−9.8	−9.2	−9
8	Withanolide A	11294368	−8.6	−9.8	−9.6	−9.7	−9.5
9	Withaphysalin N	11752064	−8.6	−9.7	−9.8	−11.3	−10.1
10	Withanolide B	14236711	−8.9	−9.6	−10.1	−10.7	−9.6
11	Withanone	21679027	−8.1	−7.7	−10	−9.3	−9.5
12	Withaphysalin F	44566968	−8.2	−8.5	−10.4	−11.2	−9.7
13	Withacnistin	54606507	−7.5	−8	−8.2	−9	−9.4
Standard inhibitors							
14	O-6 benzylguanine	4578	−7.9	-	-	-	-
15	Caffeine	2519	-	−5.8	-	-	-
16	LY2606368	46700756	-	-	−7.6	-	-
17	AZD2461	44199317	-	-	-	−11.8	-
18	MLS000552981	698490	-	-	-	-	−7

MGMT: Mismatch and Errors Repair; Chk1: Cell cycle checkpoint proteins; Chk2: Cell cycle checkpoint proteins; APE1: BER; PARP1: BER.

TABLE 20.6 Molecular Drug Properties of *W. somnifera* Phytochemicals.

S. No.	Ligands	PubChem ID	Drug-likeness (Lipinski's rule of five)	BBB penetration	Mutagenicity (Ames test)	(HIA%)
1	Withanone	21679027	S	BBB⁻	NM	94.740
2	Withanolide B	14236711	S	BBB⁺	NM	96.650
3	Withaphysalin C	191450	S	BBB⁺	NM	95.003
4	Withaphysalin M	10096775	S	BBB⁺	NM	96.885
5	Withanolide A	11294368	S	BBB⁻	NM	94.740
6	Tropine	449293	S	BBB⁺	M	99.457
7	Anaferine	443143	S	BBB⁺	M	90.023
8	Withaferin A	265237	S	BBB⁺	NM	94.740
9	Withafastuosin E	387980	S	BBB⁻	NM	84.858
10	Scopoletin	5280460	S	BBB⁻	M	93.924
11	Withacnistin	54606507	S	BBB⁺	NM	97.473
12	Withaphysalin N	11752064	S	BBB⁺	NM	96.340

TABLE 20.6 *(Continued)*

S. No.	Ligands	PubChem ID	Drug-likeness (Lipinski's rule of five)	BBB penetration	Mutagenicity (Ames test)	(HIA%)
13	Cuscohygrine	441070	S	BBB⁺	M	100.00
14	Withanolide D	161671	S	BBB⁻	NM	94.739
15	Stigmasterol	5280794	S	BBB⁺	NM	100.00
16	Chlorogenic Acid	1794427	S	BBB⁺	M	20.427
17	Withanolide E	301751	S	BBB⁻	NM	90.403
18	Dulcitol	11850	S	BBB⁺	M	12.812
19	Withasomnine	442877	S	BBB⁺	M	100.00
20	Withaphysalin D	180584	S	BBB⁺	NM	97.376
21	Pelletierine	92987	S	BBB⁺	M	94.193
22	Beta-Sitosterol	222284	S	BBB⁺	NM	100.00
23	Withaphysalin O	10436447	S	BBB⁺	NM	97.525
24	Withaphysalin F	44566968	S	BBB⁺	NM	94.540
25	Calystegine B2	124434	S	BBB⁺	M	36.118

HIA: Human Intestinal Absorption; NM: non-mutagen; M: mutagen, BBB⁺: penetrable to Blood-Brain Barrier; BBB⁻: not penetrable to Blood–Brain Barrier; S: Suitable.

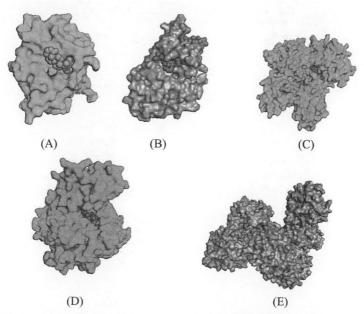

(A)   (B)   (C)

(D)   (E)

FIGURE 20.4 (See color insert.) Surface structure of the different DNA repair proteins and *W. somnifera* phytochemicals; (A) 1EH8 (cyan) and withanolide B (deep salmon), (B) 2WMW (smudge)-withanolide A (red) and D (slate), (C) 3I6U (lime green) and withaphysalin F (red),(D) 3L3L (green) and withaphysalin M (marine blue), (E) 3U8U (light teal), and withaphysalin N (orange).

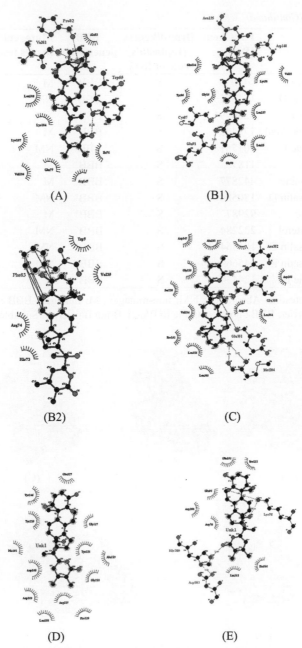

FIGURE 20.5   (See color insert.) Interaction of various amino acids of target proteins with *W. somnifera* phytochemicals and type of interaction; (A) withanolide B_1EH8, (B1) withanolide A_2 WMW, (B2) withanolide D_2WMW, (C) withphysalin F_3I6U, (D) withaphysalin M_3L3L, (E) withaphysalin N_3U8U.

ACKNOWLEDGMENT

PPK acknowledges financial support from University Grants Commission, India in the form of CSIR-UGC Junior Research fellowship. SK acknowledges Department of Science and Technology, India, for providing financial support in the form of DST-SERB Grant [EEQ/2016/000350]. SK also acknowledges the Central University of Punjab, Bathinda for providing necessary infrastructure facility.

KEYWORDS

- *Withania somnifera*
- cancer stem cells
- DNA repairs
- phytochemicals
- stemness modulation

REFERENCES

Cardnell, R. J.; Feng, Y.; Diao, L.; Fan, Y. H.; Masrorpour, F.; Wang, J.; Shen, Y.; Mills, G. B.; Minna, J. D.; Heymach, J. V.; Byers, L. A. Proteomic Markers of DNA Repair and PI3K Pathway Activation Predict Response to the PARP Inhibitor BMN 673 in Small Cell Lung Cancer. *Clin. Cancer Res.* **2013,** *19,* 6322–6328.

Carotenuto, F.; Albertini, M. C.; Coletti, D.; Vilmercati, A.; Campanella, L.; Darzynkiewicz, Z.; Teodori, L. How Diet Intervention via Modulation of DNA Damage Response Through MicroRNAs May have an Effect on Cancer Prevention and Aging, an in Silico Study. *Int. J. Mol. Sci.* **2016,** *17*(5), 752.

Chen, Y.; Chow, J. P.; Poon, R. Y. Inhibition of Eg5 Acts Synergistically with Checkpoint Abrogation in Promoting Mitotic Catastrophe. *Mol. Cancer Res.* **2012,** *10,* 626–635.

Coates, A. S.; Winer, E. P.; Goldhirsch, A. Tailoring Therapies – Improving the Management of Early Breast Cancer: St Gallen International Expert Consensus on the Primary Therapy of Early Breast Cancer. *Ann. Oncol.* **2015,** *26*(8), 1533–1546.

Colak, S.; Medema, J. P. Cancer Stem Cells – Important Players in Tumor Therapy Resistance. *FEBS J.* **2014,** *281*(21), 4779–4791.

Faragó, N.; Fehér, L. Z.; Kitajka, K.; Das, U. N.; Puskás, L. G. MicroRNA Profile of Polyunsaturated Fatty Acid Treated Glioma Cells Reveal Apoptosis-Specific Expression Changes. *Lipids Health Dis.* **2011,** *10*(1), 173.

Grogan, P. T.; Sleder, K. D.; Samadi, A. K.; Zhang, H.; Timmermann, B. N.; Cohen, M. S. Cytotoxicity of Withaferin A in Glioblastomas Involves Induction of an Oxidative

Stress-mediated Heat Shock Response While Altering Akt/mTOR and MAPK Signaling Pathways. *Invest. New Drugs* **2013**, *31*, 545–557.

Heinen, C. D.; Schmutte, C.; Fishel, R. DNA Repair and Tumorigenesis: Lessons from Hereditary Cancer Syndromes. *Cancer Biol. Ther.* **2002**, *1*, 477–485.

Heyninck, K.; Lahtela-Kakkonen, M.; Van der Veken, P.; Haegeman, G.; Vanden Berghe, W. Withaferin A inhibits NF-kappa B Activation by Targeting Cysteine 179 in IKK beta. *Biochem. Pharmacol.* **2014**, *91*, 501–509.

Jadeja, R. N.; Urrunaga, N. H.; Dash, S.; Khurana, S.; Saxena, N. K. Withaferin-A Reduces Acetaminophen Induced Liver Injury in Mice. *Biochem. Pharmacol.* **2015**, *97*, 122–132.

Kingsley, K.; Truong, K.; Low, E.; Hill, C. K.; Chokshi, S. B.; Phipps, D.; West, M. A.; Keiserman, M. A.; Bergman, C. J. Soy Protein Extract (SPE) Exhibits Differential in Vitro Cell Proliferation Effects in Oral Cancer and Normal Cell Lines. J. Diet Suppl. **2011**, *8*, 169–188.

Krichevsky, A. M.; Gabriely, G. MiR-21: a Small Multifaceted RNA. *J. Cell Mol. Med.* **2009**, *13*(1), 39–53.

Krishnakumar, R.; Kraus, W. L. The PARP Side of the Nucleus: Molecular Actions, Physiological Outcomes, and Clinical Targets. *Mol. Cell* **2010**, *39*, 8–24.

Kumazoe, M.; Sugihara, K.; Tsukamoto, S.; Huang, Y.; Tsurudome, Y.; Suzuki, T.; Suemasu, Y.; Ueda, N.; Yamashita, S.; Kim, Y.; Yamada, K.; Tachibana, H. 67-kDa Laminin Receptor Increases cGMP to Induce Cancer-Selective Apoptosis. *J. Clin. Invest.* **2013**, *123*, 787–799.

Lainchbury, M.; Matthews, T. P.; McHardy, T.; Boxall, K. J.; Walton, M. I.; Eve, P. D.; Hayes, A.; Valenti, M. R.; de Haven Brandon, A. K.; Box, G.; Aherne, G. W.; Reader, J. C.; Raynauld, F. I.; Eccles, S. A.; Garrett, M. D.; Collins, I. Discovery of 3-alkoxyamino-5-(pyridin-2-ylamino)pyrazine-2-Carbonitriles as Selective, Orally Bioavailable CHK1 Inhibitors. *J. Med. Chem.* **2012**, *55*, 10229–10240.

Ma, C. X.; Cai, S.; Li, S.; Ryan, C. E.; Guo, Z.; Schaiff, W. T.; Lin, L.; Hoog, J.; Goiffon, R. J.; Prat, A.; Aft, R. L.; Ellis, M. J.; Piwnica-Worms, H. Targeting Chk1 in p53-deficient triple-negative Breast Cancer is Therapeutically Beneficial in Human-in-mouse Tumor Models. *J. Clin. Invest.* **2012**, *122*, 1541–1552.

Mandal, C. C.; Ghosh-Choudhury, T.; Dey, N.; Choudhury, G. G.; Ghosh-Choudhury, N. miR-21 is Targeted by Omega-3 Polyunsaturated Fatty Acid to Regulate Breast Tumor CSF-1 Expression. *Carcinogenesis* **2012**, *33*, 1897–1908.

Mathur, R.; Gupta, S. K.; Singh, N.; Mathur, S.; Kochupillai, V.; Velpandian, T. Evaluation of the Effect of Withania Somnifera Root Extracts on Cell Cycle and Angiogenesis. *J. Ethnopharmacol.* **2006**, *105*, 336–341.

Min, K. J.; Choi, K.' Kwon, T. K. Withaferin A Down-regulates Lipopolysaccharide-induced cyclooxygenase-2 Expression and PGE2 Production Through the Inhibition of STAT1/3 Activation in Microglial Cells. *Int. Immunopharmacol.* **2011**, *11*(1), 137–1142.

Mohan, R.; Hammers, H. J.; Bargagna-Mohan, P.; Zhan, X. H.; Herbstritt, C. J.; Ruiz, A.; Zhang, L.; Hanson, A. D.; Conner, B. P.; Rougas, J.; Pribluda, V. S. Withaferin A is a Potent Inhibitor of Angiogenesis. *Angiogenesis* **2004**, *7*, 115–122.

Moore, N.; Lyle, S. Quiescent, Slow-Cycling Stem Cell Populations in Cancer: a Review of the Evidence and Discussion of Significance. *J. Oncology* **2011**, 1–11.

Plaks, V.; Kong, N.; Werb, Z. The Cancer Stem Cell Niche: How Essential is the Niche in Regulating Stemness of Tumor Cells? *Cell Stem Cell.* **2015**, *16*(3), 225–238.

Rah, B.; Ur, R. R.; Nayak, D.; Yousuf, S. K.; Mukherjee, D.; Kumar, L. D.; Goswami, A. PAWR-mediated Suppression of BCL2 Promotes Switching of 3-azido Withaferin A (3-AWA)-induced Autophagy to Apoptosis in Prostate Cancer Cells. *Autophagy 11*, 314–331.

Ramos, A. A.; Azqueta, A.; Pereira-Wilson, C.; Collins, A. R. Polyphenolic Compounds from Salvia Species Protect Cellular DNA from Oxidation and Stimulate DNA Repair in Cultured Human Cells. *J. Agric. Food Chem.* **2010,** *58,* 7465–7471.

Saha, S.; Islamm, M. K.; Shilpi, J. A.; Hasan, S. Inhibition of VEGF a Novel Mechanism to Control Angiogenesis by Withania Somnifera's Key Metabolite Withaferin A. *In Silico Pharmacol.* **2013,** *1,* 11.

Scapagnini, G.; Colombrita, C.; Amadio, M.; D'Agata, V.; Arcelli, E.; Sapienza, M.; Quattrone, A.; Calabrese, V. Curcumin Activates Defensive Genes and Protects Neurons Against Oxidative Stress. *Antioxid. Redox Signaling* **2006,** *8,* 395–403.

Shammas, M.; Neri, P.; Koley, H.; Batchu, R. B.; Bertheau, R. C.; Munshi, V.; Prabhala, R.; Fulciniti, M.; Tai, Y. T.; Treon, S. P.; Goyal, R. K.; Anderson, K. C.; Munshi, N. C. Specific Killing of Multiple Myeloma Cells by (-)-epigallocatechin-3-gallate Extracted from Green Tea: Biologic Activity and Therapeutic Implications. *Blood* **2006,** *108,* 2804–2810.

Shohat, B.; Gitter, S.; Abraham, A.; Lavie, D. Antitumor Activity of Withaferin A (NSC-101088). *Cancer Chemother Rep.* **1967,** *51,* 271–276.

Siegel, R. L.; Miller, K. D.; Jemal, A. Cancer Statistics. *CA Cancer J. Clin.* **2016,** *66*(1), 7–30.

Singh-Gupta, V.; Zhang, H.; Yunker, C. K.; Ahmad, Z.; Zwier, D.; Sarkar, F. H.; Hillman, G. G. Daidzein Effect on Hormone Refractory Prostate Cancer in Vitro and in Vivo Compared to Genistein and Soy Extract: Potentiation of Radiotherapy. *Pharm. Res.* **2010,** *27,* 1115–1127.

Sporn, M. B.; Dunlop, N. M.; Newton, D. L.; Smith, J. M. Prevention of Chemical Carcinogenesis by Vitamin A and Its Synthetic Analogs (retinoids). *Fed. Proc.* **1976,** *35,* 1332–1338.

Tachibana, H.; Koga, K.; Fujimura, Y.; Yamada, K. A. Receptor for Green tea Polyphenol EGCG. *Nat. Struct Mol. Biol.* **2004,** *11,* 380–381.

Tili, E.; Michaille, J. J.; Alder, H.; Alder, H.; Volinia, S.; Delmas, D.; Latruffe, N.; Croce, C. M. Resveratrol Modulates the Levels of MicroRNAs Targeting Genes Encoding Tumor Suppressors and Effectors of TGFβ Signaling Pathway in SW480 Cells. *Biochem. Pharmacol.* **2010,** *80*(12), 2057–2065.

Tili, E.; Michaille, J. J.; Gandhi, V.; Plunkett, W.; Sampath, D.; Calin, G. A. MiRNAs and Their Potential for use Against Cancer and Other Diseases. *Future Oncol.* **2007,** *3*(5), 521–537.

Widodo, N.; Kaur, K.; Shrestha, B. G.; Takagi, Y.; Ishii, T.; Wadhwa, R.; Kaul, S. C. Selective Killing of Cancer Cells by Leaf Extract of Ashwagandha Identification of a Tumor-inhibitory Factor and the First Molecular Insights to Its Effect. *Clin. Cancer Res.* **2007,** *13,* 2298–2306.

Wu, J.; Izpisua Belmonte, J. C. Stem Cells: A Renaissance in Human Biology Research. *Cell.* **2016,** *165*(7), 1572–1585.

Yadav, B.; Bajaj, A.; Saxena, M.; Saxena, A. K. In Vitro Anticancer Activity of the Root, Stem and Leaves of Withania Somnifera against Various Human Cancer Cell Lines. Indian. *J. Pharm. Sci.* **2010,** *72,* 659–663.

Yu, Y.; Hamza, A.; Zhang, T.; Gu, M.; Zou, P.; Newman, B.; Li, Y.; Gunatilaka, A. A.; Zhan, C. G.; Sun, D. Withaferin A targets Heat Shock Protein 90 in Pancreatic Cancer Cells. *Biochem. Pharmacol.* **2010,** *79,* 542–551.

Zhang, W.; Bai, W. MiR-21 Suppresses the Anticancer Activities of Curcumin by Targeting PTEN Gene in Human Non-small Cell Lung Cancer A549 cells. *Clin. Transl. Oncol.* **2014,** *16,* 708–713.

CHAPTER 21

TARGETING CANCER CELL CARBOHYDRATE METABOLISM BY PHYTOCHEMICALS

SWASTIKA DASH, PREM PRAKASH KUSHWAHA, and
SHASHANK KUMAR*

*School of Basic and Applied Sciences, Department of Biochemistry
and Microbial Sciences, Central University of Punjab, Bathinda,
Punjab 151001, India, Tel.: +91 9335647413*

*Corresponding author. E-mail: shashankbiochemau@gmail.com,
shashank.kumar@cupb.edu.in
ORCID: https://orcid.org/0000-0002-9622-0512*

ABSTRACT

Carbohydrate metabolism in cancer cells is linked to the "Warburg Effect" which states that, under aerobic conditions, cancer cells metabolize approximately 10-fold more glucose to lactate in a given time than normal cells; typically altered glycolytic pathway regulation. This has made the blocking of glycolytic pathway enzymes, a fascinating strategy to find treatment for cancer. This chapter addresses in a comprehensive manner the main glycolytic enzymes accounting for high-rate glycolysis in cancer cells. In addition, highlights of inhibitors that can be used to target the particular enzymes to decrease proliferation have also been done. Furthermore, besides the known inhibitors, molecular docking of certain methylated flavonoids was performed with the proteins (isozymes of carbohydrate metabolic pathway enzymes) to find the lead inhibitors. The compounds 2-(3,4-dimethylphenyl)-5,7-dimethyl-4H-chromen-4-one and 6-hydroxy-3,5,7,8-tetramethoxy-2-(3,4,5-trimethoxyphenyl)-4H-chromen-4-one showed potential binding against lactate dehydrogenase A and enolase 2 enzymes, respectively.

21.1   INTRODUCTION

The formation, breakdown, and interconversion of carbohydrates in living organisms are known as carbohydrate metabolism. Since ages, carbohydrates have played a significant role in being the most essential component of the body by providing the requisite energy for different metabolic purposes. Digestion breaks down the ingested complex carbohydrates to form simpler quintessential products such as glucose, fructose, and galactose. Ultimately, glucose serves to be the major product of carbohydrate breakdown which channeled through various pathways to provide energy to the cells or gets stored as glycogen in the mammalian body. To be precise, the way of glucose into the cells is basically mediated by facilitated diffusion through a family of hexose transporters termed as glucose transporter (GLUT) (1–4) transporters. The glucose that enters undergoes various enzymatic reactions to produce pyruvate as the major product while storing energy released during this process as adenosine triphosphate (ATP) and nicotinamide adenine dinucleotide (NADH) by the process of glycolysis. This glycolysis occurs mainly in the cytosol of the cell. The pyruvate thus produced, under anaerobic conditions gets converted into lactate and production of further energy. While in the presence of oxygen, the pyruvate is converted to acetyl-CoA molecules. These acetyl-coenzymeA molecules then enter the citric acid cycle (tricarboxylic acid cycle [TCA] cycle or Kreb's cycle) where large (most) of the ATP molecules are generated through a number of enzymatic reactions. Ultimately, the NADH and CO_2 produced by TCA cycle are channelized to the oxidative phosphorylation (electron transport) pathway which involves various enzymes and uses the chemical energy to produce ATP through the involvement of ATP synthase. This occurs mainly in the mitochondria. The pentose phosphate pathway is a different method of oxidizing glucose where the intermediate of glycolytic pathway (glucose-6-phosphate) serves as the precursor. This is divided into oxidative and non-oxidative phases and leads to the release of NADPH and pentose (5-carbon sugars) as well as ribose-5-phosphate (major precursor of nucleotide metabolism).

21.2   CARBOHYDRATE METABOLISM: ANTICANCER TARGETS

Carbohydrate metabolism in normal cells and cancer cells has shown remarkable differences to be studied upon, in general. In normal cells, where glucose metabolism takes place through glycolysis under anaerobic conditions; in cancer cells, glucose metabolism is marked by accelerated aerobic glycolysis (Zhao et al., 2013). The discovery of high rates of aerobic glycolysis in cancer cells by Otto Warburg in late 1920s led to the assumption that respiration, through the process of oxidative phosphorylation is impaired or damaged in cancer cells. This phenomenon was termed to be "Warburg effect" (Hay, 2016). Since cancer cells need to produce enough energy to survive when supplies and waste disposals are limited and to divert metabolic intermediates from energy production to the biosynthetic pathways supporting cell proliferation; enhanced aerobic glycolysis takes place to fuel sufficient energy to the tumor cells (Calvaresi and Hergenrother, 2013). There occur various changes in glucose metabolism in cancer cells, mainly in the glycolytic pathway, through the involvement of a number of committed steps in the pathway. The description of various committed pathways is henceforth described.

21.2.1 INHIBITORS OF GLUCOSE TRANSPORTERS

GLUT1 (Fig. 21.1) belongs to the GLUT family of transporters required for glucose shuttling across membranes. They have a high affinity for glucose and thus ensure sufficient glucose uptake by the cells (Shibuya et al., 2015). Usually, there are 14 GLUTs isoforms, with different affinities for glucose. But GLUT1 tends to be overexpressed in many cancers because of their nature of irreversibility and high affinity for glucose. Overexpression of GLUT1 in various types of cancer has provided a strong cause for the anticancer use of GLUT inhibitors. Studies have led to the finding of 2-deoxyglucose as a GLUT inhibitor and as an anti-cancer drug. Although individually its efficacy has failed to give results, it has proven efficacy in normalizing human osteosarcoma and non-small cell lung cancers to adriamycin and paclitaxel. A natural flavonoid and a competitive GLUT inhibitor, Phloretin has also been studied to retard tumor and cancer cell growth. Silybin, an additional natural flavonoid has recently been revealed as a GLUT inhibitor and is undergoing clinical trials for prostate cancer. The compound Cytochalasin B and Forskolin (naturally occurring) which binds at the GLUT1 sugar export site or close to it are well known bound inhibitors of human GLUT1 (Pinksofsky et al., 2000). Cytochalasin B is a mycotoxin that is cell permeable and displays a macrocyclic ring structure (Kapoor et al., 2016). Two more inhibitors are also studied, that is, GLUT-inhibitor 1 and GLUT-inhibitor 2 based on a phenylalanine-amide core scaffold.

A novel small molecule, WZB117, has been studied to kill lung and breast cancer cells by inhibiting GLUT1-mediated glucose transport

(Ojelabi et al., 2016). WZB117 inhibits uptake of the non-metabolizable sugar, 3-o-methylglucose by red blood cells and is a competitive inhibitor of GLUT1-mediated zero-trans sugar uptake and exchange transport but is a non-competitive inhibitor of zero-trans exit (Liu et al., 2012). This molecule binds at or near the exofacial sugar-binding site of GLUT1. Further, a small molecule inhibitor, fasentin has been studied to inhibit the intracellular domain of GLUT1 and thereby restricting glucose uptake by GLUT1. Thus, the inhibition of function or expression of GLUT1 can be considered a way of exclusively targeting cancer cells that rely upon a high rate of uptake of glucose for anaerobic glycolysis (Lu et al., 2015).

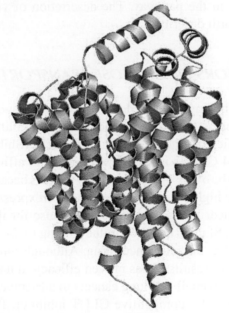

FIGURE 21.1 **(See color insert.)** Structure of glucose transporter 1 protein (PDB=4PYP)[1].

21.2.2 INHIBITORS OF HEXOKINASE 2

Hexokinase-2 (Fig. 21.2) belongs to the hexokinase family of enzymes that control the first rate-limiting step of glycolysis. They perform the phosphorylation of glucose to glucose-6-phosphate which involves the transfer of phosphate from ATP. The phosphorylated form of glucose, that

---

[1]PDB=4PYP (Protein Data Bank = Entry 4PYP).

is, glucose-6-phosphate gets entrapped inside the cell and fuels glycolysis as well as pentose phosphate pathway (Porporato et al., 2011). Usually, there are four main hexokinases isoforms in mammalian cells – HK1, HK2, HK3, and HK4. All are high-affinity hexokinases, but HK1 and HK2 have the unique ability to bind to mitochondria in a voltage-dependent anion channel (VDAC) – dependent manner. HK2 is a hypoxia-inducible factor-1 (HIF-1) target gene product and exists bound to the outer mitochondrial membrane with VDAC channel as compared to other isoforms (Evans et al., 2008). This particular presence of HK2-VDAC interaction provides preferential access to ATP (permeating VDAC). This also prevents the negative feedback inhibition by glucose-6-phosphate, which makes sure that enough glucose is utilized by tumor cells expressing mitochondria-bound HK2 (Mathupala et al., 2006). The interaction of HK2 and VDAC further interferes with the binding of pro-apoptotic proteins to VDAC which would otherwise have had triggered apoptosis. Thus, HK2 binding to VDAC offers both metabolic advantages as well as protection against apoptosis. The overexpression of HK2 has been found in many cancer types compared with normal tissues and cells (Wang et al., 2016).

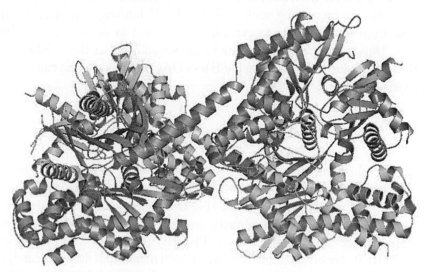

FIGURE 21.2 **(See color insert.)** Structure of hexokinase 2 protein (PDB=2NZT).

Since HK2 has been widely characterized to upregulate glycolysis and a repressor of apoptosis in numerous types of cancers; efforts have been made to study its specific inhibitors and target for anticancer drug discovery. Lonidamine has been studied widely as a specific inhibitor of mitochondria-bound hexokinase (Lin et al., 2016). The current leading compound is 3-bromopyruvate (3-BP), an alkylating agent reacting with cysteine residues in proteins. It is thus considered to be an HK inhibitor and exerts antitumor activities (including metastatic suppression) in quite a lot of types of cancers. Moreover, it may cause unavoidable side effects since it may affect multiple enzymes and is unstable. It also exhibits restriction of glycolysis at a high concentration only (Zhang et al., 2014). Metformin, a commonly used anti-diabetic drug and 2-deoxyglucose are also reported to be potent HK2 inhibitors. A decarboxylase inhibitor (Food and Drug Administration [FDA]-approved) that is usually used for the treatment of Parkinson's disease, benserazide, is also reported to hold back tumor growth by inhibiting hexokinase 2 (Kochel et al., 2017). It has been found in studies that the glucose-binding pocket of benserazide is occupied by its pyrogallol moiety through H-bond interactions and adopted a similar conformation of the substrate glucose and thus competitively inhibits it. The identification of benserazide as an HK2 inhibitor will definitely pave way for the development of more Benz analogs as novel antitumor agents (Li et al., 2017). Moreover, the azole derivative analogs such as clotrimazole and bifonazole that perform by interfering with an HK-VDAC binding that releases the enzyme from mitochondria to cytosol can be used as an inhibitor of HK activity. Thus, to suppress glycolysis in cancer cells either direct inhibition of HK2 can be done or disrupting the HK-VDAC interaction that can induce apoptosis.

21.2.3 INHIBITORS OF PHOSPHOFRUCTOKINASE 2

Fructose-2,6-bisphosphate is an important regulatory point of glycolysis acting as an allosteric activator of PFK1, one of the rate-controlling enzymes of glycolysis. Fructose-2,6-bisphosphate (F-2,6-BP) is produced from fructose-6-phosphate by a family of homodimeric enzymes known as 6-phosphofructo-2-kinase/fructose-2,6-bisphosphatases (PFKFB) (Fig. 21.3) (Porpora et al., 2011). PFKFBs are bifunctional enzymes which means that they can catalyze either the ATP-dependent phosphorylation of F6P to F2,6BP (PFK2 activity) or the de-phosphorylation of F2,6BP to F6P (FBPase activity). The various isoforms of PFKFB comprise of four members, that is, PFKFB1, PFKFB2, PFKFB3, and PFKFB4. PFKFB1, PFKFB2, PFKFB4 show the same amount of PFK2 and FBPase activity whereas PFKFB3 has high PFK2 activity and almost negligible FBPase activity. PFKFB3 gene is a target of HIF-1 and thus is seen as a major induction in hypoxia. Hypoxic stimulation of PFK2 activity of PFKFB3 is henceforth exaggerated through phosphorylation of a serine residue at position 462 of human sequence, a process involving AMP-activated protein kinase. Thus, PFKFB3 is considered to be highly expressed in many human tumors and sustains high-rate glycolysis (Hay, 2016). Till now, 3-(3-pyridinyl)-1-(4-pyridinyl)-2-propen-1-one (3PO) has been studied to be the only specific inhibitor of PFKFB3. It has been studied and found to decrease the concentration of Fructose-2,6-bisphosphate in tumor cells, leading to less glucose uptake and suppression of growth of cancer cells. However, there are clinical trials going on where there have been studies where, treatment with lapatinib, an FDA-approved HER2 inhibitor (human epidermal growth factor receptor-2), also decreased PFKFB3 expression and thus glucose metabolism in HER2$^+$ cells (O'Neal et al., 2016). Studies have also been done to find PFK15 (1-(4-pyridinyl)-3-(2-quinolinyl)-2-propen-1-one), as an inhibitor of PFKFB3, against gastric cancer. Results showed that PFK15 retarded the proliferation, leading to cell cycle arrest by blocking signaling pathways. Thus, PFK15 has been established to be a promising anticancer drug by targeting aerobic glycolysis (Zhu et al., 2016).

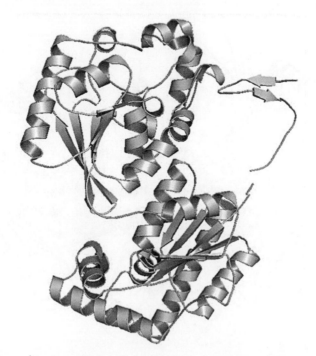

FIGURE 21.3 Structure of phosphofructokinase 2 protein (PDB=2AXN).

21.2.4 INHIBITORS OF PYRUVATE KINASE M2

Pyruvate kinase (PK) (Fig. 21.4) is an enzyme of the glycolytic pathway which catalyzes a rate-limiting step of glycolysis. The de-phosphorylation of phosphoenolpyruvate (PEP) into pyruvate to produce ATP is accomplished by this enzyme (Porpora et al., 2011). There are four PK isoforms in mammalian cells – PKM1, PKM2, PKR, and PKL which are encoded by two separate genes. The same gene, PKLR, encodes PKR and PKL through the use of alternative promoters. PKR expression is restricted to red blood cells, whereas PKL is expressed at elevated levels in the liver and to some extent in the kidney. PKM1 and PKM2 are encoded by another gene, PKM, through alternative splicing. Selection of isozymes causes the uncontrolled proliferation observed in cancer. PKM2 reexpression and down-regulation of PKM1 is associated with tumorigenesis. The active PKs are tetramers, whereas PKM1 is a constitutively active tetramer, the tetrameric active form of PKM2 is allosterically regulated by various metabolites. High-yield ATP production is provided by the tetrameric

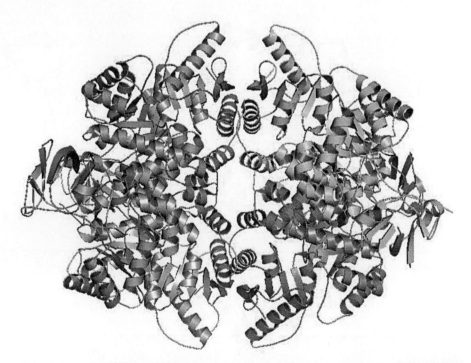

FIGURE 21.4   **(See color insert.)** Structure of pyruvate kinase M2 protein (PDB=3GQY).

configuration, whereas it's dimeric conformation allows the intermediates of glycolysis to be channelized toward biosynthesis. The tetrameric form is elevated by the accumulation of the glycolytic intermediate F-1,6-BP and by the biosynthetic byproduct serine. The phosphorylation of tyrosine 105 in response to several oncogenic tyrosine kinases further accelerates the formation of dimmers. The transfer of a non-ATP-producing phosphate to a histidine residue of phosphoglycerate mutase plays a critical role in controlling the accumulation of PEP. Most cancer cells express PKM2, thereby achieving a fine balance between promoting ATP production or cell proliferation (Iqbal et al., 2014). Moreover, the glycolysis and tumor angiogenesis is further promoted by PKM2 cooperation with HIF-1 that transactivates the associated genes (Hay, 2016).

Since a major role is played by PKM2 in cancer cell metabolism and proliferation, development of a potent anticancer drug that targets PKM2 may be of great significance. Inhibitors of PKM2 are based on the fact that proliferating cells are highly dependent on energy and lessening the activity of PKM2 would inhibit energy regeneration (Wong et al., 2013). Natural products, such as Shikonin and its analog alkannin, belonging to a family of necroptotic inducers, displayed potent and promising selective inhibition of PKM2 by not inhibiting PKM1 and PKL. Ribonucleic acid (RNA) interference targeting PKM2 has also been studied to induce growth and caspase-dependent apoptosis in numerous cancer cell lines. Moreover, the peptide aptamers, which inhibit PKM2 and not the homologous PKM1, has been seen to induce a significant decrease in cell proliferation and size under conditions where glucose metabolism is disrupted. An enormous library of diverse compounds was screened to ultimately identify two small molecule inhibitors (water soluble) which have potential to inhibit PKM2 versus PKM1 selectivity. Both molecules were reported to presumably block the allosteric F-1,6-BP-binding site of PKM2 absent in PKM1. Numerous PKM2 inhibitors have been established, comprising TT-232, VK3, VK5, and compound 3. Compound 3 possess the ability to cause PKL inhibition, whereas VK3 and VK5 selectively inhibit PKM2 to reduce glycolysis in cancer cells (Heiden et al., 2011). Recently, one of the studies reported that a natural compound namely oleanolic acid, found widely in plants which shows its excellent anticancer properties by constraining aerobic glycolysis process by shifting PKM2 to PKM1. Besides energy, cells having proliferative potential strictly depend on the cell building blocks synthesis that is favored by less active dimeric PKM2. Thus, a tetrameric form of PKM2 activation (highly active) may also inhibit cell proliferation because of the total deficiency of precursors for the synthesis of cell building blocks. Two representative compounds, namely thieno (3,2b) pyrrole (3,2d) pyridazinone and substituted N, N-diarylsulfonamide, were found to be potent activators of PKM2. Both the compounds behave as cell permeable analogs. These compounds also resemble the Fructose bisphosphate-allosteric activator of PKM2. Activation of PKM2 regulates both metabolism of cancer cell (in vitro) and tumor growth (xenograft). Another study showed that 2-oxo-N-aryl-1,2,3,4-tetrahydroquinoline-6-sulfonamides also activated PKM2 for the reduction of aerobic glycolysis. Altogether, various studies signify that PKM2 is an effective target for curative approaches. However, the only problem lies in the existence of PKM2 in normal cells also and the metabolic escape it undergoes (Dong et al., 2016). Nonetheless, the curative activation of PKM2 seems promising in restricting the metabolism of proliferative cells in cancer.

21.2.5   INHIBITORS OF LACTATE DEHYDROGENASE A

Pyruvate is at the central point between different metabolic pathways. It is the product of glycolysis, the product of oxidation of malate in proliferating cells, the main component of the Kerb's cycle, the alanine precursor in a reversible transamination reaction (nitrogen donated by glutamate) and the substrate producing lactate by redox reaction. The latter reaction that involves the simultaneous reduction of pyruvate and the oxidation of NADH into NAD^+, allows the sufficient availability of the NAD^+ pool necessary for self-sufficiency of glycolysis. NAD^+ is definitely mandatory for the oxidative phosphorylation of glyceraldehyde-3-phosphate into 1,3-diphosphoglycerate by GAPDH. Reduction of pyruvate into lactate also allows glycolytic cells to maintain the levels of pyruvate low enough to avoid cell death (Porpora et al., 2011). This reversible reaction is catalyzed by the LDH family of tetrameric enzymes. Lactate Dehydrogenases (LDHs) are encoded by four separate genes (LDHA, LDHB, LDHC, and LDHD). The two highly expressed isozymes, LDHA (Fig. 21.5) and LDHB can form either homotetramers or heterotetramers. LDHA has a higher affinity for pyruvate and LDHB has a higher affinity for lactate; LDHA favors the forward reaction and LDHB favors the reverse reaction. Thus, LDHA is the predominantly expressed LDH in cancer cells (Hay, 2016).

By restoring the NAD^+ pool required for the GAPDH reaction, LDHA plays an essential role in the accentuation of high-rate glycolysis and is therefore recognized as a therapeutic target for cancer (Allison et al., 2014). Inhibition of LDHA expression by using RNA interference impairs tumor initiation, maintenance, and progression.

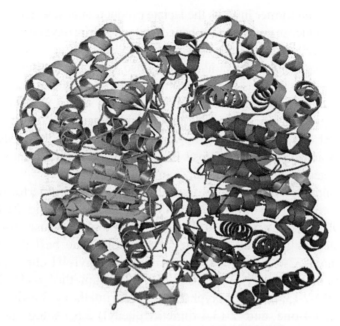

FIGURE 21.5 (See color insert.) Structure of lactate dehydrogenase A protein (PDB=4AJP).

3-dihydroxy-6-methyl-7-(phenylmethyl)-4-propylnaphthalene-1-carboxylic acid (FX11), a selective inhibitor (competitive in nature) has been recognized through screening a varied number of compounds obtained from gossypol, a natural compound and a known malarial LDH inhibitor. FX11 induced oxidative stress and cell senescence in vitro, which led to progression inhibition of human lymphoma and pancreatic cancer xenografts in vivo. Recently, N-Hydroxy-2-carboxy-substituted indole compounds have been recognized as LDHA-specific inhibitors (Miao et al., 2013). Gossypol (AT-101), a natural product found in cottonseed, is a non-selective inhibitor of LDH that blocks the binding of NADH (Fang et al., 2017). However, gossypol also inhibits glyceraldehyde 3-phosphate dehydrogenase (GAPDH), which is an NAD$^+$-dependent enzyme, and thus its antitumor activity may also include the inhibition of GAPDH. Another compound was identified which constraints both LDH isoforms (LDHA and LDHB), initiates apoptosis of hepatocellular carcinoma cell lines and destructs proliferation of breast cancer cells at rather high concentration, namely galloflavin. Other potent and selective LDHA inhibitor include GSK 2837808A (3-[{3-(cyclopropylamino) sulfonyl-7 (2,4-dimethoxy-5-pyrimidinyl)-4-quinolinyl] amino)-5-(3,5-difluorophenoxy) benzoic acid and NHI-2 (methyl 1-hydroxy-6-phenyl-4-(trifluoromethyl)-1H-indole-2 carboxylate). The former inhibits the lactate production in selected cancer cell lines, reduces glucose uptake and enhances mitochondrial oxygen consumption in carcinoma cells whereas the later inhibits cell growth and lactate production in HeLa cells (Doherty et al., 2013). Also, oxamate (sodium oxamate), an inhibitor of LDHA, has been identified to be a potential anticancer agent (Yang et al., 2014). Oxamate treatment of cells has shown to induce protective autophagy in gastric cancer cell lines. Inhibition of LDH by oxamate also caused G2/M cell cycle arrest through downregulation of the CDK1/cyclin B1 pathway and supported apoptosis through augmentation of mitochondrial reactive oxygen species generation (Zhao et al., 2015).

Beside already known inhibitors of LDHA, we hereby performed an in silico study to find out some potent methylated flavonoids (Fig. 21.6) active against LDHA enzyme. Various offline and online tools were used for docking study (protein, ligand and structure preparation). The best doc score of four flavonoids 2-(3,4-dimethylphenyl)-5,7-dimethyl-4H-chromen-4-one; 2-(3,4-dimethoxyphenyl)-3-hydroxy-5,6,7,8-tetramethoxy-4H-chromen-4-one; (2S)-2-(3,4-dimethoxyphenyl)-5,6,7-trimethoxy-3,4-dihydro-2H-1-benzopyran-4-one and 2-(3,4-dimethylphenyl)-5,6,7,8-tetramethyl-4H-chromen-4-one were -7.14, -6.94, -7.04 and -6.69, respectively. Interaction pattern of these methylated flavonoids and the target protein is depicted in Figure 21.7.

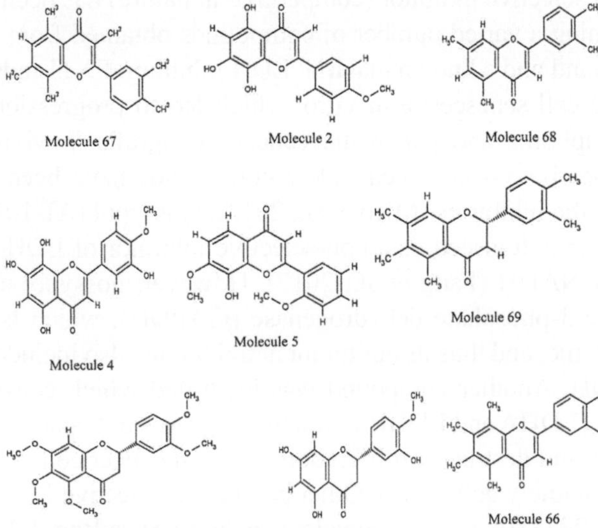

Molecule 67   Molecule 2   Molecule 68

Molecule 4   Molecule 5   Molecule 69

Molecule 64   Molecule 65   Molecule 66

FIGURE 21.6 Structure of methylated flavonoids used as anticancer phytochemicals targeting cancer cell carbohydrate metabolism pathway.

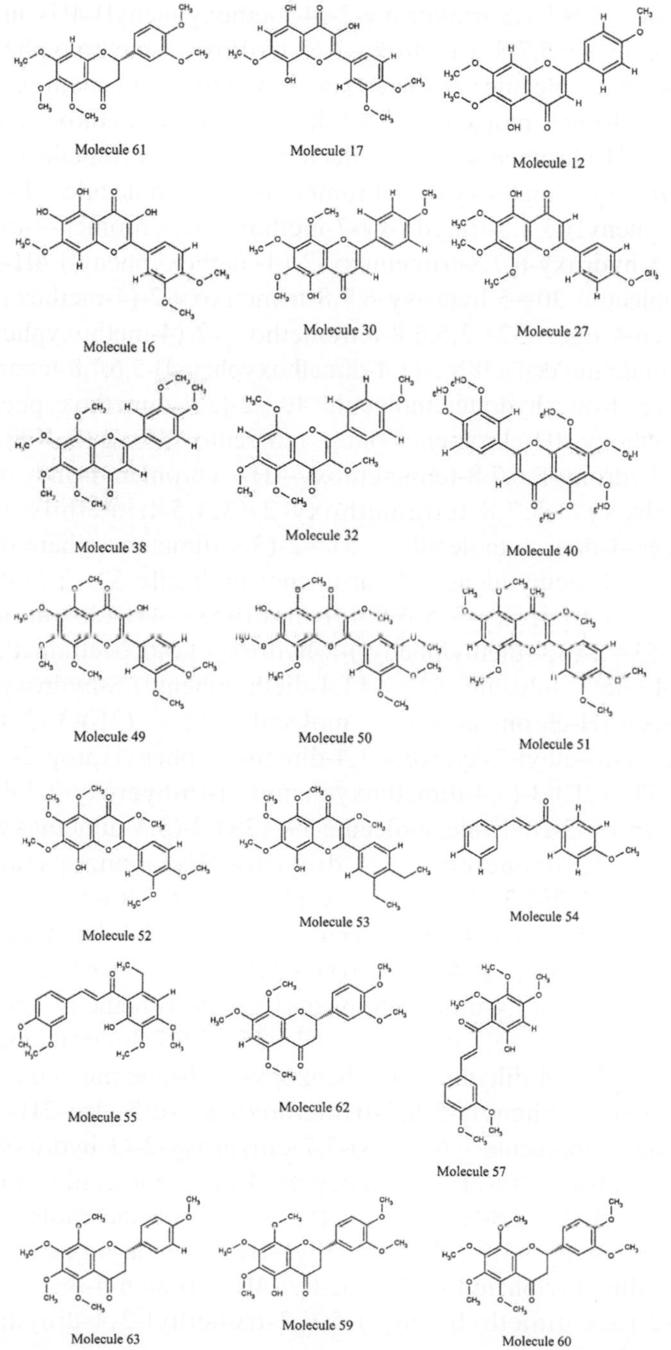

Molecule 61

Molecule 17

Molecule 12

Molecule 16

Molecule 30

Molecule 27

Molecule 38

Molecule 32

Molecule 40

Molecule 49

Molecule 50

Molecule 51

Molecule 52

Molecule 53

Molecule 54

Molecule 55

Molecule 62

Molecule 57

Molecule 63

Molecule 59

Molecule 60

FIGURE 21.6 *(Continued)*

Molecule   2 = 5,7,8-trihydroxy-2-(4-methoxyphenyl)-4H-chromen-4-one; molecule   4 = 5,7,8-trihydroxy-2-(3-hydroxy-4-methoxyphenyl)-4H-chromen-4-one; molecule 5 = 8-hydroxy-7-methoxy-2-(2-methoxyphenyl)-4H-chromen-4-one; molecule   12 = 5-hydroxy-6,7-dimethoxy-2-(4-methoxyphenyl)-4H-chromen-4-one; molecule 16 = 2-(3,4-dimethoxyphenyl)-3,5,6-trihydroxy-7-methoxy-4H-chromen-4-one;   molecule   17 = 2-(3,4-dimethoxyphenyl)-3,5,8-trihydroxy-7-methoxy-4H-chromen-4-one; molecule 27 = 5-hydroxy-6,7,8-trimethoxy-2-(4-methoxyphenyl)-4H-chromen-4-one; molecule 30 = 5-hydroxy-6,7,8-trimethoxy-2-(4-methoxyphenyl)-4H-chromen-4-one, 32 = 3,5,6,8-tetramethoxy-2-(4-methoxyphenyl)-4H-chromen-4-one; molecule38 = 2-(3,4-dimethoxyphenyl)-5,6,7,8-tetramethoxy-4H-chromen-4-one hydrate; molecule 40 = 2-(3,4-dimethoxyphenyl)-5,6,7,8-tetramethoxy-4H-chromen-4-one; molecule 49 = 2-(3,4-dimethoxyphenyl)-3-hydroxy-5,6,7,8-tetramethoxy-4H- chromen-4-one; molecule 50 = 6-hydroxy-3,5,7,8-tetramethoxy-2-(3,4,5-trimethoxyphenyl)-4H-chromen-4-one;   molecule   51 = 2-(3,4-dimethoxyphenyl)-3,5,6,8-tetramethoxy-4-methylidene-4H-chromene; molecule 52 = 2-(3,4-dimethoxyphenyl)-8-hydroxy-3,5,6,7-tetramethoxy-4H-chromen-4-one; molecule 53 = 2-(3,4-diethylphenyl)-8-hydroxy-3,5,6,7-tetramethoxy-4H-chromen-4-one; molecule 54 = 2-(3,4-diethylphenyl)-8-hydroxy-3,5,6,7-tetramethoxy-4H-chromen-4-one;   molecule   55 = (2E)-3-(3,4-dimethoxyphenyl)-1-(6-ethyl-2-hydroxy-3,4-dimethoxyphenyl) prop-2-en-1-one; molecule 57 = (2E)-3-(3,4-dimethoxyphenyl)-1-(6-hydroxy-2,3,4-trimethoxyphenyl) prop-2-en-1-one; molecule 59=(2S)-2-(3,4-dimethoxyphenyl)-5-hydroxy-6,7,8-trimethoxy-3,4-dihydro-2H-1-benzopyran-4-one; molecule   60=(2S)-2-(3,4-dimethoxyphenyl)-5,6,7,8-tetramethoxy-3,4-dihydro-2H-1-benzopyran-4-one;molecule61 = (2S)-2-(3,4-dimethoxyphenyl)-5,6,7-trimethoxy-3,4-dihydro-2H-1-benzopyran-4-one; molecule62=(2S)-2-(3,4-dimethoxyphenyl)-5,7,8-trimethoxy-3,4-dihydro-2H-1-benzopyran-4-one;   molecule   63=(2S)-5,6,7,8-tetramethoxy-2-(4-methoxyphenyl)-3,4-dihydro-2H-1-benzopyran-4-one; molecule 64=(2S)-2-(3,4-dimethoxyphenyl)-5,6,7-trimethoxy-3,4-dihydro-2H-1-benzopyran-4-one;   molecule   65=(2S)-5,7-dihydroxy-2-(3-hydroxy-4-methoxyphenyl)-3,4-dihydro-2H-1-benzopyran-4-one; molecule 66 = 2-(3,4-dimethylphenyl)-5,6,7,8-tetramethyl-4H-chromen-4-one; molecule 67 = 2-(3,4-dimethylphenyl)-3,5,7,8-tetramethyl-4H-chromen-4-one;   molecule 68 = 2-(3,4-dimethylphenyl)-5,7-dimethyl-4H-chromen-4-one;   molecule 69=(2S)-2-(3,4-dimethylphenyl)-5,6,7-trimethyl-3,4-dihydro-2H-1-benzopyran-4-one.

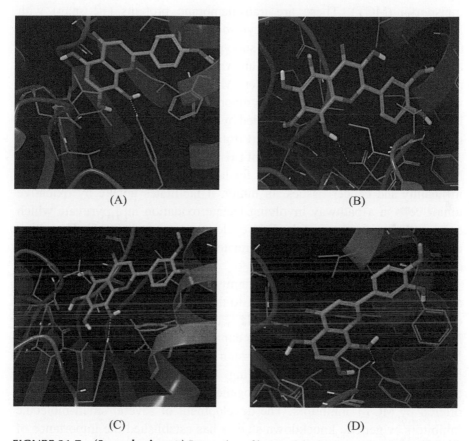

FIGURE 21.7 **(See color insert.)** Interaction of lactate dehydrogenase A protein with lead methylated flavonoids.

(A) 2-(3,4-dimethylphenyl)-5,7-dimethyl-4H-chromen-4-one (B) 2-(3,4-dimethoxyphenyl)-3-hydroxy-5,6,7,8-tetramethoxy-4H-chromen-4-one (C) (2S)-2-(3,4-dimethoxyphenyl)-5,6,7-trimethoxy-3,4-dihydro- 2H-1-benzopyran-4-one (D) 2-(3,4-dimethylphenyl)-5,6,7,8-tetramethyl-4H-chromen-4-one.

21.2.6 INHIBITORS OF MONOCARBOXYLATE TRANSPORTER

The LDHA reaction yields lactate and protons (from NADH). To avoid the death of cells and acidification, several systems have been developed that can combat these situations. These systems are called monocarboxylate transporter (MCT). These are transmembrane proteins (12 span) with N-terminus and C-terminus in the cytosolic domain and are proton-coupled (Fig. 21.8). There are in total 14 subtypes of MCTs but not all of these are currently characterized. There are various isoforms of the transporter, namely monocarboxylate transporter (MCT)1, MCT2, MCT3, and MCT4 which are passive lactate–proton symporters. Among these, MCT4 has the lowest-affinity for lactate and is coded by a HIF-1 target gene. That is why it is modified for the lactic acid export from glycolytic cancer cells and plays an important role in the regulation of pH inside the cells. On the other hand, MCT1 has an intermediate affinity for lactate and is universally expressed in healthy and cancer tissues. In tumor, it facilitates uptake by oxidative tumor cells in a pathway involving lactate oxidation into pyruvate which helps in the maintenance of the TCA cycle (Gurrapu et al., 2015). Thus, high expression of MCT1 and MCT4 is related to proliferation and invasion of cancer cells.

Cochaperone immunoglobulin family single membrane pass proteins are required for the transfer of MCT to the surface of the cell membrane is considered to be quite an exploitable feature of these transporters. MCT1, MCT3, and MCT4 bind to CD147 for expression on the cell surface, whereas MCT2 binds to embigin. The expression of a CD147 thus also requires an MCT protein that stabilizes the binding. The opportunity to simultaneously target tumor metabolism and angiogenesis within the same molecule is offered by MCT1 inhibitors. The development of several small-molecule inhibitors by genetic knockdown studies has established the importance of targeting lactate transporters in cancer therapeutics. Knockdown of MCT1 or inhibition of MCTs with the small molecule Alpha-cyano-4-hydroxy-cinnamate impairs tumor cell proliferation, migration, and survival. Further, it also impairs tumorigenic potential of glioblastoma cells in intracranial xenografts. It is supposedly a specific MCT1 inhibitor. AR-C117977, an additional MCT inhibitor has been found to have properties that suppress the immune system which will significantly prolong skin graft and heart allograft survival in mice (Kennedy et al., 2010). Recently, a small molecule inhibitor of MCT1 has been studied known as AZD3965. It is an explicit MCT1 inhibitor and is able to restrict transport of lactate both into and out of the cell. The greater effect, however, has been seen on the uptake of lactate. It was also able to produce statistically significant inhibition of cancer cell growth. AZD3965 would be particularly helpful at killing the hypoxic areas of the tumor, as these are the areas that would lack glucose when the aerobic fraction is unable to use lactate as a metabolic substrate (Bola et al., 2014). A small molecule, AR-C117977, has also been developed as a specific MCT1 inhibitor for mild immunosuppression.

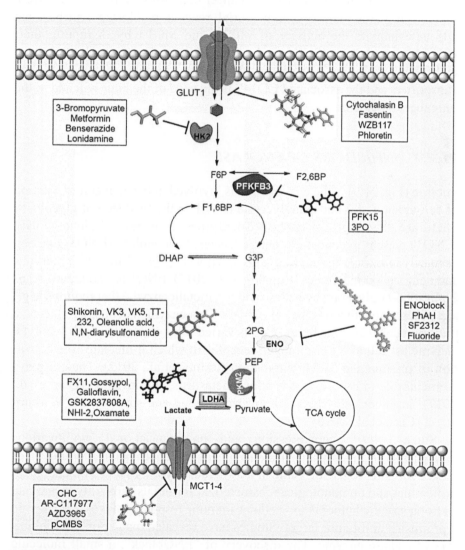

FIGURE 21.8 Anticancer targets in cancer cell carbohydrate metabolic pathway and their natural inhibitors.

Targeting CD147 is also an attractive antitumor strategy because they are essential for the stabilization and localization of MCTs to the cell membrane. One approach involves the generation of humanized anti-CD147 antibodies that can induce antibody-dependent-cell-mediated cytotoxicity. Such anti-bodies may also be utilized to deliver the drugs to CD147/MCT expressing cancer cells, which will destroy the cancer cells irrespective of their MCT expression status. The organomercurial reagent p-chloromercuribenzene sulfonate inhibits the activity of MCT1 and MCT4 by disrupting their association with CD147 (Kennedy et al., 2010). Thus, developing more such potent inhibitors that possess the ability to inhibit monocarboxylate transporters and the associated CD147 is the need of the hour will add to the anticancer armament.

21.2.7 INHIBITORS OF ENOLASE

Enolase (Fig. 21.9) is the enzyme that is involved in the conversion reaction of dehydration of 2-phosphoglycerate to PEP in the final step of glycolysis. There are three types of enolase isoenzymes in mammals: alpha-enolase (ENO1) present in almost all mature tissues; beta-enolase (ENO3) existing primarily in muscle tissues and gamma-enolase (ENO2) mainly in nervous and neuroendocrine tissues (Capello et al., 2017). ENO1 is also identified as 2-phospho-D-glycerate hydrolase and is a metalloenzyme that requires Mg^{2+} ion as a metal activator (Ji et al., 2016). This enzyme is considered to be a multifunctional enzyme because of its varied roles such as being a glycolytic enzyme as well as a plasminogen receptor in which it mediates the activation of plasmin and ECM degradation (Ramos et al., 2012). Thus, it plays a crucial role in cancer proliferation, metastasis, and invasion (Qian et al., 2017). In tumor cells, ENO1 is over-expressed and supports the Warburg effect (Chen et al., 2016).

Since ENO1 overexpression and post-translational modifications (acetylation and methylation) is prominent in cancer cells, it could be of diagnostic and prognostic value in many cancer types. ENO1's biochemical, proteomics and immunological characterization and its capability to activate a strong specific humoral and cellular immune response, makes this enzyme a promising anti-tumor target. Studies have revealed many potential inhibitors of enolase enzyme. The discovery of "ENOblock", a small molecule inhibitor has been made which is the first non-substrate analog of the enzyme (Jung et al., 2013). It directly binds to ENO1 and inhibits its activity and can also inhibit cancer cell metastasis in vivo. Thus, it is capable of being used in biological assays (Lung et al., 2017). The use of phosphonoaceto-hydroxamic acid was done to target the translational ability of ENO1. It is a pan-enolase transition-state analog inhibitor for various cancer types. It inhibits both the enolase enzymatic activity and proliferation of cancer cells. Another inhibitor has been studied in which an antibiotic is called SF2312. It is produced by the actinomycete *Micromonospora* and is active against a range of bacteria. It is the first reported phosphonate natural product inhibitor of enolase. It is an effective inhibitor of enolase with mixed competitive and non-competitive kinetics (Leonard et al., 2016). For most enolases, fluoride acts as an inhibitor and binds to enolase at the active center of the enzyme, forming a complex. This complex then blocks the binding of substrates to the enzyme, thereby exerting an inhibitory effect. The inhibition is mostly of competitive type (Qin et al., 2006). Other chemical inhibitors of enolase include D-tartonate and 3-aminoenolpyruvate-2-phosphate. Thus, altogether the inhibition of ENO1 acts as a potential anticancer target since it represses glycolytic pathway (Granchi et al., 2014). All the above-mentioned ENO1 inhibitors are very promising candidate compounds for pharmacokinetic and pharmacodynamic studies to assess their potential as anticancer drugs.

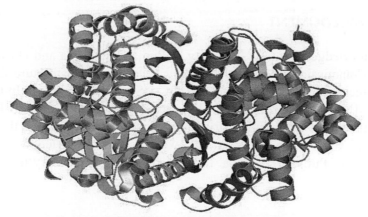

FIGURE 21.9 **(See color insert.)** Structure of enolase 2 protein (PDB=5IDZ).

Beside already known inhibitors of ENO2, we hereby performed in silico study to find out some potent methylated flavonoids (Fig. 21.6) active against ENO2 enzyme. Various offline and online tools were used for docking study (protein, ligand and structure preparation). The best doc score of two flavonoids   6-hydroxy-3,5,7,8-tetramethoxy-2-(3,4,5-trimethoxyphenyl)-4H-chromen-4-one   and   2-(3,4-dimethylphenyl)-5,6,7,8-tetramethyl-4H-chromen-4-one were -5.88 and -5.86 respectively. Interaction pattern of these methylated flavonoids and the target protein is depicted in Figure 21.10.

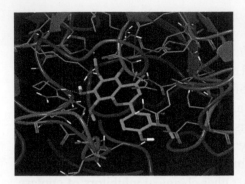 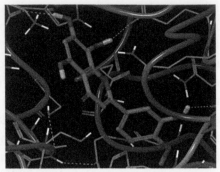

FIGURE 21.10   (See color insert.) Interaction of enolase two protein with lead methylated flavonoids.

(A)   6-hydroxy-3,5,7,8-tetramethoxy-2-(3,4,5-trimethoxyphenyl)-4H-chromen-4-one   (B)   2-(3,4-dimethylphenyl)-5,6,7,8-tetramethyl-4H-chromen-4-one.

ACKNOWLEDGMENT

SK acknowledges Central University of Punjab, Bathinda and University Grants Commission, India for providing necessary infrastructure facility and financial support in the form of UGC-BSR Research Start-Up-Grant, GP: 87 [No. F.30–372/2017 (BSR)], respectively. PPK acknowledges financial support from University Grants Commission, India in the form of CSIR-UGC Junior Research fellowship. SD acknowledges Central University of Punjab, Bathinda, India for providing necessary infrastructure facility.

KEYWORDS

- **Warburg effect**
- **carbohydrate**
- **cancer**
- **methylated flavonoids**
- **glycolytic enzymes**

REFERENCES

Allison, S. J.; Knight, J. R. P.; Granchi, C.; Rani, R.; Minutolo, F.; Milner, J.; Phillips, R. M. Identification of Ldh-A as a Therapeutic Target for Cancer Cell Killing Via (I) P53/Nad(H)-Dependent and (II) P53-Independent Pathways. *Oncogenesis.* **2014,** *3,* e102.

Bola, B. M.; Chadwick, A. L.; Michopoulos, F.; Blount, K. G.; Telfer, B. A.; Williams, K. J.; Smith, P. D.; Critchlow, S. E.; Stratford, I. J. Inhibition of Monocarboxylate Transporter-1 (Mct1) by Azd3965 Enhances Radiosensitivity by Reducing Lactate Transport. *Mol. Cancer Ther.* **2014,** *13*(12), 2805–2816.

Calvaresi, E. C.; Hergenrother, P. J. Glucose Conjugation for the Specific Targeting and Treatment of Cancer. *Chem Sci.* **2013,** *4*(6), 2319–2333.

Capello, P.; Principe, M.; Bulfamante, S.; Novelli, F. Alpha-Enolase (Eno1), a Potential Target in Novel Immunotherapies. *Front Biosci.* **2017,** *22,* 944–959.

Chen, X.; Li, L.; Guan, Y.; Yang, J.; Cheng, Y. Anticancer Strategies Based on the Metabolic Profile of Tumor Cells: Therapeutic Targeting of the Warburg Effect. *Acta Pharmacol. Sin.* **2016,** *37*(8), 1013–1019.

Doherty, J. R.; Cleveland, J. L. Targeting Lactate Metabolism for Cancer Therapeutics. *J. Clin. Invest.* **2013,** *123*(9), 3685–3692.

Dong, G.; Mao, Q.; Xia, W.; Xu, Y.; Wang, J.; Xu, L.; Jiang, F. Pkm2 and Cancer: the Function of Pkm2 Beyond Glycolysis. *Oncol. Lett.* **2016,** *11*(3), 1980–1986.

Evans, A.; Bates, V.; Troy, H.; Hewitt, S.; Holbeck, S.; Chung, Y. L.; Phillips, R.; Stubbs, M.; Griffiths, J.; Airley, R. Glut-1 as a Therapeutic Target: Increased Chemoresistance and Hif-1-Independent Link with Cell Turnover is Revealed Through Compare Analysis and Metabolomic Studies. *Cancer Pharmacol.* , **2008,** *61*(3), 377–393.

Fang, A.; Zhang, Q.; Fan, H.; Zhou, Y.; Yao, Y.; Zhang, Y.; Huang, X. Discovery of Human Lactate Dehydrogenase a (Ldha) Inhibitors as Anticancer Agents to Inhibit the Proliferation of Mg-63 Osteosarcoma Cells. *Med. Chem. Comm.* **2017,** 8.

Granchi, C.; Fancelli, D.; Minutolo, F. An Update on Therapeutic Opportunities offered by Cancer Glycolytic Metabolism. *BMCL* **2014,** *24,* 21.

Gurrapu, S.; Jonnalagadda, S. K.; Alam, M. A.; Nelson, G. L.; Sneve, M. G.; Drewes, L. R.; Mereddy, V. R. Monocarboxylate Transporter 1 Inhibitors as Potential Anticancer Agents. *ACS Med. Chem. Lett.* **2015,** *6*(5), 558–561.

Hay, N. Reprogramming Glucose Metabolism in Cancer: Can it Be Exploited for Cancer Therapy. *Nat. Rev. Cancer.* **2016,** *16,* 635-649.

Heiden, V.; Matthew, G.; Christofk, H. R.; Schuman, E.; Subtelny, A. O.; Sharfi, H.; Harlow, E. E.; Xian, J.; Cantley, L. C. Identification of Small Molecule Inhibitors of Pyruvate Kinase M2. *Biochem. Pharmacol. PMC* **2011**.

Iqbal, M. A.; Gupta, V.; Gopinath, P.; Mazurek, S.; Bamezai, R. Pyruvate Kinase M2 and Cancer: An Updated Assessment. *FEBS Lett.* **2014,** *588*(16), 2685-292.

Ji, H.; Wang, J.; Guo, J.; Li, Y.; Lian, S.; Guo, W.; Yang, H.; Kong, F.; Zhen, L.; Guo, L.; Liu, Y. Progress in the Biological Function of Alpha-Enolase. Animal. *Nutrition* **2016,** *2,* 12–17.

Jung, D. W.; Kim, W. H.; Park, S. H.; Lee, J.; Kim, J.; Su, D.; Ha, H. H.; Chang, Y. T.; Williams, D. R. A Unique Small Molecule Inhibitor of Enolase Clarifies Its Role in Fundamental Biological Processes. *ACS Chem. Biol.* **2013,** *8*(6), 1271–1282.

Kapoor, K.; FinerMoore, J. S.; Pederson, B. P.; Caboni, L.; Waight, A.; Hillig, R. C.; Bringmann, P.; Heisler, I.; Muller, T.; Siebeneicher, H.; Stroud, R. M. Mechanism of Inhibition of Human Glucose Transporter GLUT1 is Conserved between Cytochalasin B and Phenylalanine Amides. *PNAS* **2016,** *113*(17), 4711–4716.

Kennedy, K. M.; Dewhirst, M. W. Tumor Metabolism of Lactate: the Influence and Therapeutic Potential for MCT and CD147 Regulation. *Future Oncol.* **2010,** *6*(1), 127.

Kochel, K.; Tomczyk, M. D.; Simoes, R. F.; Fraczek, T.; Sobon, A.; Oliviera, P. J.; Walczak, K. Z. Evaluation of Biological Properties of 3,3′,4,4′-Benzophenonetetracarboxylic Dianhydride Derivatives and Their Ability to Inhibit Hexokinase Activity. *Bioorg. Med. Chem.* **2017,** *27*(3), 427–431.

Leonard, G. P.; Satani, N.; Maxwell, D.; Lin, Y.; Hammoudi, N.; Peng, Z.; Pisaneschi, F.; Link, T. M.; Lee, G. R.; Sun, D.; Francesco, M. E. D.; Czako, B.; Asara, J. M.; Wang, Y. A.; Bornmann, W.; DePinho, R. A.; Muller, F. L. Sf2312 is a Natural Phosphonate Inhibitor of Enolase. *Nat. Chem. Biol.* **2016,** *12,* 1053–1058.

Li, W.; Zheng, M.; Wu, S.; Gao, S.; Yang, M.; Li, Z.; Min, Q.; Sun, W.; Chen, L.; Xiang, G.; Li, H. Benserazide, a Dopadecarboxylase Inhibitor, Suppresses Tumor Growth by Targeting Hexokinase 2. *J. Exp. Clin. Cancer* **2017,** *36,* 58.

Lin, H.; Zeng, J.; Xie, R.; Schulz, M. R.; Tedesco, R.; Qu, J.; Erhard, K. F.; Mack, J. F.; Raha, K.; Rendina, A. R.; Szewzuck, L. M.; Kratz, P. M.; Jurewicz, A. J.; Cecconie, T.; Martens, S.; Martin, J. D.; Chen, S. B.; Jiang, Y.; Nickels, L.; Schwartz, B. J.; Smallwood, A.; Zhao, B.; Campobasso, N.; Qian, Y.; Briand, J.; Rominger, C. M.; Oleykowski, C.; Hardwicke, M. A.; Luengo, J. I. Discovery of a Novel 2,6-disubstituted Glucosamine Series of Potent and Selective Hexokinase 2 Inhibitors. *ACS Med. Chem. Lett.* **2016,** *7*(3), 217–222.

Liu, Y.; Cao, Y.; Zhang, W.; Bergmeier, S.; Qian, Y.; Akbar, H.; Colvin, R.; Ding, J.; Tong, L.; Wu, S.; Hines, J.; Chen, X. A Small-molecule Inhibitor of Glucose Transporter 1 Downregulates Glycolysis, Induces Cell-Cycle Arrest, And Inhibits Cancer Cell Growth *in vitro* and *in vivo*. *Mol. Cancer Thera.* **2012,** *8,* 11.

Lu, Q. Y.; Zhang, L.; Yee, J. K.; Go, V. W.; Lee, W. N. Metabolic Consequences of Ldha Inhibition by Epigallocatechin Gallate and Oxamate in Mia Paca-2 Pancreatic Cancer Cells. *Metabolomics.* **2015,** *11*(1), 71–80.

Lung, J.; Chen, K. L.; Hung, C. H.; Chen, C. C.; Hung, M. S.; Lin, Y. C.; Wu, C. Y.; Lee, K. D.; Shih, N. Y.; Tsai, Y. H. In Silico-based Identification of Human α-enolase Inhibitors to Block Cancer Cell Growth Metabolically. *Dovepress* **2017,** *11,* 3281—3290.

Mathupala, S. P.; Ko, Y. H.; Pedersen, P. L. Hexokinase II Cancer's Double-Edged Sword Acting as Both Facilitator and Gatekeeper of Malignancy When Bound to Mitochondria. *Oncogene* **2006,** *25,* 4777–4782.

Miao, P.; Sheng, S.; Sun, X.; Liu, J.; Huang, G. Lactate Dehydrogenase a in Cancer: a Promising Target for Diagnosis and Therapy. *IUBMB Life.* **2013,** *65*(11), 904–910.

O'Neal, J; Clem, A.; Reynolds, L.; Dougherty, S.; Imbert-Fernandez, Y.; Telang, S.; Chesney, J.; Clem, B. F. Inhibition of 6-Phosphofructo-2-Kinase (Pfkfb3) Suppresses Glucose Metabolism and the Growth of Her2+ Breast Cancer. *Breast Cancer Res. Treat.* **2016,** *160*(1), 29–40.

Ojelabi, O.; DeZutter, J.; Lloyd, K.; Carruthers, A. Novel Small Molecule, Wzb117, Competitively Inhibit Glut1-Mediated Glucose Transport to Halt Cancer Growth. *FASEB J.* **2016,** 30.

Pinksofsky, H. B.; Dwyer, D. S.; Bradley, R. J. The Inhibition of Glut1 Glucose Transport and Cytochalasin B Binding Activity by Tricyclic Antidepressant. *LifeSci.* **2000,** *66*(3), 271–278.

Porporato, P. E.; Dhup, S.; Dadhich, R. K.; Copetti, T.; Sonveaux, P. Anticancer Targets in the Glycolytic Metabolism of Tumors: a Comprehensive Review. *Front Pharmacol.* **2011,** *2,* 49.

Qian, X.; Xu, W.; Xu, J.; Shi, Q.; Li, J.; Weng, Y.; Jiang, Z.; Feng, L.; Wang, X.; Zhou, J.; Jin, H. Enolase 1 Stimulates Glycolysis to Promote Chemoresistance in Gastric Cancer. *Oncotarget.* **2017,** *8*(29), 47691–47708.

Qin, J.; Chai, G.; Brewer, J. M.; Lovelace, L. L.; Lebioda, L. Fluoride inhibition of Enolase: Crystal Structure and Thermodynamics. *BioChemistry 2006, 45*(3), 793–800.

Ramos, A. D.; Borrellas, A. R.; Melero, A. G.; Alemany, A. L. A-Enolase, a Multifunctional Protein: Its Role on Pathophysiological Situations. *J. Biomed. Biotechnol.* **2012.**

Shibuya, K.; Okada, M.; Suzuki, S.; Seino, S.; Takeda, H.; Kitanaka, C. Targeting the Facilitative Glucose Transporter Glut1 Inhibits the Self-Renewal and Tumor-Initiating Capacity of Cancer Stem Cells. *Oncotarget* **2015,** *2,* 651–661.

Wang, H.; Wang, L.; Zhang, Y.; Wang, J.; Deng, Y.; Lin, D. Inhibition of Glycolytic Enzyme Hexokinase II (HK2) Suppresses Lung Tumor Growth. *Cancer Cell Int.* **2016,** *16,* 9.

Wong, N.; Melo, J. D.; Tang, D. Pkm2, a Central Point of Regulation in Cancer Metabolism. *Int. J. Cell Biol.* **2013,** 242513.

Yang, Y.; Su, D.; Zhao, L.; Zhang, D.; Xu, J.; Wan, J.; Fan, S.; Chen, M. Different Effects of Ldh-A Inhibition by Oxamate in Non-Small Cell Lung Cancer Cells. *Oncotarget.* **2014,** *5*(23), 11886–11896.

Zhang, Q.; Zhang, Y.; Zhang, P.; Chao, Z.; Xia, F.; Jiang, C.; Zhang, X.; Jiang, Z.; Liu, H. Hexokinase II Inhibitor, 3-Brpa Induced Autophagy by Stimulating ROS Formation in Human Breast Cancer Cells. *Genes Cancer* **2014,** *5*(3–4), 100–112.

Zhao, Y.; Butler, E. B.; Tan, M. Targeting Cellular Metabolism to Improve Cancer Therapeutics. *Cell Death Dis.* **2013,** *4,* e532.

Zhao, Z.; Han, F.; Yang, S.; Wu, J.; Zhan, W. Oxamate-Mediated Inhibition of Lactate Dehydrogenase Induces Protective Autophagy in Gastric Cancer Cells: Involvement of the Akt-Mtor Signaling Pathway. *Cancer Lett.* **2015,** *358*(1), 17–26.

Zhu, W.; Ye, L.; Zhang, J.; Yu, P.; Wang, H.; Ye, Z.; Tian, J. Pfk15, a Small Molecule Inhibitor of Pfkfb3, Induces Cell Cycle Arrest, Apoptosis and Inhibits Invasion in Gastric Cancer. *PLoS One.* **2016,** *11*(9), e0163768.

CHAPTER 22

HERBAL DRUG DISCOVERY: THE ENVISION BIOTECHNOLOGY APPROACH

ANIKO NAGY

Envision Biotechnology, https://envisionbiotechnology.com/, Grandville, MI, USA.

E-mail: aniko.nagy@envisionbiotechnology.com

ABSTRACT

Herbal drug discovery is an essential step in the discovery of new drugs for the treatment of diseases. For many years, natural products of plant origin in its crude form have been a source of remedy against diseases especially to those in the developing countries. The traditional knowledge of herbs has proven to be invaluable even with the advent of evidence-based medicine. It is on record that about 80% of plant-derived drugs are linked to their ethnobotanical uses. To complement this, there is a need for an organized curative platform to provide reliable knowledge on herbal medicine which paves way for safer and more efficient use of plant-based medicines. The Envision Biotechnology is an organized curative herbal database platform which presents ideal information convergence of pharmaco-chemistry, absorption, distribution, metabolism, and excretion properties, drug-likeness, drug targets, associated diseases and interaction networks of herbal medicine. This chapter is a brief overview of herbal drug discovery by the Envision Biotechnology approach.

22.1 INTRODUCTION

The relevance of traditional knowledge on natural products (herbs, marine organisms, traditional therapies) of developing world has still been underestimated, principally because of the incomplete evidence-based understanding of their mechanism of action. However, more and more scientists become open to using information from natural products to develop new drugs, in addition to the western medicine. Therefore, it has a huge role to ensure evidence-based, scientifically correct data, which is a giant challenge.

Today, the Internet is the first choice of information for scientists, physicians, and other healthcare professionals. With respect to the field of botanical drug research, several investigations of commercial websites have found heterogeneous quality regarding the content presented, which might lead the scientists to a wrong direction. As a consequence, several independent initiatives have been started to assist researchers. Over the last decade, one application of modern information technology is the establishment of specialized databases. Unfortunately, information about these databases is controversial and often not known to researchers in the field. Thus, there is a basic need to give an overview of published database resources for natural product research.

22.2   ENVISION BIOTECHNOLOGY SOLUTION

Most databases were created to collect the molecular content of traditional Chinese medicine plants primarily to connect the ancient knowledge to western medicine. One of the biggest Chinese herbal databases is Traditional Chinese Medicine Integrative Database (TCMID) (Li et al., 2008), which integrate data of Chinese databases, like TCM, TCM-Taiwan, and herb ingredients' target (HIT) and build the relations between the herbal ingredients and their effects. Chinese databases contain the detailed information for preparation (Ehrman et al., 2007; Yuen et al., 2011). In addition, chemical structures of the herbs are added, which is related to diseases through targets from DrugBank (https://www.drugbank.ca/) and OMIM databases (https://mirror.omim.org/). Moreover, there are integrated data from text mining books (e.g., Encyclopedia of Traditional Chinese Medicines) and published articles, which are specifically valuable for western medicine. TCMID is a great beginning to make the Chinese data and herbal ingredient more usable for western medicine and drug development, but some details are missing, which could be better developed, for instance, to show the number of studies with compounds and effects or to filter the study type.

Another important region of traditional medicinal knowledge is Africa. African biodiversity has huge potential for drug discovery and development;

however, it has been limited to random screening of extracts based on ethnobotanical information (Novick et al., 2013). AfroDb contains information about African medicinal plants and their effects with the geographical region of plant and phytochemical data. The database includes maximum 10 tautomers per compound in the dataset with some other chemical properties like the logarithm of the octanol/water partition coefficient representing the lipophilicity factor (log P) and Lipinski violations. Moreover, it contains data from published articles, theses, textbook chapters as well as unpublished conference presentations from communication with the authors.

As one of the 12 mega-biodiversity hotspots of the world, India is another important data provider with more than 45,000 plant species, many of which associated with the use of medicinal plants in the form of traditional systems of medicine including Ayurveda. In India, there is a huge amount of well-recorded and traditionally practiced knowledge of herbal medicine; however, this kind of data needs integration with western medicine knowledge to use all their benefit. There are approximately 8000 species of plants with known medicinal uses in India, of which 3000 have been used in traditional medicine for over 1000 years (Shanmughanandhan et al., 2016). Many plants are being examined for their beneficial use in diabetes and reports occur in numerous scientific journals of the merits of using such plants (Tota et al., 2013). Furthermore, there are many data about the effectiveness of Ayurvedic formulations on rheumatoid arthritis (Mohamed et al., 2017) or data of ethnomedicinal studies on plants used by Yanadi tribe of Chandragiri reserve forest area.

It is necessary to use these databases as widely as possible, for example, adapt them to different techniques to increase the efficacy of drug discovery and development. There are many research groups, who utilize computer-aided drug design on natural products, including in silico screening, while a detailed mechanism of action with the target protein is known just for a few natural products. These studies could support the cost and time optimization of these research projects and the better understanding of the complexity of natural products. It is noteworthy, that the adequate quality of the data is prerequisite as the success of any computational technique is dependent on the quality of the data at the first place (Keum et al., 2016).

22.3 GLOBAL SCIENTIFIC HERBAL DATABASE

According to our vision, it is necessary to integrate the already existing databases and new, well-curated information to understand the mechanism behind the action of natural products. With the deep study of natural products and with the utilization of this knowledge, new target proteins and new chemical structures could be investigated. Moreover, new pharmacological models could be evolved, in this case, these new processes together could not just increase the speed of drug development but also decrease their cost.

22.4   HERBAL DISCOVERY PLATFORM

Envision Biotechnology's Herbal Discovery Platform (https://envision-biotechnology.com/dicovery-platform/) is an online platform to provide reliable knowledge on herbal medicine and dietary supplements paving the way to safer and more efficient use of plant-based dietary supplements and medicine. It contains all the chemicals that are related to one plant and their specific chemical structures as well. For visualization, a map was built to better understand and investigate the mechanism of action, for example, relationships between plants, chemicals, target proteins, and effects (Fig. 22.1). Moreover, a chemical search function was developed, in which searching is available according to substructures as well.

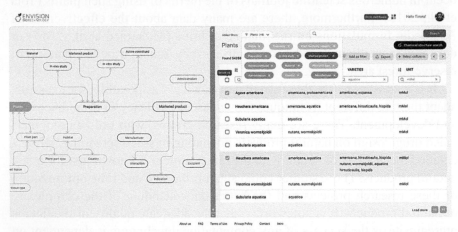

FIGURE 22.1   Screenshot of using the visual map and multiple filtering options to observe complex synergies.

With the automatic data annotation combined with manual data curation by a team of PhD scientists together with our novel visual representations of complex herbal data, Envision Biotechnology establishes the essential and necessary knowledge and scientific informatics toolkits to discover new drugs from natural products and to discover new natural products by reverse pharmacology. We can afford integrated dataset from smaller, local databases; furthermore, we work with data provider partners from different places (Africa, South and North America, India, etc.), who give us nonpublished data too. Table 22.1 shows the integrated databases in General Scientific Herbal Database version 1.0.

TABLE 22.1 Databases integrated in General Scientific Herbal Database version 1.0.

Name of the database	Description	Website
Dr. Duke's Database	Dr. Duke's Phytochemical and Ethnobotanical databases facilitate in-depth plant, chemical, bioactivity, and ethnobotany searches using scientific or common names.	https://phytochem.nal.usda.gov/phytochem
A corpus for plant–chemical relationships	Relationships between medical plants and chemicals	http://210.107.182.73/plantchemcorpus.htm
Mpd3	Medicinal Plant Database for Drug Designing	http://bioinform.info/
UNDP	Universal Natural Products Database	http://pkuxxj.pku.edu.cn/UNPD
SWEETLEAD	Highly curated resource for chemical structures	https://simtk.org/projects/sweetlead
Herding	Herb recommendations system to treat diseases using genes and chemicals	http://210.107.182.73/TCMID-WebService/herdingDemo.jsp
GlobInMed	Traditional and complementary medicine	http://globinmed.com/
TCMSP	Traditional Chinese medicine systems pharmacology database and analysis platform	http://ibts.hkbu.edu.hk/LSP/tcmsp.php
TIPDB	Traditional Chinese medicine (focus on Taiwan)	http://cwtung.kmu.edu.tw/tipdb
TCMID	Traditional Chinese medicine	www.megabionet.org/tcmid
STREPTOMEDB	Natural products produced by *Streptomyces*	www.pharmaceutical-bioinformatics.de/streptomedb
NPCARE	Natural products for cancer gene regulation	http://silver.sejong.ac.kr/npcare
SANCDB	South African natural compound database	http://sancdb.rubi.ru.ac.za
Plantlist.org	Accepted Latin name of plants	http://www.theplantlist.org/

Plant names from different databases according to The Plant List (http://www.theplantlist.org/) are harmonized. The creator of this working list collaborates with the Royal Botanic Gardens, Kew and Missouri Botanical Garden, and more other collaborators to make a complete list with accepted Latin names.

22.5 CONCLUSION

Envision Biotechnology works with a continuously growing Scientific Advisory Board (https://envisionbiotechnology.com/about-us/)with well-educated, experienced scientists from many countries (e.g., Nigeria, Cameroon, Mexico, India, Switzerland, Germany, England, Austria) to ensure different knowledge, opinions, and views.

By maintaining some healthy skepticism, we feel that the time is ripe for (re)discovering and exploiting computational natural product analysis for chemical biology and drug discovery.

KEYWORDS

- herbal drug discovery
- ethnobotanical
- traditional medicine
- envision biotechnology
- phytochemical database

REFERENCES

Ehrman, T. M.; Barlow, D. J.; Hylands, P. J. Phytochemical Databases of Chinese Herbal Constituents and Bioactive Plant Compounds with Known Target Specificities. J. Chem. Inf. Model. 2007, 47, 254–263. https://doi.org/10.1021/ci600288m.

Keum, J.; Yoo, S.; Lee, D.; Nam, H. Prediction of Compound-Target Interactions of Natural Products Using Large-Scale Drug and Protein Information. BMC Bioinf. 2016, 17(Suppl. 6), 219. https://doi.org/10.1186/s12859-016-1081-y.

Li, S.; Han, Q.; Qiao, C.; Song, J.; Cheng, C. L.; Xu, H. Chemical Markers for the Quality Control of Herbal Medicines: An Overview. Chin. Med. 2008, 3, 7. https://doi.org/10.1186/1749-8546-3-7.

Mohamed, T. A. A. M.; Agrawal, A.; Sajitha, L. S.; Mohana, P. A.; Vino, S. RAACFDb: Rheumatoid Arthritis Ayurvedic Classical Formulations database. *J. Ethnopharmacol.* **2017,** *197,* 87–91. DOI: 10.1016/j.jep.2016.06.047.

Novick, P. A.; Ortiz, O. F.; Poelman, J.; Abdulhay, A. Y.; Pande, V. S. SWEETLEAD: An in Silico Database of Approved Drugs, Regulated Chemicals, and Herbal Isolates for Computer-Aided Drug Discovery. *PLoS One* **2013,** *8,* 1–9. https://doi.org/10.1371/journal.pone.0079568.

Shanmughanandhan, D.; Ragupathy, S.; Newmaster, S. G.; Mohanasundaram, S.; Sathishkumar, R. Estimating Herbal Product Authentication and Adulteration in India Using a Vouchered, DNA-Based Biological Reference Material Library. *Drug Saf.* **2016,** *12,* 1211–1227.

Tota, K.; Rayabarapu, N.; Moosa, S.; Talla, V.; Bhyravbhatla, B.; Rao, S. InDiaMed: a Comprehensive Database of Indian Medicinal Plants For Diabetes. *Bioinformation* **2013,** *7,* 378–380. DOI: 10.6026/97320630009378.

Yuen, J.; Tse, S.; Yung, J. Traditional Chinese Herbal Medicine–East Meets West in Validation and Therapeutic Application. In *Recent Advances in Theories and Practice of Chinese Medicine;* Kuang, H., ed.; InTech, 2011; pp 239–266, DOI: 10.5772/26606.

PART IV
Phytochemical Research

GAS CHROMATOGRAPHY–MASS SPECTROMETRY ANALYSIS AND IN VITRO ANTICANCER ACTIVITY OF *TECTONA GRANDIS* BARK EXTRACT AGAINST HUMAN BREAST CANCER CELL LINE (MCF-7)

ARUL PRIYA R.[1], K. SARAVANAN[1,*], and UMARANI B.[1]

[1]PG and Research Department of Zoology, Nehru Memorial College (Autonomous), Puthanampatti, Tiruchirappalli 621007, India

*Corresponding author. E-mail: kaliyaperumalsaravanan72@gmail.com
ORCID: *https://orcid.org/0000-0003-4082-3143

ABSTRACT

This chapter presents an investigation of the presence of secondary metabolites in the ethyl acetate extract of *Tectona grandis* bark extract and the cytotoxic effect against MCF-7 cell lines. Phytochemical compounds were determined by gas chromatography–mass spectrometry (GC-MS) analysis. The cytotoxic activity, morphological assessment of cell death, potential of mitochondrial membrane potential and deoxyribonucleic acid (DNA) damage pattern were evaluated by MTT assay, acridine orange/ethidium bromide (AO/EB) staining technique, JC-1 staining method and comet assay, respectively. GC-MS chromatogram showed the presence of five major phytochemical compounds in ethyl acetate extract of *T. grandis* bark which includes flavonoids, phenols, and tannins. The inhibition concentration (IC_{50}) of ethyl acetate extract of *T. grandis* bark was calculated as 1.57 mg/mL for MCF-7 cell line and induced significant DNA damage. Thus, the present study concludes that the ethyl-acetate extract of *T. grandis* bark possesses potent antibreast cancer activity.

23.1   INTRODUCTION

Cancer is a disease which is caused by many external, internal and hereditary factors. Among the different types of cancer, breast cancer is very common in women around the world and also leading cause of death (American Cancer Society, 2012). It is most difficult to cure due to several distinct classes of tumors that exhibit different treatment responses (Ferguson et al., 2004).The common treatments of cancer were chemotherapy, radiotherapy, hormonal therapy, or surgery, which cause many side effects (Stopeck and Thompson, 2012). Thus, the identification of novel anticancer agents without side effects is urgently needed (Lachenmayer et al., 2010). Medicinal plants possess tremendous pharmacological significance in producing drugs for various disease (Baker et al., 2007; Harvey, 2008) including cancer (Newman and Cragg, 2012; Kuno et al., 2012). The vast number of drugs such as paclitaxel, etoposide, camptothecin, vinca and indole alkaloids, podophyllotoxin derivatives, etoposide, and teniposide, were currently used in chemotherapy, which originally came from plants. *Tectona grandis* (Verbenaceae) is commonly known as teak. Traditionally, it is used in treatment of many diseases such as diabetes, lipid disorders, inflammation, ulcer, and bronchitis (Warrier, 1994) and also reported to have many biological processes such as antimicrobial and antiulcer activities (Pandey et al., 1982). Khan and Miungwana (1999) reported that a compound 5-hydroxylapachol isolated from *T. grandis* had potent cytotoxic activity. However, no studies were available on anti-breast cancer activity. The present investigation was undertaken to examine the anticancer activity of ethyl acetate extract of *T. grandis* bark against MCF-7 cell lines (human breast cancer cell line).

23.2   MATERIALS AND METHODS

23.2.1   COLLECTION OF PLANT MATERIAL

The bark of *T. grandis* was selected for this study. The barks were collected from Kunnathur, (Latitude 11.2667°N and Longitude 77.4090°E), Tirupur, Tamilnadu, India. They were thoroughly washed with tap water and dried under shadow. Then they were ground well using domestic grinder.

23.2.2 PREPARATION OF EXTRACTS

According to the standard methodology (Harborne, 1988), the powdered *T. grandis* bark material was extracted by Soxhlet apparatus using ethylacetate solvent for 48 h. Then the extract was concentrated to dryness and the residues were obtained. The residues were stored in a pre-weighed sample container until further use.

23.2.3 PHYTOCHEMICAL SCREENING OF TECTONA GRANDIS BARK EXTRACT

The extracts of *T. grandis* bark were used for qualitative screening of phytochemicals such as alkaloids, carbohydrates, flavonoids, cardiac glycosides, proteins, phenols, saponins, steroids, tannins, and terpenoids by standard biochemical procedure (Kokate, 1997).

23.2.4 GAS CHROMATOGRAPHY MASS SPECTROMETRY (GC-MS) ANALYSIS

Gas chromatography–mass spectrometry (GC-MS) analysis was performed to identify the bioactive compounds in the *T. grandis* extract. The GC-MS analysis was performed using a JEOL GC MATE II instrument employing the following conditions: front inet temperature 220°C; column HP 5Ms; helium gas (99.99%) was utilized as carrier gas at a constant flow rate of 1 mL/min. In the case of oven temperature, it was 50–250°C at 10°C/min. The ion chamber temperature and gas chromatography (GC) interface temperature was 250°C. Mass analysis was done with the help of quadruple double focusing analyzer; for detection, the photon multiplier tube was used. At 70 eV, mass spectra were taken. The necessary data were gathered by the full-scan spectra within the scan range of 50–600 amu. Percentage peak area was noted and it is nothing but the per cent composition of constituents of the extract.

23.2.5 IDENTIFICATION OF COMPONENTS

On the basis of GC retention time, characterization of chemical compounds in ethyl acetate extract was identified. The mass spectra were matched with the standard mass spectra available in libraries. By employing National Institute

Standard and Technology's database (having large number of patterns) and Wiley spectra libraries, mass spectrum GC-MS interpretation was made. The unknown spectrum components were compared with the known spectrum components which were stored in NIST library. The compound name, weight of molecule and its formula and compound structure of the test materials were ascertained from NIST and PubChem libraries.

23.2.6 ANTICANCER ACTIVITY

23.2.6.1 PROCUREMENT OF CELL LINES

Cell lines of human breast cancer (MCF-7) were obtained from National Center for Cell Science, Pune, India. These cells were stored in Dulbecco's-modified Eagle's medium supplemented with 10% FBS (Sigma-Aldrich, St.Louis, Missouri, USA). Penicillin at 100 U/mL and streptomycin at 100 μg/mL were used as antibiotics (Himedia, Mumbai, India). At humidified atmosphere, the culture was kept at 5% CO_2 level in a CO_2 incubator at 37°C (Forma, Thermo Scientific, USA).

23.2.6.2 CELL VIABILITY ASSAY

The MTT tetrazolium salt colorimetric assay, described by Mosmann (1983) was performed to measure the cytotoxicity of ethyl acetate extract of *T. grandis*. The plant extract was dissolved in 100% dimethyl sulfoxide (DMSO) to prepare a stock. The stock solution was diluted separately with fresh medium to get various concentrations from 0 to 0.6 mg. About 96-well plates at plating density of 5000 cells/well were seeded after 24 h. Exactly 100 μL of sample was added to wells. DMSO (0.02%) was used as the solvent control. After 24 h, 20 μL of MTT solution (5 mg/mL in phosphate buffer solution [PBS]) was added to each well and the plate was wrapped with aluminum foil and incubated for 3 h at 37°C. By adding 100 μL of DMSO to each cell the purple formazan product was dissolved. The absorbance was observed at 570 nm (measurement) and 630 nm (reference) using a 96-well plate reader (Bio-Rad, iMark, USA). In order to calculate the respective mean values, data were collected for triplicates each. The following formula was used to calculate the percentage of growth inhibition.

$$Growth\,inhibition\,(\%) = \frac{Mean\,OD\,of\,control\,cells - Mean\,OD\,of\,treated\,cells}{Mean\,OD\,of\,Control} \times 100$$

From the obtained values, inhibition concentration (IC_{50}) for 24 h for MCF-7 cells was computed by probit analysis using SPSS windows-based software.

23.2.7 ACRIDINE ORANGE/ETHIDIUM BROMIDE STAINING FLUORESCENT ASSAY FOR CELL DEATH

Apoptotic morphology was investigated by acridine orange/ethidium bromide (AO/EB) double staining technique as described by Spector et al (1998). MCF-7 cells were cultured separately in six-well plates and treated with IC_{50} concentration of the plant extracts for 24 h, when DMSO (0.02%) was used as solvent control. The cells of treated and untreated (25 µL of suspension containing 5000 cells) were incubated with the solution of AO/EB (1 part of 100 µg/mL each of acridine orange and ethidium bromide in PBS) and examined in a fluorescent microscope (Carl Zeiss, Jena, Germany) using a UV filter (450–490 nm). For each sample, three hundred cells were counted, in triplicate, for each time point and scored as viable or dead cells by apoptosis or necrosis as judged from the nuclear morphology and cytoplasmic organization and percentages were calculated for apoptotic and necrotic cells. Morphological features of dead cells were photographed (Kumar et al., 2008).

23.2.8 ASSESSMENT OF MITOCHONDRIAL POTENTIAL (JC1 STAINING)

Mitochondrial membrane potential ($\Delta\psi m$) was assessed using the fluorescent probe JC-1, which produces orange-red fluorescence when accumulated in the mitochondria of healthy cells but fluoresces green when leached out into the cytosol due to loss of $\Delta\psi m$ resulting in a negative internal potential (Reers et al., 1991). The MCF-7 cells were grown in glass coverslips (22×22 mm) placed in the wells of 6-well plates and treated with the ethyl acetate extract of *T. grandis* at 24 h IC_{50} concentration, and 0.02% DMSO was used as solvent control. The cells were stained with JC-1 dye after 12 h exposure. In the fluorescent microscope, the cells' mitochondrial depolarization was observed and the pathological changes in the cells were also observed and recorded. The mean and standard deviation (SD) were calculated from the collected data of the three replicates each.

23.2.9 SINGLE CELL GEL ELECTROPHORESIS (COMET ASSAY)

Deoxyribonucleic acid (DNA) damage was detected using the comet assay of (Singh et al., 1988). The MCF-7 cells were treated with the complex at its 24 h IC_{50} concentration for 12 h, with 0.02% DMSO as the solvent control. The harvested cells were suspended in low melting point agarose in PBS and pipette out to microscope slides pre-coated with a layer of normal melting point agarose. The chilled slides on ice for 10 min and then immersed in lysis solution (2.5 M·NaCl, 100 mM·Na_2EDTA, 10 mM Tris, 0.2 mM·NaOH [pH 10.01], and Triton X-100) and was incubated overnight at 48°C in order to lyse the cells and permit DNA unfolding. Thereafter, the slides were exposed to alkaline buffer (300 mM·NaOH, 1 mM·Na_2EDTA, [pH >13]) for 20 min to allow DNA unwinding. The slides were washed with buffer (0.4 M Tris, pH 7.5) to neutralize the excess alkali and to remove the detergents before staining with ethidium bromide (20 mL in 50 mg/mL). Photomicrographs were obtained using the fluorescent microscope. About 150 cells from each treatment group were digitized and analysed using CASP software. The images were used to determine the DNA content of individual nuclei and to evaluate the degree of DNA damage representing the fraction of DNA in the tail, so as to assign the cells among the five categories: dead, highly damaged, damaged, slightly damaged, and intact. Data were gathered for three replicates each and used to compute the values for means and the SDs.

23.2.10 STATISTICAL ANALYSIS

Data from each of the three experiments are expressed as mean ± SD. IC_{50} values were calculated by probit analysis using windows-based SPSS statistical software.

23.3 RESULTS AND DISCUSSION

23.3.1 PRELIMINARY PHYTOCHEMICAL SCREENING

Preliminary phytochemical analysis exhibited the existence of major classes of secondary metabolites such as carbohydrate, flavonoids, phenols and tannins (Table 23.1). Flavonoids are potent water-soluble antioxidants and free radical scavengers, which prevent oxidative cell damage, have strong anticancer activity (Del-Rio et al., 1997; Okwu, 2004).

TABLE 23.1 Phytochemical Screening of Ethyl Acetate Extract of *Tectona grandis*.

S/No.	Phytocompounds	Test name	Results
1	Alkaloids	Hager's test	Negative
		Mayer's test	Negative
		Wagner's test	Negative
2	Carbohydrates	Barfoed's test	Positive
		Benedict's test	Positive
		Fehling's test	Positive
3	Cardiac glycosides	Bromine water test	Negative
4	Flavonoids	Alkaline test	Positive
		Ferric chloride	Positive
		Lead acetate test	Positive
		Shinoda test	Positive
		Mg turning test	Negative
		Zinc test	Negative
5	Phenols	Alkaline reagent test	Positive
		Ferric chloride test	Positive
		Lead acetate	Positive
6	Protein	Millions test	Negative
		Nitric acid test	Negative
		Xanthoproteic test	Negative
7	Saponin	Bubble test	Negative
		Emulsion test	Negative
		Foam test	Negative
8	Steroids	Libermann–Burchards	Negative
9	Tannin	Lead acetate test	Positive
		Ferric chloride test	Positive
10	Terpenoids	Concentrated H_2SO_4	Negative
		Libermann–Burchards	Negative

23.3.2 GC-MS ANALYSIS OF ETHYLACETATE EXTRACT OF TECTONA GRANDIS BARK

The ethylacetate extract of *T. grandis* bark was subjected to GC-MS analysis. Totally, five major phytochemical compounds were identified in ethyl acetate extract of *T. grandis* bark through GC-MS spectrum profile (Fig. 23.1 and Table 23.2). They were 4'5,7-trihydroxy isoflavone, psi-baptigenin, 4H-1-benzopyran-4-one, 5,7-dihydroxy 2(4-hydroxypheyl)-6-methoxy-, E-11-Octadecen-1-ol acetate and 11,13-Eicosadienoic acid, methyl ester with their retention time of 17.23, 18.08, 18.97, 20.02 and 20.95, respectively. A very high percentage of peak area was obtained for $C_{16}H_{12}O_6$ (40.17%). They belonged to flavonoids. Flavonoids are effective in inhibiting xanthine oxidase, COX, or LOX55 (Chang et al., 1993) and therefore which inhibits tumor cell proliferation and they were also reported to possess anticancer activity (Chandrappa et al., 2014).

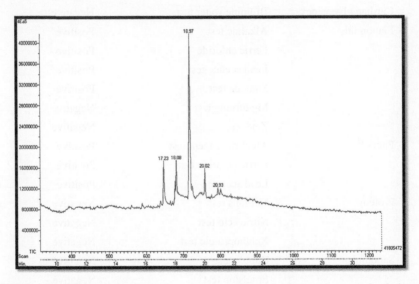

FIGURE 23.1   Gas chromatography–mass spectrometry chromatogram of ethylacetate extract of *Tectona grandis* bark.

23.3.3   EFFECT OF ETHYLACETATE EXTRACT OF T. GRANDIS TREATMENT ON THE VIABILITY OF BREAST CANCER CELL LINE (MCF-7)

MTT assay is a rapid and high accuracy colorimetric approach that widely used to determine the growth of cell and cytotoxicity of the cell, specifically in the growth of new drug (Akhir et al., 2011). The decreasing of optical density value in MTT assay was found to be positive correlation with the growth inhibitory rate and negatively correlated with proliferative rate (Andrew et al., 2008). The inhibitory effect of the ethyl acetate extract of *T. grandis* at different concentrations for 24 h on MCF-7 cells was investigated by MTT assay. The higher concentration of 3.0 mg/mL was exhibited

TABLE 23.2 Details of Compounds Identified from Ethyl acetate Extract of *T. grandis* Bark by Gas Chromatography–Mass Spectrometry Analysis.

S/No.	RT	Compound name	Molecular formula	Molecular structure of the compound	Molecular weight (g/mol)	Peak area (%)
1	17.23	4'5,7-trihydroxy isoflavone	$C_{15}H_{10}O_5$		270	16.65
2	18.08	psi-baptigenin	$C_{16}H_{10}O_5$		282	16.82
3	18.97	4H-1-benzopyran-4-one, 5,7-dihydroxy 2(4-hydroxypheyl)-6-methoxy-	$C_{16}H_{12}O_6$		300	40.17
4	20.02	E-11-cctadecen-1-ol acetate	$C_{21}H_{40}O$		308	15.29
5	20.95	11,13-eicosadienoic acid, methyl ester	$C_{21}H_{38}O_2$		323	11.06

79.1±3.93% of cell death and very minimum inhibitory concentration was obtained at 0.3 mg/mL. The IC_{50} of *T. grandis* bark extract was about 1.57 mg/mL for MCF-7 cell line (Fig. 23.2 and Table 23.3).

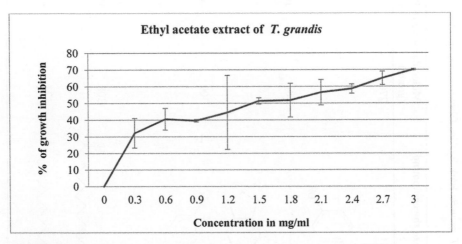

FIGURE 23.2 Cytotoxic activity of *T. grandis* bark extracts against MCF-7 breast cancer cell line by MTT assay.

TABLE 23.3 Ethylacetate Extract of *T. grandis* MTT Assay.

Concentration (mg/mL)	Cell inhibition (%) (Mean ± standard deviation [SD])	Cell viability (%) (Mean ± SD)
Control	0.0±0.00	100.0±0.00
	(0.0–0.0)	(100.0–100.0)
0.3	32.1±8.85	67.9±8.85
	(25.9–38.4)	(61.6–74.1)
0.6	40.5±6.48	59.5±6.48
	(35.9–45.0)	(55.0–64.1)
0.9	39.6±0.76	60.4±0.76
	(39.1–40.2)	(59.8–60.9)
1.2	44.5±22.15	55.5±22.15
	(28.9–60.2)	(39.8–71.2)
1.5	51.4±1.85	48.6±1.85
	(50.1–52.7)	(47.3–49.9)
1.8	51.8±10.07	48.2±10.07
	(44.7–58.9)	(41.1–55.3)
2.1	56.5±7.60	43.5±7.60
	(51.1–61.9)	(38.2–48.9)

TABLE 23.3 *(Continued)*

Concentration (mg/mL)	Cell inhibition (%) (Mean ± standard deviation [SD])	Cell viability (%) (Mean ± SD)
2.4	58.6±2.76	41.5±2.76
	(56.6–60.0)	(40.0–43.4)
2.7	65.0±4.01	35.0±4.01
	(62.0–68.0)	(32.0–38.0)
3.0	70.1±0.45	30.0±0.45
	(69.3–70.0)	(28.7–30.0)

23.3.4 MORPHOLOGY OF NORMAL AND EXTRACT TREATED MCF-7 CELLS

MCF-7 cells treated with *T. grandis* extracts exhibited notable morphological changes with regard to apoptosis-like blebbing formation, nuclear formation and apoptotic bodies (Fig. 23.3). The treatment with ethyl acetate extract apoptotic cells showed early apoptotic cells (perinuclear chromatin condensation is shown as bright green patches.) The mean percentage of apoptosis was found to be high (64.0%) (Table 23.4) in the MCF-7 cells treated with ethylacetate extract of *T. grandis*.

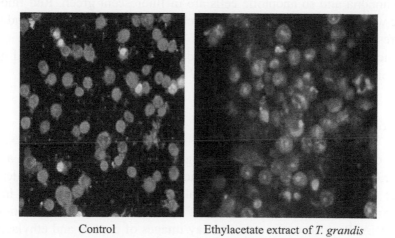

Control   Ethylacetate extract of *T. grandis*

FIGURE 23.3 **(See color insert.)** Morphological changes observed for control ethylacetate extract of *T. grandis*-treated MCF-7 cells stained with acridine orange and ethidium bromide. (1) viable cells have uniform bright green nuclei with organized structure; (2) early apoptotic cells have green nuclei, but perinuclear chromatin condensation is visible as bright green patches or fragments; (3) late apoptotic cells have orange to red nuclei with condensed or fragmented chromatin.

TABLE 23.4 Percentage of Normal, Apoptotic and Necrotic Cells on Human Breast Cancer Cell Line (MCF-7) After the Treatment of *T. grandis* Bark Powder Extract.

S.No.	Type of extracts	Normal cells (%)	Mode of cell death	
			Apoptosis (%)	Necrotic (%)
1	Control	90.3±2.08	5.3±2.52	4.3±1.53
		(88.0–92.0)	(3.0–8.0)	(3.0–6.0)
2	Ethylacetate extract of *Tectona grandis*	23.3±1.53	64.0±4.00	12.7±2.52
		(22.0–25.0)	(60.0–68.0)	(10.0–15.0)

23.3.5 ASSESSMENT OF MITOCHONDRIAL MEMBRANE POTENTIAL BY JC-1 STAINING TECHNIQUE

The loss in mitochondrial membrane potential ($\Delta\psi$m) is an early event in apoptosis. To detect the changes in mitochondrial function, JC-1 staining assay was employed. The JC-1 stain is fluorescent cation which emits red fluorescence when sequestered into the mitochondria of healthy cells with high $\Delta\psi$m. When the apoptotic cells are stained with JC-1, the red fluorescence turned into green fluorescence due to $\Delta\psi$m. Because the cells undergoing apoptosis are no longer able to retain the JC-1 cation into the mitochondria and so apoptotic cells are in fluorescent green. Red fluorescence was observed in the control (untreated healthy MCF-7 cells) and they are presented in Figure 23.4.

Since the *T. grandis* bark possessed many flavonoids, it showed good antiproliferative activity against MCF-7 lines.

23.3.6 COMET ASSAY

In the comet assay, DNA of the damaged single cell is considered as the appearance of a comet with the tail region. Since the tail length and density reflect the extent of DNA strand breaks, the percentage of DNA in the tail provides a quantitative measure of the DNA damage as a fraction of total DNA. Representative comet assay images of control and ethylacetate extract of *T. grandis*-treated cells are presented in Figure 23.5. As denoted in the image, there was an increased DNA damage in the extracts treated cells (72.5±0.29% DNAs are fully damaged and 27.5±0.60% are intact) compared to the control (4.8±0.10% DNAs are fully damaged and

94.2±0.87% are intact). Cellular stresses, such as growth factor deprivation, DNA damage, and oncogene expression, lead to stabilization are activation of the p53 tumor suppressor protein.

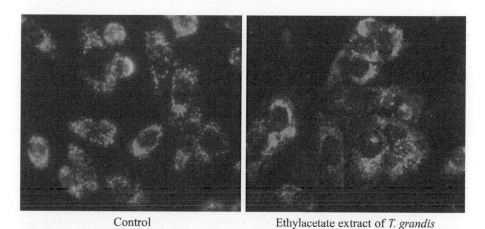

Control   Ethylacetate extract of *T. grandis*

FIGURE 23.4   (See color insert.) Photomicrographs of MCF-7 breast cancer cells, JC-1 dye accumulated in the mitochondria of healthy cells as aggregates (red–orange fluorescing); in cells treated with ethyl acetate extract of *T. grandis*, due to collapse of mitochondrial membrane potential, the JC-1 dye remained in the cytoplasm its monomeric form, which fluoresced green.

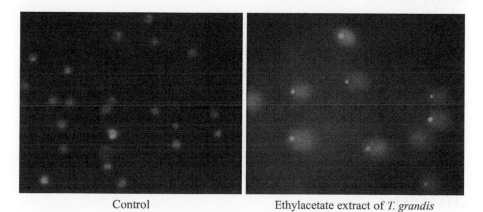

Control   Ethylacetate extract of *T. grandis*

FIGURE 23.5   (See color insert.) Deoxyribonucleic acid damage in ethylacetate extract of *T. grandis* treated MCF-7 cells is revealed in the comet assay. Comet images of DNA strand breaks at 12 h treatment of the ethylacetate extract of *T. grandis*.

23.4 CONCLUSION

The bark extract of *T. grandis* examined in this study possess varying levels of in vitro anticancer activity. Different anticancer effects were examined and found to take part in the present study. The first is cytotoxicity (decreased number of live cells), measurement of cell death by apoptosis, mitochondrial membrane potential by fluorescent probe, and measurement of DNA deterioration by comet assay. The ethyl acetate extract of *T. grandis* has possessed all of the above effects with varying degrees.

ACKNOWLEDGMENT

We would like to thank the Management, the Principal and HOD of Zoology, Nehru Memorial College, Puthanampatti, Tiruchirappalli district, Tamilnadu, India for their encouragements and for providing necessary facilities. We also thank Dr. M. Akbarsha, Director, Mahatma Gandhi Doerenkamp Centre for alternatives to use of animals in life science education, Bharathidasan University, Tiruchirappalli for giving permission to do cell line work at his centre. The first author wishes to thank the University Grants Commission, New Delhi, for financial support.

KEYWORDS

- **phytochemistry**
- **cytotoxicity**
- *Tectona grandis*
- **MCF-7 cell line**
- **comet assay**

REFERENCES

American Cancer Society. Breast Cancer Facts and Figures 2011–2012. American Cancer Society, Inc.: Atlanta, 2012.

Akhir, N.; Chua, L. S.; Majid, F. A. A.; Sarmidi, M. R.Cytotoxicity of Aqueous and Ethanol Extracts of *Ficus deltoidea* on Cell Line. *Br. J. Med. Med. Res.* **2011**, *1*, 397–409.

Andrew, L. N.; Richard, A. M.; Terry, L. R. Update on in Vitro Cytotoxicity Assays for Drug Development. *Expert. Opin. Drug Discovery* **2008,** *3,* 655–669.

Baker, D. D.; Chu, M.; Oza, U.; Rajgarhia, V. The Value of Natural Products to Future Pharmaceutical Discovery. *Nat. Prod. Rep.* **2007,** *24,*1225–1244.

Chang, W. S.; Lee, Y. J.; Lu, F. J.; Chiang, H. C. Inhibitory Effects of Flavonoids on Xanthine Oxidase. Anticancer Res.**1993,** *13,* 2165–2170.

Chandrappa, C. P.; Govindappa, M.; Anil Kumar, N. V.; Channabasava, R.; Chadrasekar, N.; Umashankar, T.; Mhabaleshwara, K. Identification and Separation of Quercetin from Ethanol Extract of *Carmonaretusa* by Thin Layer Chromatography and High Permance Liquid Chromatography with Diode Array Detection. *World J.Pharm. Pharm.Sci.* **2014,** *3,* 2020–2029.

Del-Rio, A.; Obdululio, B. G.; Casfillo, J.; Marin, F. G.; Ortuno, A. Uses and Properties of Citrus Flavonoids. *J. Agric. Food Chem.* **1997, 45,** 4505–4515.

Ferguson, P. J.; Kurowska, E.; Freeman, D. J.; Chambers, A. F.; Koropatnick, D.J.A Flavonoid Fraction from Cranberry Extract Inhibits Proliferation of Human Tumor Cell Lines. *J. Nutr.* **2004,** *134,* 1529–1535.

Harborne, J. B. *Phytochemical Methods: A Guide to Modern Techniques of Plant Analysis;* 2nd Ed.; Chapman and Hall: London, 1998.

Harvey, A. L. Natural Products in Drug Discovery. *Drug Discovery Today* **2008,** *13,* 894–901.

Khan, R. M.; Miungwana, S. M.5-Hydroxylapachol: A Cytotoxic Agent from Tectona *grandis. Phytochem* **1999,** *50,* 439–442.

Kokate, K.C. Practical Pharmacognosy, 4th Ed.; Vallabh Prakashan: New Delhi, India. 1997.

Kumar, R. S.; Arunachalam, S.; Periasamy, V. S.; Preethy, C. P.; Riyasdeen, A.; Akbarsha, M. A.Synthesis, DNA Binding and Antitumor Activities of Some Novel Polymer-cobalt (III) Complexes Containing 1, 10-phenanthroline Ligand. *Polyhedron* **2008,** *27,* 1111–1120.

Kuno, T.; Testuya, T.; Akira, H.; Takuji, T. Cancer Chemoprevention Through the Induction of Apoptosis by Natural Product. *J. Biophysical. Chem.* **2012,** *3,* 156–173.

Lachenmayer, A.; Alsinet, C.; Chang, C. Y.; Llovet, J. M.Molecular Approaches to Treatment of Hepatocellular Carcinoma. *Dig. Liver Dis.* **2010,** *42,* S264–S272.

Mosmann, T. Rapid Colorimetric Assay for Cellular Growth and Survival: Application to Proliferation and Cytotoxicity Assays. *J. Immunol. Methods* **1983,** *65,* 55–63.

Newman, D. J.; Cragg, G. M. Natural Products as Sources of New Drugs Over the 30 Years from 1981 to 2010. *J. Nat. Prod.* **2012,** *75,* 311–335.

Okwu, D. E. Phytochemicals and Vitamin Content of Indigenous Spices of Southeastern Nigeria. *J. Sustainable Agric. Environ.* **2004,** *6,* 30–37.

Pandey, B. L.; Goel, R. K.; Pathak, N. K. R.; Biswas, M.; Das,P.K. Effect of *Tectonagrandis* Linn. (Common teak tree) on Experimental Ulcers and Gastric Secretion. *Indian. J. Med. Res.***1982,** *76,* 89–94.

Reers, M.; Smith, T. W.; Chen, L. B.J-aggregate Formation of a Carbocyanin as a Quantitative Fluorescent Indicator of Membrane Potential. *Biochem.* **1991,** *3,* 4480–4486.

Singh, N. P.; McCoy, M. T.; Tice, R. R.; Schneider, E. L.A. Simple Technique for Quantization of Low Levels of DNA Damage in Individual Cells. *Exp. Cell Res.* **1988,** *175,* 184–191.

Spector, D. L.; Goldman, R. D.; Leiwand, L. A.A Simple Technique for Quantitation of Low Levels of DNA Damage in Individual Cells. *Exp. Cell Res.* **1998,** *175,* 184–191.

Stopeck, A. T.; Thompson, P.A. Breast Cancer Treatment and Management. **2012.** http://emedicine.medscape.com/article/1947145-treatment.

Warrier, P. S. *Indian Medicinal Plants,*1st ed.; Orient Longman Private Limited: New Delhi, 1994.

CHAPTER 24

PHYTOCHEMICAL ANALYSIS OF *NIGELLA SATIVA* L. SEEDS AQUEOUS EXTRACT BY GAS CHROMATOGRAPHY–MASS SPECTROSCOPY AND FOURIER-TRANSFORM INFRARED

SHAISTA JABEEN N.[1,*], JAGAPRIYA L.[1],
SENTHILKUMAR BALASUBRAMANIAN[2], DEVI K.[1],
and JAISON JEEVANANDAM[3]

[1]*Department of Zoology, PG and Research Unit, Dhanabagyam Krishnaswamy Mudaliar College for Women (Autonomous), Sainathapuram, RV Nagar, Vellore, Tamil Nadu 632001, India, Tel.: 919600636818*

[2]*Department of Zoology, Thiruvalluvar University, Serkadu, Vellore, Tamil Nadu, India*

[3]*Department of Chemical Engineering, Faculty of Engineering and Science, Curtin University CDT 250, 98009 Miri Sarawak, Malaysia*

**Corresponding author. E-mail: sj2khan16@gmail.com
ORCID: https://orcid.org/0000-0003-3796-8755*

ABSTRACT

Plants including herbs serve as a unique source of bioactive compounds that possess therapeutic benefits in the treatment of several diseases. Among herbal species, *Nigella sativa* possess enormous bioactive compounds and their aqueous seed extract is a significant way to isolate crude bioactive compounds which can later be separated using different techniques. The study reported in this chapter focuses on the extraction of bioactive components from *N. sativa* seeds and characterize them through gas chromatography–mass spectrometry (GC-MS) and Fourier-transform infrared (FTIR) spectroscopy. Preliminary phytochemical screening studies revealed the presence of pharmaceutically substantial phytochemicals. GC-MS analysis identifies 11 bioactive compounds with therapeutic property based on their molecular mass retention time and peak values, whereas FTIR spectra indicate the presence of different functional groups that correspond to various significant phytochemicals. These bioactive components from *N. sativa* seed extracts are highly beneficial as a curative agent for several diseases ranging from cancer to acquired immune deficiency syndrome in future.

24.1   INTRODUCTION

Plants especially herbs serves as a unique and significant source of novel biological compounds that has the potentiality to cure a range of diseases from cancer to digestion problems (Zhou et al., 2017). In 2005, World Health Organization reported that there is an increased dependence on the use of herbal drugs and over 80% of the world population rely on herbs for the treatment of various diseases due to their superior accessibility, price, and lack of side effects, compared to chemical-based drugs (Benzie and Wachtel-Galor, 2011). Herbal medicines have been utilized as a complementary and an alternative medicine for centuries and recent advances in the pharmaceutical industry leads to the standardization and regulation of these herbal drugs. Recently, progressive development of new and sophisticated chromatographic techniques such as thin-layer chromatography, high-performance liquid chromatography, gas chromatography coupled with mass spectrometry, nuclear magnetic resonance techniques helps in the identification, isolation, and characterization of compounds present in herbs. These advanced characterization techniques play a major role in discovering novel compounds and phytoconstituents from herbs that possess enhanced medicinal properties.

Among different herbal species, *Nigella sativa* is an exceptional herb which has been cultivated for their less toxic drug compounds (Tavakkoli et al., 2017). The scientific classification of *N. sativa* is shown in Table 24.1. In different countries, it is called by distinct names such as *kalonji*, black cumin, black caraway, *kala jeera*, *nigella* (Spanish), *pivorette* (French), *Nigella* (Italian), *Habat et Baraka* (Egyptian), *kalonji* (Africa and India), and Habba Soda (Oman). *N. sativa* is an annual herbaceous plant with bicolor flowers of pale blue and white. The capsule of the flower contains seeds as shown in Figure 24.1 and grows up to the height of 20 in. It is initially grown in Mediterranean, Middle East, Africa (Egypt), and later brought to India by some travelers. It is now cultivated in North Indian regions such as Punjab, Gujarat, Rajasthan, and some parts of south India (Nergiz and Ötleş, 1993; Hyam and Pankhurst, 1995). Among the plant parts, the seeds of *N. sativa* attracted numerous researches due to the presence of phytochemicals with superior therapeutic properties (Saadia et al., 2017; Butt et al., 2018). Historically, the seeds of *N. sativa* possess high therapeutic benefits that attract ancient Egyptians because of which the seeds were placed in the tomb of Tutankhamun. Similarly, Roman surgeon Dioscorides cured dog and crocodile bites by using a mixture of *N. sativa* and vinegar (Osbaldeston and Wood, 2000). Recent literatures also suggested that the phytochemicals and essential oil present in *N. sativa* seed extracts are attributed to possess many medicinal potentials such as carminative (Babayan et al., 1978), immunomodulator (Salem, 2005), antimicrobial (Bakal et al., 2017), antibacterial (Ashraf et al., 2017), cardiovascular (Hebi et al., 2016), hepatoprotective (Adam et al., 2016), nephro-protective (Benhelima et al., 2016), neuro-protective (Sedaghat et al., 2014), and antitumor (Ait Mbarek et al., 2007) activities. This chapter reports about the phytochemical analysis of *N. sativa* aqueous seed extract using gas chromatography–mass spectroscopy (GC-MS) and Fourier-transform infrared (FTIR) spectroscopy. Additionally, the possible biomedical applications of phytochemicals present in *N. sativa* seed extract were also presented.

TABLE 24.1 Scientific Classification of *Nigella sativa*.

Kingdom	Phylum	Class	Order	Family	Genus	Species
Plantae	Magnoliophyta	Magnoliopsida	Ranunculales	Ranunculaceae	*Nigella*	*sativa*

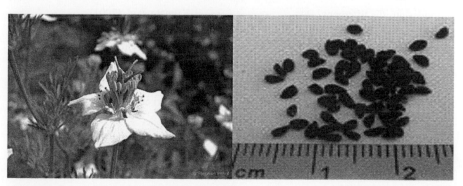

FIGURE 24.1 *Nigella sativa* flower and seeds.

24.2 CHEMICAL COMPOSITION OF *NIGELLA SATIVA* SEEDS

N. sativa seeds are enriched with various therapeutic phytochemicals such as thymoquinone (TQ), dithymoquinon, dihydrothymoquinone (DHTQ), thymol α and β pinene, carvacrol, and d-limonene. Additionally, these seeds are rich in essential oil with a 0.4% saturated fatty acids (Ali et al., 2003). It is reported that the presence of phytochemicals such as alkaloids, terpenoids, phenolic compounds, steroids, and flavonoids are responsible for various pharmacological activities of the plant. Though the seeds consist of numerous phytocompound, only four major compounds such as TQ dithymoquinone DHTQ, and thymol are proved to be important for the biomedical and pharmaceutical application. Table 24.2 lists the quantity of phytochemicals present in *N. sativa* seed extracts (Ali et al., 2003). Figure 24.2 shows the molecular structure of four major phytochemicals present in *N. sativa* seed extract.

TABLE 24.2   List of Phytochemicals and Their Quantity Present in *N. sativa* Seed Extract.

Phytochemicals	Quantity (%)	References
Fixed oils	36–38	Lautenbacher (1997)
Essential oils	0.4–2.5	
Thymoquinone	27.8–57	El–Dakhakhny (1963); Ali et al. (2003)
ρ-cymene	7.1–15.5	
Carvacrol	5.8–11.6	
t-anethole	0.25–2.3	
4-terpineol	2–6.6	
Longifoline	1–8	
Alkaloids such as nigellicine, nigellidine, nigellimine, and N-oxide	–	Malik et al. (1985a); Malik et al. (1985b); Malik et al. (1992); Malik et al. (1995)
Monodesmosidic triterpene saponin, α-hederin	–	Kumara et al. (2001)
Monounsaturated fatty acid	18–29	Nickavar et al. (2003); Cheikh-Rouhou et al. (2007); Sultan et al. (2009)
Polyunsaturated fatty acid	60.1±1.5	
Saturated fatty acids	12–25	
Proteins	20.8–31.2	Takruri et al. (1998); Atta (2003)
Total carbohydrates	24.9–40	
Linoleic acid	57.3±1.5	Sultan et al. (2009)
Dihydrothymoquinone	3.84±0.1	
Thymol	2.32±0.26	
Thymohydroquinone	0.7–1.1	Benkaci–Ali et al. (2007)

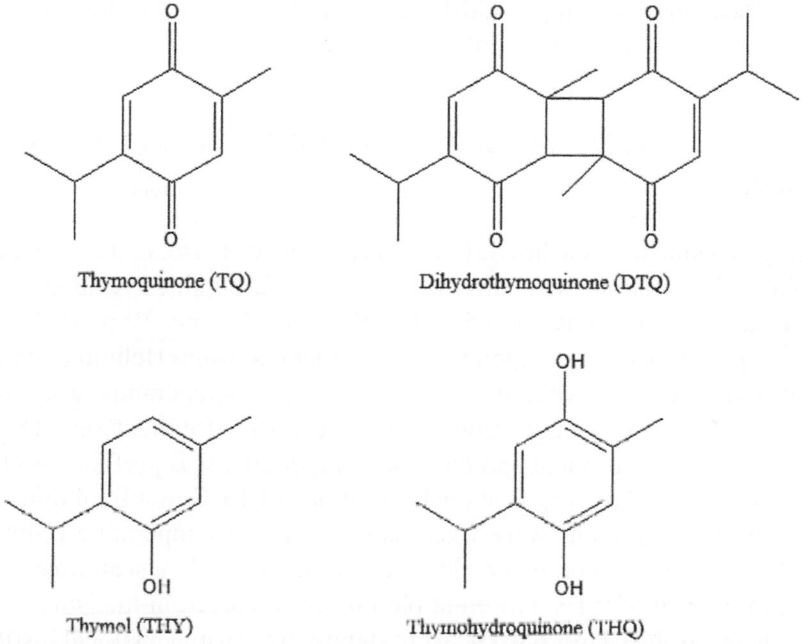

FIGURE 24.2   Molecular structure of four major phytochemicals present in *N. sativa* seeds.

24.3   MATERIALS AND METHODS

24.3.1   SAMPLE COLLECTION AND PROCESSING

The seeds of *N. sativa* were purchased from the local market of Vellore. These seeds were washed with clean water, shade dried, and ground with an electric grinder. Exactly 50 g of *N. sativa* seed powder was measured and diluted in 500 mL of double-distilled water to isolate crude extract by using Soxhlet extractor. Later, the crude aqueous extract was stored in a refrigerator at 4°C for further qualitative analysis.

24.3.2   QUALITATIVE AND QUANTITATIVE PHYTOCHEMICAL SCREENING OF N. SATIVA SEEDS

To detect, identify, and isolate the different phytochemical constituents from the crude aqueous extract, qualitative tests were carried out using standard procedures as described in previous literature (Harborne, 1973; Sofowora, 1982; Trease and Evans, 1989). The quantitative analysis of phytochemicals was carried out by using GC-MS and FTIR to identify the bioactive compounds with biomedical applications.

24.3.3 GAS CHROMATOGRAPHY-MASS SPECTROMETRY ANALYSIS

The phytochemicals from the crude aqueous extract were isolated using Clarus 680 GC. The isolation was carried out using a fused silica column, filled with Elite-5MS (5% biphenyl 95% dimethylpolysiloxane, 30 m × 0.25 mm ID × 250 μm df) and the components were separated using Helium as carrier gas at a constant flow of 1 mL/min. The injector temperature was set at 260°C during the chromatographic run. The 1 μL of extract sample was injected into the instrument and the oven temperature was prefixed as 60°C for 2 min; followed by 300°C at the heating rate of 10°C/min for 6 min. The mass detector conditions were fixed as transfer line temperature (240°C); ion source and ionization mode electron impact at 70 eV, a scan time 0.2 s, and scan interval of 0.1 s. Different parameters involved in the isolation of phytochemicals by Clarus 680 GC were standardized using National Institute of Standards and Technology (NIST) data. The spectrums of the components were compared with the spectrum database of known components in the GC-MS NIST (2008) library.

24.3.4 IDENTIFICATION OF COMPOUNDS

The percentage of each compound was calculated by comparing the peak value area and the total area. The identification of the components in the extracts was based on the comparison of their retention indices and mass spectra fragmentation patterns along with the previous literature. The compounds – their name, molecular structure, and molecular weight were identified by matching their spectra with the known component spectra from the GC-MS NIST library.

24.3.5 FOURIER-TRANSFORM INFRARED SPECTROSCOPY ANALYSIS

Infrared spectroscopy is one of the powerful analytical tool used to identify organic, polymeric, and inorganic materials such as sample composition, additives, contaminants, and unknown materials. The technique is based on the chemical substances that exhibit selective absorption in the infrared region. When the sample is exposed to infrared, the sample molecules selectively absorb radiation of a specific wavelength which gives rise to absorption spectrum. A pinch of sample powder was placed on infrared spectrometer with constant pressure applied to collect the data of infrared absorbance over wave number ranges from 650 to 4000/cm and computerized for analysis by using the OMNIC software. All FTIR spectra were collected with a resolution of 4/cm.

24.4 RESULTS AND DISCUSSION

In the present study, qualitative phytochemical screening test results of *N. sativa* seed extract as shown in Table 24.3 revealed the presence of secondary metabolites such as alkaloids, tannins, flavonoids, terpenoids, phenols, cardiac glycosides, saponins, diterpenes, and steroids. Each of these phytochemicals are known to possess therapeutic potentials (Tiwari et al., 2002). Previously, it was reported that tannins were present in the methanolic extract of *N. sativa* seeds (Eloff, 1998). Tannins form complexes binding with proteins through hydrophobic, hydrogen, and covalent bonding and thus, act as an antibacterial agent by deactivating cell adhesions, enzymes, and transport proteins (Hashem et al., 1982). Similarly, saponins possess enormous beneficial effects ranging from anti-inflammatory effect (Lin et al., 2016), anticarcinogenic properties (Oh and Sung, 2001) to inhibit HIV infection (Nakashima et al., 1989; Singh et al., 2017). Literature also suggest that flavonoids help in the prevention of cardiovascular diseases (Majewska-Wierzbicka et al., 2012), neurodegenerative diseases (Macready et al., 2009), and cancer (Kozlowska et al., 2014). Other phytochemicals present in *N. sativa* possess significant benefits including terpenoids as antioxidants (Grassmann, 2005), steroids in enhanced seed dormancy, and germination in agriculture (Vriet et al., 2012), alkaloids as a drug for Alzheimer's disease (Ng et al., 2015) and glycosides for the treatment of congestive heart failure and cardiac arrhythmias (Begum et al., 2015). It is evident from the literature and results as shown in Table 24.3 that the *N. sativa* seed extract would have vast beneficial effects on human health due to the presence of the pharmaceutically significant phytochemicals.

TABLE 24.3 Qualitative Phytochemical Screening on *N. Sativa* Seeds.

Secondary metabolites	Results	Type of test
Tannins	+	Gelatin test
Saponins	+	Froth's test
Flavonoids	+	Alkaline reagent test
Anthroquinones	+	Barntrager's test
Terpenoids	+	Salkowski test
Steroids	+	Leibermann–Burchard test
Alkaloids	+	Mayer's test
Glycosides	+	Salkowski's test
Carbohydrates	+	Molisch's test
Pholobotanins	+	Pholobotanins test

Note: + = Presence; – = absence.

GC-MS study reveals the presence of various bioactive compounds in the crude seed extract of *N. sativa*. The GC-MS chromatogram revealed several peaks out of which 12 high-level peaks were studied and their molecular structure as well as their significant therapeutic activities were depicted in Table 24.4.

The functional groups present in the seed extract were studied using FTIR spectroscopic analysis and the results were summarized in Table 24.5. The FTIR spectra of the *N. sativa* aqueous seed extract is shown in Figure 24.3. The FTIR spectral chart for the functional groups identified the presence of alcohol, hydroxyl, alkynes, alkene, alkanes, alkyl, amine, carboxylic acid, esters, ethers ketones, aldehydes, and a carbonyl group in the aqueous seed extracts. These functional groups indicate the presence of alkaloids, polyphenols, terpenoids, tannins, flavonoids, and saponins in the crude seed extract (Jeevanandam et al., 2017). FTIR spectra further confirm the presence of pharmaceutically significant phytochemicals that are isolated in the qualitative phytochemical screening test. The functional groups revealed by FTIR spectra helps in the formulation of these phytochemicals for pharmaceutical and nutraceutical applications.

TABLE 24.4 Bioactive Compounds with Their Molecular Structure by Gas Chromatography–Mass Spectrometry Analysis and Their Possible Therapeutic Activity.

Bioactive compounds	Molecular structure	Therapeutic activities
Leucinyl glycine hydrazine, N-[2,4-dinitrophenyl]		Antitumor activity, antimicrobial activity (Saini and Saini, 2011)
1,3-Diazetidine, 2,4-bis (hexafluoroisopropylideno) -1,3-diphenyl- 1,3-diphenyl-2,4-bis [2,2,2-trifluoro-1-(trifluoromethyl) ethylidene		Anti-microbial, antifungal activity (Tsoungas et al., 1987)
Quinazoline, 6-methoxy-4-methylthio-2-phenyl		Anti-inflammatory, antioxidant (Kumar et al., 2011)

TABLE 24.4 (*Continued*)

Bioactive compounds	Molecular structure	Therapeutic activities
Glucitol, d-Glucitol		Antidiuretic, laxative (El-Kabbani et al., 2004)
4-hydroxyphenyllactic acid, ethyl ester, di-TMS		Laxative activity (Conforti et al., 2006)
Propanedioic acid, mononitrile, 2-[tetrahydro-4-(4-fluorophenyl)-2,2-dimethyl-4-pyranyl]-, ethyl ester Ethyl cyano [4-(4-fluorophenyl)		Anti-oxidant activity (Al-Marzoqi et al., 2015)
Pentasiloxane, 1,1,3,3,5,5,7,7,9,9-decamethyl-1,1,3,3,5,5,7,7,9,9-decamethylpentasiloxane		Antiaging, skin-emolients, anti-allergic, contraceptive, antidiuretic, anti-dermatophytic activity (Sulaiman et al., 2016)

TABLE 24.4 *(Continued)*

Bioactive compounds	Molecular structure	Therapeutic activities
3-Phenyl-2H-chromene		Anti-HIV, anti-allergic (Kusumoto et al. 1995), anti-inflammatory, antibacterial, anti-cancer, antifungal (Sarpangala et al., 2017)
Pyridine, 1,2,3,6-tetrahydro-1-methyl-4-[4-chloro-phenyl]- $$4-(4-chlorophenyl)-1-methyl-1,2,3,6-tetrahydropyridine		Antioxidant, antitumor activity, anti-inflammation activity, neuroprotective (Hu et al., 2014)

TABLE 24.4 *(Continued)*

Bioactive compounds	Molecular structure	Therapeutic activities
p-cyanophenyl p-(2-propoxyethoxy) benzoate 4-cy-anophenyl 4-(2-propoxyethoxy) benzoate		Antimicrobial, chemoprotective, antibacterial activity (Nicas et al., 1989)
Trimethylsilyl-di (trimethylsiloxy)-silane 1,1,1,5,5,5-hexamethyl-3-(trimethylsilyl) trisiloxane		Anti-allergic, antioxidant activity pharmaceuticals (1999)

TABLE 24.5 Fourier-transform infrared analysis of *N. sativa Seeds Extract.*

S/No.	Peak value	Bond	Functional group
1	3417.86	O–H stretch	Alcohols
2	3377.36	-OH stretch	Hydroxyl
3	3346.5	C–H stretch	Alkynes
4	3305.99	C–H stretch	Alkene
5	3008.95	-C–H stretch	Alkyl
6	2926.01	-NH$_2$ stretch	Amine
7	2856.58	-NH stretch	Amine
8	1710.86	C=O strech	Carboxylic acids, esters, ketones, aldehydes
9	1654.92	C=O stretch	α carbonyl group α, β-unsaturated ketones, aldehydes
10	1548.84	C=O stretch	α, β-unsaturated ketones, aldehydes
11	1458.18	C–H bend	Alkanes
12	1419.61	C–H bend	Alkanes
13	1244.09	C–O stretch	Alcohols, carboxylic acids, esters, ethers
14	1163.08	C-O stretch	Alcohols, carboxylic acids, esters, ethers
15	1053.13	C–H bend	Alkanes
16	719.45	C–H bend	Alkanes
17	621.08	C–H bend	Alkanes

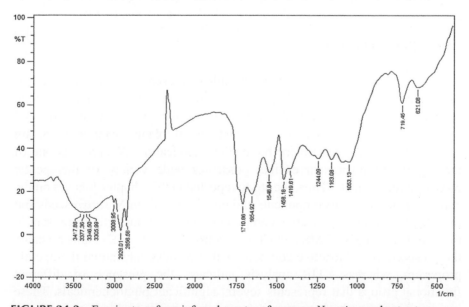

FIGURE 24.3 Fourier-transform infrared spectra of aqueous *N. sativa* seed extract.

24.5   FUTURE PERSPECTIVE

GC-MS and FTIR help in the identification and isolation of bioactive compounds and metabolites, especially phytochemicals present in the crude aqueous extract of *N. sativa* seed extract. These isolated bioactive compounds and phytochemicals are highly beneficial in the treatment of various diseases and also as nutrients for nutrition deficient patients. Thus, these bioactive compounds have attracted several pharmaceutical and nutraceutical industries for drug formulation (Chan et al., 2010). *N. sativa* seed extracts have been extensively used for the nanoparticle synthesis. Gold (Fragoon et al., 2012), silver (Ranjan et al., 2013), reduced graphene oxide (Awad et al., 2017), zinc oxide (Al-Shabib et al., 2016) nanoparticles and reduced graphene oxide silica nanocomposites (Awad et al., 2016) are recently synthesized using *N. sativa* seed extracts. The present study will help in identifying the phytochemical responsible for nanoparticle formation and in fine-tuning their morphology and physicochemical properties to use them in the desired biomedical application. Further, the present study will also help in the isolation and purification of bioactive compounds that can be encapsulated using nano-based formulation such as dendrimers and micelles. In future, these nano-formulations will occupy pharma-industry and help in the targeted and controlled delivery of therapeutic phytochemicals to enhance their bioactivity and bioavailability in biofluids (Jeevanandam et al., 2017).

24.6   CONCLUSION

The bioactive compounds and phytochemicals present in plants have gained biomedical application, as they possess enormous beneficial therapeutic properties against several diseases. The isolation, identification, and purification of these bioactive components of plants from extracts are important in utilizing them for biomedical application. *N. sativa* is one of the significant plant sources that possesses wide variety of therapeutic bioactive components. Thus, the study reported in this chapter focuses on the extraction of bioactive components and metabolites from *N. sativa* seeds and investigates about the bioactive compounds and functional groups present in the extract through GC-MS and FTIR spectroscopy. GC-MS results revealed the presence of 11 bioactive compounds that possess substantial therapeutic properties, whereas FTIR analysis indicates the presence of different functional groups that represents several significant phytochemicals. These bioactive components from *N. sativa* seed extracts are highly beneficial as a curative agent for several diseases and can be used in the treatment of diseases ranging from cancer to acquired immune deficiency syndrome in future.

KEYWORDS

- **phytochemicals**
- ***Nigella sativa* seeds**
- **thymoquinone**
- **gas chromatography–mass spectrometry**
- **Fourier-transform infrared**

REFERENCES

Adam, G. O.; Rahman, M. M.; Lee, S. J.; Kim, G. B.; Kang, H.-S.; Kim, J. S.; Kim, S. J. Hepatoprotective Effects of Nigella Sativa Seed Extract Against Acetaminophen-induced Oxidative Stress. *Asian Pac. J. Trop. Med.* **2016,** *9*(3), 221–227.

Ait Mbarek, L.; Ait Mouse, H.; Elabbadi, N.; Bensalah, M.; Gamouh, A.; Aboufatima, R.; Benharref, A.; Chait, A.; Kamal, M.; Dalal, A. Anti-Tumor Properties of Blackseed (Nigella sativa L.) Extracts. *Braz J. Med. Biol. Res.* **2007,** *40*(6), 839–847.

Ali, B.; Blunden, G. Pharmacological and Toxicological Properties of Nigella Sativa. Phytother. Res. **2003,** *17*(4), 299–305.

Al-Marzoqi, A. H.; Hameed, I. H.; Idan, S. A. Analysis of Bioactive Chemical Components of Two Medicinal Plants (Coriandrum sativum and Melia azedarach) Leaves Using Gas Chromatography-mass Spectrometry (GC-MS). *Afr. J. Biotechnol.* **2015,** *14*(40), 2812–2830.

Al-Shabib, N. A.; Husain, F. M.; Ahmed, F.; Khan, R. A.; Ahmad, I.; Alsharaeh, E.; Khan, M. S.; Hussain, A.; Rehman, M. T.; Yusuf, M. Biogenic Synthesis of Zinc Oxide Nanostructures from Nigella Sativa Seed: Prospective Role as Food Packaging Material Inhibiting Broad-spectrum Quorum Sensing and Biofilm. *Sci. Rep.* **2016,** 636761.

Ashraf, S.; Anjum, A. A.; Ahmad, A.; Firyal, S.; Sana, S.; Latif, A. A. In Vitro Activity of Nigella Sativa Against Antibiotic Resistant Salmonella Enterica. *Environ. Toxicol. Pharmacol.* **2017.**

Atta, M. B. Some Characteristics of Nigella (Nigella sativa L.) Seed Cultivated in Egypt and its Lipid Profile. *Food Chem.* **2003,** *83*(1), 63–68.

Awad, M. A. G.; Hendi, A. A.; Ortashi, K. M. O.; Laref, A. Green Synthesis of Reduced Graphene Oxide Silica Nanocomposite Using Nigella Sativa Seeds Extract. **2016.** Google Patents.

Awad, M. A. G.; Hendi, A. A.; Ortashi, K. M. O.; Laref, A. Green Synthesis of Reduced Graphene Oxide Using Nigella Sativa Seed Extract **2017.** Google Patents.

Babayan, V.; Koottungal, D.; Halaby, G. Proximate Analysis, Fatty Acid and Amino Acid Composition of Nigella Sativa L. Seeds. *J. Food Sci.* **1978,** *43*(4), 1314–1315.

Bakal, S. N.; Bereswill, S.; Heimesaat, M. M. Finding Novel Antibiotic Substances from Medicinal Plants—Antimicrobial Properties of Nigella Sativa Directed Against Multidrug Resistant Bacteria. *Eur. J. Microbiol. Immunol.* **2017,** *7*(1), 92–98.

Begum, H. A.; Hamayun, M.; Zaman, K.; Hussain, A.; Ruaf, M. Phytochemical Evaluation of Ethnobotanically Selected Medicinal Plants of Mardan. *Pakistan. J. Adv. Bot. Zool.* **2015,** 31–35.

Benhelima, A.; Kaid-Omar, Z.; Hemida, H.; Benmahdi, T.; Addou, A. Nephroprotective and Diuretic Effect of Nigella Sativa L Seeds Oil on Lithiasic Wistar Rats. *Afr. J. Tradit. Complementary Altern. Med. (AJTCAM)* **2016,** *13*(6), 204–214.

Benkaci–Ali, F.; Baaliouamer, A.; Meklati, B. Y.; Chemat, F. Chemical Composition of Seed Essential oils from Algerian Nigella Sativa Extracted by Microwave and Hydrodistillation. *Flavour Fragrance J.* **2007,** *22*(2), 148–153.

Benzie, I. F.; Wachtel-Galor, S. Herbal Medicine: Biomolecular and Clinical Aspects. CRC Press: Boca Raton (FL), 2011.

Butt, U. J.; Shah, S. A. A.; Ahmed, T.; Zahid, S. Protective Effects of Nigella Sativa L. Seed Extract on Lead Induced Neurotoxicity During Development and Early Life in Mouse Models. *Toxicol. Res.* **2018.**

Chan, E.; Tan, M.; Xin, J.; Sudarsanam, S.; Johnson, D. E. Interactions Between Traditional Chinese Medicines and Western. *Curr. Opin. Drug Discovery Dev.* **2010,** *13*(1), 50–65.

Cheikh-Rouhou, S.; Besbes, S.; Hentati, B.; Blecker, C.; Deroanne, C.; Attia, H. Nigella Sativa L.: Chemical Composition and Physicochemical Characteristics of Lipid Fraction. *Food Chem.* **2007,** *101*(2), 673–681.

Conforti, F.; Statti, G.; Uzunov, D.; Menichini, F. Comparative Chemical Composition and Antioxidant Activities of Wild and Cultivated Laurus Nobilis L. Leaves and Foeniculum Vulgare Subsp. Piperitum (Ucria) Coutinho Seeds. *Biol. Pharm. Bull.* **2006,** *29*(10), 2056–2064.

El–Dakhakhny, M. Studies on the Chemical Constitution of Egyptian Nigella Sativa l. Seeds. ii1) the Essential Oil. *Planta Med.* **1963,** *11*(04), 465–470.

El-Kabbani, O.; Darmanin, C.; Chung, R. T. Sorbitol Dehydrogenase: Structure, Function and Ligand Design. *Curr. Med. Chem.* **2004,** *11*(4), 465–476.

Eloff, J. Which Extractant Should be Used for the Screening and Isolation of Antimicrobial Components from Plants? *J. Ethnopharmacol.* **1998,** *60*(1), 1–8.

Fragoon, A.; Li, J.; Zhu, J.; Zhao, J. Biosynthesis of Controllable Size and Shape Gold Nanoparticles by Black Seed (Nigella sativa) Extract. *J. Nanosci. Nanotechnol.* **2012,** *12*(3), 2337–2345.

Grassmann, J. Terpenoids as Plant Antioxidants. *Vitam. Horm.* **2005,** 72505–72535.

Harborne, J. Phytochemical Methods, a Guide to Modern Techniques of Plant Analysis; Harborne, J. B., Ed.; Chapman and Hall Ltd.: London, 1973.

Hashem, F.; El-Kiey, M. *Nigella Sativa* Seeds of Egypt. *J. Pharm. Sci. United Arab Republic* **1982,** 3121–3133.

Hebi, M.; Zeggwagh, N.; Hajj, L.; El Bouhali, B.; Eddouks, M. Cardiovascular Effect of Nigella Sativa L. Aqueous Extract in Normal Rats. *Cardiovascular Haematol. Disorders-Drug Targets.* **2016,** *16*(1), 47–55.

Hu, Y.; Zhang, J.; Yu, C.; Li, Q.; Dong, F.; Wang, G.; Guo, Z. Synthesis, Characterization, and Antioxidant Properties of Novel Inulin Derivatives with Amino-pyridine Group. *Int. J. Biol. Macromol.* **2014,** 7044–7049.

Hyam, R.; Pankhurst, R. Plants and Their Names: A Concise Dictionary. Oxford University Press: New York, 1995.

Jeevanandam, J.; Aing, Y. S.; Chan, Y. S.; Pan, S.; Danquah, M. K. Nanoformulation and Application of Phytochemicals as Antimicrobial Agents. Antimicrobial Nanoarchitectonics: From Synthesis to Applications. Elsevier **2017**, *1,* 62–82.

Jeevanandam, J.; San Chan, Y.; Danquah, M. K. Biosynthesis and Characterization of MgO Nanoparticles from Plant Extracts Via Induced Molecular Nucleation. *New J. Chem.* **2017**, *41*(7), 2800–2814.

Kozlowska, A.; Szostak-Wegierek, D. Flavonoids-food Sources and Health Benefits. *Rocz. Państw. Zakł. Hig.* **2014**, 65(2), 79–85.

Kumar, A.; Sharma, P.; Kumari, P.; Kalal, B. L. Exploration of Antimicrobial and Antioxidant Potential of Newly Synthesized 2, 3-disubstituted Quinazoline-4 (3H)-ones. *Bioorg. Med. Chem. Lett.* **2011**, *21*(14), 4353–4357.

Kumara, S. S. M.; Huat, B. T. K. Extraction, Isolation and Characterisation of Antitumor Principle, α-hederin, from the Seeds of Nigella Sativa. *Planta Med.* **2001**, *67*(01), 29–32.

Kusumoto, I. T.; Nakabayashi, T.; Kida, H.; Miyashiro, H.; Hattori, M.; Namba, T.; Shimotohno, K. Screening of Various Plant Extracts Used in Ayurvedic Medicine for Inhibitory Effects on Human Immunodeficiency Virus Type 1 (HIV-1) Protease. *Phytother Res.* **1995**, *9*(3), 180–184.

Lautenbacher LM Schwarzkummelöl: eine neue quelle ungesattigter fettsauren. Deutsche Apothekcr-Zeitung. **1997**, *137*(50), 68–69.

Lin, J.; Cheng, Y.; Wang, T.; Tang, L.; Sun, Y.; Lu, X.; Yu, H. Soyasaponin Ab Inhibits Lipopolysaccharide-induced Acute Lung Injury in Mice. *Int. Immunopharmacol.* **2016**, 30121–30128.

Macready, A. L.; Kennedy, O. B.; Ellis, J. A.; Williams, C. M.; Spencer, J. P.; Butler, L. T. Flavonoids and Cognitive Function: A Review of Human Randomized Controlled Trial Studies and Recommendations for Future Studies. *Genes Nutr.* **2009**, *4*(4), 227–242.

Majewska-Wierzbicka, M.; Czeczot, H. Flavonoids in the Prevention and Treatment of Cardiovascular Diseases. Polski Merkuriusz Lekarski: Organ *Polskiego Towarzystwa Lekarskiego* **2012**, *32*(187), 50–54.

Malik, S.; Zaman, K. Nigellimine: A New Isoquinoline Alkaloid from the Seeds of Nigella Sativa. *J. Nat. Prod.* **1992**, *55*(5), 676–678.

Malik, S.; Ahmad, S.; Chaudhary, I. Nigellimine N-oxide-a New Isoquinoline Alkaloid from the Seeds of Nigella Sativa. *Heterocycles* **1985a**, *23*(4), 953–955.

Malik, S.; Cun-Heng, H.; Clardy, J. Isolation and Structure Determination of Nigellicine, a Novel Alkaloid from the Seeds of Nigellasativa. *Tetrahedron Lett.* **1985b**, *26*(23), 2759–2762.

Malik, S.; Hasan, S. S.; Choudhary, M. I.; Ni, C. Z.; Clardy, J. Nigellidine—a New Indazole Alkaloid from the Seeds of Nigella Sativa. *Tetrahedron Lett.* **1995**, *36*(12), 1993–1996.

Nakashima, H.; Okubo, K.; Honda, Y.; Tamura, T.; Matsuda, S.; Yamamoto, N. Inhibitory Effect of Glycosides Like Saponin from Soybean on the Infectivity of HIV in Vitro. *Aids* **1989**, *3*(10), 655–658.

Nergiz, C.; Ötleş, S. Chemical Composition of Nigella Sativa L. Seeds. *Food Chem.* **1993**, *48*(3), 259–261.

Ng, Y. P.; Tsun, T. C.; Ip, N. Y. Plant Alkaloids as Drug Leads for Alzheimer's Disease. *Neurochem. Int.* **2015**, 89260–89270.

Nicas, T. I.; Wu, C.; Hobbs, J.; Preston, D.; Allen, N. Characterization of Vancomycin Resistance in Enterococcus Faecium and Enterococcus Faecalis. *Antimicrob. Agents Chemother.* **1989**, *33*(7), 1121–1124.

Nickavar, B.; Mojab, F.; Javidnia, K.; Amoli, M. A. R. Chemical Composition of the Fixed and Volatile Oils of Nigella Sativa L. from Iran. *Z. Naturforsch. C.* **2003**, *58*(9–10), 629–631.

Oh, Y. J.; Sung, M. K. Soybean Saponins Inhibit Cell Proliferation by Suppressing PKC Activation and Induce Differentiation ofHT-29 Human Colon Adenocarcinoma Cells. *Nutr. Cancer* **2001,** *39*(1), 132–138.

Osbaldeston, T. A.; Wood, R. P. Dioscorides: De Materia Medica. Ibidis: Johannesburg, 2000.

Pharmaceuticals, E. D.-G. Cosmetics Legislation Cosmetic Products **1999.** Comisión europea.

Ranjan, P.; Das, M. P.; Kumar, M. S.; Anbarasi, P.; Sindhu, S.; Sagadevan, E.; Arumugam, P. Green Synthesis and Characterization of Silver Nanoparticles from Nigella Sativa and Its Application Against UTI Causing Bacteria. *J. Acad. Ind. Res.* **2013,** 245–249.

Saadia, M.; Rehman, S.; Robin, S.; Ruby, T.; Sher, M.; Siddiqui, W. A.; Khan, M. A. Potential of Nigella Sativa Seed Aqueous Extract in Ameliorating Quinine-induced Thrombocytopenia in Rats. *Pak. J. Pharm. Sci.* **2017,** *30*(5), 1679–1690.

Saini, D. K.; Saini, M. R. Evaluation of Radioprotective Efficacy and Possible Mechanism of Action of Aloe Gel. *Environ. Toxicol. Pharmacol.* **2011,** *31*(3), 427–435.

Salem, M. L. Immunomodulatory and Therapeutic Properties of the Nigella Sativa L. Seed. *Int. Immunopharmacol.* **2005,** *5*(13), 1749–1770.

Sarpangala, K. B.; Ashwin, D.; Sarpangala, M. Analgesic, anti-inflammatory and Wound Healing Properties of Arecanut, Areca Catechu l.: A Review. Int. J. Ayurveda Pharma Res. **2017,** 4(12).

Sedaghat, R.; Roghani, M.; Khalili, M. Neuroprotective Effect of Thymoquinone, the Nigella Sativa Bioactive Compound, in 6-hydroxydopamine-induced Hemi-parkinsonian Rat Model. *IJPR* **2014,** *13*(1), 227.

Singh, B.; Singh, J. P.; Singh, N.; Kaur, A. Saponins in Pulses and Their Health Promoting Activities: A Review. *Food Chem.* 2017.

Sofowora, A. Medicinal Plants and Traditional Medicine in Africa. John Wiley and sons LTD: New York, 1982.

Sulaiman, W.; Azizi, W. M.; Azad, A. K.; Daud, N. A.; Sunzida, N. K. Evaluation of Skin Elasticity After Used Different Seaweed Containing Products by DermaLab® Combo. *Asian J. Pharm Pharmacol.* **2016,** *3*(2), 72–76.

Sultan, M. T.; Butt, M. S.; Anjum, F. M.; Jamil, A.; Akhtar, S.; Nasir, M. Nutritional Profile of Indigenous Cultivar of Black Cumin Seeds and Antioxidant Potential of Its Fixed and Essential Oil. *Pak. J. Bot.* **2009,** *41*(3), 1321–1330.

Takruri, H. R.; Dameh, M. A. Study of the Nutritional Value of Black Cumin Seeds (Nigella sativa L). *J. Sci. Food Agric.* **1998,** *76*(3), 404–410.

Tavakkoli, A.; Ahmadi, A.; Razavi, B. M.; Hosseinzadeh, H. Black Seed (Nigella sativa) and Its Constituent Thymoquinone as an Antidote or a Protective Agent Against Natural or Chemical Toxicities. *Iran. J. Pharm. Res.* **2017,** 162–123.

Tiwari, A. K.; Rao, J. M. Diabetes Mellitus and Multiple Therapeutic Approaches of Phytochemicals: Present Status and Future Prospects. *Curr. Sci.* **2002,** 30–38.

Trease, G. E.; Evans, W. C. Pharmacognosy. Bailliere Tindall: London, 1989; pp 45–50.

Tsoungas, P. G.; Tsiamis, C.; Michael, C.; Sigalas, M. Theoretical Justification of Structure-reactivity Correlation of 1, 2-benzisoxazole 2-oxides. *Tetrahedron* **1987,** *43*(4), 785–790.

Vriet, C.; Russinova, E.; Reuzeaua, C. Boosting Crop Yields with Plant Steroids. *Plant Cell.* **2012,** *24*(3), 842–857. DOI: 10.1105/tpc.111.094912. Epub 2012 Mar 20 (Advance Publication March).

Zhou, Z. H.; Yang, J.; Kong, A. N. Phytochemicals in Traditional Chinese Herbal Medicine: Cancer Prevention and Epigenetics Mechanisms. *Curr. Pharmacol. Rep.* **2017,** *3*(2), 77–91.

CHAPTER 25

PHYTOCHEMICAL STUDIES ON FIVE NIGERIAN INDIGENOUS VEGETABLES

FALEYIMU, O. I.[1,*], SOLOMON T.[2], and AJIBOYE JOHN ADEBAYO[3]

[1]Department of Forestry, Wildlife and Environmental Management, Ondo State University of Science and Technology, Okitipupa, Nigeria

[2]Department of Biological Sciences, Ondo State University of Science and Technology, Okitipupa, Nigeria

[3]Department of Chemical Sciences, Ondo State University of Science and Technology, Okitipupa, Nigeria

*Corresponding author. E-mail: orimoloyespecial@gmail.com
ORCID: *https://orcid.org/0000-0001-7766-9173

ABSTRACT

Vegetables have been an important source of food and medicine since time immemorial. They have been reported to be beneficial in the treatment of various diseases. The potentials of vegetables to be used as medicines have been attributed to their phytochemical compositions. This chapter is an account of the investigation of the phytochemical constituents of five indigenous vegetables from Okitipupa local government area of Ondo State, Nigeria: *Crassocephalum rubens, Solanum nigrum, Gongronema latifolium, Senecio biafrae,* and *Clerodendrum volubile.* The vegetables were analyzed following standard procedures. *C. rubens, S. biafrae, S. nigrum, and C. volubile* possesses the highest ascorbic acid (++) while *G. latifolium* had the least ascorbic acid (+). The presence of some minerals is an indication that the vegetables contain mineral elements that may be useful in nutrition. Also, the presence of other phytochemicals attests to the potential therapeutic effects of the vegetables while serving as food for man.

25.1   INTRODUCTION

Inadequate information on the available nutrients and phytochemicals in our native vegetable species with which Nigeria is blessed is partly responsible for their under exploitation especially in areas where they are found and consumed. There are large arrays of laxatives, sedatives, and soporifics or sleep-inducing components in the vegetable kingdom.

Vegetables like *Senecio biafrae* belonging to the family of Asteraceae (local name: worowo) act as a tonic and are excellent for the nerves (Ahmed and Chaudhary, 2009). *S. biafrae* belong to this group of vegetables that grow in large quantity as undercover in tree crop plantation. Some of these leafy vegetables are also considered for their high medicinal value as the juice extracted from the leaves are wholly applied to fresh wounds or cuts as styptic in the rural community for man and animal use (Gulliice et al., 2004). The high edible mucilaginous fiber, leaves, and stem are used to treat indigestion or as laxative and as purgative. Moreover, fresh succulent leaves of *S. biafrae* are used as a leafy vegetable in Sierra Leone, Ghana, Benin, Nigeria, Cameroon, and Gabon. Some vegetables are highly beneficial in the treatment of various diseases.

Clerodendrum volubile, an understudied indigenous vegetable, belongs to the family Lamiaceae (Verbenaceae) and it is one of the widely distributed plants in the tropical regions of the world. The vegetables are popularly known as "marugbo" or "eweta" among the Ikale, Ilaje, and Apoi people found in Ondo State, Nigeria. The leaf of *C. volubile* is commonly consumed as vegetable soups mostly blended with other vegetables. Locally, the vegetable can be blended either fresh or dried and applied as spices in cooking (Adefegha, 2011). Interestingly, the dried leaves produce the darker soup content. Commonly referred to as "eweta" by the Ikales (majorly the people in Okitipupa local government area (LGA) of Ondo State, Nigeria), the leaves of *C. volubile* have great nutritional value as well as herbal and medicinal value. According to Dansi et al. (2008), many traditional leafy vegetables possess the ability to cure, regulate, and stimulate properties besides food qualities and are used as a nutraceutical. Though most of the traditional leafy vegetables is water, they are sometimes a veritable natural pharmacy of minerals (calcium, magnesium, potassium, iron, and sodium), vitamins, and phytochemicals (alkaloids, flavonoids, glycosides, and tannins). However, some studies revealed that some vegetable species are potentially toxic to humans and animals (Agbaire et al., 2013).

The genus *Crassocephalum rubens* popularly known as èfó-ebúre or ẹfọ ébòlò is a dicotyledonous plant that belongs to the family Asteraceae. For tropical Africa, 24 species were reported with 15 of these species in

West Africa. In Nigeria, nine species were identified. *C. rubens* occurs in rainforest, deciduous, and secondary forests, and also in mangrove and disturbed roadside forest. Some communities semi-cultivate the vegetable in home gardens or on fertile land portions near homesteads. The leaves are slightly laxative. They are used in traditional medicine to treat a range of complaints. They are given to women after childbirth for their laxative effect; they are used as a treatment for "belly palava" (stomach ache); when eaten in quantity they are used to treat liver complaints; they are used as an infusion against colds. Applied externally, they are made into poultices to treat burns. The leaf sap is applied to sore eyes and is also instilled into the eye to remove filarial parasites. They are crushed in water and rubbed into the ear to treat an earache.

Gongronema latifolium is the botanical name for a local leaf/herb called "utazi" by the eastern part (Igbo/Ibo) of Nigeria, belonging to the family of Asclepiadaceae. The western part of Nigeria call this leaf "arokeke" and it is a tropical rainforest plant mainly used as vegetable, medicine, or spice by the people. *G. latifolium* (iteji) is a climbing shrub that reaches up to 5-m long with woody base, hollow stems, and fleshy roots. The plant is highly medicinal in nature, which suggests why its health benefits cannot be over-emphasized. It is has anti-sickling, antioxidant, antiasthmatic, antipyretic, hypoglycemic, and anti-inflammatory properties (Stevels, 1990).

The plant *Solanum nigrum* Linn (Family name: Solanaceae) commonly called black nightshade. The Solanaceae or nightshades are an economically important family of flowering plants. It ranges from annual and perennial herbs to vines, lianas, epiphytes, shrubs, and trees, and includes a number of important agricultural crops, medicinal plants, spices, weeds, and ornamentals. Many members of the family contain potent alkaloids, and some are highly toxic, but many cultures eat nightshades, in some cases as staple foods.

This study was carried out to evaluate the phytochemical and the nutritional composition of common indigenous vegetables in Okitipupa LGA of Ondo State, Nigeria so as to put into literature the significance of consuming these common vegetables.

25.2 MATERIALS AND METHODS

25.2.1 STUDY AREA

This study was carried out in Okitipupa LGA of Ondo State, Nigeria (Fig. 25.1).

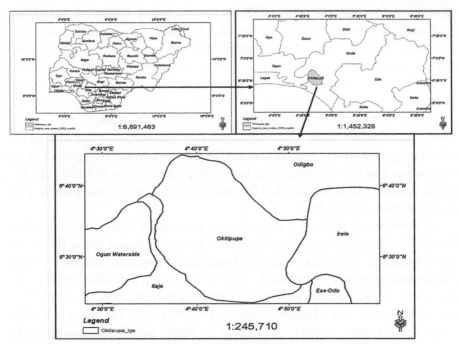

FIGURE 25.1 Map of the study area (Okitipupa local government area of Ondo State, Nigeria).

25.2.2 COLLECTION OF SAMPLES

Some vegetable samples were purchased from popular local markets within Okitipupa, while others were collected at local home gardens/backyard gardens in Okitipupa. Samples collected were identified by Mr. Samuel A. in the herbarium unit of the University of Science and Technology, Okitipupa. During collection, samples were kept aseptically in a sterile foil paper and a sterilized container, tied and labeled appropriately in readiness for phyto-chemical and nutritional analysis.

25.2.3 PREPARATION OF EXTRACTS

The analysis determined the active compounds that contribute to the flavor, color, and other characteristics of the vegetables. A 100 g of the vegetable samples were washed with deionized water to remove dust particles, the leaves were dried under shade for 3–4 days. The leaves were then milled to obtain the powder using an electric blender, the powder was soaked in 360 mL of sterile distilled methanol and 240 mL of sterile distilled water in a ratio of 3:2 for 4 days at 30–32°C. The plant extracts were filtered through a millipore filter (0.25 μm). The resulting filtrates were concentrated under reduced pressure at 50°C and then transferred into a well labeled sterile bottle as described by Kumar et al. (2009).

25.2.4　PHYTOCHEMICAL SCREENING

25.2.4.1　TEST FOR ALKALOIDS

About 1% HCl and six drops of Meyer's reagent and Dragendroff's reagent was added to the extract. The organic precipitate indicates the presence of alkaloids (Kumar et al., 2009).

25.2.4.2　TEST FOR FLAVONOIDS

About 5 mL of dilute ammonia solution was added to the extract of each sample, followed by addition of concentrated H_2SO_4. A yellow coloration confirms the presence of flavonoids which disappeared immediately.

25.2.4.3　TEST FOR SAPONIN

Exactly 20 mL of distilled water was measured in a graduated cylinder for 15 min, the formation of foam (about 1-cm layer of foam) indicated the presence of saponin (Kumar et al., 2009).

25.2.4.4　TEST FOR TANNINS

Few drops of lead acetate were added to about 5 mL of the extract, the formation of a yellow precipitate indicated the presence of tannin (Edeoga et al., 2005).

25.2.4.5　TEST FOR CARBOHYDRATE

About two drops of Molisch was added to 2 mL of the sample extract in a test tube and mixed thoroughly, while the 2 mL of concentrated H_2SO_4

was added. A reddish violet color appeared immediately which indicated the presence of carbohydrates.

25.2.4.6 TEST FOR PROTEIN

Exactly 2 mL of protein solution and 40% NaOH solution and 1–2 drops of 1% CuSO4 solution was added. A violet color indicated the presence of peptide linkage of the molecule.

25.2.4.7 TEST FOR ASCORBIC ACID

About 10 drops of starch solution were added to the filtrate with the aid of a pipette and it was stirred. Iodine solution was added in drops until a color that persisted longer than 20 s which is the endpoint. The color change showed the presence of Vitamin C (Omaha, 2011).

25.2.5 DETERMINATION OF MINERAL CONTENT

Milled samples (5 g) were dry ashed in a furnace at 550°C for 24 h. The resulting ash was cooled in a desiccator. Two milliliters of concentrated HCl was added to dissolve the ash and a few drops of concentrated HNO_3 were added. The solution was placed in a boiling water bath and evaporated almost to dryness. The contents were then transferred to a 100-mL volumetric flask and diluted to volume with deionized water and appropriate dilutions were made for each sample before analysis. Magnesium, calcium, and iron contents were determined using atomic absorption spectrophotometer, while sodium and potassium were quantified with a flame photometer (AOAC, 1990).

25.3 RESULTS

In Table 25.1, the result of the study revealed that the *C. rubens* and *S. biafrae* had alkaloid that is highly present (++) unlike *G. latifolium* where alkaloid was not found present (−), while studies on *S. nigrum* and *C. volubile* revealed the presence of alkaloid (+). Flavonoid was present in *C. rubens, S. nigrum,* and *C. volubile* but moderately present while it was observed to be absent in *S. biafrae* and *G. latifolium*. The *C. rubens* indicate the presence of all the constituents except saponin, though alkaloid was highly present (++) while flavonoid and tannin were found in moderate form (+). *S. biafrae* revealed the presence of alkaloids and tannin in abundance (++) while flavonoid and saponin were absent (−). In *G. latifolium* alkaloid and flavonoid were absent (−) while saponin was present (+) but tannin was highly present (++).

TABLE 25.1 Phytochemical Screening of the Selected Vegetable Samples.

Samples	Alkaloid	Flavonoid	Saponin	Tannin	Carbohydrate	Protein	Ascorbic Acid
Crassocephalum rubens	++	+	−	+	++	++	++
Senecio biafrae	++	−	−	++	++	I+	++
Gongronema latifolium	−	−	+	++	++	+	+
Solanum nigrum	+	+	++	+	++	+	++
Clerodendrum volubile	+	+	++	+	++	++	+I

Present = (+); Highly present = (++); Absent = (−).

Although *S. nigrum* and *C. volubile* were shown to possess the three secondary metabolites, saponin was found to be highly present (++).

All the nutritional constituents (carbohydrate, protein, and ascorbic acid) tested was found present in all the vegetable samples, although some were highly present (++) while some were moderately present (+), whereas all the samples showed that carbohydrate is highly present (++).

Though all the samples are proteinous but *C. rubens, S. biafrae,* and *C. volubile* are highly proteinous among the samples because of their high presence (++). The study also revealed high presence of ascorbic acid in all the samples (++) except *G. latifolium* which was moderately present (+).

Five mineral elements were established in the analysis. The elements are calcium (Ca), potassium (K), magnesium (Mg), iron (Fe), and sodium (Na). The *S. biafrae* had the highest Ca (49.5 mg/100 g) content among other vegetable samples while the least content was recorded in *C. rubens* and *S. nigrum* which were of the same concentration (18.5 mg/100 g), (Fig. 25.2).

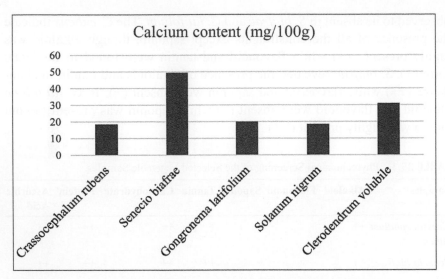

FIGURE 25.2   Calcium concentration of the selected indigenous vegetables.

The iron content was maximum in *C. volubile* "eweta" when compared with other vegetables (Fig. 25.3).

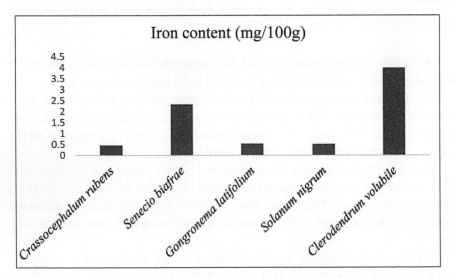

FIGURE 25.3   Iron concentration of the selected indigenous vegetables.

Although the minimum potassium content was recorded in *C. rubens* (9.17 mg/100 g) (Fig. 25.4), the *S. biafrae* recorded the highest (31.91 mg/100g).

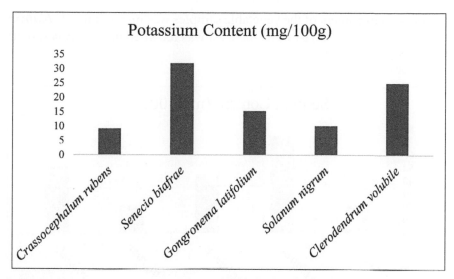

FIGURE 25.4   Potassium concentration of the selected indigenous vegetables.

The magnesium content of the vegetable was found to be maximum in *G. latifolium* "Iteji" and *C. volubile* "eweta" (0.60 mg/100 g), while the least magnesium content was obtained in *S. nigrum* "efo odu" (0.50 mg/100 g), (Fig. 25.5).

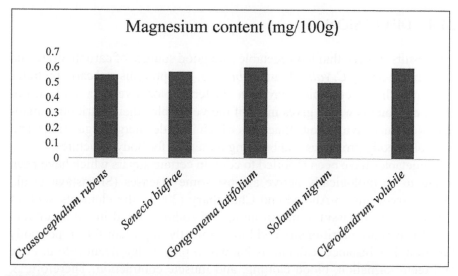

FIGURE 25.5   Magnesium concentration of the selected indigenous vegetables.

The sodium content of the vegetable samples was maximum in *S. biafrae* "worowo" (74.4 mg/100 g) while the least was recorded in *S. nigrum* (20.70 mg/100 g), (Fig. 25.6).

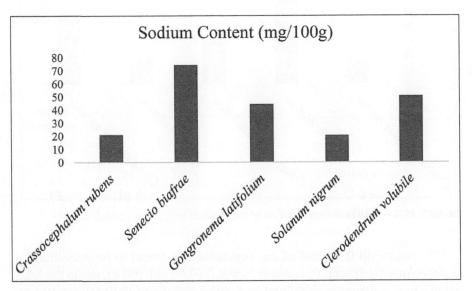

FIGURE 25.6 Sodium concentration of the selected indigenous vegetables.

25.4 DISCUSSION

The results showed that the vegetables are good sources of carbohydrate and protein, especially *C. volubile* and *S. biafrae*. The proteins and carbohydrates present in these vegetables may be a cluster of bioactive sugars, glycoproteins, or proteins which gives most of the vegetables their nutritional qualities. Nutrients have various functions which include energy, regulations, and control of body processes and building materials for body structures.

Vegetables have been reported to contain certain sugars which have been found to be biologically active against some diseases (Srivastava et al., 1989). According to Ahmed and Chaudhary (2009), the elements such as calcium, iron, potassium, magnesium, and sodium found in small amount in the leaves are nutritionally and biochemically important for proper body function. For instance, calcium is known to play a significant role in bone and teeth formation, blood clotting, and muscle contraction. Therefore, *S. biafrae* exhibiting the maximum content of calcium (49.5 mg/100 g) is the best among the vegetable studied for bone and teeth formation, blood clotting, and muscle contraction. Minerals like magnesium are needed as a cofactor in enzyme catalysis in the body (Ahmed and Chaudhary, 2009). Potassium and sodium which are available in the intracellular and extracellular fluid, aid in maintaining electrolyte balance and membrane fluidity. Iron is one of the component of some metalloenzymes, myoglobin, and hemoglobin (Ahmed and Chaudhary, 2009), that is essential in the transport of oxygen and carbon dioxide during respiration or cellular metabolism. This hemoglobin carrying iron serves as a buffer to regulate changes in blood pH (Kamshilov and Zaprudnova, 2009). It is known that inorganic mineral elements such as potassium, calcium play crucial roles in the maintenance of normal glucose tolerance and in the release of insulin from β-cells of islets of Langerhans (Choudhary and Bandyopadhyay, 1999). Iron plays a very important role in hemoglobin formation and normal functioning of the central nervous system (Adeyeye and Otokiti, 1999).

Specific plants have been used in the treatment of diseases long before history was written and they have proved to be invaluable as sources for pharmaceutical preparations. The availability of secondary metabolites such as alkaloids, flavonoid, saponin, and tannins in the vegetables may contribute to its medicinal value. Some of these compounds are well documented to exhibit hypoglycemic activity in animals (Akhtar et al., 1981).

C. volubile is a plant that has been used for the treatment of various ailments in traditional medicine. However, claims of treatment successes have been made without any scientific basis. The results confirm the presence of constituents which are known to exhibit medicinal as well as physiological activity (Sofowora, 1993). S. biafrae and G. latifolium oil are acidic having phenolic groups which could be attributed to the abundant presence of tannins which are soluble in water and hence there is partial solubility of the oil extract in water. Though the bulk of the weight of traditional leafy vegetables is water, they represent a veritable natural source for minerals, vitamin, and phytochemical compounds such as alkaloids, flavonoids, glycosides, and tannins.

25.5 CONCLUSION

The vegetables sampled for analysis exhibited some forms of nutritional values which enable the plant to be known for having therapeutic values. It is to be noted that vegetables contain some certain nutritional elements which make the plants to be a source of nourishment for the body, promote good health and proper functional mechanism in the body system. The results revealed the presence of medicinally active constituents in the five vegetable plants studied. The phytochemical compounds identified in this study have earlier been proved to be bioactive. The presence of some of these compounds have been confirmed by previous workers to have medicinal as well as physiological activity and, therefore, could be said to be responsible for the efficacy of the leaves of the plants studied in the treatment of different ailments. The continued traditional medicinal use of these plants is, therefore, encouraged while it is suggested that further work should be carried out to isolate, purify, and possibly characterize the active constituents responsible for the activity of these plants that make them edible for nutritional value and treatment of different ailments.

KEYWORDS

- indigenous vegetables
- phytochemical constituents
- flavonoids
- alkaloids
- saponins

REFERENCES

Adefegha, S. A.; Oboh, G. Medicinal Plants. *J. Food Process. Technol.* **2011**, *2*(1), 2157–7110.

Adeyeye, E.; Otokiti, M. K. O. Proximate Composition and Some Nutritional Valuable Minerals of Two Varieties of Capsicum Annum (Bell and Cherry Peppers). *Discovery Innovation* **1999**, *11*, 75–81.

Ahmed, D.; Chaudhary, M. A. Medicinal and Nutritional Aspects of Various Trace Metals Determined in Ajuga Bracteosa. *J. Appl. Sci. Res.* **2009**, *5*(7), 864–886.

Akhtar, M. S.; Athar, M. A.; Yaqub, M. Effect of Momordica Charantia on Blood Glucose Level of Normal and Alloxan-Diabetic Rabbits. *Planta Med.* **1981**, *42*, 205–212.

AOAC. *Official Methods of Analysis*, 15th edn.; Association of Official Analytical Chemists: Washington DC, 1990.

Choudhary, K. A.; Bandyopadhyay, N. G. Preliminary Studies on the Inorganic Constituents of Some Indigenous Hyperglycaemic Herbs on Oral Glucose Tolerance Test. *J. Ethnopharmacol.* **1999**, *64*, 179–184.

Dansi, A. A.; Adoukonou-Sagbadja, H.; Faladé, V.; Yedomonhan, H.; Odou, D.; Dossou, B. Traditional Leafy Vegetable and Their use in the Benin Republic. *Genet. Resour. Crop Evol.* **2008**, *55*, 1239–1256.

Edeoga, H. O.; Okwu, D. E.; Mbaebie, B. O. Phytochemical Constituents of Some Nigerian Medicinal Plants. *Afr. J. Biotechnol.* **2005,** *4*(7), 685–688.

Gulliice, M.; Aigiizel, A.; Ogiiteu, H.; Segul, M.; Karaman, I.; Sahin, F. Antimicrobial Effect of Quercus Ilex L. extract. *Phytother. Res.* **2004,** *18,* 208–211.

Kamshilov, I. M.; Zaprudnova, R. A. Interspecies Differences of Hemoglobin Buffer Properties and of Ion Environment in Some Freshwater Fish. *J. Evol. Biochem. Physiol.* **2009,** *45*(2), 242–244.

Kumar, A.; Ilavarsan, P.; Jayachandran, T.; Decaraman, M.; Aravindhan, P.; Padmanaban, N.; Krishnan, M. R. V. Phytochemical Investigation on a Tropical Plant. *Pak J. Nutr.* **2009,** *8*(1), 83–85.

Omaha, T. 2011; U.S. Department of Energy: Iodine and Vitamin C Test, Jun 14, 2011.

Sofowora, A. Medicinal Plants and Traditional Medicine in Africa. Spectrum Books Ltd: Ibadan, Nigeria, 1993; p 289.

Srivastava, R.; Kulshreshtha, D. K. Bioactive Polysaccharides from Plants. Phytochem **1989,** *28*(11), 2877–2883.

Stevels, J. M. C. Légumes traditionnels du Cameroun: une étude agrobotanique. *Wageningen Agricultural University Papers No 90-1.* Wageningen University: Wageningen, Netherlands, **1990**; p 262.

INDEX

A

Abiotic stress, 233–235, 238
  mechanism, 234
  tolerance, 233, 234, 238
Abscisic acid, 102, 213
Absorbance
  accuracy, 318, 321, 341
  fluorescence, 361
Acarbose, 148
Accelerated solvent extraction (ASE), 269
Accuracy, 296, 316, 317, 322, 341,
  352–354, 358, 361, 578
Acetate
  malonate pathway, 49
  test, 394, 396, 577
Acetic
  acid, 139, 157, 295, 300, 385, 396, 398,
    401, 406, 410
  anhydride, 396, 397, 400
Acetoacetyl-CoA, 45
Acetonitrile, 90, 272, 275, 297, 300, 301,
  329, 351
Acetylcholine receptors, 134
Acetyl-CoA, 45, 66, 538
  carboxylase, 45
Acetylsalicylic acid, 7
Achnatherum robustum, 301
Achyrocline satureioides, 269
Acifluorfen, 87
Aconitic acid, 201
Acridine orange, 471, 571, 575, 581
  ethidium bromide (AO/EB), 571, 575
Acrocarpia, 212
Actinoplanes spp, 148
Activator protein 1 (AP-1), 518, 523, 527
  AP endonuclease, 521
Active agents/surfactants, 126
Adenosine triphosphate (ATP), 513, 529,
  538, 540–542, 544, 545
  ATP molecules, 538
Adrenaline, 154

Adsorption chromatography, 254
Aerobic
  fraction, 552
  glycolysis, 539, 543, 545
Aerosol formulation, 474
Aesculus hippocastanum L, 128
Aflatoxins, 332
Agilent Mass Hunter Workstation Data
  acquisition software, 500
Aglycon, 63
Aglycone, 61, 63, 124–128, 135–137, 139,
  162, 166, 209
  aglycone nature, 125
Aglycones, 127, 141
Agrobacterium rhizogenes, 98
Ajmalicine, 58, 71
Alanine, 232, 234, 237, 433, 441, 546
Alcohol, 12, 85, 94, 121, 133, 141, 164,
  209, 390, 394, 399, 404, 408, 419, 594
Alcoholic potassium hydroxide test, 399
Aldehyde glycosides, 63
Aldehydes, 17, 18, 594, 599
Aldoximes, 65
Alfalfa saponins, 126
Aliphatic
  aldehydes, 17
  diones, 91
Alium sativum, 171
Alkaline
  buffer, 576
  picrate, 405
  reactions, 410
Alkaloids, 6, 11, 17, 29, 37, 39, 41, 43, 44,
  47, 48, 54, 56–58, 119–122, 129–135,
  148, 153, 154, 156, 158, 170, 199, 201,
  204, 208, 209, 213, 230, 232, 249, 263,
  267, 295, 299, 301, 345, 346, 393, 394,
  404, 406, 407, 465, 466, 524, 572, 573,
  577, 590, 593, 594, 606, 607, 609–611,
  615, 616
Alkylation, 436, 520

Allantoin, 234

Allergic
  diseases, 124
  reactions, 124

Allicin, 190

Allium cepa, 91

Allophycocyanin, 211

Allosteric inhibition, 144

Alloxan, 436, 437

Alpha-enolase (ENO1), 554

Alternaria
  brassicicola infection, 87
  cassia, 103

Aluminum chloride, 404

Alzheimer's disease, 593

Amaranthus caudatus, 147

Ameliorate, 430, 449–451

Amine transferase, 44

Amino acid, 11, 41, 51, 56, 70, 120, 145,
  154, 158, 181, 99, 201, 202, 208, 209,
  213, 230, 232, 234, 236, 245, 288, 295,
  335, 400, 441, 522, 532
  metabolism, 236

Aminotransferase, 433

Ammodaucus leucotrichus, 487

Ammonia
  borate complex, 414
  gas, 416
  hydroxide, 397, 407, 409, 410
  layer, 397, 398
  thiocyanate solution, 410

Amorphous
  compounds, 122
  powders, 121

AMP-activated protein kinase, 543

Amylase inhibitors, 119, 120, 147

Amyloplasts, 202

Amyotrophic lateral sclerosis, 441

Anabasis aphylla, 131

Anaerobic
  conditions, 538
  metabolism, 144

Anaferine, 524

Anagallis, 215

Analgesics, 130

Analysis of variance (ANOVA), 24,
  481–485, 487–491

Analyte, 267, 290, 297, 298, 308, 313, 315,
  322, 323, 326, 328–336, 340, 351, 357,
  362, 363
  concentrations, 311
  groups, 326
  molecules, 332, 333

Analytical
  laboratories, 356
  method, 104, 352, 354
    measures, 352
    validation, 362
  procedure, 352, 354, 355, 382
  separation, 271
  technique, 19, 27, 226, 231, 254, 276,
    346, 368, 373, 377, 430
  tools, 296, 343, 346, 363
  weighing balance, 412, 414, 417, 421

Anatomy, 22, 198

Ancestral species, 431

Anecdotal claims, 428

Anhydride, 92, 396, 524

Animal
  model, 164, 427, 429–435, 439, 440, 442,
    454, 472, 473
    human diseases, 430
  species, 208, 434
  scientific investigation, 429

Anion/cation exchange, 329, 330

Antheraxanthin, 211

Anthocyanidins, 37, 41, 49, 53, 54, 122,
  139, 141, 142, 162, 205

Anthocyanin, 40, 41, 45, 138, 141, 153,
  154, 158, 159, 162, 186, 191, 205, 234,
  249, 267, 326, 344, 399

Anthracyclines, 465

Anthraquinone, 37, 41, 45, 63, 66–68, 71,
  136, 214, 215, 397, 403, 404

Anti-allergenic, 164

Anti-allergic, 51, 128, 596, 597
  anti-allergic activity, 124

Anti-allergy, 12

Anti-anxiety calmative, 526

Antiarrhythmic, 134

Anti-arthritic, 165, 526

Antiasthmatic, 138, 607

Antiatheromatous, 185

Anti-atherosclerosis, 12, 185, 189

Antibacterial, 12, 15, 96, 100, 119, 120, 128, 589, 593, 597, 598
Antibiotics, 70, 80, 206, 213, 555, 574
Anticancer, 14, 28, 80, 81, 120, 125, 128, 145, 169, 183, 186, 207, 209, 465, 476, 513, 518, 539, 541, 543, 545, 548, 554, 555, 572, 578, 584, 597
  activators, 164
  activity, 186, 572, 574, 576
  agents, 128, 142
  drugs, 28, 465, 555
  targets, 538
Anticancerous
  drugs delivery, 28
  effects, 28
Anticarcinogenic, 14, 54, 80, 593
Antidiabetic, 12, 13, 80, 119, 141, 183, 185, 433
Antidotal treatment, 120
Antiestrogenic, 90, 162
Antifeedant effect, 17
Antifoam, 419, 420
Antifungal, 12, 14, 18, 96, 99, 100, 129, 454, 595, 597
Antiglaucoma agent, 130
Antihelminthic, 12
Anti-hyperglycemic properties, 164
Antihypertension, 12, 58
Antihypertensive drugs, 134, 154, 185, 209
Anti-infective, 207, 209
Anti-inflammatory, 13, 15, 16, 24, 51, 53–55, 63, 81, 96, 127, 139, 146, 154, 158, 159, 162, 163–166, 168, 185, 189, 190, 205, 433, 475, 526, 529, 597, 607
  activity, 15, 124, 142, 157, 158
  effect, 593, 162
  functions, 12
  property, 146
Antimalarial, 12, 14, 15, 57, 129, 130, 207, 209
  activity, 12
  agent, 134
  compound, 57, 207
  drug, 129
Antimicrobial, 13–15, 23, 51, 53, 63, 79, 80, 81, 87, 90, 91, 106, 135, 138, 141, 146, 185, 204, 206, 344, 433, 434, 483, 487, 488, 489, 491, 572, 589, 595

  activities, 79, 124, 487
  agents, 12
  antioxidant properties, 487
  compounds, 54
  effects, 128
  property, 146
  substances, 81
Antimutagenic, 12, 63, 128, 148
Antineoplastic
  agent, 146
  effects, 185
Anti-nutrients, 10
Anti-oncogenic property, 518
Antioxidant, 5, 10, 13–15, 19, 51, 53–55, 61, 80, 81, 91, 96, 119, 120, 124, 127, 138, 141, 146, 148, 155, 158, 162, 185–187, 190, 205, 230, 232, 235, 236, 454, 487, 490, 526, 527, 576, 593, 595, 598, 607
Antipyretic, 128, 607, 209
Antiseptic, 123, 207
Antispasmodic, 55, 128, 138, 164
Anti-trypanocidal agents, 12
Antitumor, 28, 51, 55, 81, 90, 96, 119, 129, 134, 154, 169, 191, 207, 433, 469, 542, 547, 553, 589, 597
Antitumorigenic properties, 528
Anti-tussive, 526
Antiulcer, 55, 154, 185, 572
Antiviral, 12, 14, 15, 63, 128, 129, 135, 139, 146, 154, 164, 185, 474
  activities, 119
  property, 146
Anxiety, 435, 526
  disorders, 435
Apigenin, 139, 183, 213
Apigeninidin (2-(4-hydroxyphenyl) benzo-pyrilium chloride, 91, 98
Apocynaceae, 133, 199, 208, 209, 230
Apoptosis, 20, 166, 471, 513, 515, 518, 528, 541, 542, 545, 547, 548, 575, 581, 582, 584
Aporphine, 131
Apurinic/apyrimidinic endonuclease-1 (APE1), 520, 523, 527, 529, 530
Aqueous phase, 270
Arabidopsis/Brassicaceae species, 87
Arabinose, 42, 50, 63

Arachidonic acid pathways, 159
Arachis hypogaea, 80, 91, 300
Arogenate, 43, 44
Aromatic hydrocarbon, 54, 204
Aromaticity, 133
Artemisia annua, 70
Artemisinin, 207, 325, 331
Artichokes, 142
Artificial food additives, 40
Arvicanthis niloticus, 438
Asbestos, 439
Ascorbic acid metabolism, 143
Ashing temperature, 372
Asparagus racemosus, 155
Aspartate, 433, 522
Aspergillus
    flavus, 86
    sojae, 86
Asteraceae, 133, 155, 199, 209, 215, 606
Asthma, 135, 156, 435
Asthmatic patients, 135
Astringent, 18, 40, 121, 123
Ataxia-telangiectasia mutated (ATM), 527,
    528
Atomic
    absorption spectroscopy (AAS), 373, 377
    emission spectroscopy (AES), 373
    spectroscopy techniques, 373
Atraric acid, 213
Atropa belladonna, 129, 131
Atropine, 131, 134, 209
    injections, 134
Attention deficit hyperactivity disorder, 435
Autism-related disorder, 432
Autoimmune
    diabetes, 436
    disorders, 188
    model, 437
Automatic
    calculation, 333
    cell changer, 318
    transfer, 333
Automatized extraction process, 269
Autophagy, 548
Autosamplers, 104, 318, 328, 333, 336, 341
Ayurvedic medicine, 6, 497, 498
Azadirachta indica, 267

B

Bacillariophyceae, 211
Bacillus
    anthracis, 135
    cereus, 100
    pumilus, 100
    subtilis, 135
Bacteria, 18, 46, 58, 66, 70, 80, 81, 83,
    129, 145, 154, 164, 170, 210, 248, 445,
    487–489, 555
Bacterial
    growth, 103
    pneumonia, 434
Barfoed's
    reagent, 401
    test, 401, 577
Base excision repair (BER), 520–522, 529,
    530
Beer–Lambert's law, 256, 307
Belly palava, 607
Benedict's
    reagent, 401
    test, 401, 577
Benzoic acid, 90, 547
Benzopyrrole, 131
Berberidaceae, 133, 208
Berberine, 131, 133, 156
Berberis amurensis, 301
Beryllium, 439
Betacyanin, 399
Beta-enolase (ENO3), 554
Betaine, 133, 233, 237
Betulinic acid, 164
Bidentate ligand, 142
Bifurcaria, 212
Binary solvent system, 360
Bioactive
    components, 252, 255, 267, 454, 588, 600
    compounds, 5, 8, 200, 207, 247, 252,
        253, 256, 257, 268, 428, 573, 587, 588,
        592, 594, 600
    constituents, 200, 257
    molecules, 199, 247, 258, 465
    PhA compounds, 79
    properties, 191
Bioactivity, 51, 52, 54, 55, 57, 61, 63, 65,
    68, 162, 232, 453, 465, 504, 565, 600
Bioactivity of,

alkaloids, 57
anthocyanins, 54
anthraquinones, 68
flavonoids, 51
glycoside, 65
lignans, 52
phenolics, 55
saponins, 63
steriods, 68
terpenoids, 61
Bioassays, 271, 433, 466
Bioavailability, 138, 600
Biochemical
    activities, 38, 440
    analysis, 19, 144
    cellular targets, 236
    physiological evidence, 105
    parameters, 472, 473, 475
Biodiversity, 5, 463, 464, 562, 563
Bioindicators, 213
Bioinformatics, 6, 231, 467, 468, 499, 500
Biological
    activity, 37, 38, 63, 81, 119, 127, 185,
        186, 207, 212, 428, 454, 466, 506
    assays, 554
    effects, 120
    function, 12, 124, 134, 148
    molecules, 291
    processes, 144, 170, 226, 572
    roles of tannins, 123
    system, 382, 391, 476
Biologically active
    components, 249
    constituents, 248
Biomarkers, 232, 234, 237
Biomedical sciences, 482
Biomolecules, 5, 12, 257, 430, 508
Bioprospecting, 200
Bioremediation, 9, 235
Biostatistics, 4, 22–25, 481–484, 487–491,
    493
Biosynthesis, 17, 37, 40, 41, 44–51, 53, 54,
    56, 58, 61, 63–68, 71, 79, 83, 86, 93, 95,
    96, 98, 100, 102, 103, 105, 130, 186, 202,
    217, 229, 230, 545
Biosynthesis of
    alkaloids, 56
    anthocyanins, 53

anthraquinones, 66
flavonoids, 49
glycosides, 63
lignan, 51
phenolics, 54
phytochemicals, 40
saponins, 61
steroids, 68
terpenoids, 58
Biosynthetic pathway, 4, 7, 10, 37, 38,
    49–53, 55, 57, 59, 60, 64, 66, 71, 83,
    95–97, 99, 101, 204, 217, 218, 232, 288,
    539
Biotechnology, 7, 8, 10, 27, 106
Biotic/abiotic agents, 81
Biuret reagent, 400
Bivariate statistics, 481, 484
Blood samples, 440
Blue reagent, 400
Boerhaavia diffusa, 227
Bonding type, 350
Bone morphogenetic protein, 514
Boraginaceae, 133
Boric acid solution, 414–416
Borntrager's test, 397, 398
Botrytis cinerae, 100
Bowman–Birk inhibitor, 145
Brassica vegetables, 80
Bronchiolus epithelial cells, 474
Bronchitis, 135, 435, 572
Bronchoconstriction, 134
Bronchopulmonary dysplasia, 135
Buchner funnel, 419, 420
Bumping chips, 415
Butanol, 271, 295, 397, 401, 407

C

Caenorhabditis elegans, 429
Caffeine, 11, 47, 57, 129, 131, 135, 530
    citrate, 135
    consumption, 135
    metabolite, 135
Calcium
    chloride solution, 410
    oxalate, 142, 143, 144, 199, 201, 202,
        214, 410
    poisoning, 120
Calibration

curves, 313, 333, 338
  method, 339
  standards, 318
Camalexin, 39, 87
Camellia sinensis, 191
Campesterol, 11, 68, 70, 191, 331
Camptotheca acuminata, 58, 465
Camptothecin, 58, 465, 572
Cancer, 6, 7, 20, 28, 52, 53, 81, 119, 124,
    138, 139, 141, 142, 144, 159, 164, 166,
    169, 183, 188, 190, 191, 229, 431, 435,
    439, 445, 454, 471, 513–518, 520–523,
    527–529, 533, 537–548, 552, 553–556,
    565, 571, 572, 574, 580, 583, 588, 593,
    601
  cell metastasis, 554
  stem cells (CSCs), 513, 514
  tumor initiation, 190
Cannabinoid levels, 308
Cannabinoids, 326
Cannabis sativa, 129
Canthaxanthin, 185
Capillary
  fragility, 138
  tube, 293
Capsaicinoids, 326
Capsaicins, 333
Capsanthin, 138
Capsicum annuum L, 129, 130
Carbohydrate, 50, 56, 63, 147, 170, 232,
    236, 401, 422, 436, 537, 538, 548, 553,
    556, 576, 611, 614
Carbohydrate metabolism, 537, 538
Carbohydrates, 10, 42, 121, 148, 170, 202,
    203, 212, 231, 233, 277, 344, 401, 498,
    538, 573, 590, 610, 614
Carbon skeleton, 139, 164, 205
Carboxylic groups, 54
Carcinogen actions, 439
Carcinogenic, 16, 431, 474, 475
Carcinogenicity tests, 472
Carcinoma cells, 548
Cardenolides, 398
Cardiac
  arrhythmias, 593
  glycosides, 63, 68
  ischemia, 435
Cardiovascular

diabetic complications, 54
disease, 6, 139, 158, 179, 190, 191, 431,
    593
  problems, 191
  protective activities, 80
Carica papaya, 93, 301
Carotenoids, 11, 58, 182, 183, 185, 186,
    208, 210, 213, 235, 295, 428
Cassia obtusifolia, 103
Castanea sativa, 123
Catechin, 49, 50, 51, 53,122, 123, 138, 139,
    141, 146, 147, 159, 183, 191
Catechol, 122
Catharanthus roseus, 58, 71, 227, 230
Caulocystis, 212
Cecil Instruments, 307, 309, 322
Cell
  cultures, 70, 98, 101, 189, 430
  cycle
    inhibition, 20
    phase, 522
  division, 474
  membrane, 128, 469, 470, 552, 553
  pluripotency, 514
  proliferation, 52, 162, 170, 183, 514, 518,
      528, 539, 545, 552, 578
  proteases, 144
  stirring, 318
  vacuoles, 201
  viability assay, 574
  wall, 79, 81, 101, 102
Cellular
  contents disorganization, 81
  cytoplasmic damage, 139
  growth, 469
  stresses, 583
Cellulose, 201, 203, 263, 269
Central
  nervous system (CNS), 134, 502, 615
  processing unit (CPU), 499
Centrifugal partition chromatography
    (CPC), 279
Ceratocystis clavigera, 90
Cetrelia olivetorum, 214
Chalcone, 49, 50, 53, 96, 138, 139, 141,
    159, 205
  isomerase, 50, 54, 96
  synthase, 54

Charaka Samhita, 498
Charophyceae, 211
Chelate forms, 371
Chelating agent, 402
Chelidonium majus, 156, 157, 301
Chemical
  agents, 200, 302
  bonds, 257, 282
  classification, 130
  compositions, 5, 489
  compounds, 6, 19, 20, 85, 119, 120, 136,
    199, 201, 217, 343, 344, 382, 463, 464,
    467, 573
  constituents, 197–200, 253
  defense, 65
  electronic environment, 280
  element, 382
  formula (C II OH), 54
  induction model, 436
  interactions, 19
  nature, 84, 182, 290
  poisoning, 134
  polymorphism, 482
  reagents, 294
  reduction, 217
  stability, 248
  structure, 54, 83, 122, 159, 184, 204, 257,
    278, 279, 281, 466
  substances, 198, 217, 382, 593
  synthesis approach, 70
  transformations, 126
  variability, 10
Chemical
  properties, 133, 143
  reduction, 217
  variability, 217
Chemistry of
  flavonoids, 139
  glycosides, 136
  oxalates, 143
  saponins, 125
  tannins, 121
Chemodiversity, 299
Chemomicroscopy, 262, 282
Chemoprevention, 28, 527
Chemoprofiles, 343
Chemotaxonomic
  characters, 217

  classification, 203
  study, 216, 262, 263
  values, 211
Chemotaxonomists, 198, 199, 210, 215, 263
Chemotaxonomy, 197–201, 212, 214–218,
  261, 262, 282
  lower plants classification, 212
    algae, 212
    bryophytes, 214
    higher plants classification, 216
    lichens, 215
Chemotherapeutic drug, 142, 514
Chemotypes, 216, 483
Chemoxanomical classifications, 213
Chinese data and herbal ingredient, 562
Chitinases, 81, 99
Chloral hydrate solution, 262
Chlorhydric acid solution, 419
Chloroform, 104, 121, 143, 295, 347,
  394–397, 399, 403, 406
Chlorogenic acid, 11, 123, 148, 160, 216
Chlorophyceae, 210, 211
Chlorophyll, 183, 186, 210, 213, 277, 294,
  315, 345, 348
Chlorophytes, 211
Cholesterol
  binding properties, 124
  lowering effect, 128
Choline, 524
Chorismate mutase, 44
Chorismic acid, 66, 67
Chromatogram, 293, 298, 302, 323–326,
  333, 335, 340, 358–360, 500, 571, 578,
  594
Chromatographic
  data, 333
  fingerprint, 19, 357
  method, 255, 299
  parameters, 355, 360
  separation, 223, 231, 271, 272, 351, 357,
    362
  technique, 19, 253, 255, 271, 277, 287,
    299, 302, 588
Chromatography, 6, 19, 214–216, 226–228,
  235, 238, 248, 253–255, 261, 262,
  271–274, 277–279, 287, 289–291, 293,
  296, 299–301, 307, 322, 323, 333, 335,

343, 346–350, 355, 394, 395, 434, 467, 483, 501, 571, 573, 578, 588, 589
Chromophore, 309, 315, 331
Chromosome, 444, 474, 522
Chrysanthemum, 61
Chrysophanol, 66
Chrysophyceae, 211
Chrysophytes, 211
Chrysopogon zizanioides, 228, 237
Cicer arietinum, 98, 228
Cinchona, 6, 129, 131
Cinchona officinalis, 7
Cinnamaldehyde, 17
Cinnamate, 43, 95, 96, 205, 232
Cinnamic acid 4-hydroxylase (CA4H), 54, 99
Cinnamomum zeylanicum, 488
Cistus
  incanus, 474
  limon, 93
Claviceps purpurea, 131
Clerodendrum volubile, 605, 606
C-linkage bond, 139
Cocaine, 134
Cochliobolus heterostrophus, 86
Co-elution detection, 334
Coffea arabica, 131
Colander washing, 369
Colchicine, 131, 134, 404
Colchicum autumnale, 131
Coldextraction, 249
Colletotrichum
  circinans, 18
  graminicola, 92
  lindemuthianum, 82
  musae, 92
  sublineolum, 86
  gloesporides, 100
Colloidal solutions, 122
Column
  categories, 330
  chromatography, 248, 253, 261, 262, 273, 290, 299, 346
  dimensions, 334, 349
  heater/chillers, 331, 333
Column
  heater/chillers, 331
  temperature, 352, 355

chromatography, 254
Contemporary analytical techniques, 373
  inorganic elemental analysis, 373
    atomic spectroscopy techniques, 373
    inductively coupled plasma mass spectrometry, 374
    inductively coupled plasma optical emission spectroscopy, 374
    neutron activation analysis, 375
    X-ray fluorescence, 374
  organic elemental analysis techniques, 375
Comet assay, 571, 576, 582, 583, 584
Complementary and alternative
  medicine therapy, 498
  medicine, 8
Complex sample matrices, 339
Compound annual growth rate (CAGR), 27, 182
Computational
  phytochemistry, 4, 498, 503
  tools, 497, 499, 509
Computer languages, 509
Conductivity detector, 296, 351
Conductivity detectors, 332
Conventional systems, 273
Convolvulaceae, 85, 93, 94
Copper acetate test, 397
Coptis chinensis, 301
Coronary heart disease, 40, 188
Costus speciosus, 90
Coumarin, 11, 18, 43, 44, 63, 85, 93, 135, 232, 249, 399
Countercurrent chromatography (CCC), 271, 278, 292
Crassocephalum rubens, 605, 606
Cratylia mollis, 171
Crop
  breeding program, 226
  enhancement program, 231
  plantation, 606
Cryptophyceae, 211
Cryptoxanthin, 138, 185
Crystalline precipitate, 394
Crystallizable catechins, 123
Crystallization, 278
C-terminus, 552
Cucumis sativus, 92

Cuminaldehyde, 18
Cupressus torulosa, 483, 487, 488
Curcuma longa, 160, 518
Curcumin, 160, 294, 518, 523, 528
Cuscohygrine, 524
Cutaneous carcinoma, 28
Cuvettes, 309–311
Cyanide, 65, 405, 409
Cyanidin, 139, 163
Cyanobacteria, 199, 211, 212
Cyanogenic glycoside, 44, 63, 65, 136, 209, 308, 405, 409
Cyanophyceae, 211, 212
Cyclic dehydroquinate compound, 43
Cyclization, 62, 96, 100, 101, 207
Cycloartenol, 68
Cyclohexene ring, 148
Cyclopentanopyran monoterpenoid, 402
Cyclophosphamide, 438
Cylindrospermum, 212
Cymbopogon
  citratus, 488
  flexuosus, 488, 489
Cystoseira, 212
Cytochalasin, 539
Cytokines, 166, 169, 170, 514, 518
Cytoplasm, 95, 136, 516, 517, 583
Cytosol, 45, 60, 102, 516, 538, 542, 575
Cytotoxic, 51, 469
  action, 518
  activity, 55, 164, 168, 571, 572
Cytotoxicity, 83, 469, 487, 489, 554, 574, 578, 584

D

Dactylis, 216
Daidzein, 139, 183, 523
Danio rerio, 429
Daucus carota, 186
Daunorubicin, 465
Decarboxylation, 44
Decoction, 265
Degassing, 329
Deionized
  distilled water, 369
  water, 370, 383, 404, 608, 610
    demineralized water, 383
Delphinidin, 139, 162, 163

Dementia, 435, 441
Densitometry scanning, 360
Deoxyribonucleic acid (DNA), 83, 470, 571, 576
Deoxyxylulose, 56
Derivatization, 328
Dermal administration, 473
Dermatological signs, 473
Desiccator, 407, 408, 412, 417, 418, 421, 422, 610
Designerfoods, 179–182, 192
Detectors, 276, 278, 296, 298, 316, 317, 323, 331–334, 351
Determination of triterpenes, 403
Detoxify heavy metals, 201
Deuterium, 309
Deuterium lamps, 318
D-glucose, 42, 50, 209
Diabetes, 29, 119, 147, 148, 158, 188, 190, 191, 229, 431, 432, 435–438, 445, 563, 572
Diabetes mellitus, 148, 432, 435
Diagonal chromatography, 299
Diallyl disulfide, 190
Diaphoresis, 134
Dicotyledonous plant species, 68
Dicotyledons, 90, 92, 94
Dietary
  saponins, 127
  supplements, 180, 182, 465, 500, 564
Diethyl ether, 141, 407, 417–419
Diethyleneglycol, 237
Diffuse reflectance measurements, 318
Digestion, 265, 368, 371–374, 413, 415, 527, 588
Digestive system, 527
Dihydro
  derivatives, 49
  flavonol, 49, 53,90
  kaempferide, 230
  phenanthrenes, 84, 85
  thymoquinone (DHTQ), 590
Dimeric phenylpropanoids, 51
Dimethyl
  allyl diphosphate (DMAPP), 46, 47, 58, 59
  polysiloxane, 592
  sulfoxide (DMSO), 574–576

Dimocarpus longan, 300
Dinitrophenylhydrazine, 401
Dinoflagellates, 210, 211
Dinophyceae, 211
Diode array detector, 254, 298
Dioscorea collettii, 128
Dioscoreaceae, 91, 215
Diosgenyl 2-amino-2-deoxy-β-D-
   glucopyranoside, 128
Disease
   management, 40, 429
   resistance, 80, 87, 92, 103, 105, 106, 232
Dissolution
   accessories, 318
   vessels, 318
Distillation methods, 269
Diterpene, 7, 84, 95, 99, 100, 164, 204, 207,
   397, 593
Diterpenes/Sesterterpenes, 207
Diterpenoids, 60, 92, 99
   biosynthesis pathway, 95
DNA
   dependent protein kinase (DNAPK), 522,
      527
   glycosylate, 521
   repair, 527, 533
      genes, 527
      mechanism, 520
   strand breaks, 582, 583
Docetaxel, 465
Docosahexaenoic acid (DHA), 182, 188
Double
   indicator, 414, 415
   stranded helix, 516
Doxorubicin, 465
Dracocephalum moldavica, 489
Dragendroff's
   reagent, 394, 609
   test, 394
Drechslera longirostrata, 90
Drosophila, 427–429, 443, 446–449, 451,
   452, 454
   development, 451, 454
   melanogaster, 427, 429, 446–448
Drug
   application, 472
   design, 506, 509, 563
   designing, 19, 498, 499, 500, 503, 504

molecule, 502, 505, 506
   relevant properties, 502
Drugs source, 28
Dulbecco's modified Eagle's medium, 574
D-xylose, 63
Dye exclusion method, 469

E

E-bioprospecting, 19
E-cadherin mutations, 516
Echinacea spp, 300
Edema, 161, 165, 473, 474
Egg yolks, 187
Eicosanoid synthesis, 158
Eicosapentaenoic acid (EPA), 188, 500
Electrical conductivity, 332, 383
Electrochemical detectors, 333
Electromagnetic radiation, 267
Electron transport, 190, 538
Electronic structure, 257
Electrophoresis, 215, 261–263, 282
Electrophoretic patterns, 215
Electrospray ionization, 104, 227, 230
Elemental profiling, 367, 377
Ellagitannin, 122, 123
Elucidation technology, 466
Embryonic development, 452
Emesis symptoms, 134
Emodin, 66
Emphysema, 135
Emulsifying agents, 126
Endcapping, 350
Endophytes, 210
Endoplasmic reticulum, 467
Energy
   minimizations, 504
   spectrum, 375
   yielding compounds, 4
Ent-copalyl-diphosphate (ent-CDP), 95
Enteritis, 124
Environmental
   contaminants, 308
   hazards, 4, 10
   influence, 217
   pollution, 9, 235
   stress, 5, 185
Environment-friendly technology, 237
Envision biotechnology, 566, 561

Enzymatic reactions, 41, 538
Enzyme
    acetoacetyl-CoA thiolase, 45
    aldose reductase, 185
    catalyzed reactions, 43, 47, 68
    inhibitors, 81, 185
    pinoresinol reductase, 51
    ribulose phosphate epimerase, 43
    squalene synthetase, 68
Ephedra
    type, 466
    vulgaris, 130
Ephedrine, 130, 199, 466
Epicatechin, 49, 139, 183
Epilepsy, 435
Epirubicin, 465
Epistatic interactions, 451
Ergonovine, 130
Ergosines, 333
Ergosterol, 331
Ergotamine, 131
Erigeron bonariensis, 199, 215
Eriodictyol, 139
Erlenmeyer flask, 414, 417
Erucastrum canariense, 90
Erythema, 473, 474
Erythrose 4-phosphate, 43
Erythroxylon coca, 131
Erythroxylum subsessile, 301
Escherichia coli, 100, 103, 135, 521
Esophagitis, 124
Essential oils, 17, 18, 25, 206, 212, 215,
    253, 264, 269, 270, 326, 400, 453,
    481–483, 487–491, 589, 590
Estrogen receptors (ERs), 90
Estrogenic
    activities, 138
    properties, 90
Ethanoic/glacial acetic acid, 400
Ethanol, 104, 143, 250, 268, 295, 300, 385,
    390, 396, 404, 406, 407, 414, 415
Ethnobotanical, 6, 561, 563, 566
Ethnobotany, 8
Ethnomedicinal formulations, 20
Ethnomedicine, 8, 20
Ethyl acetate, 104, 121, 147, 250, 300, 359,
    399, 408, 571–575, 577, 578, 581–584
Eucalyptus, 17, 122, 199, 206, 215

Euglenophyceae, 211
Eukaryotes, 58, 516
Euphorbia lathyris, 300
Euphorbiaceae, 85, 93, 94, 198
Euphorbieae, 199
European Food Safety Authority, 465
Evaporative light scattering detector, 296,
    351
Extraction
    method, 247, 251–253, 258, 265
        accelerated solvent extraction, 252
        cold extraction, 253
        hydrodistillation, 253
        microwave-assisted extraction, 252
        serial exhaustive extraction, 251
        solvent extraction method, 250
        supercritical fluid extraction, 252
        ultrasound-assisted extraction/sonica-
            tion, 252
    procedures, 263, 452
    solvent, 266
    techniques, 261, 371, 377
        dry ashing, 371
        microwave digestion, 372
        wet digestion, 372

F

Fabaceae, 84, 133, 184, 199, 208, 209, 234
Fatty
    acid, 188, 202, 203, 211, 212, 232, 249,
        399, 518, 519, 590
    chain, 416
    composition, 211, 212
    acyl chains, 70
Ferric
    acid, 160, 216
    chloride test, 395
Festuca
    rubra, 216
    versuta leaf, 91
Fibroblast growth factor, 514
Filter paper, 250, 269, 393, 407, 408, 410,
    415, 418, 420, 453
Filtration, 269, 320, 327, 338, 341, 347
Final method optimization (FDA), 348, 451,
    542, 543
Flame ionization detector, 104, 278
Flash chromatography (FC), 272, 275

Flavanols, 139
Flavanone, 39,49, 50, 85, 90, 91, 139, 141,
    148, 158, 159,205, 215
    3-hydroxylase, 54
Flavanonol, 183, 215
Flavones, 49, 138, 139, 141, 158, 159, 183,
    205, 215, 249
Flavonoids, 11, 14, 29, 37, 39, 41, 43, 44,
    45, 49–51, 99, 119, 122, 138–141, 148,
    153, 154, 158, 159, 161, 162, 182–186,
    191, 199, 204, 205, 215, 216, 232, 235,
    249, 263, 288, 295, 333, 345, 346, 382,
    394, 404, 524, 527, 537, 548, 551, 555,
    556, 571, 573, 576–578, 582, 590, 593,
    594, 606, 609, 615, 616
    aglycones, 141
    containing
        celery, 142
        chocolate/cocoa, 141
    reaction pathway, 49
    immunomodulation, 159
Flavonol, 39, 49, 148, 158, 183, 205, 249
Flavonolignans, 53
Flavopunctelia, 214
Flavylium cation, 162
Floridean, 211
Fluorescence
    associated with β-particle ionization, 332
    detectors, 332
Fluorescent
    cation, 582
    detector/diode array, 296
    microscope, 575, 576
Folin–ciocalteu test, 395
Food
    chain, 4, 236
    containing phytochemicals, 11
    Drug Administration, 522, 542
    Quality Protection Act, 17
Fourier-transform infrared, 255, 261, 262,
    588, 589, 599, 601
    spectroscopy (FTIR), 248, 255, 256, 588,
        589, 592–594, 600
        FTIR analysis, 592, 600
        FTIR spectra, 588, 594
Fractional crystallization, 278
Fragaria X ananassa, 228
Free-fatty acids, 135

Frizzled receptors, 514
Fructose, 43, 137, 209, 233, 538, 542
    6-phosphate, 43
    bisphosphate-allosteric activator, 546
Fruit ripening, 238
Frullania, 213, 216
Functional groups, 281, 330, 594, 600
Fungal
    infection, 92, 232
    inoculation, 103
    sources, 154
    spore germination, 18
Fungicidal, 18, 138
Funtumia latifolia, 131
Furano and dimethyl pyranocoumarins, 215
Furastanol saponins, 128
Fusarium
    graminearum, 86
    moniliforme, 18
    oxysporum, 100
    proliferatum, 99
    solani, 100
    thapsinum, 99
    wilt, 101

G

Galacto-oxylipins, 90
Galactose, 42, 50, 538
Gallic acid, 11, 55, 122, 123, 204, 269, 406,
    409
Gallocatechin, 230, 519
Gallotannin, 122, 123
Gamma
    enolase (ENO2), 554
    ray energies, 375
Garryaceae, 215
Gas chromatography (GC), 19, 104,
    226–228, 230–234, 236, 237, 248,
    253–255, 261, 262, 277, 278, 281, 290,
    291, 299, 500, 571, 573, 574, 577, 588,
    589, 592, 594, 600
    GC-mass spectrometry (GCMS), 290,
        299, 300, 577, 601
Gastric cancer cell, 548
Gastritis, 124, 208
Gastrointestinal
    disorders, 435
    motility, 134

Gel
  chromatography, 277
  permeation, 277, 330
Gelatin test, 395
Gene
  expression, 159, 162, 224, 431, 516, 518
  function, 223, 229, 449
Genes encoding PhA detoxifying enzymes,
  83
Genetic
  disorders, 449
  engineering approaches, 223, 225, 235
  information, 522
  interactions, 450
  mechanism, 449
  modification, 436
Genistein, 139, 183, 523, 528
Genome, 20, 105, 226, 430, 444, 445, 527
Genomic
  information, 105
  instability, 527
Genotoxic, 439
Genotoxicity, 472, 489
Geographic range, 217
Geometry optimization, 508
Geranyl diphosphate, 59
Germ tube elongation, 81
Germination inhibition, 81
Gibberella pulicaris, 103
Gingerol derivatives, 205
Ginkgo biloba, 90
Glioblastoma cells, 552
Gliomas, 518
Global
  markets, 357
  mechanization, 235
  positioning system information, 377
Glucanases, 81
Gluconate 6-phosphate, 43
  dehydrogenase, 43
Glucorhamnose, 42, 50
Glucose
  6-phosphate, 538, 540, 541
    dehydrogenase, 42
  hydroxycarboxylic acids, 54
  metabolism, 538, 539, 543, 545
  tolerance, 438, 615
  transporter (GLUT), 538, 539

family of transporters, 539
  inhibitor, 539
  isoforms, 539
Glucoside, 91, 93, 137
Glucosinolates, 201, 204
Glucuronic acid, 137
Glucuronide, 137
Glutamate, 234, 522, 546
Glutathione, 98, 232, 236
Glyceollin production, 102
Glyceraldehyde 3-phosphate dehydrogenase
  (GAPDH), 546, 547
  GAPDH reaction, 546
Glyceric acid, 237
Glycerol, 121, 135, 233, 237, 416
Glycine, 142, 143, 233, 263, 595
Glycitein, 139
Glycogen synthase kinase-3 β (GSK-3β),
  516
Glycolysis, 43, 202, 537–546, 554
Glycolytic
  enzymes, 537, 556
  pathway, 537–539, 544, 555
Glycone, 135, 137, 209
Glycopeptides, 102
Glycoproteins, 84, 330, 614
Glycosides, 37, 39, 42, 43, 63–65, 68, 70,
  93, 119, 120, 135–139, 141, 159, 162,
  164, 184, 201, 204, 209, 263, 274, 276,
  288, 295, 345, 398, 409, 464, 573, 577,
  593, 606, 615
Glycosidic, 50, 124–126, 135, 136, 139,
  147, 148, 184, 209, 521
  compounds, 12, 125, 14, 125
Glycosylation, 62
Glycyrrhiza glabra, 127, 167
Glyphosate, 102, 103
Gongronema latifolium, 605, 607
Gradient
  elution, 297, 326, 330
  extraction, 264, 266, 269
Graminicola, 98
Graphics processing unit (GPU), 499
Gravitational movements, 291
Green tea extract possesses, 518
Grinding extraction sample, 264
Gymnosperms, 90, 91, 201, 214

H

Hager's
    reagent, 393
    test, 393, 577
Halogenated coumarins, 18
Hamelia patens, 227, 230
Haussknechtia elymatica, 155
Health
    beneficial compounds, 225
    promoting foods, 182
Heating
    element, 250
    period, 265
Heat-labile compounds, 266, 278
Heat-stable compounds, 278
Heavy metals (HMs), 235, 236
Hematopoietic system, 439
Hemoglobin formation, 615
Hemolytic activity, 124, 126, 128
Hemostatic, 123
Hepatocellular carcinoma cell, 547
Hepatoprotective, 12, 15, 53, 63, 139, 185,
    589
Herbal
    based targeted drug delivery, 497
    discovery platform, 564
    drug discovery, 561, 566
    drugs, 9, 344, 381, 382, 500, 588
    formulations, 370
    medicinal research, 498
    products, 29, 182, 302, 346, 465, 498
    species, 587, 588
Herbivores, 4, 10, 18, 41, 120, 138, 144,
    209
Herbivory, 201, 203, 208
Herbs, 11, 123, 164, 465, 475, 498, 509,
    561, 562, 587, 588, 607
Hesperidin, 138
Hesteretin, 139
Heterocyclic alkaloids, 131
Heterocyclic ring, 130, 131, 154, 158, 184
    pyrane, 139
Heterodimer, 522
Heteronuclear multiple-bond correlation
    (HMBC), 280, 281
Hevea brasiliensis, 93
Hexadecatrienoic acid, 211
Hibiscus rosa sinensis, 155

High-performance
    liquid chromatography (HPLC), 103,
        104, 226, 230, 253–255, 262, 272, 275,
        276, 290, 292, 296–302, 307, 322–324,
        326–329, 331, 334, 335, 339–342,
        346–348, 351, 353, 355, 363, 500
        analysis method, 348
        column, 330, 355
        instrumentation, 341
        instrumentations and analysis, 307
        making, 296
        method, 104, 348, 352
        software, 298
        system, 297, 322, 338
    thin-layer chromatography(HPTLC), 253,
        255, 290, 355–358, 361–363
        design and development, 362
        development, 357
        validation, 362
Hispidol, 139
Histamine, 332
Histidine, 130, 545
Histological examination, 473, 474
Histone, 84, 528
Histopathological studies, 475
Histopathology, 450, 473, 474
Homeostasis, 236, 437, 438, 445, 514, 526
Homesteads, 607
Homogeneous, 353, 383, 406, 415, 453
    mixture, 330
    samples, 327
Homologous recombination (HR), 520, 522,
    528
Homotetramers/heterotetramers, 546
Hordeum vulgare, 130
Hotcontinuous extraction, 266
Human
    animal studies, 128
    cholesterol, 68
    chronic diseases, 119
    consumption, 106, 125
    disorder, 431, 450
    lymphoma, 547
Huntington' disease, 441
Hybridization, 133, 200
Hydrastis canadensis, 131
Hydrocarbon, 99, 164, 350

Hydrochloric acid, 393, 394, 396, 397, 403, 406, 408, 410, 414
Hydrodistillation, 249, 253, 270
Hydrogen
  atom, 279, 280
  bonding, 148, 505
  peroxide, 87, 142, 437
Hydrolysis, 43, 61, 122, 124, 126, 127, 135, 136, 139, 144, 147, 402, 416, 419
Hydrolyzable tannins, 122, 123, 184, 396
Hydrolyzed mixture, 420
Hydrophilic interaction liquid chromatography, 330
Hydrophobic, 124, 190, 272, 348, 350, 529, 593
Hydroquinone, 63
Hydroxycinnamic acid, 54, 204
Hydroxycinnamoyl alcohols, 51
Hydroxyester wyerol, 103
Hydroxyharmane, 213
Hydroxyl
  group, 43, 54, 62, 66, 92, 80, 158
  radicals, 437
Hydroxylated polyphenolic compounds, 138
Hydroxylation, 96, 183
Hydroxymethyl anthraquinones, 68
Hyoscyamine, 209
Hyperglycemia, 435, 437
Hyperlipidemia, 147
Hyperoxaluria, 142
Hyperproteinemia, 147
Hypocotyl, 102

I

Idarubicin, 465
Illicium verum, 17
Imidazole, 130, 131
Immiscible phases mix, 278
Immune
  modulatory effects, 159
  system, 12, 81, 153, 154, 164, 166, 169, 170, 190, 498, 514, 552
Immunity, 86, 87, 155, 169, 444
Immunoadjuvants, 153, 154
Immunological
  agent, 166
  characterization, 554
Immunomodulating

functions, 153
  property, 153, 154
Immunomodulation, 159
Immunomodulators, 153, 154, 159, 169, 170
Immunomodulatory, 12, 13, 153–155, 159, 164, 166, 169, 170
  effects, 154, 164
  properties, 12
Immunopathology, 154
Immunostimulant efficacies, 166
Immunostimulatory, 128, 185
Immunosuppressants, 153, 154
Immunosuppression, 154, 553
In vitro
  systems, 463, 475
  toxicological tests, 469
In vivo
  models, 466, 473
  systems tests, 476
  tests, 472, 476
  toxicity evaluation, 463, 466
  toxicological studies, 472
Indigenous vegetables, 605, 607, 612–614, 616
Indigofera, 214
Indole, 94, 130, 131, 209
  alkaloids, 58, 130, 208, 209
Inductively coupled plasma optical emission spectroscopy (ICP-OES), 373, 376
Infections, 47, 80, 90, 119, 128, 153, 170, 205, 247, 518
  endocarditis, 434
  microbes, 438
Inflammatory
  bowel disease, 435
  mediator-related pathways, 527
  signs, 473
Infrared
  spectrometer, 296, 593
  spectroscopy (IR), 212, 225, 227, 248, 255, 256, 258, 279. 281, 528, 592
  ultraviolet spectroscopy, 281
Infusion, 261, 264, 265, 607
Inhibitors of glucose transporters, 539
Inoculum, 103
Inorganic/organic molecule, 382
Inosine monophosphate (IMP), 47

Inositol hexakisphosphate (IP6)/inositol polyphosphate, 402
Insecticidal property and defense mechanism, 146
Insoluble tannates, 120, 122
Installation qualification (IQ), 321, 340
Instrument validation process, 318, 321
Instrumentation, 326, 327, 333, 340, 355, 356
Insulin production, 436
Integrating spheres, 318
Interconversion/degradation, 202
Interferons (IFN), 160, 166, 171
Interglycosidic bonds, 127
International Organization for Standardization (ISO), 353
Intestinal absorption, 502
Intracellular pathways, 467, 476
Intraperitoneal infection, 434
Ionic charge, 332
Ionization, 104, 227, 278, 300, 351, 592
Ipecacuanha, 123
Ipomoea batatas, 95
Iridiods, 402
Iron chloride, 410
Islets of Langerhans, 615
Isochlorogenic acids, 148
Isocratic, 274, 297, 326, 330
   elution, 297, 326
Isoegomaketone, 483, 488
Isoflavanones, 85, 205
Isoflavone, 49, 50, 85, 93, 139, 142, 159, 183–185, 577, 579
   hydroxylase, 99
   O-methyl transferase, 99
   reductase, 99
Isoflavonoid, 11, 84, 95, 96, 99, 102, 205, 232
Isolate crude bioactive compounds, 587
Isolation
   characterization, 261, 282
   phytochemicals, 247, 253
   plantmetabolites, 288
   processes, 203
   purification, 271
Isolettetierine, 524
Isoliquiritigenin, 139
Isomeric forms, 330

Isopentane, 206
Isopentenyl
   diphosphate (IPP), 46, 47, 58, 59, 66–68, 95
   pyrophosphate, 62
Isoprene, 58, 164, 206–208
Isoprenoid, 17, 58, 62, 68, 95, 164, 185, 204, 205
Isoquinoline, 131, 208
Isorhamnetin, 139, 216
Isotopic masses/fingerprints, 374

J

Jaceidin, 230

K

Kaempferol, 49, 139, 183
Kala jeera, 588
Karyopherin superfamily, 517
Kauralexin
   induction, 92
   regulation, 92
Kauralexins, 79, 85, 92
Kaurene synthase, 92
Kerb's cycle, 546
Keto group, 44
Ketone, 17, 295, 483, 488, 594, 599
Kidney disorders, 445
Kinetic
   energy, 252
   information, 434
   parameter, 434
Kjeldahl
   flask, 414
   method, 413
Kollman-united atom charges, 504
Kunitz trypsin inhibitor, 145

L

Laboratory
   atmosphere, 331
   environment types, 324
   information management system, 333
Lactate
   dehydrogenase (LDH), 144, 469, 470, 546–548, 551
   protons, 551

Landsburgia, 212
Lanosterol, 68, 331
Laphophora williamsii, 130
Lariciresinol, 51
Larval tissues, 452
Lauraceae, 199, 215, 488
Laurus nobilis, 488
LDHA inhibitor, 547
Lectins, 153, 154, 170
Lemongrass, 489, 490
Lens culinaris, 228
Leptin receptor, 438
Lethal dose, 440, 448, 450, 472
Leucoanthocyanidin
    dioxygenase, 54
    reductase, 50
Leucoanthocyanidins, 50, 53
Leucoanthocyanins, 399
Leukotrienes, 159
L-fructose, 63
Lichexanthone, 214
Liebermann
    burchard test, 396
    test, 395
Liebig condenser, 414–416
Ligand
    based drug designing, 506
    binding, 330
    structure-based drug designing, 500
Lignan, 11, 37, 39, 41, 43, 44, 51–53, 63,
    90, 183, 203, 205, 403
Lilium maximowiczii, 91
Limit of,
    detection (LOD), 349, 352, 354, 355
    quantitation (LOQ), 352, 354, 355
Limonene, 11, 213, 308, 487, 590
Linalool, 213
Linearity, 310, 322, 341, 352–354
Linoleic acid, 188, 189, 211, 212, 518
Linum usitatissimum, 189
Lipid synthesis, 232
Lipophilicity factor, 563
Lipopolysaccharides, 84
Lipoproteins cholesterol, 191
Liquid
    chromatography, 19, 214, 226, 248,
        253–255, 261, 262, 276, 278, 290, 346,
        467, 500, 588

    mass spectrometry (LC-MS), 226, 230,
        500
liquid
    chromatography, 292
    partition chromatography, 271
    phase, 254, 276, 292
    sample, 256, 310, 326, 412, 421
    solid/adsorption chromatography, 272
Liquorice, 127, 136
Liver cholesterol levels, 128
Local government area (LGA), 606, 607
Long-lasting compounds, 294
Low-density lipoprotein (LDL), 40
Low-pressure liquid chromatography, 272
L-rhamnose, 50, 63, 209
Lupeol, 164, 207, 208
Lupinine, 131
Lupinus luteus, 131
Lutein, 182, 185–187
Luteolin, 49, 139, 183, 523
Luteolinidin, 85, 91, 92, 98, 99
Lycopene, 11, 138, 182, 186, 187, 210
Lymphomas and sarcomas tumors, 439
Lymphorization, 370
Lymphorized samples, 370
Lysergic acid, 332
Lysine, 56, 130, 208, 522

M

Maceration, 261, 264, 265, 288, 327, 347
Machine washing, 369
Macromibiuma ferriei, 212
Macromolecules, 21, 201, 504
Macrophomina phaseolina, 18
Macroscopic swelling, 473
Magnaporthe
    grisea, 232
    oryzae, 100
Magnetic field, 257, 279
Mahonia manipurensis, 301
Malic acid, 11, 332
Malonyl coenzyme, 184
Malonyl-CoA, 37, 41, 50, 53, 66, 87
Malonyl-coa pathway, 45
Malvaceae, 85, 93, 94, 155, 215
Malvidin, 139, 162
Mammalian
    cells, 541, 544

metabolism, 453
species, 432
systems, 451
Mandragora officinarum, 129
Mangifera indica, 227, 300
Manufacturer's specifications, 321, 340, 341
Marine
derived compounds, 8
environments, 5
Mass spectrometry (MS), 19, 104, 226–228, 230–234, 236, 237, 255, 257, 276, 278, 279, 281, 290, 291, 300, 333, 334, 373, 374, 467, 489, 500, 501, 571, 573, 574, 577, 578, 588, 589, 592, 594, 600
Matairesinol, 213
Matrix preparation techniques, 368
cleaning, 368
drying, 370
milling storage, 370
Mayer's test, 393, 577, 594
MCF-7 cell line, 571, 580, 584
Medicago
sativa L, 99
truncatula, 63
Medical
evaluation, 181
foods, 181
pharmaceutical industries, 4
Medicinal
plant/herb, 6
plants, 6, 19, 20, 119, 199, 200, 205, 226, 229–231, 248, 463, 466, 563, 572, 607
legumes, 119
metabolomics resource, 226
values, 344, 428
Meloidogyne incognita, 233
Meningitis, 434
Menopausal-related symptoms, 185
Menstruum, 264
Mentha pulegium, 227, 230
Metabolic
activity, 19, 469
pathway, 41, 48, 70, 229, 235, 237, 537, 553
reactions, 19
stability, 27
Metabolite complexity, 223, 231

Metabolomics, 8, 10, 19, 105, 223–227, 229–238
Metal
elements, 367, 371, 372, 375
interaction, 505
Methanol, 147, 268, 272, 295, 300, 301, 329, 347, 351, 358, 359, 394–396, 404, 406, 407, 440, 609
Methyl
orange, 390
protogracillin, 128
protoneogracillin, 128
red
indicator, 390, 415
methylene blue combination, 414
vanillin, 312
Methylate/hemimethylate, 521
Methylated flavonoids, 556
Methylation, 68
Methylene dichloride, 359
Methylerythritol phosphate (MEP), 95
Mevalonate kinase, 45
Mevalonate
monophosphate, 45
pathway, 37, 41, 45–47, 95
Mevalonic
acid, 45, 58, 60, 67, 68
independent pathway, 58, 60, 61
pathway, 59, 68
Mice model, 430, 431, 454
Microbial
activity, 126
attack, 164, 204
growth, 124, 369
infection, 79, 203
Microcapillary tube, 272
Microcephaly, 445
Micro-fractionation, 19
Microliters, 330
Micromonospora, 555
Micronucleus assay, 474
Micronutrients, 410
Microorganisms, 4, 81, 129, 146, 248, 344
Micropipette, 293
Microporous matrix, 268
Microwave
digestion, 372

assisted extraction, 19, 247, 252, 264, 267, 288
Million's reagent, 400
Milton Technical Centre, 307, 309, 322
Mirabilis jalapa, 5
Mismatch repair (MMR), 520, 521
Mitochondrial
   depolarization, 575
   disorders, 190
   function, 513, 582
   membrane, 190, 541, 571, 582–584
   oxygen consumption, 548
Mitotic cell division, 474
Mitragyna speciosa, 129
Mobile phase, 254, 255, 271–278, 289–292, 294, 296, 297, 322, 323, 326–330, 334, 344, 346, 350–353, 355, 358–360, 362, 394–397, 399–401
   changes, 297
   composition, 351, 352, 355
   optimization, 359
Modular instrumentation components, 327
Modulation of detoxifying enzymes, 12
Molecular
   approaches, 79
   biology, 83, 94, 105, 106, 449
   cellular levels, 466
   compound, 466
   docking, 6, 21, 22, 27, 499, 503, 505, 508, 529, 537
   docking procedures, 6
   dynamics (MD), 505
      programming/studies, 508
   mass, 281, 347, 386, 588
   mechanics, 504
   modeling program, 504
   simulation, 508
   structures, 266, 279
   system, 505
   weight, 54, 81, 121–124, 147, 154, 206, 257, 330, 350, 502, 592, 466
Molecule inhibitors, 545, 552
Molisch's
   reagent, 401
   test, 136, 401, 594
Molluscicidal activity, 271
Momilactone A, 82, 83, 92, 99
Monocarboxylate, 551, 552, 554

transporter (MCT), 552, 554
Monochromator, 309, 315, 316
Monocotyledons, 90, 91, 216
Monographs, 357, 377
Monolayers, 290
Monomeric bonding, 350
Monosaccharide, 63, 127, 137, 169, 401
Monosaccharide/disaccharide, 63
Monoterpenes, 7, 18, 164, 204, 206, 213, 235
Monoterpenoid
   indole alkaloids (MIAs), 230
   oxindole alkaloids (MOAs), 230
Morphine, 6, 7, 11, 57, 130, 209, 271
Morphological/anatomical characters, 198, 201, 215, 218
Morphology, 19, 198, 199, 214, 470, 575, 600
Mouse infection models, 474
Mucous membrane, 134
Multicell changers, 319
Multi-component
   mixtures, 257
   plant extract samples, 276
   samples, 346, 349
Multidetector sequential analysis, 341
Multidimensional hyphenated systems, 341
Multilevel molecular, 430
Multiple-drug-resistant strains, 248
Mus musculus, 429
Musa acuminata, 92
Muscular defects, 450
Mutagenic agents, 522
Mutagenicity, 502
Mycelial growth inhibition, 81
Mycolaminaran, 102
Mycosphaerella pinodes, 102
Mycotoxins, 308, 331
Myricetin, 139, 183
Myristic acid, 211, 233
Myrobalans, 122
Myxoxanthin, 211
Myxoxanthophyll, 211

N

NADPH-dependent enzyme dihydrofla-vonol 4-reductase, 50
Nano cell holders, 318

Nano-flow chip integrated circuit miniatur-
    ization, 341
Nanogram range, 361
Nanoparticle (NP), 27, 28, 469
Nanoscale, 330
Nanotechnology, 28
NaOH test, 394, 398, 399
Naphthoquinone, 212
Naringenin, 49, 92, 139
National Institute of Standards and Tech-
    nology (NIST), 500, 574, 592
Natural
    derived compounds, 463, 466, 476
    killer (NK), 166, 170, 171, 438
    products, 4, 7, 8, 12, 19, 20, 22, 26, 70,
        84, 159, 198, 203, 229, 263, 271, 278,
        346, 382, 439, 464–467, 475, 476, 509,
        561–565
    sources, 84, 119, 367, 368
    sun-drying methods, 370
Nematodes, 80, 81, 84, 231
Neoxanthin, 185
Nephrolithiasis, 142
Neuaralgia, 130
Neurobehavioral conditions, 431
Neuroblastoma, 515, 523
Neurochemical transmitters, 430
Neurocognitive function, 451
Neurodegenerative
    disorders, 435, 439, 445
Neuro inflammation, 440
Neuronal growth, 431
Neutron activation analysis, 373
Newtonian equations, 508
N-Hydroxy-2-carboxy-substituted indole
    compounds, 547
Nicotiana tabacum, 71, 95, 209
Nicotinamide adenine dinucleotide
    (NADH), 538
Nicotine, 57, 133, 319–321
Nigella sativa, 155, 587–589, 601
Ninhydrin test, 400
Nitric oxide (NO), 155–157, 159, 165, 168
Nitrogen
    atom, 133, 208
    phosphorous detector–flame photometric
        detector, 278
    containing compounds, 92, 129, 231

N-methyltransferase, 47
Noller's test, 397
Nonalcoholic beverages, 47
Noncarbohydrate moiety, 63
Non-ER-mediated mechanisms, 90
Non-genotoxic, 439
Non-heterocyclic alkaloids, 130
Non-homologous end joining (NHEJ), 520,
    522, 528
Nonionizing energy, 372
Nonobese diabetic (NOD), 437, 438
Nonoxidative phase, 43
Nonpolar
    analyte, 252
    hydrogens, 504
    polar components, 296
    solvents, 251
Nonprotein amino acids, 201
Non-vitamin A precursors, 185
Norlupinane, 131
Normalization, 340
Normal-phase chromatography, 272
Notorious disease, 28
N-oxide, 133, 590
N-terminus, 552
Nuclear
    damage, 467
    formation, 581
    magnetic resonance (NMR), 19, 21, 218,
        226–230, 232–234, 238, 248, 255–257,
        261, 262, 279, 280, 333, 334, 467, 476,
        500, 501, 504, 588
        profiling approaches, 19
        techniques, 257, 467
    magnetic resonance spectroscopy, 218,
        248, 256, 279
    overhauser effect spectroscopy (NOESY),
        280
Nucleic acids, 12, 54, 203, 263, 504, 506
Nucleotide excision repair (NER), 520–522
Nucleotide metabolic, 37, 47
Nucleotide
    excision repair, 521
    metabolic pathway, 47
Null hypothesis, 361
Nutraceutical, 4, 10, 12, 13, 37, 40, 71, 179,
    180, 182, 183, 185, 186, 191, 192, 465,
    466, 476, 594, 600, 606

Nutraceuticals and their therapeutic activity, 182
  carotenoids
    biological activity of carotenoids, 186
    phytochemistry of carotenoids, 185
  coenzyme Q10, 190
  flavonoids, 183
  lutein and zeaxanthin, 187
  organosulfur compounds, 190
  other phytonutraceuticals, 191
  phenolics, 183
    biological activity of flavonoids, 185
    phytochemistry of flavonoids, 184
  polyunsaturated fatty acids, 188
    alpha-linolenic acid, 189
    linolenic acid, 189
Nutraceutics, 40, 428
Nutrient
  analysis, 410
  availability/deficiency, 217
  content, 181, 411
Nutritional
  effect, 465
  requirements, 181
Nux vomica, 123

O

Obesity, 147, 190, 431, 438
Ocimum basilicum oils, 487
Octadecatetraenoic acid, 212
Octaketide acyl chain, 66
Oil/volatile compounds, 270
Oleanolic acid, 128
Oleic acid, 211
Oligosaccharides, 84, 147, 148, 332
Omega 6 fatty acid, 189
Omic's approaches, 238
One-dimensional NMR, 280
Operating qualification (OQ), 321, 341
Ophiorrhiza pumila, 58
Ophthalmic functions, 134
Ophthalmology, 134
Optimization of lead phytochemicals, 22
Optimized potentials for liquid simulations-all atom (OPLS-AA), 505
Optimum performance laminar chromatography (OPLC), 253, 255

Optional accessory hardware configurations, 318
Oral
  bioavailability, 27
  supplementation, 190
Organic
  chemistry, 8, 288
  compounds, 120, 135, 203, 224, 235, 257, 295
  elemental analyses, 375
  plants, 371
  solvents, 121, 136, 263, 268
Organization for Economic Co-operation and Development (OECD), 472
Organoleptic properties, 4
Organomercurial reagent, 554
Organometallic, 375
Organophosphate containing insecticide, 134
Organophosphorous compounds, 375
Organ-specific toxicity, 475
Origanum
  majorana, 230
  vulgare, 488
Ormocarpum kirkii, 300
Ornithine, 130, 208, 234
Orobanche cernua, 18
Orthovanadate/verapamil, 102
Oryza sativa, 92, 99, 227
Osmoprotectants, 236, 237
Ostrinia nubilalis, 86
Oxalate, 142–144
  crystals, 199, 201, 214
  metabolism, 142
Oxalates, 119, 120, 142, 144, 201, 214, 400
Oxalic acid, 11, 142–144, 201, 237, 332, 410
Oxalyl chloride, 143
Oxidation, 43, 44, 51, 62, 139, 183, 202, 205, 207, 333, 437, 546, 552
  reaction, 43
Oxidative
  cell damage, 159, 576
  coupling, 53
  nonoxidative, 42
  phosphorylation, 124, 538, 539, 546
    related pathways, 236
Oxidizing agents, 81, 295, 372

Oxidosqualene cyclase, 62
Oxygen
  atoms, 357
  species, 87, 162, 186, 437, 469, 529, 548

P

Pachypodol, 139
Paclitaxel, 207, 465, 539, 572
Paddles, 318
Palmitic acid, 211, 233
Palynology, 198
Papaver somniferum, 56, 71, 130, 199
Papaveraceae, 94, 133, 208
Parasympathetic nervous system, 134
Paraxanthine, 135
Parenteral administration, 474
Parkinson's disease, 441
Particle
  shape, 349
  size, 275, 346, 349
Pathogenesis-related (PR) proteins, 81
Pathogenic
  mechanisms, 439
  nonpathogenic fungus, 83
  organisms, 86
  prokaryotes, 47
Pathogenicity, 83, 86
Pathogens, 4, 10, 12, 17, 18, 20, 79, 80, 81,
  83, 84, 86, 92, 95, 96, 99, 102, 104–106,
  120, 209, 231, 232
Peganum harmala, 301
Pelagophytes, 211
Pelargonidin, 49, 139, 162
Penicillium ulaiense, 17
Pentacyclic triterpene acid, 308
Pentadecanoic acid, 212
Pentose phosphate, 37, 41–43, 50, 63, 538,
  541
Peonidin, 139, 162, 163
Peptide aptamers, 545
Peptides, 451, 504
Percolation, 261, 264–266
Performance qualification (PQ), 321, 341
Perilla frutescens, 483, 488, 489
Perillaldehyde, 17
Perinuclear chromatin condensation, 581
Pest and disease management, 17

Petroleum ether, 143, 267, 300, 403, 406,
  408, 417–420
Petunidin, 139, 162
Peumus boldus, 131
PH range, 147, 351
Phaeophyceae, 210, 211
Pharma research, 24
Pharmaceutical
  chemistry, 6
  companies, 8, 498
  development, 468
  grade, 465
  industries, 4, 21, 232, 362
  ingredient, 318
  nutraceutical applications, 594
Pharmaceutics, 20, 37, 40, 71, 428
Pharmaco-chemistry, 561
Pharmacodynamics, 451
Pharmacognosists, 202, 262
Pharmacognosy, 8, 79, 119, 197, 261
Pharmacokinetic, 230, 362, 451, 475, 503,
  555
Pharmacological
  activity, 123, 129, 136, 207, 435, 503,
    590
  applications, 8, 129
  biochemical properties, 134
  characteristics, 130
  properties, 126
Pharmacology, 23, 129, 467, 565
  drug development, 23
Pharmafoods, 179, 180, 192
Phaseolus vulgaris, 82
Phelan-McDermid syndrome, 432
Phenol red, 390
Phenolic
  acids, 158, 183, 204, 216
  compounds, 14, 18, 56, 85, 123, 158,
    159, 183, 191, 201, 204, 205, 216, 230,
    236, 298, 345, 590
  content, 215, 403
  glycosides, 63
  group, 141
  solution, 403
  structure, 162
Phenolics, 10, 11, 25, 26, 37, 39–41, 43, 54,
  55, 85, 92, 153, 154, 183, 199, 204, 205,

215, 231, 263, 269, 288, 297, 298, 300, 403, 428
Phenolphthalein
 indicator, 390
 solution, 402
Phenones, 249
Phenotype, 233, 449–451, 453
Phenylalanine, 43, 44, 51, 54, 63, 95, 233, 539
 ammonia-lyase (PAL), 54, 63, 95, 96, 98, 99, 101–103
Phenylethylamine alkaloids, 130
Phenylpropanoid, 17, 138, 184, 204, 232
 pathway, 53, 54
Phenylpropanoids (PPs), 92
Phlobaphenes, 122
Phlobatannins, 122, 396
Phocomelia, 7
Phosphate
 buffer solution (PBS) 574–576
 groups, 43
Phosphodiester bonds, 521
Phosphoenolpyruvate (PEP), 43, 544, 545, 554
Phosphonoacetohydroxamic acid, 554
Phosphorylation, 43, 236, 516, 540, 542–545
Photoluminescent agents, 28
Photomicrographs, 576, 583
Photomultiplier detector, 316, 317
Photosynthesis, 38, 185, 186, 210, 213
Photosynthetic algae, 210, 213
Phthalideisoquinoline alkaloid, 216
Phycobilins, 210, 211
Phycoerythrin, 211
Phylloxanthins Xanthos, 186
Phylogenetic
 classification system, 217
 relationships, 200, 218
 system, 216
Physical
 parameters, 475
 properties, 126, 186, 292
Physiological
 biochemical functions, 139
 stress conditions, 86
Phytoalexin (PhA), 11, 15, 79–88, 90–93, 95, 96, 98–106, 232

degradative enzyme inhibitors (PhA synergists), 81
 detection methods, 104
 inhibitor/suppressor/degradation/detoxification mechanisms, 83
 mechanism, 104
 production, 79, 82, 90, 95, 102
 regulation, 101
 synergists, 81
 synthesis, 82, 84, 95, 103
Phytocassanes, 85, 92, 99, 104
Phytochemical,
 characterization, 499, 500
 compounds, 307
 constituents, 605, 616
 database, 566
 dataset, 21
 elimination processing, 308
 experiments, 491
 groups, 251
 markers, 197, 201
 mirna regulation, 516
 research, 23, 27
 screening, 302, 381, 609
 screening test, 594
 Society of
  Asia (PSA), 25, 26
  Europe (PSE), 25
  North America (PSNA), 25
Phytochemicokinetics, 434
Phytochemistry, 1, 3, 4, 6–9, 21, 25–27, 29, 119, 179, 197–200, 218, 288, 482, 484, 495, 497–499, 500, 503, 506, 509, 511, 584, 600
Phytochemists, 4, 19, 20, 26
Phytochemotaxonomy, 218
Phytocompound, 201, 590
Phytoconstituents, 25, 68, 252, 261–263, 268–271, 343, 344, 346, 382, 513, 525, 529, 588
Phytoestrogens, 184
Phytolaccaceae, 93, 94
Phytomedicinal products, 367
Phytomedicine, 22, 28, 435
Phytonutrients, 10, 58
Phytopathogenic fungi, 18, 146
Phytopharmacological studies, 452
Phytopharmacology, 390, 428, 454

Phytophthora
  cambivora, 101
  infestans, 80
  megasperma var *sojae*, 82
Phytoremediation, 9, 10, 223, 225, 228,
  235, 237, 238
Phytosterol, 11, 68, 70, 126, 166, 169, 190,
  191, 202, 326
Phytotoxicity, 18
Phytotoxins, 10
Picrotoxin, 7
Pinobanksin, 215
Pinoresinol, 51
Pinosylvin, 101
Pinus
  contorta, 90
  sylvestris, 101
Piper cabralanum, 469
Piperidine, 130, 131, 208
Planar chromatography, 360
Plant
  alkaloids, 209
  biochemistry, 105
  classification, 198, 200, 218, 262
  defense, 18, 79, 86, 104, 106, 224, 288
  derived
    compounds, 27, 223
    metabolites, 224, 225, 238
    molecules, 476
    product, 19
  development, 201, 224
  disease management, 17
  growth, 185, 203, 224, 234, 236, 238
  improvements, 226
  kingdom, 5, 183, 198, 202, 204, 224, 382
  maceration, 104
  material, 154, 249, 251, 257, 266, 267,
    269, 270, 369
  metabolites, 288
  metabolomics, 19, 223, 226
  molecular biology, 83
  natural-based drugs, 464
  oriented drugs, 464
  parasitic nematodes, 232
  pathogen interactions, 18, 223, 224, 231,
    233, 238
  pathology, 10
  pest interactions, 231

pigments, 183
species, 104, 124, 182, 198, 204, 205,
  209, 483, 488, 563
systematics, 200
taxonomists, 198
taxonomy, 198, 376
tissue homogenization, 266
Plants nonnitrogenous, 61
Plasma protein, 502
Plastic/aluminum, 272
Plastids, 43, 60, 95
Platanus acerifolia, 93
Platelet aggregations, 12
Poaceae plants, 84
Podophyllum species, 465
Polar
  compounds, 207, 268
  metabolites, 230
  organic solvent, 329
  polarizable molecules, 267
  solutes, 351
  solvents, 251, 266, 269
Poly (ADP-ribose) polymerase (PARP),
  520, 522, 527
  PARP recognizing protein, 522
Polyacetylenes, 84, 85, 249
Polyacrylamide, 263
Polyalcohols, 332
Polychromator disperses, 317
Polyfluorinated compounds, 376
Polygonaceae, 66, 123
Polyketide, 17, 66, 67
Polylysine, 84
Polymeric bonding, 350
Polyols, 213, 234, 237, 275
Polypeptides, 249, 277
Polyphenol compounds, 121
Polyphenolic
  compound, 518
  nature, 124, 148
Polyphenols, 183, 204, 249, 474, 527, 594
Polyphylloides, 212
Polysaccharides, 54, 84, 99, 153, 154, 169,
  211, 213
Polyunsaturated fatty acids (PUFA), 188,
  189, 211, 212, 518, 520
Porphyridium Näg, 212
Post-column derivatization, 341

Postmenopausal osteoporosis, 142
Potassium
  dichromate solution, 122
  ferricyanide, 122
  iodide, 393, 409
  mercuric iodide, 393
  permanganate, 319, 320, 399
Potato tubers, 103, 104
Potent molecules, 104
Prasinophytes, 211
Premenstrual syndrome, 189
Primary
  metabolism, 201, 203, 288
  metabolites, 10, 38, 81, 197, 199, 202,
    203, 213, 288
Principal component analysis (PCA), 483
Proanthocyanidin, 122, 142, 148, 182, 184,
  406
Probiotics, 182
Pro-inflammatory
  gene transcription, 159
  mediators, 159, 165
    synthesis inhibition, 158
Proline-rich protein (PRP), 98
Prophylactic, 134, 191
Prosapogenins, 127
Prostaglandins, 159
Prostephanus truncatus, 17
Protease inhibitors, 119, 120, 144–146
Protein
  aceous molecules, 147
  containing plant organs, 263
  ligand complexes, 504
Proteolytic
  cleavage, 146
  degradation, 144
Protoalkaloid, 56, 154, 158
Protodioscin, 128
Protoneodioscin, 128
Proximate
  analysis, 410, 422
  composition, 382, 410, 411, 422
Prunella sp, 300
Psammomys obesus, 438
Pseudoalkaloids, 154, 158
Pseudomonas
  ovalis, 100
  syringae pv. *glycinea*, 96

Pseudotannins, 123
Pseudotropine, 524
Psidium guajava, 147
Ptychomitrium sinense, 212
Puccinia striiformis, 231
Pulmonary fibrosis, 435
Punica granatum, 160, 191
Purine, 131, 135
PyMOL molecular visualization system,
  529
Pyricularia
  oryzae, 99
  sativa, 90
Pyridine, 131, 597
Pyrrolidine, 130, 131, 521
Pyrrolizidine, 131, 135
  alkaloid (PA), 135
  ring, 131
Pyruvate, 46, 144, 470, 538, 544, 546, 552
Pytochemical screening, 436

Q

Qualitative
  analysis, 362, 381, 402, 422, 591
  changes, 224
  method, 348, 363
  phytochemical analysis, 393
  profiling, 343, 346
  quantitative
    analysis, 358
    analytical and separation techniques,
      226
    estimation, 345
    identification, 224
    metabolite data, 224
  tests, 591
Quantification, 104, 253, 299, 307, 308,
  335, 342, 346, 382, 383
  limits, 322, 341
Quantitative
  analysis, 238, 272, 381–383, 422, 591
  estimation, 343, 346, 356, 422
  methods, 224
  qualitative
    composition, 217
    measurements, 224
  structure–activity relationship (QSAR),
    499, 506, 508

Quaternary
  compounds, 133
  gradient, 326
  solvent systems, 360
Quercetin, 138, 139, 183, 185, 190, 216,
  269, 404, 528
  dimethyl ether, 230
Quercus robur, 123
Quillaja saponaria, 127
Quinine, 6, 7, 57, 129–131, 134, 209
Quinoline, 131
Quinone, 43, 398

R

Radical
  related diseases, 55
  scavengers, 576
Radioactive
  isotopes, 375
  nucleoside, 474
Radio
  activity, 474
  chemical detectors, 332
  labelled material, 332
Ranunculaceae, 133, 155, 208, 589
Raphanus sativus, 228, 236
Raphides, 197, 199, 201, 215
Rat model, 53, 432, 454
Rattus norvegicus, 429
Rauvolfia
  nukuhivensis, 301
  serpentina, 58, 131
Reagent preparation, 382, 384, 422
Recreational drugs, 129, 208
Refractive index detector, 296, 332, 351
Renal insufficiency, 435
Respiratory passages, 474
Resuscitation, 134
Resveratrol, 11, 85, 87, 91, 138, 518, 523,
  528
Retinoic acid, 164, 514
Reversed phase high performance chroma-
  tography (RP-HPLC) separation, 351
Rhamnetin, 216
Rhizobium leguminosarum, 103
Rhizoctonia
  infection, 231
  solani, 18, 231

Rhizomes, 128, 202, 465
Rhizopus
  microspores, 86, 92
  stolonifera, 99
Rhizoremediation, 236
Rhodiola imbricata, 155
Rhodophyceae, 210, 211
Rhubarb, 122, 123, 136, 144
Ribonucleic acid (RNA), 201, 441,
  448–450, 516, 517, 545, 546
Ribose phosphate isomerase, 43
Ribosome-inactivating proteins, 129
Ribulose phosphate, 43
Rice blast fungal pathogen, 232
Ricinus communis, 131
Rishitin metabolism, 103, 104
Robustness, 322, 341, 352, 355
Rootknot nematodes (RKNs), 232
Rosaceae, 85, 94, 209
Rosmarinic acid, 148, 216
Rotary evaporator, 250
Rotavirus, 129
Rubiaceae, 94, 133, 155, 199, 208, 230
Rutaceae, 85, 93, 94, 133, 199, 215

S

Sabinene, 487
Saccharum officinarum, 91, 92, 300
S-adenosyl-L-methionine (SAM), 47
Salicylate-dependent induction, 87
Salicylic acid, 204
Salinity stress, 228, 234
Salivation, 134
Salkowski test, 396, 594
Salvation parameters, 504
Sample
  application, 358
  diffusion, 349
  inlet/injectors, 328
  preparation, 269, 297, 341, 344, 347, 348,
    355, 357, 362, 367, 371, 377
Sapogenin, 61–63, 124
Saponin, 11, 37, 39, 58, 61–63, 119,
  124–129, 135, 146, 148, 153, 154, 164,
  166–168, 209, 249, 271, 345, 395, 404,
  407, 408, 428, 573, 577, 590, 593, 594,
  609, 611, 615, 616
  glycosides, 63

lysed erythrocytes, 128
rich diets, 128
Satureja thymbra, 18
Scapania undulata, 213
Schizophrenia, 435
Scopolamine, 209
Secologanin, 56, 59, 61, 209
Secondary metabolites, 3, 4, 10, 17, 37–41, 61, 70, 79, 81, 95, 104, 120, 129, 136, 138, 164, 183, 197–199, 201–204, 212–214, 217, 218, 226, 230, 231, 233–235, 237, 238, 288, 296, 299, 346, 363, 428, 571, 576, 593, 611, 615
Sedum alfredii, 228, 237
Seed germination, 81, 238
Semantides, 199, 201, 214
Senecio
  biafrae, 605, 606
  vulgaris, 131
Senecionine, 131
Sennosides, 326
Septicemia, 434
Sesquiterpenes, 11, 59, 60, 84, 85, 95, 204, 206, 207, 299
Sesquiterpenoids, 85, 93, 213
Shikimate, 37, 43, 49, 63, 103
  acid, 41, 43, 54, 66, 67, 184, 204
Shinado's test, 394
Silver nitrate, 397, 402, 409
Single-beam spectrophotometers, 315, 316
Sipettes, 319
Sitophilus granarius, 17
Sitosterol, 11, 68, 70, 166, 169, 191
Skin
  histology, 473
  soft tissue infection, 434
  toxicity, 473
Sodium
  bicarbonate solution, 400
  carbonate/ammonia, 133
  chloride, 256, 395, 407
  hydroxide, 319, 320, 398, 399, 402, 404, 409, 414, 419
  nitroprusside, 398
  oxamate, 548
Solanaceae, 84, 85, 93, 94, 129, 133, 199, 208, 209, 215, 233, 513, 524, 607
Solanum

dulcamara, 129
nigrum, 605, 607
tuberosum, 80
Solid
  filters/solutions, 318
  phase extraction (SPE), 327, 341
  stationary phase, 290
Solubilization, 320
Solvent
  evaporation, 360
  extraction methods, 19
  system, 267, 273, 274, 297, 360, 399, 401
Somniferine, 524
Somnine, 524
Sophora flavescens, 301
Sorghum bicolor, 81
Soy isoflavones, 182, 523
  isoflavones treatment, 523
Soybean plants, 232
Soybean's metabolism, 232
Spearman's *mum basilicum*, 488
Spectrophotometer (SM), 276, 281, 307–309, 311–313, 315–321, 338, 374, 409, 434, 610
Spectroscopic technique, 257
Sphagnic acid, 213
Sphagnum rubellum, 213
Sphytochemicodynamic, 433
Spinal cord injury, 431
Split-beam spectrophotometers, 317
Squalene, 62, 68, 164
  synthase, 62
Stachys tuberifera, 131
Standard
  additions, 339
  deviations (SD), 487, 489, 556, 575, 576, 580, 581
STATA software, 485
Stationary phase, 254, 255, 271–293, 296, 322, 323, 346, 357–359, 362
Statistical
  Analysis Software (SAS), 481, 482, 484, 487, 488
  applications, 483–485
  methods, 482
  package, 481, 482
  software, 485, 491
  test/analysis, 23

Steam distillation, 264, 270
Steel head adaptor, 414
Stem cell technologies, 443
Stephania sinica, 301
Stereochemistry, 7, 464
Steroid, 68, 69, 85, 126, 158, 164, 406, 408
Steroidal
  drugs, 191
  saponins, 128
  sugar moieties, 125
Steroids, 37, 39, 41, 45, 58, 68, 164, 209,
  216, 295, 346, 396, 406, 408, 428, 573,
  590, 593
Sterols, 68, 126, 153, 154, 190, 191, 249
Stigmasterol, 68, 70, 191
Stilbene synthase, 101
Storage techniques, 371
Streptococcus aureus, 487
Streptomyces spp, 147, 465
Streptozotocin, 55, 436
Strictosidine, 56, 57, 209
Strophanthus, 209
Structural elucidation, 218, 257, 279, 281
Structure-based drug designing, 504
Styloids, 201
Succinylbenzoic acid, 66
Sugar molecule, 209
Suitable stationary phase, 357
Sulfuric acids reagent, 396, 400
Supercritical fluid extraction (SFE), 247,
  249, 252, 253, 264, 268, 269, 288
Supersaturation, 278
Surface area, 262, 264, 276, 290, 346, 349,
  350, 357, 371, 412
Systemic lupus erythematosus, 435
Syzygium
  aromaticum, 17
  cumini, 147
  jambos, 488, 489

T

Tangeritin, 139
Tannic acid, 11, 121, 124, 394, 405, 409
Tannin, 11, 15, 18, 40, 54, 55, 119–124,
  148, 183, 184, 204, 214, 216, 249, 267,
  288, 332, 345, 395, 396, 405, 409, 571,
  573, 576, 593, 594, 606, 609, 611, 615
Taraxanthin, 211

Taxifolin, 183
Taxol, 28, 465, 476
Taxonomic
  distribution, 130
  features, 211
  study, 202, 263
Taxonomy, 129, 197–200, 211, 216, 218,
  263, 344
Taxus brevifolia, 465
Tea catechins, 182
Tectonagrandis, 584
Tectorigenin, 183
Teratogenic effects, 7
Terpene synthase, 7
Terpenes, 7, 10, 11, 13, 29, 40, 45, 58–61,
  148, 164, 182, 204–207, 231, 295, 397
Terpenoids, 7, 37, 39, 41, 45, 59, 85, 92,
  153, 154, 164, 201, 205, 215, 249, 263,
  299, 345, 396, 573, 590, 593, 594
Test for
  carboxylic acids, 400
  coumarin, 399
  cyanogenic glycosides, 398
  diterpenes, 397
  emodins, 402
  essential oils, 399
  fatty acids, 399
  oxalate, 400
  phlobatannins, 396
  phytate, 402
  reducing sugar, 401
  resins, 400
  terpenes, 397
  terpenoids, 396
Tester sinkers/baskets, 318
Tests for
  alkaloids, 393
  anthocyanin, 399
  anthraquinone, 397
  carbohydrate, 401
  cardiac glycosides, 398
  glycosides, 398
  proteins and aminoacids, 400
  quinone, 398
  saponins, 395
  steroids, 396
  tannins, 395
  terpenoids, 396

triterpenoids, 397
Tetrahedron structure, 357
Tetrahydrocannabinols, 326
Tetrahydrofuran (THF), 351
Tetranychus cinnabarinus, 17
Tetrapleura tetraptera, 271
Tetraprenyl toluquinols, 212
Tetrapyrrolic, 211
Tetrazolium salts-based assays, 470
Thalidomide, 7
Thea sinensis, 131
Theanine, 146
Theobroma cacao, 93, 131, 191
Theobromine, 47, 135
Theophylline, 135
Therapeutic
    effect on rheumatoid arthritis, 142
    mydriatic, 134
    nutraceuticals, 191
    phytochemicals, 600
Thermal conductivity detector, 278
Thermolabile drugs, 264
Thiazolidinediones, 436
Thymbra spicata, 18
Thymoquinone (TQ), 590, 601
Thymus vulgaris, 488
Thyroid gland, 439
Tiliaceae, 93, 94, 215
Tissue
    remodeling, 146
    repair, 144
Titration, 414, 416
Toxic compounds, 235
Toxicants, 449
Toxicity, 9, 15, 55, 80, 129, 154, 236, 248,
    249, 381, 382, 433, 435, 437, 440, 441,
    453, 463, 465–467, 472–475, 489, 499,
    502, 503
    evaluation, 502
    investigation, 473
    natural products, 466
Toxicological
    assay, 433
    profile, 469
Traditional
    Chinese Medicine Integrative Database
        (TCMID), 562, 565
    medicine, 563, 566

Tranquilizers, 526
Trans-caryophyllene, 483, 488
Tribolium castaneum, 17
Tricarboxylic acid cycle(TCA), 405, 406,
    538, 552
Trichoderma viride, 101
Triglycerides, 332, 416
Triterpene units, 59
Triterpenes, 59, 95, 164, 204, 207
Triterpenoid
    aglycone, 124
    saponins, 124, 126
Triterpenoids, 164, 207, 397
Triticum aestivum, 227
Tropane, 131
Tropino, 524
Tryptophan, 43, 56, 63, 130, 208, 209
T-tests, 24, 483
Tubocurarine, 134
Tumor
    initiation, 546
    suppressive
        effects, 129
        gene, 518
Tungsten, 309
    halogen lamps, 319
Two-dimensional techniques (2D-NMR),
    280
Types of chromatography, 290
    adsorption chromatography, 290
    counter current chromatography, 292
    gas chromatography, 291
    high-performance liquid chromatography,
        296
        columns, 297
        detectors, 298
        mobile phase selection, 297
        sample preparation and loading, 297
    ion-exchange chromatography, 291
    loading of sample, 293
        developing agents, 294
        loading of sample, 293
        resolution, 296
        RF value, 296
        running of TLC, 294
    size exclusion chromatography, 291
    thin-layer chromatography (TLC),
        253–255, 262, 272–275, 279, 290,

292–297, 299, 301, 302, 343, 355, 357,
    359, 361, 394–397, 399–401
Typhoid, 208
Tyrosine, 43, 44, 51, 56, 130, 208, 545

U

Ubiquitous peroxidase enzymes, 51
Ulcer, 435, 572
Ulmus americana, 95
Ultrasonic water baths, 329
Ultrasound-assisted extraction (UAE), 249,
    252, 264, 266, 267
Ultraviolet (UV), 10, 80, 84, 90, 101, 104,
    185, 205, 214, 255, 256, 275, 281, 294,
    295, 298, 307–309, 315, 317, 332, 334,
    338, 341, 351, 372, 520, 528, 575
    facilitated radicals, 372
    region, 310
    spectroscopy, 248
    visible
        chromophore, 309, 315, 331
        detector, 331, 341
        spectrophotometer, 296, 298, 309, 315,
            342
        spectroscopy, 256
Uncaria tomentosa, 155
Urbanization, 235
Urinary tract infection, 434
Urination, 134
Urogenital dysfunction, 435
Urolithiasis, 142
Ursolic acid, 11, 125, 165, 207, 208, 403
US Food and Drug Administration, 333, 465
Usnic acid, 213, 214
Ustilago maydis, 86

V

Vaccines, 128, 166, 167, 432
Vaccinium oxycoccos, 191
Vacuum liquid chromatography (VLC), 272,
    274, 275
Validation, 27, 318, 321, 348, 352, 354,
    363, 451, 469, 508
Vanilla bean, 205
Vanillin, 205
Vascular
    endothelial growth factor (VEGF), 529
    plants, 211, 214

tissue factor expression, 189
Vasodilator effects, 80
Verbenaceae, 94, 202, 215, 572, 606
Vetiver, 490
    plants, 237
Vicia, 103, 215
    faba, 103
Vinblastine, 134, 209, 465
Vinca
    minor, 227, 230
    rosea, 465
Vincristine, 134, 209, 465
Vindesine, 465
Vinorelbine, 465
Violaxanthin, 185, 211
Viruses, 81, 84, 145, 170, 231, 445, 516
Virus-induced models, 438
Viscosity, 248, 352
Viscous mobile phases, 349
Viscum album, 171
Vitamin, 10, 11, 128, 146, 181, 183, 185,
    213, 401, 412, 498, 527, 606, 615
Vitex negundo, 24
Vitis
    labrusca, 269
    vinifera, 81, 191
Volatile
    components, 291
    elements, 371
    liquid, 293
    materials, 371
    poisonous, 65
Voltage-dependent anion channel (VDAC),
    541, 542
Volumetric flask, 403–405, 610

W

Wadelia calendulacea, 253
Wagner's
    reagent, 393
    test, 393, 577
Warburg effect, 539, 554, 556
Ward's method, 488
Water
    impurities, 383
    insoluble additional products, 126
    soluble
        blue, 211

green product, 319
Wavelength, 307, 309, 310, 317–319, 331, 332, 374
   accuracy, 318, 321, 341
   scanning, 311
Wavenumber, 256
Web resources, 446
Whatman filter paper, 403–408, 410, 419
Withania somnifera, 169, 513, 523–533
World Health Organization (WHO), 5, 20, 26, 417, 464, 497
Wound
   healing, 12, 15, 16, 438
   model, 128

X

Xanthine skeleton, 47
Xanthomonas oryzae, 232
Xanthophylls, 186, 187, 210, 211, 232
Xanthoproteic test, 400, 577
Xanthosine monophosphate, 47
Xanthoxylin, 85, 93, 94
Xanthyletin, 93
X-axis, 298, 311, 392
Xenografts, 547, 552
Xenon, 309
   lamps, 319

X-ray, 257, 282, 374, 375
   absorption fluorescence, 334
   characteristic signatures, 374
   crystallography, 255, 257, 282, 504
   diffraction, 278, 282, 334
   excitation, 257
   fluorescence (XRF), 373–375
   radiation, 374
Xylulose-5-phosphate, 43

Y

Yam, 124
Y-axis, 298, 311, 313, 392
Yohimbine, 58, 134

Z

Zea mays L, 187
Zealexins, 79, 85, 92
Zeathanin, 11, 182, 185–187, 211, 235
Zebra fish, 429
Zinc and ring finger 3 (ZNRF3), 514
Zingiber officinale, 227
Zingiberaccae, 230
Ziziphus jujuba, 128
Zucker diabetic fatty rat, 438
Zygophyllum, 215
Zymoseptoria tritici, 227

Printed and bound by CPI Group (UK) Ltd, Croydon, CR0 4YY

23/10/2024

01777703-0020